Lecture Notes in Computer

Edited by G. Goos, J. Hartmanis, and J. van Leeuwen

Springer
Berlin
Heidelberg
New York
Hong Kong
London
Milan
Paris
Tokyo

Takeyoshi Dohi   Ron Kikinis (Eds.)

Medical Image Computing and Computer-Assisted Intervention – MICCAI 2002

5th International Conference
Tokyo, Japan, September 25-28, 2002
Proceedings, Part I

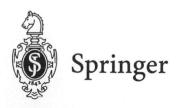 Springer

Series Editors

Gerhard Goos, Karlsruhe University, Germany
Juris Hartmanis, Cornell University, NY, USA
Jan van Leeuwen, Utrecht University, The Netherlands

Volume Editors

Takeyoshi Dohi
Department of Mechano-informatics
Graduate School of Information Science and Technology
University of Tokyo, 7-3-1 Hongo Bunkyo-ku, 113-8656 Tokyo, Japan
E-mail: dohi@miki.pe.u-tokyo.ac.jp

Ron Kikinis
Department of Radiology, Brigham and Women's Hospital
75 Francis St., MA, 02115 Boston, USA
E-mail: kikinis@bwh.harvard.edu

Cataloging-in-Publication Data applied for

Die Deutsche Bibliothek - CIP-Einheitsaufnahme

Medical image computing and computer assisted intervention :
5th international conference ; proceedings / MICCAI 2002, Tokyo, Japan,
September 25 - 28, 2002. Takeyoshi Dohi ; Ron Kikinis (ed.). - Berlin ;
Heidelberg ; New York ; Hong Kong ; London ; Milan ; Paris ; Tokyo :
Springer
Pt. 1 . - (2002)
  (Lecture notes in computer science ; Vol. 2488)
  ISBN 3-540-44224-3

CR Subject Classification (1998): I.5, I.4, I.3.5-8, I.2.9-10, J.3

ISSN 0302-9743
ISBN 3-540-44224-3 Springer-Verlag Berlin Heidelberg New York

Springer-Verlag Berlin Heidelberg New York
a member of BertelsmannSpringer Science+Business Media GmbH

http://www.springer.de

© Springer-Verlag Berlin Heidelberg 2002
Printed in Germany

Typesetting: Camera-ready by author, data conversion by Olgun Computergrafik
Printed on acid-free paper   SPIN: 10870635   06/3142   5 4 3 2 1 0

Preface

The fifth international Conference in Medical Image Computing and Computer Assisted Intervention (MICCAI 2002) was held in Tokyo from September 25th to 28th, 2002. This was the first time that the conference was held in Asia since its foundation in 1998. The objective of the conference is to offer clinicians and scientists the opportunity to collaboratively create and explore the new medical field. Specifically, MICCAI offers a forum for the discussion of the state of art in computer-assisted interventions, medical robotics, and image processing among experts from multi-disciplinary professions, including but not limited to clinical doctors, computer scientists, and mechanical and biomedical engineers. The expectations of society are very high; the advancement of medicine will depend on computer and device technology in coming decades, as they did in the last decades.

We received 321 manuscripts, of which 41 were chosen for oral presentation and 143 for poster presentation. Each paper has been included in these proceedings in eight-page full paper format, without any differentiation between oral and poster papers. Adherence to this full paper format, along with the increased number of manuscripts, surpassing all our expectations, has led us to issue two proceedings volumes for the first time in MICCAI's history. Keeping to a single volume by assigning fewer pages to each paper was certainly an option for us considering our budget constraints. However, we decided to increase the volume to offer authors maximum opportunity to argue the state of art in their work and to initiate constructive discussions among the MICCAI audience.

It was our great pleasure to welcome all MICCAI 2002 attendees to Tokyo. Japan, in fall, is known for its beautiful foliage all over the country. The traditional Japanese architectures always catches the eyes of visitors to Japan. We hope that all the MICCAI attendees took the opportunity to enjoy Japan and that they had a scientifically fruitful time at the conference. Those who could not attend the conference should keep the proceedings as a valuable source of information for their academic activities.

We look forward to seeing you at another successful MICCAI in Toronto in 2003.

July 2002   DOHI Takeyoshi and Ron Kikinis

Organizing Committee

Honorary Chair

Kintomo Takakura — Tokyo Women's Medical University, Japan

General Chair

Takeyoshi Dohi — The University of Tokyo, Japan
Terry Peters — University of Western Ontario, Canada
Junichiro Toriwaki — Nagoya University, Japan

Program Chair

Ron Kikinis — Harvard Medical School and Brigham and Women's Hospital, USA

Program Co-chairs

Randy Ellis — Queen's University at Kingston, Canada
Koji Ikuta — Nagoya University, Japan
Gabor Szekely — Swiss Federal Institute of Technology, ETH Zentrum, Switzerland

Tutorial Chair

Yoshinobu Sato — Osaka University, Japan

Industrial Liaison

Masakatsu Fujie — Waseda University, Japan
Makoto Hashizume — Kyushu University, Japan
Hiroshi Iseki — Tokyo Women's Medical University, Japan

Program Review Committee

Alan Colchester	University of Kent at Canterbury, UK
Wei-Qi Wang	Dept. of E., Fudan University, China
Yongmei Wang	The Chinese University of Hong Kong, China
Jocelyne Troccaz	TIMC Laboratory, France
Erwin Keeve	Research Center Caesar, Germany
Frank Tendick	University of California, San Francisco, USA
Sun I. Kim	Hanyang University, Korea
Pierre Hellier	INRIA Rennes, France
Pheng Ann Heng	The Chinese University of Hong Kong, China
Gabor Szekely	Swiss Federal Institute of Technology Zurich, Switzerland
Kirby Vosburgh	CIMIT/MGH/Harvard Medical School, USA
Allison M. Okamura	Johns Hopkins University, USA
James S. Duncan	Yale University, USA
Baba Vemuri	University of Florida, USA
Terry M. Peters	The John P. Robarts Research Institute, Canada
Allen Tannenbaum	Georgia Institute of Technology, USA
Richard A. Robb	Mayo Clinic, USA
Brian Davies	Imperial College London, UK
David Hawkes	King's College London, UK
Carl-Fredrik Westin	Harvard Medical School, USA
Chris Taylor	University of Manchester, UK
Derek Hill	King's College London, UK
Ramin Shahidi	Stanford University, USA
Demetri Terzopoulos	New York University, USA
Shuqian Luo	Capital University of Medical Sciences, USA
Paul Thompson	UCLA School of Medicine, USA
Simon Warfield	Harvard Medical School, USA
Gregory D. Hager	Johns Hopkins University, USA
Kiyoyuki Chinzei	AIST, Japan
Shinichi Tamura	Osaka University, Japan
Jun Toriwaki	Nagoya University, Japan
Yukio Kosugi	Tokyo Institute of Technology, Japan
Jing Bai	Tsinghua University, China
Philippe Cinquin	UJF (University Joseph Fourier), France
Xavier Pennec	INRIA Sophia-Antipolis, France
Frithjof Kruggel	Max-Planck-Institute for Cognitive Neuroscience, Germany

Ewert Bengtsson   Uppsala University, Finland
Ève Coste Maniére   INRIA Sophia Antipolis, France
Milan Sonka   University of Iowa, USA
Branislav Jaramaz   West Penn Hospital, USA
Dimitris Metaxas   Rutgers University, USA
Tianzi Jiang   Chinese Academy of Sciences, China
Tian-ge Zhuang   Shanghai Jiao tong University, China
Masakatsu G. Fujie   Waseda University, Japan
Takehide Asano   Chiba University, Japan
Ichiro Sakuma   The University of Tokyo, Japan
Alison Noble   University of Oxford, UK
Heinz U. Lemke   Technical University Berlin, Germany
Robert Howe   Harvard University, USA
Michael I Miga   Vanderbilt University, USA
Hervé Delingette   INRIA Sophia Antipolis, France
D. Louis Collins   Montreal Neurological Institute,
                               McGill University, Canada
Kunio Doi   University of Chicago, USA
Scott Delp   Stanford University, USA
Louis L. Whitcomb   Johns Hopkins University, USA
Michael W. Vannier   University of Iowa, USA
Jin-Ho Cho   Kyungpook National University, Korea
Yukio Yamada   University of Electro-Communications, Japan
Yuji Ohta   Ochanomizu University, Japan
Karol Miller   The University of Western Australia
William (Sandy) Wells   Harvard Medical School, Brigham and
                               Women's Hosp., USA
Kevin Montgomery   National Biocomputation Center/Stanford
                               University, USA
Kiyoshi Naemura   Tokyo Women's Medical University, Japan
Yoshihiko Nakamura   The University of Tokyo, Japan
Toshio Nakagohri   National Cancer Center Hospital East, Japan
Yasushi Yamauchi   AIST, Japan
Masaki Kitajima   Keio University, Japan
Hiroshi Iseki   Tokyo Women's Medical University, Japan
Yoshinobu Sato   Osaka University, Japan
Amami Kato   Osaka University School of Medicine, Japan
Eiju Watanabe   Tokyo Metropolitan Police Hospital, Japan
Miguel Angel Gonzalez Ballester INRIA Sophia Antipolis, France
Yoshihiro Muragaki   Tokyo Women's Medical University, Japan

Local Organizing Committee

Ichiro Sakuma   The University of Tokyo, Japan
Mitsuo Shimada   Kyushu University, Japan
Nobuhiko Hata   The University of Tokyo, Japan
Etsuko Kobayashi   The University of Tokyo, Japan

MICCAI Board

Alan C.F. Colchester   University of Kent at Canterbury, UK
(General Chair)

Nicholas Ayache   INRIA Sophia Antipolis, France
Anthony M. DiGioia   UPMC Shadyside Hospital, Pittsburgh, USA
Takeyoshi Dohi   University of Tokyo, Japan
James Duncan   Yale University, New Haven, USA
Karl Heinz Höhne   University of Hamburg, Germany
Ron Kikinis   Harvard Medical School , Boston, USA
Stephen M. Pizer   University of North Carolina, Chapel Hill, USA
Richard A. Robb   Mayo Clinic, Rochester, USA
Russell H. Taylor   Johns Hopkins University, Baltimore, USA
Jocelyne Troccaz   University of Grenoble, France
Max A. Viergever   University Medical Center Utrecht,
                             The Netherlands

Table of Contents, Part I

Robotics in Image-Guided Surgery

Robotics – Tele-operation

Robotics – Device

Robotics – System

Validation

Brain-Tumor, Cortex, Vascular Structure

Brain – Imaging and Analysis

Segmentation

Cardiac Application

Computer Assisted Diagnosis

Table of Contents, Part II

Interventions – Navigation

Simulation

Modeling

Statistical Shape Modeling

Registration – 2D/D Fusion

Registration – Similarity Measures

Non-rigid Registration

Visualization

Novel Imaging Techniques

Using an Endoscopic Solo Surgery Simulator for Quantitative Evaluation of Human-Machine Interface in Robotic Camera Positioning Systems

Atsushi Nishikawa[1], Daiji Negoro[1], Haruhiko Kakutani[1], Fumio Miyazaki[1],
Mitsugu Sekimoto[2], Masayoshi Yasui[2], Shuji Takiguchi[2], and Morito Monden[2]

[1] Department of Systems and Human Science,
Graduate School of Engineering Science, Osaka University
1-3 Machikaneyama-cho, Toyonaka City, Osaka 560-8531, Japan
[2] Department of Surgery and Clinical Oncology,
Osaka University Graduate School of Medicine
2-2 Yamadaoka, Suita City, Osaka 565-0871, Japan

Abstract. An endoscopic solo surgery simulator was designed to quantitatively evaluate human-machine interface in robotic camera positioning systems. Our simulator can assess not only the quantitative efficiency of laparoscopic cameraworks but also the influence of cameraworks upon the accuracy of surgical actions. Two human-machine interfaces: a face motion navigation system and a voice activated system were developed and compared. As a result, the face control interface was more efficient in cameraworks than the voice control, even under a stress to control the instruments. However, it was also found that the face motion may have bad influence on precise surgical actions.

1 Introduction

In laparoscopic surgery, the vision of the operating surgeon depends on a camera assistant responsible for guiding the laparoscope. Recently, several robotic camera positioning systems have been devised towards the realization of "solo surgery" in which the operating surgeon directly controls all of the interventional procedure including the laparoscope guiding task. In such robotic systems, the human(surgeon)-machine(robot) interface is of paramount importance because it is the means by which the surgeon communicates with and controls the robotic camera assistant.

These days comparative experimental studies evaluating the performance of laparoscope positioning systems with different human-machine interfaces are reported[1–7]. These studies can be classified into two types.

- In [1–4], typical laparoscopic cameraworks such as pan/tilt/zoom movements and their combinations were objectively and quantitatively assessed. However, no instrument operation was included in the assessment tasks.
- In [5–7], a standard intervention task with the regular use of instruments such as laparoscopic cholecystectomy was performed/simulated on a phantom model or a pig(in vivo). However, the task procedure time, the number of camera control commands, and the subjective judgement such as rating on the comfort were only used as criteria for assessment.

T. Dohi and R. Kikinis (Eds.): MICCAI 2002, LNCS 2488, pp. 1–8, 2002.

The purpose of this project is not only to comparatively evaluate the quantitative efficiency of laparoscopic cameraworks under a lot of stress to control surgical instruments such as forceps and foot pedal, but also to investigate the influence of cameraworks through the human-machine interface upon the accuracy of instrument operation. To date, there has been no research to accomplish this.

We have developed two human-machine interfaces for controlling a laparoscope positioner: a face-motion navigation system and a voice-activated system. These two "real" human-machine interfaces are directly connected with our computer-based assessment system, "Endoscopic Solo Surgery Simulator (ESSS)", that simulates a laparoscope, the patient's body and tissues, surgical instruments such as left/right forceps and a camera-holding robot manipulator. We implemented three basic intervention tasks on the simulator for the comparative experiment. These tasks include the model of motions in laparoscopic surgery such as removing the gallbladder. We recorded a lot of data such as the time to complete the task, the camera moving time, the frequency of the surgeon's commands, the number of errors of the instrument operation, the total moving distance of the tip of the virtual laparoscope, and the total moving distance of the tip of the virtual instruments, then we analyzed them.

2   Overview of Laparoscope Control Interface

First of all, we briefly explain our laparoscope control interface. The details of the system can be found in [8].

2.1   Face Control Interface(FAce MOUSe)

One of our laparoscope control interface, FAce MOUSe system, generates the robot manipulator control commands based on the operating surgeon's face motion. It mainly consists of a CCD camera placed just over the TV monitor, and a Linux PC with a video capturing board. The core system in the PC can detect and track the surgeon's face features in real-time from a sequence of video images captured through the CCD camera. The system estimates the position and the pose of the surgeon's face in real-time from the image processing result and then recognizes the surgeon's face gestures.

2.2   Voice Control Interface

The other interface forms a voice-controlled laparoscope positioning system, which is based on the commercial voice recognition engine, ViaVoice(IBM Corporation). It mainly consists of a microphone worn by the surgeon and a Windows PC with a USB device, and generates the manipulator control commands by interpreting the surgeon's simple Japanese words inputted through the USB device from the microphone.

3   Endoscopic Solo Surgery Simulator

In order to compare the above two human-machine interfaces for positioning the laparoscope, we developed a computer-based assessment system, the Endoscopic Solo Surgery Simulator(ESSS), which mainly consists of an instrument control interface and a main computer. The hardware configuration of our assessment system is shown in Fig. 1(a).

3.1   Instrument Control Interface (VLI)

The Virtual Laparoscopic Interface (VLI) (Immersion Corporation) was utilized as the instrument simulation device. The VLI tracks the motion of a pair of laparoscopic surgical instruments simultaneously, each moving in 5 degrees of freedom (a 1st and 2nd D.O.F. for pivoting about its insertion point, i.e., pitch and yaw motions, a 3rd D.O.F for insertion/retraction, a 4th D.O.F. for spinning about its insertion axis, i.e., roll motion, and the rest for open-close motion of the instrument handle). The latency is less than 1 ms, resulting in sampling rates of 1000Hz. The VLI also monitors the on/off signals of a foot switch in real-time.

3.2   Main Computer

A Windows PC with AMD Athlon 1.4 GHz processor was used as a main computer. It generates three-dimensional computer graphics (3DCG) using the OpenGL graphics library. All of the software modules on the PC were developed by using Visual C++ version 6.0 (Microsoft Corporation). The PC has two standard RS-232 serial ports for respectively connecting to the laparoscope/instrument control interfaces, and also has a graphic card.

The software system configuration is shown in Fig. 1(b). The system has a laparoscopic camera model, a robot manipulator kinematics model, a patient body model, and surgical instrument(forceps) shape/structure models. Analyzing the inputs from the laparoscope/instrument control interfaces based on these models, the simulator in real-time calculates:

1. the position and orientation of the laparoscopic camera,
2. the position and orientation of the two surgical instruments, and the open-close state of their handle,
3. the distance between the tip of the laparoscope/instrument and the center of gravity of the target object(corresponding to the virtual tissue), and
4. the angle between the direction from the tip of the laparoscope/instrument to the centroid of the target point and the direction of the longitudinal axis of the laparoscope/instrument.

Based on the above informations, the simulator decides the state of the target object such as *"appropriately captured by the laparoscope (can be touched/grasped with the instrument)"*, *"in touch with the instrument"*, *"grasped with the instrument"*, *"sticked with the instrument(indicating an error)"*, *"attached to the*

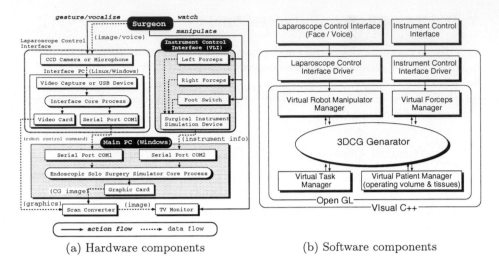

(a) Hardware components   (b) Software components

Fig. 1. System configuration.

instrument", *"can be detached from the instrument"*, and so on. As a result, the system can manage the timing of cameraworks and the number of errors (For details, see the next chapter). Finally, these calculation results are sent to the graphics software module (3DCG generator) and the virtual laparoscopic image is generated using the OpenGL library. The state of the target object is represented by its color, as a feedback information for the operator.

4   Intervention Tasks

Design of the study involved creation of a laparoscopic intervention task that accurately simulated in vivo laparoscopic surgical conditions. We chose the laparoscopic cholecystectomy (gallbladder removal) as the model operation because it is one of the standard laparoscopic interventions and nowadays performed frequently. We made the camerawork analysis of an in vivo laparoscopic cholecystectomy that had been performed[8] using our laparoscope positioning system. Finally, we worked out the following three tasks, in which the instrument operation part was designed based on that of the commercial computer-based laparoscopic trainer, MIST VR[9].

4.1   Task Setting

Fig. 2 shows comparison between the screenshots of the three basic tasks performed in an in vivo laparoscopic cholecystectomy and the corresponding images generated by our simulator. Now we briefly explain these tasks.

Task 1. It was designed to simulate basic maneuvers in the process of "retrieval of gallbladder". Notice that the target sphere and the target box in Fig. 2(a)

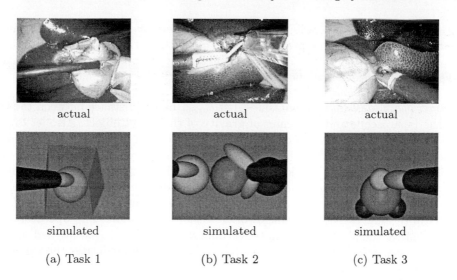

actual   actual   actual

simulated   simulated   simulated

(a) Task 1   (b) Task 2   (c) Task 3

Fig. 2. Screenshots of basic tasks. (a), Task 1: retrieval of gallbladder. (b), Task 2: dissection and ligation of cystic duct and vessel. (c), Task 3: dissection of gallbladder from liver. Upper part: real laparoscopic images taken during an actual cholecystectomy operation. Lower part: virtual laparoscopic images simulated by the ESSS system.

correspond to the gallbladder dissected from liver and the disposal bag respectively.

Task 2. It simulates a part of basic operations in the process of "dissection and ligation of cystic duct and vessel", especially "clipping of gallbladder duct". In this task, the target object, corresponding to the cystic duct, is composed of four spheres, as shown in Fig. 2(b).

Task 3. It was designed to simulate basic operations in the time segment of "dissection of gallbladder from liver". During this process, the surgeon applies a foot pedal-controlled cutting tool(diathermy) to the dissection spot in the gallbladder bed and burns the spot off by contact for a few seconds using a foot switch control. In Fig. 2(c), the main sphere and the small sub-spheres correspond to the gallbladder and the dissection/bleeding spots on the gallbladder surface respectively.

4.2 Task Management

In this section, we summarize the major points of task management in the ESSS.

Error scoring system— If at any time during these processes the instrument tip goes inside the target object, the color of the target object changes to red indicating an error which is recorded. In this case, contact with the instrument tip must be restored before the task can be continued. The judgement of errors is made based on the radius of the target sphere (r_{target}) and the distance between the instrument tip and the centroid of the target, say d_{tool}. If $d_{tool} \leq C_{error} \cdot r_{target}$ (where C_{error} is a predefined positive constant less than 1), the system will consider that the target is sticked with the instrument.

Camerawork induction mechanism— Let d_{scope} be the distance between the tip of the laparoscope and the center of gravity of the target object. Also let θ_{scope} be the angle between the direction of the longitudinal axis of the laparoscope and the direction from the tip of the scope to the centroid of the target. In the ESSS, the target under consideration can be touched/grasped if and only if it is captured with appropriate magnification in the video center, that is, $d_{scope} < T_d$ and $\theta_{scope} < T_\theta$ (where T_d and T_θ indicates predetermined thresholds). This inevitably induces regular cameraworks without exception. The operator can tell whether the above condition concerning d_{scope} and θ_{scope} is satisfied or not by confirming the color of the target (e.g., the light blue indicates the target is appropriately captured.).

Log file generation— During the task, the frame number, the coordinate of the tip point of the laparoscope, the coordinate of the tip point of the left and right surgical tools, errors if any, and the type of camera control commands are sequentially logged on a text file. After the completion, task beginning time and termination time are also logged on it.

5   Experiment

In this study, the face motion-based laparoscope control interface[8] was evaluated and compared to a voice control interface. All the tasks(Task 1–3) on the ESSS system were applied to this experiment. Camerawork time, the number of camerawork commands, camera moving distance, instrument moving distance, the number of errors, and task completion time were analyzed from the log files generated during each task execution. The task repetition number was set to two. All of the tasks involved four subjects. One of them was familiar with the face controlled interface but the rest had used the system several times before.

Experimental results are illustrated in Fig. 3. In these figures, the error bar with "×" indicates data for the face tracking based system while the "+"marked one indicates the result by voice control. Each error bar illustrates the mean("×" or "+" position) and minimum/maximum values. Although there was no significant difference between the interfaces for the task completion time (Fig. 3(f)), we got two interesting results:

- For all tasks, both the camerawork time and the laparoscope moving distance were shorter for the face motion-based interface compared to the voice control interface (Fig. 3(a)(b)). Furthermore, the number of camerawork commands in task 3 using the face control was smaller than the number with voice control interface, although there was no significant difference between the interfaces for that in task 1 and task 2 (Fig. 3(c)). In Task 3, the

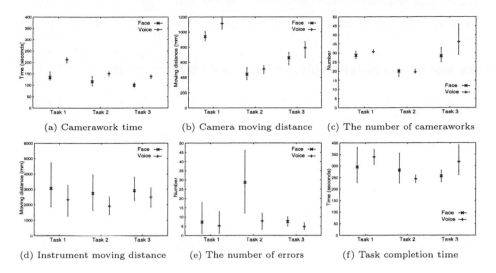

Fig. 3. Results of comparison of the two human-machine interfaces. (a), Camerawork time. (b), Laparoscope moving distance, (c), The number of camerawork commands. (d), Instrument moving distance (mean of the values for the left/right instruments). (e), The number of errors. (f), Task completion time. In these figures, the error bar with "×" indicates data for the face tracking based system while the "+"marked one indicates the result by voice control. Each error bar illustrates the mean("×" or "+" position) and minimum/maximum values.

subject had to position the laparoscope in high accuracy for removing small-sized subtargets. These results demonstrates the quantitative efficiency of laparoscopic cameraworks through face/voice commands.

− For all tasks, the instrument moving distance was longer for the face interface compared to the voice interface (Fig. 3(d)). Especially, the number of errors in Task 2 was significant greater for the face motion-based system compared to voice control system (Fig. 3(e)). In Task 2, the subject had to control the laparoscope and the instrument simultaneously and carefully. These results demonstrate the influence of face motion/vocalization upon the instrument operation.

6   Conclusion

Two human-machine interfaces for controlling the laparoscope were comparatively evaluated using a solo surgery simulator. The face control interface was more efficient in laparoscopic cameraworks than the voice control, even under a lot of stress to control the instruments. This is because the face motion can easily and flexibly represent not only the omni-direction of scope motion but also its motion velocity. As shown in the experimental results, however, in our current model it may have a bad influence on complex and precise surgical actions (may interrupt the flow of the procedure) especially in case that the laparoscope and the instrument should be simultaneously controlled. To solve this problem we are studying an improved model for guiding the laparoscope based on the visual tracking of both the surgeon's face and surgical instruments[10].

References

1. Ballester, P., Jain, Y., Haylett, K. R., McCloy, R.F.: Comparison of Task Performance of Robotic Camera Holders EndoAssist and Aesop. Computer Assisted Radiology and Surgery, Proc. of the 15th Intl. Congress and Exhibition, Elsevier Science (2001) 1071–1074
2. Yavuz, Y., Ystgaard, B., Skogvoll, E., Marvik, R.: A Comparative Experimental Study Evaluating the Performance of Surgical Robots Aesop and Endosista. Surgical Laparoscopy, Endoscopy & Percutaneous Techniques **10** (3) (2000) 163–167
3. Allaf, M.E., Jackman, S.V., Schulam, P.G., Cadeddu, J.A., Lee, B.R., Moore, R.G., Kavoussi, L.R.: Laparoscopic Visual Field. Voice vs Foot Pedal Interfaces for Control of the AESOP Robot. Surg Endosc **12** (12) (1998) 1415–1418
4. Kobayashi, E., Nakamura, R., Masamune, K., Sakuma, I., Dohi, T., Hashimoto, D.: Evaluation Study of A Man-machine Interface for A Laparoscope Manipulator. Proc. of the 8th Ann Meeting of Japan Soc Comput Aided Surg (1999) 121–122
5. Arezzo, A., Ulmer, F., Weiss, O., Schurr, M.O., Hamad, M., Buess, G.F.: Experimental Trial on Solo Surgery for Minimally Invasive therapy. Comparison of Different Systems in A Phantom Model. Surg Endosc **14** (10) (2000) 955–959
6. Buess, G.F., Arezzo, A., Schurr, M.O., Ulmer, F., Fisher, H., Gumb, L., Testa, T., Nobman, C.: A New Remote-Controlled Endoscope Positioning System for Endoscopic Solo Surgery. The FIPS Endoarm. Surg Endosc **14** (4) (2000) 395–399
7. Kobayashi, E., Masamune, K., Sakuma, I., Dohi, T., Shinohara, K., Hashimoto, D.: Safe and Simple Man-machine Interface for a Laparoscope Manipulator System. Comparison of Command Input Methods. J. Japan Soc Comput Aided Surg **3** (2) (2001) 71–78
8. Nishikawa, A., Hosoi, T., Koara, K., Negoro, D., Hikita, A., Asano, S., Miyazaki, F., Sekimoto, M., Miyake, Y., Yasui, M., Monden, M.: Real-Time Visual Tracking of the Surgeon's Face for Laparoscopic Surgery. Medical Image Computing and Computer-Assisted Intervention, Proc. of 4th Intl. Conference, Springer-Verlag (2001) 9–16
9. Wilson, M.S., Middlebrook, A., Sutton, C., Stone, R., McCloy, R.F.: MIST VR: A Virtual Reality Trainer for Laparoscopic Surgery Assesses Performance. Ann R Coll Surg Engl. **79** (6) (1997) 403–404
10. Nishikawa, A., Asano, S., Miyazaki, F., Sekimoto, M., Yasui, M., Monden, M.: A Laparoscope Positioning System based on the Real-Time Visual Tracking of the Surgeon's Face and Surgical Instruments. Computer Assisted Radiology and Surgery, Proc. of the 16th Intl. Congress and Exhibition, Springer-Verlag (2002)

Automatic 3-D Positioning of Surgical Instruments during Robotized Laparoscopic Surgery Using Automatic Visual Feedback

A. Krupa[1], M. de Mathelin[1], C. Doignon[1], J. Gangloff[1], G. Morel*,
L. Soler[2], J. Leroy[2], and J. Marescaux[2]

[1] LSIIT (UMR CNRS 7005), University of Strasbourg I, France
{alexandre.krupa,michel.demathelin}@ensps.u-strasbg.fr
[2] IRCAD (Institut de Recherche sur le Cancer de l'Appareil Digestif), France

Abstract. This paper presents a robotic vision system that automatically retrieves and positions surgical instruments in the robotized laparoscopic surgical environment. The goal of the automated task is to bring the instrument from an unknown or hidden position to a desired location specified by the surgeon on the endoscopic image. To achieve this task, a special instrument-holder is designed that projects laser dot patterns onto the organ surface which are seen on the endoscopic images. Then, the surgical instrument positioning is done using an automatic visual servoing from the endoscopic image. Our approach is successfully validated in a real surgical environment by performing experiments on living pigs in the surgical training room of IRCAD.

1 Introduction

Robotic laparoscopic systems have recently appeared, *e.g.*, ZEUS (Computer Motion, Inc.) or DaVinci (Intuitive Surgical, Inc.). With these systems, robot arms are used to manipulate the surgical instruments as well as the endoscope. The surgeon tele-operates the robot through master arms using the visual feedback from the laparoscope. This reduces the surgeon tiredness, and potentially increases motion accuracy by the use of a high master/slave motion ratio. Furthermore, teleoperation allows to perform long distance surgical procedures (see *e.g.* [1]). In a typical surgical procedure, the surgeon first drives the laparoscope into a region of interest (for example by voice, with the AESOP system of Computer Motion Inc.). Then, he or she drives the surgical instruments at the operating position. A practical difficulty lies in the fact that the instruments are generally not in the field of view at the start of the procedure. Therefore, the surgeon must either blindly move the instruments into the field of view of the endoscope, or zoom out with the endoscope as to get a larger view. Similarly, when the surgeon zoom in or moves the endoscope during surgery, the instruments may leave the endoscope's field of view. Consequently, instruments

---

* Now with the University of Paris 6 - LRP6 - Paris - France

T. Dohi and R. Kikinis (Eds.): MICCAI 2002, LNCS 2488, pp. 9–16, 2002.
© Springer-Verlag Berlin Heidelberg 2002

may have to be moved blindly with a risk of an undesirable contact between instruments and internal organs.

Therefore, in order to assist the surgeon, we propose a visual servoing system that automatically brings the instrument at the center of the endoscopic image (see, [2] and [3] for earlier works in that direction). Furthermore, when the instrument is in the field of view, the system provides a measurement of the distance between the organ and the tip of the instrument. Our system also allows to move automatically the instruments at a 3-D location chosen by the surgeon. The surgeon specifies the position in the image (with, *e.g.*, a touch-screen or a mouse-type device) and sets the distance value between the instrument and the organ at his or her convenience. Note that prior research was conducted on visual servoing techniques in laparoscopic surgery in, *e.g.*, [4],[5] and [6]. However, these systems were guiding the endoscope toward the region of interest instead of the instruments.

Our system includes a special device designed to hold the surgical instruments with tiny laser pointers. This laser pointing instrument-holder is used to project laser spots in the laparoscopic image even if the surgical instrument is not in the field of view. The image of the projected laser spots is used to automatically guide the instrument in the field of view. A major difficulty in designing this automatic instrument positioning system lies in the unknown relative position between the endoscope and the robot holding the instrument, and in the use of monocular vision that lacks depth information. In [7], the authors added an extra laser-pointing endoscope with an optical galvano scanner and a 955 *fps* high-speed camera to estimate the 3-D surface of the scanned organ. However, their method requires to know the relative position between the laser-pointing endoscope and the camera which is estimated by adding an external camera watching the whole system (OPTOTRAK system). In our approach, instead, we robustly estimate in real time the distance between instrument and organ by using images of optical markers mounted on the tip of the instrument and images of the laser spots projected by the same instrument. Then, visual feedback allows to automatically position the instrument at a desired location.

The paper is organized as follows. Section 2 describes the system configuration and the endoscopic laser pointing instrument prototype. In section 3, robust image processings leading to laser patterns and optical markers detection are briefly explained. The control scheme used to position the instrument by automatic visual feedback is described in section 4. In the final section, we present experimental results in real surgical conditions at the operating room of IRCAD.

2   System Description

2.1   System Configuration

The system configuration used to perform the autonomous positioning of the surgical instrument is shown in figure 1.a. The system includes a laparoscopic surgical robot and an endoscopic laser pointing instrument-holder. The robot allows to move the instrument across a trocar placed at a first incision point. A

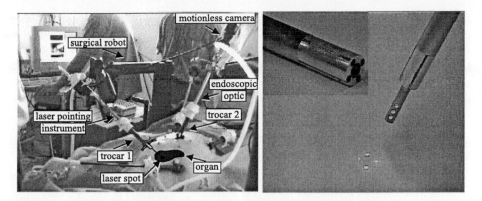

Fig. 1. (a) System configuration (b)-(c) Endoscopic laser pointing instrument-holder

second trocar is put in order to insert an endoscopic optical lens which provides the feedback view and whose relative position to the robot base frame is generally unknown.

2.2   Endoscopic Laser Pointing Instrument-Holder

We have designed the prototype of an endoscopic laser pointing instrument-holder shown in figure 1.b. It is a 30 *cm* long metallic pipe with 10 *mm* external diameter to be inserted through a 12 *mm* standard trocar. Its internal diameter is 5 *mm* so that a standard laparoscopic surgical instrument can fit inside. The head of the instrument-holder contains miniature laser collimators connected to optical fibers which are linked to external controlled laser sources. This device allows to remote laser sources which can not be integrated in the head of the instrument due to their size. The laser pointing instrument-holder mounted on a cleaning-suction instrument is shown in figure 1.c. The instrument-holder, with the surgical instrument inside, is held by the end-effector of the robot. It allows to project optical markers on the surgical scene. Three tiny light emitting diodes are fixed on the tip of the instrument to provide the optical markers needed to compute the depth information.

3   Robust Detection of Lasers Spots and Optical Markers

Robust detection of the geometric center of the projected laser spots in the image plane and detection of the image positions of the optical markers mounted on the instrument are needed in our system. Due to the complexity of the organ surface, laser spots may be occulted. Therefore a high redundancy factor is achieved by using at least four laser pointers. We have found in our experiments *in vivo* with four laser sources that the computation of the geometric center is always possible with a small bias even if three spots are occulted. Due to the viscosity of the organs, the surfaces are bright and laser spots are diffused. Therefore, the main difficulty is to precisely detect diffused laser points from the images speckle due to the ligthing conditions. A simple image binarization is not suitable. Our approach consists in synchronizing the laser sources with the image capture board in such a way that the laser spots are turned on during the even field of image frames and are turned off during the odd frames. In this manner, laser spots are visible one line out of two and can be robustly detected with a highpass spatial 2D FIR filter. Figure 2 shows images resulting

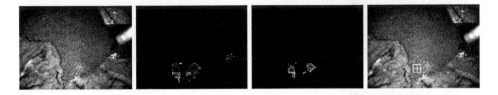

Fig. 2. Robust laser spot detection on a liver

from different steps of the image processing (original image - hightpass filtering - thresholding and erosion - detected geometric center). Coordinates of the center of mass are then computed from the filtered image. Note that the motions of organs due to heart beat and breathing may be also extracted with this spatial filtering of the image interlacing. They act like noise on the computed geometric center. Therefore a lowpass time filtering is also applied on the center of mass coordinates to reduce this noise. The optical markers mounted on the instrument are also synchronized with the image capture board. In contrast with the laser sources, the three optical markers are turned on during the odd frames and turned off during the even frames. Using the same method of detection, the image of optical markers is extracted. Coordinates of the center of the markers are then obtained using an ellipse detection algorithm (see figure 3.a).

4   Instrument Positioning with Visual Servoing

In laparoscopic surgery, instrument displacements are constrained to 4 DOF through an incision point. Only three rotations and one translation are allowed. Let R_L be a frame of reference at the tip of the instrument and R_C the camera frame (see figure 3.b). We define the instrument's velocity vector $\dot{W} = (\omega_x \quad \omega_y \quad \omega_z \quad v_z)^T$ where ω_x, ω_y and ω_z are rotational velocities of frame R_L with respect to camera frame R_C expressed in R_L and v_z is the translational velocity of the instrument along the z_L axis. In the case of a symmetrical instrument like the cleaning-suction instrument, it is not necessary to turn the instrument around its own axis to do the desired task. So only 3 DOF will be actuated for this kind of instrument and the operational space velocity vector is reduced to $\dot{W}_{op} = (\omega_x \quad \omega_y \quad v_z)^T$. For a non symmetrical instrument like a clamping instrument, the rotational speed ω_z can be kept in vector $\dot{W}_{op}$. To perform a positioning of the instrument, the surgeon specifies the target point on the screen. The required visual features are image coordinates $S_p = (u_p \quad v_p)^T$

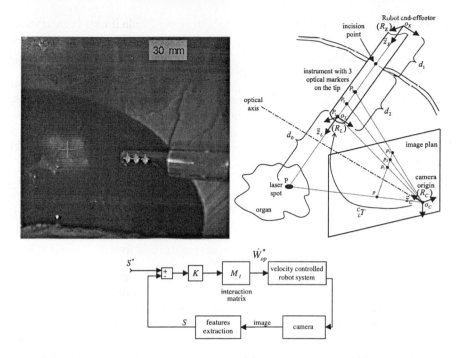

Fig. 3. (a) Robust optical markers detection (b) System geometry (c) Control scheme

of the center of mass of the projected laser spots. This center of mass is seen as the projection of the instrument axis onto the organ. Adding optical markers on the tip of the instrument allows to compute the distance d_0 between the organ and the instrument (see section 4.1). Figure 3.c shows the control scheme used for this positioning. The feature vector to control is $S = (u_p \quad v_p \quad d_0)^T$. If the classical image-based control strategy is used for visual servoing (cf. [8]), the reference velocity vector $\dot{W}_{op}^*$ is chosen proportional to the error on the features: $\dot{W}_{op}^* = M_I K (S^* - S)$ where K is a positive diagonal gain matrix, M_I is the interaction matrix, $M_I = J_S^{-1}$ in classical visual servoing where J_S is a Jacobian matrix relating the instrument velocity vector $\dot{W}_{op}$ to the image feature velocity vector $\dot{S}$, $(\dot{S} = J_S \dot{W}_{op})$. Furthermore, $S^* = (S_p^* \quad d_0^*)^T$, where $S_p^* = (u_p^* \quad v_p^*)^T$ is the desired instrument position in the image and d_0^* is the desired distance between the organ and the tip of the instrument. The distance between organ and instrument velocity can be measured only if the laser spots and the instrument markers are visible (see section 4.1). When the tip of the instrument is not in the field of view, only S_p can be controlled. Therefore, the instrument retrieval and positioning algorithm must have three stages:

Stage 1: Positioning of the laser spot at the center of the image by visual servoing of S_p only; control of $(\omega_x \quad \omega_y)^T$ only, with $\dot{W}_{op}^* = (\omega_x^* \quad \omega_y^* \quad 0)^T$.

Stage 2: Bringing down the instrument along its axis until the optical markers are in the field of view; open-loop motion at constant speed v_z^* with $\dot{W}_{op}^* = (0 \quad 0 \quad v_z^*)^T$.

Stage 3: Full visual servoing.

4.1   Depth Measurement

Adding optical markers on the tip of the instrument allows to measure the distance d_0. We put 3 markers P_1, P_2, P_3 along the instrument axis in such a way that we can assume that P_1, P_2, P_3 are collinear with the center of mass of the laser spots P (see Figure 3.a). Then, the projective cross-ratio τ (cf.[9]) is computed from points P, P_1, P_2, P_3 and their respective projection in order to estimate the depth d_0:

$$\tau = \frac{\left(\frac{\overline{pp_2}}{\overline{p_1p_2}}\right)}{\left(\frac{\overline{pp_3}}{\overline{p_1p_3}}\right)} = \frac{\left(\frac{\overline{PP_2}}{\overline{P_1P_2}}\right)}{\left(\frac{\overline{PP_3}}{\overline{P_1P_3}}\right)} \ . \quad \text{and} \quad d_0 = \overline{PP_1} = (\tau - 1)\frac{\overline{P_1P_2}.\overline{P_1P_3}}{\overline{P_1P_3} - \tau.\overline{P_1P_2}} \ . \quad (1)$$

4.2   Interaction Matrix

To control the position of the instrument in the image plane, one needs to compute the Jacobian matrix J_S which relates the visual features velocity $\dot{S}$ and the instrument velocity $\dot{W}_{op}$. This Jacobian matrix can be computed analytically if the camera is motionless and if the relative position of the instrument with respect to the camera can be measured as well as the depth variation (if the instrument is in the field of view). For safety reasons, it is not suitable that the laser spots centering error signals, $(S_p^* - S_p)$, induces depth motions ($v_z^* \neq 0$). Furthermore, when the instrument is going up or down ($v_z^* \neq 0$), this motion does not induce an error on the laser spot centering. Therefore, it is recommended to choose the interaction matrix M_I as follows:

$$M_I = \begin{pmatrix} A_{[2\times 2]} & 0_{[2\times 1]} \\ 0_{[1\times 2]} & -1 \end{pmatrix} \ . \quad \widehat{A} = \begin{pmatrix} \frac{\Delta u_p}{\omega_x^* \Delta T} & \frac{\Delta u_p}{\omega_y^* \Delta T} \\ \frac{\Delta v_p}{\omega_x^* \Delta T} & \frac{\Delta v_p}{\omega_y^* \Delta T} \end{pmatrix}^{-1} \ . \quad (2)$$

The matrix A in (2) can be analytically computed from J_S if the instrument is visible in the image. When it is not the case, as is stage 1 of the algorithm, this matrix is identified in an initial procedure. This initial identification procedure consists in applying a constant velocity reference signal $\dot{W}_{op}^* = (\omega_x^* \ \omega_y^* \ 0)^T$ during a short time interval ΔT. Small variations of laser spot image coordinates are measured and the estimation of A is given by $\widehat{A}$ in (2). The stability of the visual feedback loop is always guaranteed as long as $A\widehat{A}^{-1}$ remains positive definite [10]. Should the laser spot centering performance degrades, it is always possible to start again the identification procedure.

5   Experiments

Experiments in real surgical conditions on living pigs were conducted in the operating room of IRCAD (see Figure 1.a). The experimental surgical robotic task was the autonomous retrieval of a instrument not seen in the image and then its positioning at a desired 3-D position. We use a bi-processor PC computer (1.7 GHz) for image processing and for controlling, via a serial link, the surgical robot from ComputerMotion. A standard $50 fps$ PAL endoscopic camera hold by a second robot (at standstill) is linked to a PCI image capture board that grabs grey-level images of the observed scene. For each image the center of mass of the laser spots is detected in about 20 ms. The successive steps in the autonomous retrieval and positioning procedure are as following:

Step 1: changing the orientation of the instrument by applying rotational velocity trajectories (on ω_x^* and ω_y^*) in open loop to scan the organ surface with the laser spot until they appear in the endoscopic view.

Step 2: automatic identification of the interaction matrix A ($cf.(2)$).

Step 3: centering of the laser spots in the image by visual servoing.

Step 4: descent of the instrument by applying a velocity reference signal v_z^* in open loop until it appears in the image, keeping orientation servoing.

Step 5: real time estimation of the distance d_0 and depth servoing to reach the desired distance, keeping orientation servoing.

Step 6: new positioning of the instrument to desired 3-D locations by automatic visual servoing at the command of the surgeon. The surgeon indicates on the screen the new laser point image coordinates, $S_p^* = (u_p^* \ v_p^*)^T$, and specifies the new desired distance d_0^* to be reached. Then the visual servoing algorithm performs the positioning.

Figure 4.a-d shows experimental measurements of the laser image coordinates u_p and v_p during the identification stage of A and during the centering stage by visual servoing. For the identification procedure, four positions have been considered to relate variations of the laser image position and angular variations. We can notice a significant perturbation due to the breathing during the visual servoing. For robust identification purpose, we average several measurements of small displacements. This allows to reduce the effect of the breathing which acts like a disturbance. Figure 4.e shows the 2D trajectory obtained (in the image)

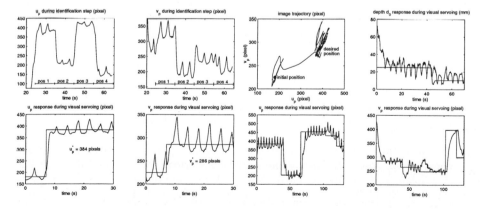

Fig. 4. (a)(b)(c)(d)-(e)(f)(g)(h) Experimental measurements

during the centering step by visual servoing. The oscillating motion around the initial and desired position are also due to the effect of breathing that acts as a periodic perturbation. Figure 4.f shows the measured distance d_0 during the depth servoing at step 5. Responses 4.g and 4.h display the laser image coordinates when the surgeon specifies new positions to be reached in the image.

Acknowledgements

The financial support of the french ministry of research ("ACI jeunes chercheurs" program) is gratefully acknowledged. The experimental part of this work has been made possible thanks to the collaboration of Computer Motion Inc. that has graciously provided the medical robots. In particular, we would like to thank Dr. Moji Ghodoussi for his technical support in the use of the medical robots.

References

1. J. Marescaux, J. Leroy, M. Gagner, and al. Transatlantic robot-assisted telesurgery. *Nature*, 413:379–380, 2001.
2. A. Krupa, C. Doignon, J. Gangloff, M. de Mathelin, L. Soler, and G. Morel. Towards semi-autonomy in laparoscopic surgery through vision and force feedback control. In *Proc. of the Seventh International Symposium on Experimental Robotics (ISER)*, Hawaii, December 2000.
3. A. Krupa, M. de Mathelin, C. Doignon, J. Gangloff, G. Morel, L. Soler, and J. Marescaux. Development of semi-autonomous control modes in laparoscopic surgery using visual servoing. In *Proc. of the Fourth International Conference on Medical Image Computing and Computer-Assisted Intervention (MICCAI)*, pages 1306–1307, Utrecht, The Netherlands, October 2001.
4. G.-Q. Wei, K. Arbter, and G. Hirzinger. Real-time visual servoing for laparoscopic surgery. *IEEE Engineering in Medicine and Biology*, 16(1):40–45, 1997.
5. G.-Q. Wei, K. Arbter, and G. Hirzinger. Automatic tracking of laparoscopic instruments by color-coding. In Springer Verlag, editor, *Proc. First Int. Joint Conf. CRVMed-MRCAS'97*, pages 357–366, Grenoble, France, March 1997.
6. A. Casals, J. Amat, D. Prats, and E. Laporte. Vision guided robotic system for laparoscopic surgery. In *Proc. of the IFAC International Congress on Advanced Robotics*, pages 33–36, Barcelona, Spain, 1995.
7. M. Hayashibe and Y. Nakamura. Laser-pointing endoscope system for intraoperative 3Dgeometric registration. In *Proc. of the 2001 IEEE International Conference on Robotics and Automation*, Seoul, Korea, May 2001.
8. F. Chaumette, P. Rives, and B. Espiau. Classification and realization of the different vision-based tasks. In *World Scientific Series in Robotics and Automated Systems, Vol. 7*, pages 199–228. Visual Servoing, K. Hashimoto (ed.), Singapore, 1993.
9. S.J. Maybank. The cross-ratio and the J-invariant. *Geometric invariance in computer vision*, Joseph L. Mundy and Andrew Zisserman, MIT press:107–109, 1992.
10. B. Espiau, F. Chaumette, and P. Rives. A new approach to visual servoing in robotics. *IEEE Trans. on Robotics and Automation*, 8(3):313–326, june 1992.

Development of a Compact Cable-Driven Laparoscopic Endoscope Manipulator

Peter J. Berkelman, Philippe Cinquin, Jocelyne Troccaz,
Jean-Marc Ayoubi, and Christian Létoublon

Laboratoire TIMC-IMAG, Groupe GMCAO
Faculté de Médecine de Grenoble
Joseph Fourier University and CNRS 38706 La Tronche, France*

Abstract. This report describes continuing development of a novel compact surgical assistant robot to control the orientation and insertion depth of a laparoscopic endoscope during abdomenal surgery. The sterilizable manipulator is sufficiently small and lightweight that it can be placed directly on the body of the patient without interfering with other handheld instruments during abdomenal surgery. It consists of a round base, a clamp to hold the endoscope trocar, and two joints which enable azimuth rotation and inclination of the endoscope pivoting about the insertion point. The robot is actuated by thin cables inside flexible sleeves which are pulled by electric motors with a rack-and-pinion drive. Operation of the robot is demonstrated using an abdomenal surgical simulation trainer and experimental results are given.

1 Introduction

We have developed a compact and lightweight endoscope manipulator to serve as a surgical assistant during laparascopic surgery. In typical minimally invasive laparoscopic surgical procedures, the principal surgeon requires an assistant to hold the endoscope and an attached video camera so that the abdomenal cavity can be viewed by the surgeon while manipulating laparoscopic instruments with both hands through keyhole incisions. To avoid occupying a second surgeon, the human assistant can be replaced by a robotic endoscope manipulator. It is a simple task for a robotic assistant to move an endoscope to a desired orientation and insertion depth inside the abdomen, as the insertion point of the endoscope at its keyhole incision is fixed so that only three degrees of freedom are required. Furthermore, speed and accuracy requirements are low, and sensitive force control is unnecessary as the endoscope does not contact internal tissues.

Several robot systems have previously been developed for laparoscopic endoscope manipulation during surgery [1–4]. The *AESOP*[5,6] from Computer Motion and *EndoAssist*[7] from Armstrong Healthcare are two examples of commercially available endoscope manipulator devices. In addition, minimally invasive complete telerobotic surgical systems include the *Da Vinci*[8] system from

---

* This work is supported under RNTL grants (Ministère de L'Industrie, ANVAR, MMM Project) under the leadership of PRAXIM Inc.

T. Dohi and R. Kikinis (Eds.): MICCAI 2002, LNCS 2488, pp. 17–24, 2002.

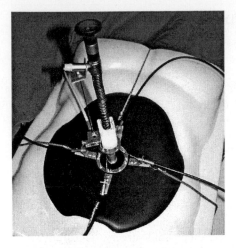

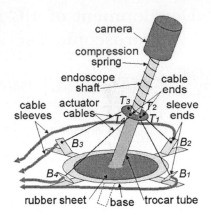

Fig. 2. Initial Endoscope Manipulator Schematic

Fig. 1. Initial Endoscope Manipulator

Intuitive Surgical Systems and *Zeus* from Computer Motion. Clinical studies [9, 10, 7] with various endoscope manipulator devices have indicated that the use of robotic endoscope assistants leads to a more stable image with no detrimental impact on efficacy or safety and a shorter duration of specific surgical interventions in many cases when compared to using a human assistant to hold the endoscope.

Although current endoscope manipulators perform well, they are generally large, heavy, complex, and expensive. In the limited space of a typical crowded operating room, the base of a conventional robot occupies a considerable amount of floor space next to the patient and the robot arm holding the endoscope may restrict full access to the abdomen of the patient. Hence it would be advantageous to have a much more lightweight, simple, and unobtrusive endoscope manipulator which would be easier to setup and use in conventional operating rooms. The novel features of our endoscope manipulator are that it is sufficiently lightweight that it can be strapped directly on the abdomen of the patient and that it is driven by cables inside flexible sleeves connected to motors in a separate module. The size and mass of our endoscope manipulator are nearly equivalent to that of the endoscope and camera.

Our first endoscope manipulator prototype used four cables connected directly between a circular base and the endoscope shaft to control endoscope orientation and a fifth cable along the endoscope shaft with compression springs to control the insertion depth. This system is described in detail in [11] and is shown in Figures 1 and 2. McKibben artificial pneumatic muscles [12, 13] attached to each cable were used for actuation.

The use of tensioned cables and sleeves to position medical instruments on a patient was proposed by Cinquin and Troccaz [14]. A cable-driven tele-echography slave robot [15] uses the same principles to manipulate an ultrasound probe on a patient.

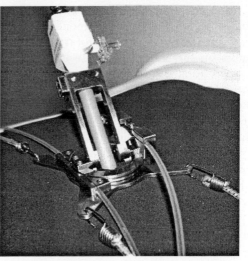

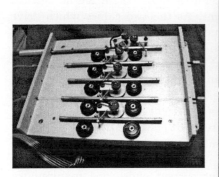

Fig. 3. Actuator Motors and Drives

Fig. 4. New Laparoscopic Endoscope Manipulator on Simulation Abdomen

2   Current Prototype

Our current endoscope manipulator prototype is of the same overall shape and size as the previous prototype, but we use motorized rack-and-pinion drives in place of the pneumatic muscle actuators and a small mechanism with two rotational joints driven by pairs of antagonistic cables in place of the arrangement of four cables working together in parallel. The cable and spring configuration used to control the insertion depth of the endoscope is essentially the same as previously. Rotation of the endoscope on its axis is currently unactuated; another cable and motor could be added for this rotation if there is demand. The actuators are shown in Figure 3 and the new prototype mechanism is shown with the endoscope and trocar on a simulated abdomen in Figure 4.

Each rotational joint is driven by a single motor and rack with a cable attached at each end to rotate the joint in both directions. The endoscope insertion is actuated by a third motor and rack. Each motor is controlled in position by an analog feedback servocontrol circuit. The new motorized actuation system is more compact, more easily controlled, and more reliable than the previous pneumatic muscle actuators. The cables are replaceable and the tension is easily adjustable to compensate for stretching from repeated use.

In our new mechanism, the endoscope trocar is rigidly clamped to a small arm which is attached to the manipulator base through two rotational joints, instead of being supported by four tensioned cables and a flexible rubber sheet as with the previous prototype. The axes of the two rotation joints intersect at the endoscope insertion point incision. The endoscope insertion actuation cable can still be released easily at any time to remove the endoscope from the trocar for replacement or cleaning of the lens.

The new endoscope orientation mechanism is more precise and more robust since there are no flexible components in the mechanism other than the actuation cables which drive the two rotational joints. Furthermore there are no vertical forces on the endoscope at its insertion point. As the two cables which drive each rotation joint are in direct opposition and the sum of their lengths remains constant throughout the motion of the joint, the ends of the cables can be attached to opposite ends of a single rack and motor, so that only one motor is necessary for each degree of freedom of the manipulator. For the same reasons, the kinematics and control of the new device is greatly simplified as well.

The mechanism is fabricated from stainless steel to be durable and easily sterilizable. The actuation cables are Teflon-coated and enclosed by Teflon sleeves. The cables and sleeves are disposable and would be replaced before each surgical procedure for sterility.

The relevant measured parameters of our current endoscope manipulator prototype are as follows:

Size:	70 mm diameter, 75 mm height
Mass:	350 g
Stiffness:	0.6 Nm/°, 0.40 N/mm
Motion Range:	360° azimuth rotation, 60° inclination, 200 mm translation
Speed:	75°/sec, 80 mm/sec

The size and mass of the device given do not include the 450 mm length and 340 g mass of the endoscope and camera. The limited stiffness in rotation is due to the elasticity of the actuator cables and in translation is due to the compression springs opposing the cable on the endoscope shaft.

3   Kinematics

The two axes of rotation of the manipulator mechanism intersect at the insertion point of the endoscope. The kinematics of the current manipulator are simple and straightforward, as the actuator cable lengths directly determine the position of the endoscope camera expressed in spherical coordinates (θ, ϕ, ρ):

$$\theta = l_1/R_1$$
$$\phi = l_2/R_2 \tag{1}$$
$$\rho = b - l_3$$

where l_1, l_2, and l_3 are the positions of the three cable actuators, R_1 and R_2 are the radii of the horizontal base ring and vertical semicircle which are rotated by the cables, and b is the length of the endoscope. The relations between the endoscope configuration expressed in Cartesian and in spherical coordinates is:

$$x = \rho \cos \theta \sin \phi,$$
$$y = \rho \sin \theta \sin \phi, \tag{2}$$
$$z = \rho \cos \phi,$$

and are inversible as:

$$\rho = \sqrt{x^2 + y^2 + z^2}$$
$$\theta = \tan^{-1}(y/x) \tag{3}$$
$$\phi = \cos^{-1}\left(\frac{z}{\sqrt{x^2 + y^2 + z^2}}\right).$$

The vertical configuration of the endoscope corresponds to a kinematic singularity as the value of θ is undefined for $\phi = 0$. The two coordinate systems are shown with a schematic of the endoscope in Figure 5.

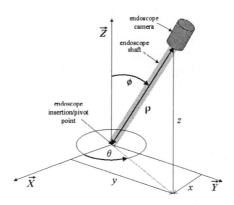

Fig. 5. Endoscope Manipulator Kinematics in Spherical and Cartesian Coordinates

If desired, noncontact 3D magnetic or optical localization systems could be used with the endoscope manipulator to provide absolute position feedback rather than the motor position feedback currently used. The localizer 3D coordinates would have to be registered to the endoscope pivot point to convert the localizer Cartesian (x, y, z) coordinates to the spherical/actuator spherical/actuator (θ, ϕ, ρ) coordinates using Equation 3.

4   Control Results

Each position variable was measured by the potentiometer on its actuator to provide the response data shown in Figures 6, 7, and 8. Each coordinate variable is shown plotted against time in seconds in response to two step commands in opposite directions.

The θ angle response is the most accurate because there is no gravity loading on this horizontal rotation joint. This 90° rotation was executed with the endoscope halfway extended at a 45° inclination. The ϕ rotation angle response is quicker in one direction than the other due to the gravity loading torque from the mass of the endoscope when it is not vertical. The translation response ρ is visibly less precise because it is actuated by only one cable with restoring forces provided by the compression springs on the shaft of the endoscope, whereas two cables operate antagonistically to actuate each of the two rotational joints. The response performance of the manipulator as shown is sufficient for a surgical assistant robot, where desired speeds are low and an surgeon operates the robot directly.

5   Current Work

Preliminary testing of our new prototype has indicated the need for several minor modifications to be done to improve the performance and practicality of the endoscope manipulator: The lever arm which clamps to the trocar should be shortened so to take up less space, reduce weight, and allow the trocar to be placed in a better position. The trocar clamp should be releasable by hand, so it could be replaced easily during surgery if required. The actuator cables and sleeves and their connection to the endoscope manipulator mechanism must be reconfigured to interfere less with the surgeon's instruments by being attached to the mechanism together in the same location and direction. To reduce the maximum required cable tension, the size of the pulley on the endoscope inclination joint should be increased and and a spring may be added to counterbalance the weight of the endoscope camera.

The currently implemented operator interfaces are rudimentary; motion commands for the endoscope manipulator can be given only by computer mouse or by rotating potentiometer dials. We have begun to investigate various possibilities for more sophisticated hands-free control which would be suitable for use in surgery, such as eye tracking, head tracking, voice commands, or multifunctional pedals. We also plan to replace the current PC control system with an embedded controller to make the complete system easily portable in a briefcase-sized package. Once these modifications are completed we plan to proceed with clinical validation.

6   Conclusion

We have developed and demonstrated a working prototype of a laparascopic surgical assistant endoscope manipulator which is especially lightweight, compact, and unobtrusive due to cable-driven actuation and being attached directly to the abdomen of the patient. The current prototype is an improvement of our previous mechanism.

Acknowledgements

The work of Eric Boidard and the expertise of Gildas de Saint Albin have significantly contributed to this project. The new prototype was designed and fabricated in cooperation with Alpes Instruments Inc. of Meylan, France.

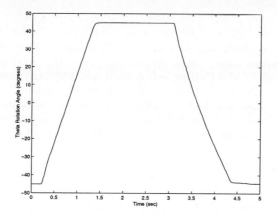

Fig. 6. Theta Response to Step Command Inputs

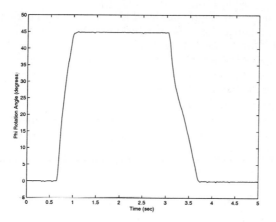

Fig. 7. Phi Response to Step Command Inputs

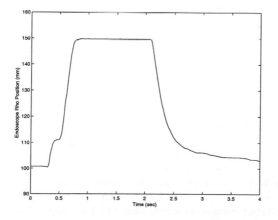

Fig. 8. Rho Response Step Command Inputs

References

1. E. Kobayashi, K. Masamune, I. Sakuma, T. Dohi, and D. Hashimoto, "A new safe laparoscopic manipulator system with a five-bar linkage mechanism and optical zoom," *Computer Aided Surgery*, vol. 4, no. 4, pp. 182–192, 1999.
2. R. H. Taylor, J. Funda, B. Eldridge, S. Gomory, K. Gruben, D. LaRose, M. Talamini, L. Kavoussi, and J. A. Anderson, "Telerobotic assistant for laparoscopic surgery," in *Computer Integrated Surgery: Technology and Clinical Applications* (R. H. Taylor, S. Lavallee, G. C. Burdea, and R. Mosges, eds.), pp. 581–592, MIT Press, 1995.
3. V. F. Munoz *et al.*, "Design and control of a robotic assistant for laparoscopic surgery," in *9th International Suymposium on Intelligent Robotic Systems*, (Toulouse, France), July 2001.
4. G. F. Buess, A. Arezzo, M. O. Schurr, F. Ulmer, H. Fisher, L. Gumb, T. Testa, and C. Nobman, "A new remote-controlled endoscope positioning system for endoscopic solo surgery–the fips endoarm," *Surgical Endoscopy*, vol. 14, pp. 395–399, 2000.
5. W. P. Geis, H. C. Kim, E. J. B. Jr., P. C. McAfee, and Y. Wang, "Robotic arm enhancement to accommodate improved efficiency and decreased resource utilization in complex minimally invasive surgical procedures," in *Medicine Meets Virtual Reality: Health Care in the Information Age*, (San Diego), pp. 471–481, 1996.
6. J. M. Sackier and Y. Wang, "Robotically assisted laparoscopic surgery: from concept to development," in *Computer Integrated Surgery: Technology and Clinical Applications*, pp. 577–580, MIT Press, 1995.
7. S. Aiono, J. M. Gilbert, B. Soin, P. A. Finlay, and A. Gordon, "Controlled trial of the introduction of a robotic camera assistant (EndoAssist) for laparoscopic cholecystectomy," in *11th Annual Scientific Meeting Society for Minimally Invasive Therapy*, (Boston), September 1999.
8. G. S. Guthart and J. K. Salisbury, "The Intuitive (TM) telesurgery system: Overview and application," in *International Conference on Robotics and Automation*, (San Francisco), pp. 618–621, IEEE, April 2000.
9. L. Mettler, M. Ibrahim, and W. Jonat, "One year of experience working with the aid of a robotic assistant (the voice-controlled optic holder AESOP) in gynaecological endoscopic surgery," *Human Reproduction*, vol. 13, pp. 2748–2750, 1998.
10. L. R. Kavoussi, R. G. Moore, J. B. Adams, and A. W. Partin, "Comparison of robotic versus human laparoscopic camera control," *Journal of Urology*, vol. 154, pp. 2134–2136, 1995.
11. P. J. Berkelman, P. Cinquin, J. Troccaz, J. Ayoubi, C. Letoublon, and F. Bouchard, "A compact, compliant laparoscopic endoscope manipulator," in *International Conference on Robotics and Automation*, (Washington D.C.), IEEE, May 2002.
12. V. L. Nickel, M. D. J. Perry, and A. L. Garrett, "Development of useful function in the severely paralyzed hand," *Journal of Bone and Joint Surgery*, vol. 45A, no. 5, pp. 933–952, 1963.
13. H. F. Schulte, "The characteristics of the McKibben artificial muscle," in *The application of external power in prosthetics and orthotics*, pp. 94–115, Washington D. C.: National academy of sciences-National research council, 1961.
14. P. Cinquin and J. Troccaz, "Système télécommandable de positionnement sur un patient d'un dispositif d'observation intervention," Patent 99 09363, France, 1999.
15. A. Vilchis-Gonzales, J. Troccaz, P. Cinquin, F. Courreges, G. Poisson, and B. Tondu, "Robotic tele-ultrasound system (TER): Slave robot control," in *IFAC*, 2001.

Flexible Calibration of Actuated Stereoscopic Endoscope for Overlay in Robot Assisted Surgery

Fabien Mourgues and Ève Coste-Manière

CHIR Team,
www.inria.fr/chir
INRIA, 2004 route des lucioles,
06902 Sophia-Antipolis Cedex, France
{fabien.mourgues,eve.coste-maniere}@inria.fr

Abstract. Robotic assistance have greatly benefited the operative gesture in mini-invasive surgery. Nevertheless, the surgeon is still suffering from the restricted vision of the operating field through the endoscope. We thus propose to augment the endoscopic images with preoperative data.

This paper focuses on the use of a priori information to initialise the overlay by a precise calibration of the actuated stereoscopic endoscope. The flexibility of the proposed method avoids any additional tracking system in the operating room and can be applied to other augmented reality systems. We present quantitative experimental calibration results with the da Vinci^{TM} surgical system, as well as the use of these results to initialise the overlay of endoscopic images of a plastic heart with a coronary artery model.

1 Introduction

Mini-invasive surgery presents many advantages for the patient: the incisions and the trauma are reduced, the post-operative recovery time is limited. It takes now advantages of robot assistance: the endoscope and the instruments are controlled by the surgeon through a master console. The comfort and the precision of the gesture are improved. In the da Vinci robot system, a stereoscopic endoscope provides the surgeon with an immersive 3D vision of the operating field thus providing good depth perception. However it still suffers from the classical constraints of the mini-invasive surgery: the keyhole vision is confined and greatly increases the difficulty of locating landmarks necessary for the operation. For example in the coronary artery bypass interventions, two difficulties are present: distinguishing the target artery among the grooves of the other arteries and locating the position of the stenosis on the latter. During the preoperative planning the surgeon visualises this information on the 3D+t model of the coronary tree built from angiography acquisitions [1] but the transposition in the endoscopic view of the operating field is not easy.

T. Dohi and R. Kikinis (Eds.): MICCAI 2002, LNCS 2488, pp. 25–34, 2002.

Thus, the enhancement of the surgeon's vision with pre or intraoperative information has become an important research challenge. It has been addressed in classical laparoscopic procedures [2] by restoring the surgeon's natural point of view, or in neurosurgery [3], by mapping endoscopic images on a preoperative brain surface. Some results of superposition in the laparoscopic view are given in [4] but no study concerns the augmentation of the 3D vision of the operating field in robot assisted surgery.

In coronary artery bypass interventions, the superposition of cartographic information (labelled arteries, direction to the target) requires new research efforts as described in [5]. The operating conditions - left lung collapse, CO_2 insufflation in the rib cage to provide space for the intervention, pericardium opening, organs motion - increase the difficulty of the registration with preoperative acquisitions (angiography, CT-scan).

We propose to address the problem in two steps:

1. use a priori information by registering the intraoperative endoscopic view and **the patient model in the preoperative situation**. This step needs:

- the calibration of the actuated endoscope (cameras parameters and position of the camera frames with respect to the actuated arm) to localise the latter in the robot frame.
- the **external** rigid registration of the patient in the operating room with respect to the preoperative acquisitions and the registration of the robot with respect to the patient. This step is solved using fiducial markers on the patient skin, segmented in CT-scan images and pointed by the robot arm [6].

This first step should give a good initialisation of the intraoperative overlay.

2. use of intraoperative acquisition. The heart deformations, displacements and motions must be considered to improve the coherency of the augmentation of the endoscopic images. The stereoscopic endoscope simplify the extraction of 3D information [7] with no need of structured light [2] and we investigate the use of appropriate landmarks for our cardiac application. The simultaneous use of other intraoperative acquisitions modalities (eg. ultrasound) could help the registration.

This paper mainly addresses the first step of the overall intraoperative registration problem: the calibration of the actuated stereoscopic endoscope by a new flexible method compatible with the operating room constraints. This method can be applied to any Augmented Reality (AR) system with cameras attached to a sensor localised with respect to a fixed reference. It presents some experimental calibration results and finally illustrates the first use of these results to initialise an endoscopic overlay.

2   Related Works and Contributions

Our endoscopic overlay system can be decomposed as a classical video-see through AR system: the two endoscopic cameras delivering the view of the real

scene on two display screens (for a 3D vision of the operating field) and a localisation system. The orientation and position of a frame attached to the rigid
endoscope is continuously computed from the articular coordinates of the robot.
The problem of calibration can be divided into two parts: the determination of
the two camera models and the estimation of the orientation and position of the
cameras with respect to the localised frame (figure 1). The camera calibration is
now well studied [8–10] and applied to the endoscopes [11, 4]. On the other hand,
the calibration of see-through display tracked with magnetic or optical technologies have been addressed for AR applications. In [12] a video see-through system
is calibrated using a 3D calibration object. The object and the Head-Mounted
Display are localised with an optical tracker and the calibration is performed
with Tsai's method [8]. The same method is used in [4] for a laparoscope. In
[13] the calibration pattern is reduced to a single 3D point fixed to the tracker
transmitter box. The method is active and adapted to the stereo case.

In our specific problem, the localisation of the endoscope is given by the
robot arm. We developed a calibration method based on a planar grid [10] which
avoids any additional tracking system to localise the pattern. This pattern, in an
arbitrary position, is observed with the actuated endoscope from unknown points
of view. The position of the grid with respect to the robot is an output of the
algorithm. The calibration protocol is flexible, in one step (camera parameters
including radial distortion, endoscope tip - camera transformation) and easily
usable in the operating room.

3   Material and Methods

After a description of the endoscope model and the protocol, the two parts of the
calibration process are developed: the first one consists of the determination of
the geometry of the two cameras: intrinsic parameters and radial distortion, rigid
transform between the two camera frames, by extending to the stereo case the
method proposed in [10]. The second one consists of computing and refining the
transformation D_{off} (see figure 1) between the camera frames and the endoscope
tip.

3.1   Actuated Endoscope Model

The stereoscopic endoscope is set on a actuated arm. Its position D_{er_i} with
respect to the fix robot-base is deduced from the articular coordinates. The
figure 1 illustrates the frames of the robot-base, the actuated endoscopic arm
and the two cameras. Each of the two cameras is described by the classical
pinhole model [14]. The intrinsic parameters matrices are noted:

$$A^{k=0,1} = \begin{bmatrix} f_u^k & \gamma^k & u_0^k \\ 0 & f_v^k & v_0^k \\ 0 & 0 & 1 \end{bmatrix} \tag{1}$$

By introducing the rigid transform D_{01} between the two camera frames, the
projection matrices can be written in the first camera frame as:

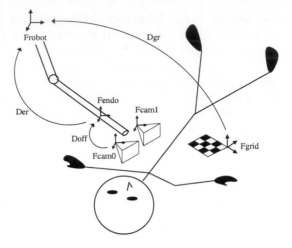

Fig. 1. Definition of the frames.

$$P^0 = A^0 [I_3|0_3] \ and \ P^1 = A^1 [R_{01}|T_{01}] \tag{2}$$

We consider the two first terms k_1^k and k_2^k of the radial lens distortion. Finally the endoscope model is completed by the rigid transform D_{off} between the right camera frame and the endoscope tip given by the articular coordinates.

3.2 Protocol

Before the introduction of the endoscope in its trocar, the focus is adjusted and a grid is set in front of the endoscope in an arbitrary position with respect to the robot and the patient. The actuated endoscope is moved around the grid and a few views are acquired. The corners of the grid are extracted and the algorithm is run. The overall process only takes a few minutes.

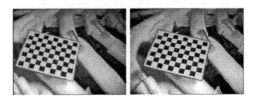

Fig. 2. Left and right view of the calibration grid.

3.3 Determination of the Parameters of the Two Cameras

This first part of the method consists of the determination of the geometry of the two cameras: intrinsic parameters and radial distortion, rigid transform between the two camera frames.

Intrinsic parameters and pose estimation. The intrinsic parameters are estimated assuming the cameras are free of distortion. As shown in [10], they are derived from the properties of the collineations between the planar grid and the projected points. With at least three views, all the five intrinsics parameters may be estimated in the generic case. For each point of view, the pose D_i of the right camera with respect to the grid is determined from the intrinsic parameters and the properties of the collineations. Then, an estimate D_{01} of the transformation between the two camera frames is derived.

Refinement. The intrinsic parameters, the poses D_i (rotation vector r_i, translation T_i) of the right camera with respect to the grid and D_{01} (rotation vector r_{01}, translation T_{01}) are refined by globally minimising the distance from the projection of the points M_j of the grid to the detected ones $m_{ij}^{0,1}$ in all available stereo pairs. We also introduce the distortion coefficients k_1^k and k_2^k, initialised at 0. This non-linear criterion is minimised using the Levenberg-Marquardt algorithm [15]:

$$\sum_i \sum_j \quad \|m_{ij}^0 - m(f_u^0, f_v^0, \gamma^0, u_0^0, v_0^0, k_1^0, k_2^0, r_i, T_i, M_j)\|^2$$
$$+ \|m_{ij}^1 - m(f_u^1, f_v^1, \gamma^1, u_0^1, v_0^1, k_1^1, k_2^1, r_i, T_i, r_{01}, T_{01}, M_j)\|^2 \tag{3}$$

Such bundle adjustment technique is commonly used in photogrammetry (see [16] for a recent review).

3.4   Determination of the Cameras - Endoscope Tip Transform

This second part of the method can be applied to any AR system with cameras attached to a sensor localised with respect to a fixed reference (optic or magnetic tracker). The absolute position of the calibration grid is simultaneously determined.

Use of the endoscope displacements. As illustrated in figure 1, the absolute position D_{gr} of the calibration grid is unknown. We overcome the difficulty by using the displacement matrices between two positions: the displacement of the endoscope with respect to the robot and the displacement of the cameras with respect to the grid. Between the positions i and $i + 1$ of the endoscope, we can write:

$$D_{m_{i \to i+1}} = D_{i+1} * D_i^{-1} = D_{off}^{-1} D_{er_{i+1}}^{-1} D_{er_i} D_{off} \tag{4}$$

id est:

$$D_{er_{i+1}} D_{off} D_{m_{i \to i+1}} = D_{er_i} D_{off} \tag{5}$$

The matrices can be parameterised using quaternions q [17] and vectors of translation, leading to the following system:

$$q_{er_{i+1}} * q_{off} * q_{m_{i \to i+1}} = q_{er_i} * q_{off} \tag{6}$$

$$\left(R_{er_{i+1}} - R_{er_i}\right) T_{off} = T_{er_i} - T_{er_{i+1}} - R_{er_{i+1}} R_{off} T_{m_{i \to i+1}} \tag{7}$$

By expanding the equation (6) for n displacements of the endoscope, we have for the rotation:

$$Aq_{off} = 0 \tag{8}$$

This last equation is solved using a singular value decomposition of the $4n \times 4$ matrix A (see [18] fro a recent review and analysis) . Then, the expansion of the equation (7) , gives for the translation:

$$BT_{off} = C \tag{9}$$

where B is a $3n \times 3$ matrix and C a vector of dimension $3n$. The problem is solved from:

$$T_{off} = \left(B^t B\right)^{-1} B^t C \tag{10}$$

The grid-robot transformation is then deduced from any endoscope position:

$$D_{gr} = D_{er_i} * D_{off} * D_i \tag{11}$$

Refinement. The position of the grid D_{gr} and the cameras - endoscope tip transform D_{off} are refined by minimising, using the Levenberg-Marquardt algorithm [15], the following criterion. The residual error is a quantitative indication of the performance of the superposition of the points in the images and the virtual view generated using the endoscope model and the state of the actuated endoscope.

$$\sum_i \sum_j \quad \|m_{ij}^0 - m_i^0(r_{off}, T_{off}, r_{gr}, T_{gr}, M_j)\|^2 \\ + \|m_{ij}^1 - m_i^1(r_{off}, T_{off}, r_{gr}, T_{gr}, M_j)\|^2 \tag{12}$$

4   Experiments and Results

The da Vinci^{TM} surgical system was used for experiments with the cardiac surgery team at Hôpital Européen Georges Pompidou, Paris, France. An acquisition system has been developed in the team to synchronously acquire the two video channels of the endoscope and the state of the robot with dedicated APIs written by Intuitive Surgical. The PC-based system serves this data through a network from the operating room of the hospital. A very high speed network allows us to collect the data and work from our lab in Sophia-Antipolis. A surgical robotics simulator previously developed [6] (see also our companion paper) is connected through the network and computes in real time the two virtual views corresponding to the endoscope position by using the calibration results.

Endoscope Calibration. We acquired several data sets and verified the stability of the result. For each data set of n endoscopic positions, we applied the algorithm on all the $n - 1$ endoscopic positions subsets.

After optimisation of the parameters of the two cameras, the reprojection error was less than half a pixel (eq. 3). We also computed the RMS error of the distance from the 2D points to the epipolar lines which measures the quality of the calibration. The residual error was around one pixel.

The transformation between the cameras and the tip of the endoscope was estimated as explained earlier. The residual error computed using the calibration results and the forward kinematics of the robot (eq. 12) was of the order of 4 pixels on the data subsets. We obtained equivalent reprojection error on the position of the endoscope non used in the calibration procedure. We hope to improve this error by using a calibration procedure that would correct the measured position of the endoscopic arm.

3D reconstruction of the operating field. As described in [5] we investigate the use of surfacic information to refine the overall registration problem. The experimental setup is composed of a plastic phantom composed of a heart and rib cage. After calibration of the actuated endoscope, the cameras parameters are used to reconstruct in 3D by stereoscopy the surface of the plastic heart. We use the cameras to endoscope transformation and the forward kinematics of the robot to fuse the surface patches corresponding to different positions of the endoscope for the fixed robot frame. Figure 3(c) depicts preliminary results of 3D reconstruction of the heart surface. These results are displayed with segmented surface of the heart from preoperative CT scan. Animal experiments are currently carried out to better validate the proposed approach and assess its adaptability.

Overlay in the endoscope. The the rib cage of the phantom is registered to preoperative CT data using a fiducial markers based pointing mechanism. On the other hand, a 3D model of the coronary arteries had been obtained from angiographic projections [1]. After calibration, the endoscope is inserted in its trocar and placed in operating position. We use the calibration results to model the cameras, find the cameras to robot transformation and perform the first augmentation of the endoscopic images with the preoperative model of the arteries. Figure 3(d) illustrates this overlay. We have observed a misalignment which can be attributed to the external registration error, the limited precision of the robot kinematics and the precision of the endoscope calibration. The different sources of error are being further investigated through a more discriminating experimental setup that we are currently building.

5   Discussion and Future Trends

This work addresses the problem of augmenting endoscopic 3D vision in robot assisted surgery. It focuses on the use of a priori information to initialise the overlay by a precise calibration of the actuated stereoscopic endoscope. The proposed method avoids any additional tracking system in the operating room. Its flexibility is compatible with the constraints of the operating theatre and it can be applied to a variety AR systems.

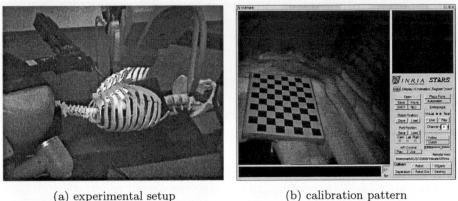

(a) experimental setup   (b) calibration pattern

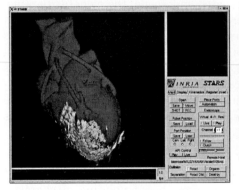

(c) surface patches of the plastic heart reconstructed from the endoscopic images
and the preoperative heart model segmented in CT-scan.

(d) superposition of the preoperative
model of the coronary arteries in the endoscopic view of the plastic heart.

Fig. 3. Experimental results

3D reconstructions of the operating field performed in an experimental setup
composed of a plastic heart inside a rib cage illustrate the quality of the results. The experiments were performed with Professor Alain Carpentier's cardiac
surgery team and the Intuitive Surgical team at the Hôpital Européen Georges
Pompidou, Paris, France. The error measured on a planar calibration pattern
observed from an unknown point of view in an operative configuration is around
4 pixels. We investigate the reduction of this error by more precisely calibrating
the mechanic of the actuated endoscope. This improvement should have conse-
quences on the use of the direct robot kinematics to initialise the overlay and
we are building an experimental setup to quantify the error of the registration
string from the preoperative acquisitions to the intraoperative overlay in the
endoscope.

Meanwhile we address, the second aspect of the registration problem: the use of intraoperative information. We investigate, on in vivo images of animals, the way to refine the displacement of the endoscope deduced from the forward robot kinematics, to deal with the dynamic aspect and to constrain the registration by using eligible landmarks for our cardiac application.

Acknowledgements

Thierry Vieville and Olivier Faugeras are gratefully acknowledged for some fruitful ideas during the development of this work. We also thank Cyril Coirier from Intuitive Surgical France and Prof. Alain Carpentier and the cardiac surgery team at the Hôpital Européen Georges Pompidou, Paris.

References

1. Mourgues, F., Devernay, F., Malandain, G., Coste-Manière, E.: 3d+t modeling of coronary artery tree from standard non simultaneous angiograms. In: Proceedings MICCAI. Volume 2208 of Lecture Notes in Computer Science., Springer (2001) 1320–1322
2. Fuchs, H., Livingston, M., Raskar, R., Colucci, D., Keller, K., State, A., Crawford, J., Rademacher, P., Drake, S., A.Meyer: Augmented reality visualization for laparoscopic surgery. In: Proc. of MICCAI'98. Volume 1496 of LNCS., Springer (1998) 934–943
3. Dey, D., Slomka, P., Gobbi, D., Peters, T.: Mixed reality merging of endoscopic images and 3-D surfaces. In: Proceedings MICCAI. Volume 1935 of Lecture Notes in Computer Science., Springer (2000) 796–803
4. Buck, S.D., Cleynenbreugel, J.V., Geys, I., Koninckx, T., Koninck, P.R., Suetens, P.: A system to support laparoscopic surgery by augmented reality visualization. In: Proceedings MICCAI. Volume 2208 of Lecture Notes in Computer Science., Springer (2001) 691–698
5. Devernay, F., Mourgues, F., Coste-Manière, E.: Towards endoscopic augmented reality for robotically assisted minimally invasive cardiac surgery. In IEEE, ed.: Proceedings of Medical Imaging and Augmented Reality. (2001) 16–20
6. Coste-Manière, È., Adhami, L., Severac-Bastide, R., Lobontiu, Adrian Salisbury, J.K.J., Boissonnat, J.D., Swarup, N., Guthart, G., Mousseaux, É., Carpentier, A.: Optimized port placement for the totally endoscopic coronary artery bypass grafting using the da Vinci robotic system. In Russ, D., Singh, S., eds.: Lecture Notes in Control and Information Sciences, Experimental Robotics VII. Volume 271., Springer (2001)
7. Mourgues, F., Devernay, F., Coste-Manière, E.: 3D reconstruction of the operating field for image overlay in 3D-endoscopic surgery. In: Proceedings of International Symposium on Augmented Reality. (2001)
8. Tsai, R.Y.: A versatile camera calibration technique for high-accuracy 3D machine vision metrology using off-the-shelf TV cameras and lenses. IEEE Journal of Robotics and Automation 3 (1987) 323–344
9. Maybank, S.J., Faugeras, O.D.: A theory of self-calibration of a moving camera. The International Journal of Computer Vision 8 (1992) 123–152

10. Zhang, Z.: Flexible camera calibration by viewing a plane from unknown orientations. In: Proceedings of the 7th International Conference on Computer Vision, Kerkyra, Greece, IEEE Computer Society, IEEE Computer Society Press (1999) 666–673

11. Khadem, R., Bax, M.R., Johnson, J.A., Wilkinson, E.P., Shahidi, R.: Endoscope calibration and accuracy testing for 3d/2d image registration. In: Proceedings MICCAI. Volume 2208 of Lecture Notes in Computer Science., Springer (2001) 1361–1362

12. Sauer, F., Khamene, A., Bascle, B., Rubino, G.: A head-mounted display system for augmented reality image guidance: Towards clinical evaluation for iMRI-guided neurosurgery. In: Proceedings MICCAI. Volume 2208 of Lecture Notes in Computer Science., Springer (2001) 707–716

13. Genc, Y., Sauer, F., Wenzel, F., Tuceryan, M., Navab, N.: Optical see-through HMD calibration: A stereo method validated with a video see-through system. In: Proceedings of International Symposium on Augmented Reality. (2000)

14. Faugeras, O.: Three-Dimensional Computer Vision. MIT Press (1993)

15. More, J.: The levenberg-marquardt algorithm, implementation and theory. In Watson, G.A., ed.: Numerical Analysis. Lecture Notes in Mathematics 630. Springer-Verlag (1977)

16. Triggs, B.: Optimal estimation of matching constraints. In Koch, R., Gool, L.V., eds.: Workshop on 3D Structure from Multiple Images of Large-scale Environments SMILE'98. Lecture Notes in Computer Science (1998)

17. Pervin, E., Webb, J.: Quaternions in computer vision and robotics. In: Proceedings of the International Conference on Computer Vision and Pattern Recognition, Washington, IEEE (1983) 382–383

18. Papadopoulo, T., Lourakis, M.: Estimating the jacobian of the singular value decomposition: Theory and applications. Research Report 3961, INRIA Sophia-Antipolis (2000)

Metrics for Laparoscopic Skills Trainers: The Weakest Link!

Stephane Cotin[1,3], Nicholas Stylopoulos[1,2,3], Mark Ottensmeyer[1,3],
Paul Neumann[1,3], David Rattner[2,3], and Steven Dawson[1,3]

[1] The Simulation Group, Massachusetts General Hospital, Boston, MA
[2] Department of Surgery, Massachusetts General Hospital, Boston, MA
[3] Harvard Medical School, Boston, MA
scotin@partners.org

Abstract. Metrics are widely employed in virtual environments and
provide a yardstick for performance measurement. The current method
of defining metrics for medical simulation remains more an art than a science. Herein, we report a practical scientific approach to defining metrics,
specifically aimed at computer-assisted laparoscopic skills training. We
also propose a standardized global scoring system usable across different
laparoscopic trainers and tasks. The metrics were defined in an explicit
way based on the relevant skills that a laparoscopic surgeon should master. We used a five degree of freedom device and a software platform
capable of 1) tracking the motion of two laparoscopic instruments 2)
real time information processing and feedback provision. A validation
study was performed. The results show that our metrics and scoring
system represent a technically sound approach that can be easily incorporated in a computerized trainer for any task, enabling a standardized
performance assessment method.

1   Introduction

Ask a surgeon whether virtual reality based simulation will be an important educational aid and the answer is predictably "yes". The rationale for this response
is that current methods of training have been recently placed under scrutiny
by experts, physicians, and the general public. As a result of the Institute of
Medicine report "To Err is Human: Building a Safer Health System" [8], the
American Board of Medical Specialties (ABMS) along with the Accreditation
Council on Graduate Medical Education (ACGME) initiated a joint outcomes
project. The aim of this project is to identify and quantify the factors that con-
stitute "medical competence" and promote the development of the appropriate
training models to improve medical performance and skills acquisition [1]. These
leading medical educators advocate the application of computer simulation in the
arena of medical training. Indeed, during the past ten years medical simulation
has progressed to a level of academic prototypes [12, 3, 18, 9, 4] or commercial
products [13, 14]. Computerized systems have enabled the recording of quantitative parameters including instrument motion and applied forces, which cannot

T. Dohi and R. Kikinis (Eds.): MICCAI 2002, LNCS 2488, pp. 35–43, 2002.

be measured with conventional instruments alone. This is a major step towards skill acquisition. As Dr David Leach, the director of ACGME said "What we measure we tend to improve" [11]. A corollary of this statement is that by creating accurate and relevant metrics we can augment the advantages offered by existing training systems and improve skills acquisition and learning. Unfortunately today, the lack of appropriate metrics represents one of the weakest links in medical simulation.

1.1 Laparoscopic Skills Training

The expanding application of laparoscopy is a factor that has reemphasized the absolute requirement for technical competency. Laparoscopic surgery is a technically demanding discipline, which imposes significant psychomotor challenges on surgeons, making it an ideal candidate for medical simulation. However, because of the need for faster and more accurate modelling algorithms, the educational and clinical aspects have been downplayed and several questions remain to be answered. Is task training important? If yes, what tasks should be simulated and what are the appropriate ways to evaluate task performance? These two questions are very familiar to all the researchers in the field of medical simulation, but few have addressed these issues. The first question has been answered by the Society of American Gastrointestinal Surgeons (SAGES), which is the first official association to officially adopt a set of skill testing modules [16]. Skills training is essential because it optimizes the learning opportunities in the operating room by increasing the level of confidence and comfort with the fundamentals of laparoscopy [21, 2, 5, 11]. The second question has been partially answered through the development of virtual environments and enhanced training boxes that permit controlled conditions under which we can elucidate the elements of skill and try to understand the underlying cognitive demands of laparoscopic surgery [20].

Until recently there was a tendency to view performance assessment and metrics in very simplistic terms [11]. The first non-computer based laparoscopic skills trainers incorporated empirical outcome metrics as an indirect way to evaluate performance and learning. Performance, however, cannot be evaluated solely on the basis of the outcome [15]. With the advent of computer simulation it became apparent that it will be possible to define specific metrics that can be used effectively and efficiently to evaluate performance [17]. An efficient metric should not only provide information about performance but also identify 1) the key success/failure factors of performance, 2) the size and the nature of the gap between expert and novice performance. Thus, it should point to the action that needs to be taken in order to resolve these gaps.

2   Material and Methods

In order to make computer simulation a stronger link in medical training, we propose a set of appropriate metrics that illustrates the relationship between the kinematic properties of the motion of laparoscopic instruments and the special cognitive and psychomotor skills that a laparoscopic surgeon should master.

Additionally, a standardized method of performance assessment is imperative to ensure comparability across different systems and training conditions. In this section we first introduce the concept of task-independent metrics for skills assessment and how it relies on kinematics analysis. We describe the various parameters used to represent the essential characteristics of any laparoscopic task, and how these parameters are combined into a standardized score. The mechanical apparatus used to record data from the laparoscopic instruments is detailed in section (2.2), followed by a description of the implementation of the kinematic analysis software and its interface in section (2.3). Finally, the experimental setup and the validation study are described in section (3) as well as the results of the study and their clinical significance.

2.1 Task-Independent Metrics

It is not clear how surgeons learn and adapt to the unusual perceptual motor relationships in minimally invasive surgery. A major part of the learning process, however, relies on an apprenticeship model according to which an expert surgeon qualitatively assesses the performance of the novice[1] [15]. In order to define a *quantitative* performance metric that is useful across a large variety of tasks, we looked at the way expert surgeons instruct and comment upon the performance of novices in the operating room. Expert surgeons are able to evaluate the performance of a novice by watching on the operating room monitor the motion of the visible part of the instruments that have been introduced into the abdominal cavity. Based on this information and the outcome of the surgical task, the expert surgeon can characterize qualitatively the overall performance of the novice on each of the key parameters that are required for efficient laparoscopic manipulations.

We identified the following components of a task that account for competence while relying only on instrument motion: compact spatial distribution of the tip of the instrument, smooth motion, good depth perception, response orientation, and ambidexterity. Time to perform the task as well as outcome of the task are two other important aspects of the "success" of a task that we decided to include [15, 11, 16]. Finally, in order to transform these parameters into quantitative metrics, we relied on kinematics analysis theory that has been successfully used in previous work to study psychomotor skills [10]. Most laparoscopic tracking devices or haptic interfaces can provide information about kinematic parameters, in particular: position of a three-dimensional point representing the tip of the instrument, rotation of the instrument about its axis, and degree of opening of the handle. All these variables are time-dependent and we will use the following notations in the remaining of the paper: $[x(t), y(t), z(t)]^T$ is the three-dimensional position of the tip of the instrument, and $\theta(t)$ is the rotation of the instrument about its axis. The five kinematic parameters we have defined so far are:

- *Time*: this is the total time required to perform the task (whether the task was successful or not). It is measured in seconds and represented as $P_1 = T$.

---

[1] The term novice connotes a surgeon in training.

- *Path Length*: it is the length of the curve described by the tip of the instrument over time. In several tasks, this parameter describes the spatial
  distribution of the tip of the laparoscopic instrument in the workspace of
  the task. A compact "distribution" is characteristic of an expert. It is measured in centimeters and represented as P_2.

$$P_2 = \int_0^T \sqrt{\left(\frac{dx}{dt}\right)^2 + \left(\frac{dy}{dt}\right)^2 + \left(\frac{dz}{dt}\right)^2} \, dt \tag{1}$$

- *Motion Smoothness*: this parameter is based on the measure of the instantaneous jerk defined as $j = \frac{d^3x}{dt^3}$ and represents a change of acceleration and
  is measured in cm/s^3. We derive a measure of the integrated squared jerk J
  from j as follows:

$$J = \sqrt{\frac{1}{2} \int_0^T j^2 dt} \tag{2}$$

The time-integrated squared jerk is minimal in smooth movements [6]. Because jerk varies with the duration of the task, J has to be normalized for
different tasks durations. This was done by dividing J by the duration T of
the task: $P_3 = J/T$.

- *Depth Perception*: we measure depth perception as the total distance trav-
  elled by the instrument along its axis. It is represented as P_4 and can easily
  be derived from P_2.
- *Response orientation*: this parameter characterizes the amount of rotation
  about the axis of the instrument and illustrates the ability to place the tool
  in the proper orientation in tasks involving grasping, clipping or cutting. It
  is represented as P_5 and measured in radians.

$$P_5 = \sqrt{\int_0^T \frac{d\theta^2}{dt} dt} \tag{3}$$

All of these parameters can be seen as cost functions where a lower value
describes a better performance. *Task-independence* is achieved by computing
the z-score [7] of each parameter P_i. The z-score z_i corresponding to parameter
P_i is defined as follows

$$z_i = \frac{P_i^N - \overline{P_i^E}}{\sigma_i^E} \tag{4}$$

where $\overline{P_i^E}$ is the mean of $\{P_i\}$ for the expert group and σ_i^E is the standard
deviation. P_i^N corresponds to the result obtained by the novice for the same
parameter. Assuming a normal distribution, 95% of the expert group should
have a z-score $z_i \in [-2; 2]$. Therefore we can limit the range of values for z_i to
$[-z_{max}; z_{max}]$ with $z_{max} > 2$. In our implementation we used $z_{max} = 10$.

A *standardized score* is computed from the independent z-scores z_i according
to the following equation

$$z = 1 - \frac{\sum_{i=1}^N \alpha_i z_i}{\sum_{i=1}^N \alpha_i z_{max}} - \alpha_0 z_0 \tag{5}$$

where N is the number of parameters, z_0 is a measure of the outcome of the task and α_0 the weight associated with z_0. There are various ways of evaluating z_0 and it can be either a binary measure ($z_0 = 0$ for success, $z_0 = 1$ for failure), or a more complex measure, as introduced by several authors [15, 16]. Similarly, α_i is the coefficient for a particular parameter P_i.

2.2 Apparatus

The subjects' position trajectories was measured with a modified Virtual Laparoscopic Interface (VLI) (Immersion Corp., San Jose, CA). The VLI includes tool handles similar to laparoscopic instruments, but there are no tool tips with which to manipulate real objects. To permit the use of the VLI as a tracking instrument, the main shafts and tool handles from the VLI were removed, and replaced with a system which allows the use of a variety of laparoscopic instruments. Figure 1

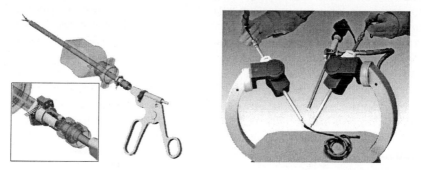

Fig. 1. (Left): modified Virtual Laparoscopic Interface to support the use of laparoscopic instruments and real objects. Inset (left): detail of bayonet connection and Hall effect/magnet arrangement. (Right): testbed for the "Cobra Rope Drill" task.

shows the modified system, including the original VLI equipment, the new main shafts, the laparoscopic instruments, and the bayonet connectors which permit rigid connection between the two. By replacing the main shaft of the VLI and modifying the laparoscopic instruments, the pitch/yaw/roll and thrust sensors can be used without modification. The gripper sensor in the original system is a Hall effect sensor that detects the motion of the actuator shaft in the tool handle. The original sensor blocks the insertion of full length instruments, so it was removed, and a new Hall sensor and rare-earth magnet combination were installed as shown in figure 1. This also simplifies interfacing the modifications to the VLI, since the signal output is electrically identical to the unmodified system.

The instrument modifications and Hall effect sensor placement were performed as precisely as possible, but due to the sensitivity of the sensor to small changes in the distance between it and the magnet, each instrument was separately calibrated. This ensures good correspondence between the true gripper axis motion and that measured by the system. Changing the calibration constants and offsets when switching tools is computed by software.

Laparoscopic trocar and cannula assemblies were also incorporated and special care was taken so that the friction at the point of entry of the instruments is realistic. For visual feedback we used a fixed surgical endoscope, camera, and light source (Telecam SL NTSC/Xenon 175, Karl Storz Endoscopy-America, Inc., Culver City, CA), to provide the same visual feedback encountered in minimally invasive procedures. The relative orientation between the endoscopic camera, the instrument axis and the monitor was approximately the same to minimize the mental effort of relating visual and instrument frames [19].

2.3 Software System

We have developed a software interface that integrates data processing as well as visualization of the instrument motion, path, parameters P_i and normalized score. Our system uses the *Virtual Laparoscopic Interface* API from Immersion Corp. as a basis for communication with the VLI. The raw data consists of time-stamped values of the position and orientation of each of the two laparoscopic instruments, recorded at a sampling rate of about 20 ms. Before computing any of the kinematic parameters, the raw data is filtered. We have implemented various low-pass filters, using mean and median filtering. The results presented in section (3) have been obtained after filtering with a median filter (window size=5). In order to compute accurately high order derivatives of the position, we used a second-order central difference method (if no filtering and/or first order methods were used, an accurate computation of the jerk would be very difficult).

We implemented the user interface using C++, FLTK[2], and OpenGL. The user interface offers real-time display of the tip of the tool, and its path (see Figure 2). Kinematics analysis and computation of the score are performed at the end of the task, providing immediate information to the user. Moreover, a visual comparison of the results of the experts group and the novice illustrates clearly what skills need to be improved in order to get a higher score. To account for the two laparoscopic instruments available in the VLI, we compute a z-score for each tool: z_{left} and z_{right}, and define the overall score as $z = (z_{left} + z_{right})/2$. The coefficients α_i are all set to 1 except for z_0 which is set to 0.5 if the goal of the task is not achieved. This illustrates the flexibility of our approach and its ability to take into account the specifics of the hardware and goals of the tasks (by allowing one to vary the weights α_i of the parameters P_i).

3   Experimental Results and Discussion

Three tasks of increasing difficulty selected from established training programs (the Yale Laparoscopic Skills and Suturing Program, the SAGES-FLS training program and the graded exercises used at Harvard Center of Minimally Invasive Surgery) were examined:

---

[2] Fast Light Toolkit, http://www.fltk.org

- *Task 1: Peg Board Transfer*: the purpose of this task is to assess eye-hand coordination, bimanual dexterity, and depth perception,
- *Task 2: Cobra Rope Drill*: the purpose of this task is to assess depth perception, two-handed choreography, and non-dominant hand development,
- *Task 3: Needle-Cap* : the purpose of this task is to assess depth perception, non-dominant hand development, and targeting.

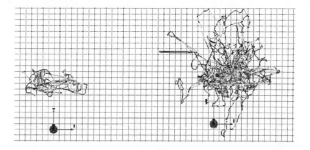

Fig. 2. Screenshot of our user interface displaying the path of the expert (left) and the novice (right) after completion of the "Cobra Rope Drill" task. The trajectory is color-coded based on velocity. A compact path is characteristic of expert's performance.

In order to validate our scoring system, we conducted a study comparing experts and novices surgeons. The expert group consisted of staff surgeons from our hospital, while the novice group consisted of 20 surgeons in training. Each of the experts was asked to perform each task several times. Each of the novices was asked to perform each task once, and was visually assessed by an expert. Most of the novices had had prior exposure to the tasks they were asked to perform. The values of the different parameters $\{P_i\}$ as well as the score z were computed using our software platform and recorded on file.

The results of the study illustrate several important aspects of our method. First, they confirm that our metrics are independent of the task being performed. Without changing any of the parameters P_i or weights α_i used in the computation of the overall score, our method still provides an efficient way of discriminating between expert and novice performance, irrespective of the task, as illustrated in table (1).

Table 1. This table presents the overall scores obtained by novices and experts in our study. It clearly highlights the gap existing between expert's and trainee's performance, irrespective of the task. None of the subjects in our novice group obtained a score above the threshold $(\overline{z^E} - 2\sigma^E)$ that distinguishes experts from non-experts.

	Task 1	Task 2	Task 3
Expert mean score (standard deviation)	1.0 (0.035)	1.0 (0.03)	1.0 (0.015)
Novice minimum score	0.22	0.38	0.04
Novice maximum score	0.69	0.58	0.72

In addition to an overall measure that discriminates between experts and non-experts, our method provides additional feedback by identifying the key factors that contribute to the overall score. For instance, we can see in Figure (3) that factors such as depth perception, smoothness of motion, and response orientation are major indicators of performance, while time and path length (often referenced in the literature) do not provide enough information to capture the magnitude of the difference. By comparing the expert's verbal assessment and the parameters P_i for which existed a significant difference between novice and expert, a high correlation was found, thus validating our choice of parameters.

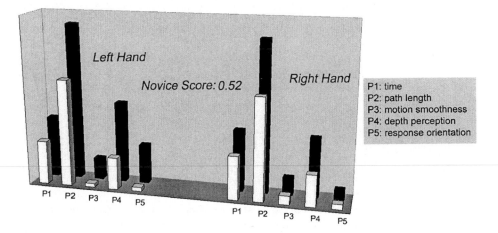

Fig. 3. This diagram illustrates the comparison between the experts group (light blue) and a novice (dark blue). The overall score given to the novice by our system was 0.52; this score can be explained by low values associated with particular parameters (P_3, P_4, P_5). Such feedback is very important to provide a meaningful interpretation of the score.

4   Conclusion

The method presented in this paper represents a work in progress. We have demonstrated that it is possible to extract meaningful information from the analysis of the motion of laparoscopic instruments only. This is a novel contribution and it allows the definition of task-independent metrics and the formulation of a standardized global scoring system for laparoscopic skills training. We have also shown that our approach can be a successful alternative to the verbal assessment scheme used in the classic apprenticeship model. Therefore it can be introduced in computer-based learning systems for surgical skills training.

Acknowledgements

This work was supported by U.S. Army Medical Research Acquisition Activity under contract DAMD17-99-2-9001. The ideas and opinions presented in this paper represent the views of the authors and do not, necessarily, represent the views of the Department of Defense.

References

1. ACGME Outcome project. Available at http://www.acgme.org/outcome/
2. Anastakis, D.J., Hamstra, S.J., Matsumoto, E.D.: Visual-spatial abilities in surgical training. Am. J. Surg. 179(6) (2000) 469–471
3. Brown, J., Montgomery, K., Latombe, J.C., Stephanides, M.: A Microsurgery Simulation System. In: Niessen, W.J., Vierger, M.A. (eds.): MICCAI 2001, vol. 2208. Springer-Verlag Berlin Heidelberg (2001) 137–144
4. Cotin, S., Delingette, H., Ayache, N.: A hybrid elastic model for real-time cutting, deformations and force feedback for surgery training and simulation. The Visual Computer 16 (2000) 437–452
5. Derossis, A.M., Fried, G.M., Abrahamowicz, M., Sigman, H.H., Barkun, J.S., Meakins, J.L.: Development of a model for training and evaluation of laparoscopic skills. Am. J.Surg. 175(6) (1998) 482–487
6. Hogan, N., and Flash, T.: Moving gracefully: Quantitative theories of motor coordination. Trends Neurosci. 10 (1987) 170–174
7. Howell D.C. (ed.). Fundamental Statistics for the Behavioral Sciences with CDRom. Duxbury Press Pacific Grove, CA (1998)
8. Kohn, L.T., Corrigan, J.M., Donaldson, M.F. (eds.): To Err is Human. Building a Safer Health System. Institute of Medicine, National Academy Press, Washington, D.C. (1999)
9. Kuhnapfel, U.G., Kuhn, C., Hubner, M., Krumm, H.G., Maa, E.H., Neisius, B.: The Karlsruhe Endoscopic Surgery Trainer as an example for virtual reality in medical education, Minimally Invasive Therapy and Allied Technologies 6 (1997) 122–125
10. Mavrogiorgou, P., Mergl, R., et al.: Kinematic analysis of handwriting movements in patients with obsessive-compulsive disorder. J. Neurol. Neurosurg. Psychiatry 70(5) (2001) 605–612
11. Metrics for objective assessment of surgical skills workshop. Scottsdale Arizona (2001). Final report. Available at: http://www.tatrc.org/
12. Picinbono, G., Delingette, H., Ayache, N. Non-linear and anisotropic elastic soft tissue models for medical simulation. In ICRA2001: IEEE International Conference Robotics and Automation, (2001)
13. Procedicus MIST. Mentice Medical Simulation, Gothenburg, Sweden
14. Reachin Laparoscopic Trainer. Reachin Technologies AB. Stockholm, Sweden
15. Rosser, J.C. Jr., Rosser, L.E., Savalgi, R.S.: Objective evaluation of a laparoscopic surgical skill program for residents and senior surgeons. Arch. Surg. 133(6) (1998) 657–661
16. Society of American Gastrointestinal Endoscopic Surgeons. Fundamentals of laparoscopic surgery. Available at: http://www.fls-test.org/
17. Satava, R.M.: Accomplishments and challenges of surgical simulation. Surg. Endosc. 15(3) (2001) 232–241
18. Szekely, G., Brechbuhler, C., Hutter, R., Rhomberg, A., Ironmonger, N. Schmid, P.: Modelling of Soft Tissue Deformation for Laparoscopic Surgery Simulation. In: Wells, W.M., Colchester, A., Delp S. (eds.): MICCAI 1998. Lecture Notes in Computer Science, vol. 1496. Springer-Verlag Berlin Heidelberg (1998) 550–561
19. Tendick, F., Jennings, R., Tharp, G., Stark, L.: Sensing and Manipulation Problems in Endoscopic Surgery: Experiment, Analysis, and Observation. Presence 2(1) (1993) 66–81
20. Tendick, F., Downes, M., Goktekin, T., Cavusoglu, M.C., Feygin, D., Wu, X., Eyal, R., Hegarty, M., Way L.W.: A Virtual Environment Testbed for Training Laparoscopic Surgical Skills. Presence 9(3) (2000) 236–255
21. Wanzel, K.R., Hamstra, S.J., Anastakis, D.J., Matsumoto, E.D., Cusimano, M.D.: Effect of visual-spatial ability on learning of spatially-complex surgical skills. Lancet 359(9302) (2002) 230–231

Surgical Skill Evaluation by Force Data
for Endoscopic Sinus Surgery Training System

Yasushi Yamauchi[1], Juli Yamashita[1], Osamu Morikawa[1], Ryoichi Hashimoto[1],
Masaaki Mochimaru[1], Yukio Fukui[1,2], Hiroshi Uno[3], and Kazunori Yokoyama[4]

[1] National Institute of Advanced Industrial Science and Technology (AIST),
Tsukuba Central 6, 1-1-1, Higashi, 305-8566 Tsukuba, Japan
{y.yamauchi,yamashita-juli,morikawa,hashimoto-r,
m-mochimaru,y.fukui}@aist.go.jp
http://unit.aist.go.jp/humanbiomed/humed_en/indexE.htm
[2] Institute of Information Sciences and Electronics, University of Tsukuba,
1-1-1, Ten-noudai, 305-8573 Tsukuba, Japan
[3] KOKEN CO., LTD., 3-14-3, Mejiro, Toshima-ku, 171-0031 Tokyo, Japan
[4] ENT clinic@Tsukuba South Avenue, 2-18-2, Takezono, 305-0032 Tsukuba, Japan
ra4k-ykym@asahi-net.or.jp

Abstract. In most surgical training systems, task completion time and error
ratio are common metrics of surgical skill. To avoid applying unnecessary and
injurious force to the tissue, surgeons must know for themselves how much
force they are exerting as they handle surgical tools. Our goal is to develop an
endoscopic sinus surgery (ESS) training system that quantitatively evaluates the
trainee's surgical skills. In this paper, we present an ESS training system with
force sensors for surgical skill evaluation. Our experiment revealed that the
integral of the force data can also be one of the useful metrics of surgical skill.

1 Introduction

Recently, endoscopic surgery has become widely used as a less invasive method than
conventional means. In endoscopic surgery, a small opening must be made for the
insertion of the endoscope and forceps, but deep lesions can be treated directly, i.e.,
without celiotomy. This provides marked advantages, such as less invasiveness and
shorter hospital stays. On the other hand, it is difficult to interpret the positions of
lesions on endoscopic images, due to the limited endoscopic visual field and the
narrowness of the spaces around the legions; in addition the long forceps used in
endoscopic surgery tend to restrict movement. It has been reported that these
limitations can cause complications such as injury to tissues around the lesions. To
solve these problems, new surgical devices and navigation systems supporting
endoscopic surgery have been developed. However, the development of training
devices to improve surgical skills has only just started, and new methods must be
developed to quantitatively and objectively evaluate improvement in surgical skills.

A variety of systems have been developed for training in various types of surgical
procedures. Most of the studies in surgical training based on virtual reality techniques
[1-3] focus on helping the trainee learn a surgical procedure by simulation and
imitation but do not mention surgical skill evaluation. These surgical 'simulation'

T. Dohi and R. Kikinis (Eds.): MICCAI 2002, LNCS 2488, pp. 44–51, 2002.
© Springer-Verlag Berlin Heidelberg 2002

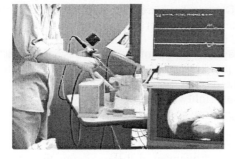 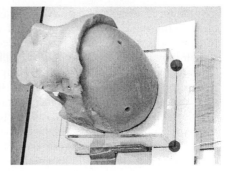

Fig. 1. Endoscopic sinus surgery training system. The endoscopic view *(lower right)* is also shown for the subject. The force output is shown on the computer display *(upper right)*.

Fig. 2. Force sensors are fixed beneath the platform of the dummy (left and right circles). These sensors detect the forces perpendicular to the surface of the desk.

systems do not provide quantitative data about the trainee's technical progress, and should not be confused with surgical 'training' systems. The most popular metrics of surgical skill are task completion time and error ratio [4,5], which are also commonly used in surgical training systems [6-11]. However, these metrics are not adequate for evaluating the quality of surgical tasks, because a fast but rough technique can damage tissues. From the qualitative point of view, a few studies on surgical skills have added force analysis as a metric. O'Toole et al. [12] applied force analysis to a surgical training system for a suturing task.

We are developing a training system that employs force analysis [13] for endoscopic sinus surgery (ESS). As the surgeon's working space in the nasal cavities is far narrower than it is in laparoscopic surgery, avoiding excessive collision between surgical tools and tissue is an essential point in ESS training. A few ESS training systems have been proposed [3,9,10], but none have succeeded in quantifying collision force as a metric of surgical skill. In this study, we examine surgical force as well as task completion time as metrics of surgical skill.

2 ESS Training System

The ESS training system that we have developed (Fig. 1) consists of a head dummy, force sensors, endoscope, position sensor, video monitoring system, and computer systems.

The dummy is an accurate reproduction made of urethane resin and based on a mold of a cranial bone specimen. Since the dummy has a modular structure consisting of a skull module and left and right nasal cavity modules, the nasal cavity modules are interchangeable for future use. To make the nasal cavity module similar to an actual nasal cavity, the urethane bone was given soft tissues made of silicone and colored to look like nasal mucosa. The face of the dummy is made of a porous urethane epidermis. CT images of the dummy showed no excessive artifact, and the average CT value of the dummy was around 250HU. This indicates that our ESS training system is also applicable in the training of image-guided sinus surgery.

Two force sensors (PS-5KA, Kyowa Dengyo Inc.) are fixed beneath the platform of the dummy (Fig. 2), one on the left and the other on the right. The output of the force sensors is digitized (5 Hz), recorded by a computer (PC-9801RX, NEC Inc.) and shown in real time on the computer display. The output of the sensors is adjusted to 0 when no external force exists. If the output of both sensors is positive, it indicates that a force perpendicular to the surface of the desk is working. If one output is positive and the other is negative, a moment to rotate rightward or leftward is working.

The endoscopic system consists of a rigid forward-oblique endoscope at 30 degrees (Shinko Optics, 4mm in diameter), a video camera, and an illuminator. The endoscopic image is displayed on a 14-inch color CRT monitor (Sony Inc.). To determine the task completion time from the movement of the endoscope tip, a probe of an optical position sensor (Hybrid Polaris, Northern Digital Inc.) is fixed to the CCD unit of the endoscope.

The dummy, endoscope, and monitors are arranged so that they can be observed simultaneously on a single video frame. The conditions of the experiments are recorded with a camcorder (Sony Inc.).

3   Experiments

In the experiments, the subjects conducted two types of surgical tasks: 'evaluation tasks' and 'training tasks'. The evaluation tasks were performed in the left nasal cavity of the dummy, and the training tasks, which were similar to the evaluation tasks, were performed in the right nasal cavity. Each trainee's performance was evaluated in each evaluation task. Kinematical learning specific to the right nasal structure occurred by repeated training, but it was useless for the left nasal cavity, in which the evaluation tasks were performed, because the left and right cavities have different structures. Therefore, the evaluation of skills in the evaluation tasks was not affected by the kinematical learning that occurred in the training tasks.

3.1   Tasks

Figure 3 shows the two task types. The evaluation tasks were to confirm the ostium of the left frontal sinus by the forward-oblique endoscope at 30 degrees, and to take the tip of the forceps to the ostium. When the endoscope is introduced into the nasal cavity, the ostium can be spontaneously seen by direct insertion because the endoscope is usually inserted looking obliquely upward. Then the endoscope was removed, the forceps was inserted into the site slightly forward from the endoscope, and the tip of the forceps was taken to the ostium while the endoscope confirmed its position. This procedure was done once in each evaluation task period.

For the training tasks, the target was the ostium of the right maxillary sinus. Although the endoscope was inserted looking obliquely upward, it had to be rotated 90 degrees anticlockwise on the way to the target, because the ostium is situated on the side. The rotated endoscope was removed from the nasal cavity, the forceps was inserted into the site slightly forward from the endoscope, and the tip of the forceps was taken to the target while the endoscope confirmed its position. In each training task period, this procedure was repeated for five minutes.

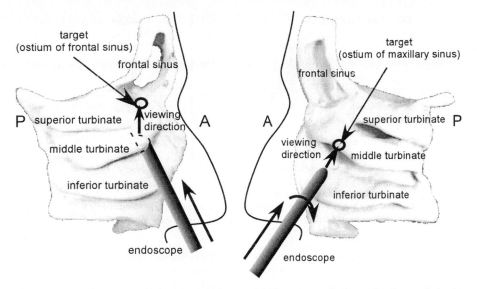

Fig. 3. The evaluation task and the training task. The target of the evaluation task is the ostium of the left frontal sinus *(left)*, whereas the target of the training task is the ostium of the right maxillary sinus *(right)*. In the training task, the endoscope should be rotated 90 degrees on the way.

3.2   Subjects

The subjects were three non-medical volunteers who had not used an endoscope and two resident physicians who had limited experience in endoscopic sinus surgery (fewer than 20 cases each). None of the five subjects had previously used the training system. Data from the evaluation tasks performed by an experienced otorhinologist who had performed endoscopic surgery in more than 200 cases were used as the expert reference data.

The output of the force sensors (5 Hz) and the position of the endoscope tip (10 Hz) were measured during the surgical and training tasks, and the camcorder synchronously recorded the conditions of the operation and the endoscopic images. The task completion time was defined as the period when the tip of the endoscope was in the nasal cavity, as measured by the position sensor.

3.3   Experiment Procedures

The experiment procedures for all subjects consisted of a pre-experiment learning session and five tasks as following steps. The total time of the experiment was around 1 hour per subject.

Pre-experiment learning: After outlines of the experiments were presented and the anatomical structures of the left and right nasal cavities were explained, the subjects studied the basic operation of the endoscope and forceps twice by watching afrom the videotape, and then actually performed the operation.

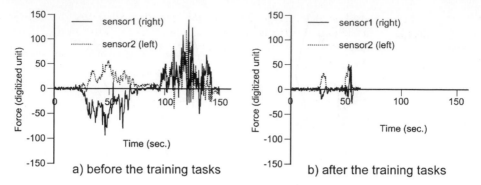

Fig. 4. Time evolutions of the output of force sensors of a resident. Before the training tasks (a), an evaluation task took over two minutes and excessive force occurred. After the training tasks (b), the task completion time was shorter and the force was lower than before.

First evaluation task: The subjects learned the evaluation tasks once by watching a videotape of the tasks being performed by an experienced ESS surgeon, then immediately performed the same tasks. Force and position data were recorded during the tasks.

First training task: Subsequently, the subjects learned the training tasks once by watching a videotape of this task as performed by the expert, then immediately performed the training tasks for five minutes. After the completion of the training tasks, his/her performance, as recorded by the video camera, was played back on the VCR and displayed on the image monitor. This was followed by a replay of the learning videotape about the training tasks. This was the feedback for the subjects.

Second evaluation task: This was the same as the first evaluation task.

Second training task: This was the same as the first training task.

Third evaluation task: This was the same as the first evaluation task.

4   Results

Fig. 4 shows the time evolutions of the output of the force sensors during a) the first and b) the third evaluation tasks performed by one of the residents. The unit of force is digitized voltage from an A/D converter.

As shown in Fig. 4a, strong and irregular forces and moments were detected. Pushing the dummy towards the platform with the forceps or endoscope caused strong positive forces, and twisting the dummy on the platform with the forceps or endoscope inserted into the nasal cavity caused strong negative forces. These forces were judged to be unnecessary, because the expert showed no such forces. In the third evaluation tasks (Fig. 4b), the forces were clearly lower than those in the first performance, indicating the training's effects on the force data.

To evaluate surgical skill, we need a kind of index for force exerted. We propose three indices: a) maximum, b) average and c) integral, based on the absolute values from the two sensors (Fig. 5). The expert's data normalize all the data in these figures. Clinically, the maximum shows the instantaneous strong force, the average indicates the average force on the tissue, and the integral shows the total force on the tissue during the tasks. For all parameters, the data obtained from the expert were the lowest (1.0), indicating that the expert can totally reduce the unnecessary load on the tissue. Fig. 5d shows the subjects' task completion times. The trend is almost the same as that of the force data.

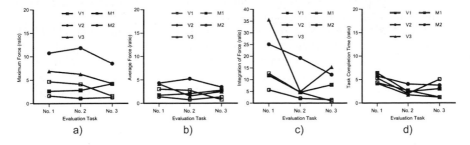

a)   b)   c)   d)

Fig. 5. Indices for the evaluation tasks: a) maximum force, b) average force, c) integration of the force, and d) completion time. V1, V2, and V3 are the non-medical volunteers, and M1 and M2 are the residents. All data are normalized by those of an expert.

5   Discussion

Of the three force indices, the integral was decreased significantly by the repeated performance of the surgery (non-parametric: Friedman's test ($p < 0.05$), Wilcoxson's coding rank test ($p < 0.05$)). The mean and maximum were reduced slightly, but the differences were not statistically significant. As the dimension of the integral is the multiplication of time and force, the characteristics of the integral can inherit those of both the task completion time and average force. Clinically, the integral reflects both the magnitude and duration of friction caused by the endoscope or forceps contacting tissues on the way to the lesions. Therefore, the integral is considered the most adequate force index of surgical skill in ESS.

The differences between the expert, the residents, and the non-medical subjects are clearly shown in Fig. 4c. The reference data obtained from the expert showed an excellent performance compared with any of the subjects. In the two residents, the initial performance was lower than that by the expert, but the integral steadily decreased with the completion of two training tasks, reaching a level close to that of the expert. On the other hand, in the three non-medical subjects, the integral decreased but did not finally reach the level of the expert. Within the limitations of the small number of subjects and the statistical analysis with the presumption of normal distribution, there was a significant difference in the integral of force between the residents and non-medical subjects (analysis of variance, $p < 0.05$).

Force indices are adequate to evaluate the interference between surgical tools and organs, and are applicable to the training of nasal, bronchoscopic, angioscopic, and gastrointestinal surgeries. Force evaluation is also valuable for tasks in microsurgery and robotic surgery, in which the surgeon does not obtain force-feedback directly. In the latter cases, the difference to an adequate force is the most meaningful metric [19]. The analysis of the surgical tool's position will also serve as a quantitative index of surgical skill [15]. The position sensors in our system will also enable such analysis.

The tasks in this study are for short-term learning. But in real applications, training occurs in periods of several days to several months. It is necessary to evaluate the usefulness of the proposed training system in such long-term training, and also to study the skill learning system over a long period.

In most of the existing systems with surgical force measurement [12,14-18], force/torque sensors are attached to the surgical tools. When the objective of training is to avoid unnecessary tool-to-dummy collision, sensors can be attached to the dummy. Doing so, the systems accept any kind of existing surgical tools. It should also be added that the sensors attached to the dummy only detect tool-to-dummy collisions.

6   Conclusions

To aid endoscopic surgical training, we have developed a training system based on a dummy of the nasal cavities that is equipped with force sensors, conducted experiments using a training protocol for surgical operations, and evaluated the metrics for the improvement of surgical skills by repeated training. It was indicated that the integral of the absolute values of the force sensor output was an adequate physical index of surgical force. Additional studies are currently under way to precisely evaluate surgical skill via a 6-DOF force sensor, and by a position sensor to analyze the motion of a surgical tool. Based on these studies, we hope to propose a new surgical training system and training protocols that would contribute to the training of endoscopic sinus surgery.

References

1. Kaufmann, C., Zakaluzny, S., Liu, A.: First Steps in Eliminating the Need for Animals and Cadavers in Advanced Trauma Life Support. In: Proc. of MICCAI 2000, Lecture Notes in Computer Science, Vol. 1935. Springer-Verlag (2000) 618-623
2. Gomes, M.P.S.F., Davies, B.L.: Computer-Assisted TURP Training and Monitoring. In: Proc. of MICCAI 2000, Lecture Notes in Computer Science, Vol. 1935. Springer-Verlag (2000) 669-677
3. Edmond, J.C.V., Heskamp, D., et al.: ENT Endoscopic Surgical Training Simulator. In: Proc. of MMVR, Studies in Health Technology and Informatics, Vol. 39. IOS Press (1997) 518-528
4. Rosser Jr, J.C., Rosser, L.E., Savalgi, R.S.: Objective evaluation of a laparoscopic surgical skill program for residents and senior surgeons. Arch. Surg. 133 (1998) 657-661
5. Hanna, G.B., Shimi, S.M., Cuschieri, A.: Task performance in endoscopic surgery is influenced by location of the image display. Ann. Surg. 227 (1998) 481-484
6. Jordan, J.A., Gallagher, A.G., McGuigan, J., McGlade. K., McClure, N.: A comparison between randomly alternating imaging, normal laparoscopic imaging, and virtual reality training in laparoscopic psychomotor skill acquisition. Am. J. Surg. 180 (2000) 208-211
7. Gallagher, A.G., McClure, N., McGuigan, J., Crothers, I., Browning, J.: Virtual reality training in laparoscopic surgery: a preliminary assessment of minimally invasive surgical trainer virtual reality (MIST VR). Endoscopy 31 (1999) 310-313

8. Derossis, A.M., Fried, G.M., Abrahamowicz, M., Sigman, H.H., Barkun, J.S., Meakins, J.L.: Development of a model for training and evaluation of laparoscopic skills. Am. J. Surg. 175 (1998) 482-487
9. Rudman, D.T.: Functional endoscopic sinus surgery training simulator. Laryngoscope 108 (1998) 1643-1647
10. Weghorst, S.: Validation of the Madigan ESS simulator. In: Proc. of MMVR, Studies in Health Technology and Informatics, Vol. 50. IOS Press (1998) 399-405
11. Yamashita, J., Yamauchi, Y., et al.: Real-Time 3D Model-Based Navigation System for Endoscopic Paranasal Sinus Surgery. IEEE Biomed. Eng. 46 (1999) 107-116
12. O'Toole, R.V., Playter, R.R., Krummel, T.M., Blank, W.C., Cornelius, N.H., Roberts, W.R., et al.: Measuring and developing suturing technique with a virtual reality surgical simulator. J. Am. Coll. Surg. 189 (1999) 114-127
13. Yamauchi, Y., Suzuki, M., et al.: A Training System for Endoscopic Sinus Surgery with Skill Evaluation. In: Proc. of CARS 2001, International Congress Series, Vol. 1230. Elsevier Science (2001) 1150
14. Rosen, J., Hannaford, B., MacFarlane, M.P., Sinanan, M.N.: Force controlled and teleoperated endoscopic grasper for minimally invasive surgery--experimental performance evaluation. IEEE Trans. Biomed. Eng. 46 (1999) 1212-1221
15. Emam, T.A., Hanna, G.B., Kimber, C., Dunkley, P., Cuschieri, A.: Effect of intracorporeal-extracorporeal instrument length ratio on endoscopic task performance and surgeon movements. Arch. Surg. 135 (2000) 62-65
16. Hanna, G.B., Shimi, S., Cuschieri, A.: Influence of direction of view, target-to-endoscope distance and manipulation angle on endoscopic knot tying. Br. J. Surg. 84 (1997) 1460-1464
17. Hanna, G.B., Drew, T., Clinch, P., Shimi, S., Dunkley, P., Hau, C., et al. Psychomotor skills for endoscopic manipulations: differing abilities between right and left-handed individuals. Ann. Surg. 225 (1997) 333-338
18. Rosen, J., Hannaford, B., Richards, C.G., Sinanan, M.N.: Markov modeling of minimally invasive surgery based on tool/tissue interaction and force/torque signatures for evaluating surgical skills. IEEE Trans. Biomed. Eng. 48 (2001) 579-591
19. Salcudean, S.E., Ku, S., Bell, G.: Performance measurement in scaled teleoperation for microsurgery. In: Proc. of CVRMed-MRCAS'97, Lecture Notes in Computer Science, Vol. 1205. Springer-Verlag (1997) 789-798

Development of a Master Slave Combined Manipulator for Laparoscopic Surgery

Functional Model and Its Evaluation

Makoto Jinno[1], Nobuto Matsuhira[1], Takamitsu Sunaoshi[1] Takehiro Hato[1],
Toyomi Miyagawa[1], Yasuhide Morikawa[2], Toshiharu Furukawa[2], Soji Ozawa[2],
Masaki Kitajima[2], and Kazuo Nakazawa[3]

[1] Corporate R&D Center, Toshiba Corporation
1, Komukai Toshiba-Cho, Kawasaki-Ku, Kawasaki 212-8582, Japan
[2] Department of Surgery, Keio University
35, Shinano-machi, Shinjyuku-ku, Tokyo 160-8582, Japan
[3] Department of System Design Engineering, Keio University
3-14-1 Hiyoshi, Kohoku-ku, Yokohama 223-8522, Japan

Abstract. Minimally invasive surgery helps patients by accelerating postoperative recovery. However, its application is impeded because it is necessary for the surgeons performing such surgery to possess surgical skills of a high order. Thus, for laparoscopic surgery, a master slave combined manipulator (MCM) has been proposed that enhances the surgeon's skill. The master grip and the slave hand with wrist joints are combined through the manipulator body, and a surgeon can perform the operation near to the patient. The slave hand is controlled by the master grip electrically and its position is directly controlled by the surgeon. The prototype model of the MCM has been developed and the function of the MCM has been verified by basic evaluation tests, and the MCM has been applied in an animal experiment. This paper describes the basic performance of the MCM.

1   Introduction

Laparoscopic surgery and other types of minimally invasive surgery (MIS) have entered widespread use in recent years. In laparoscopic surgery, a surgeon performs a surgical operation by using forceps through a few holes in the patient's abdomen, each hole being about 10 mm in diameter, while monitoring the image captured by a laparoscope. Owing to the small incision, the patient can recover earlier and suffers less pain, and the medical cost is reduced. Thus, laparoscopic surgery is highly advantageous for the patient. However, it is necessary for the surgeon performing such surgery to possess surgical skills of a high order. One of the main reasons is the lack of degrees of freedom for the free motion of the forceps. Applying techniques from robotics, we add wrist joints to the conventional forceps, and thus construct a robotic tool. The manipulator is able to enhance the surgeon's skill, reduce the demands imposed on the surgeon by laparoscopic surgery, and greatly contribute to the quality of the life (QOL) of the patient. Thus, a master slave combined manipulator has been newly developed. It was evaluated by the basic experiments such as suturing and

T. Dohi and R. Kikinis (Eds.): MICCAI 2002, LNCS 2488, pp. 52–59, 2002.
© Springer-Verlag Berlin Heidelberg 2002

ligaturing using a phantom model and applied in an animal experiment. As a result, the validity of the surgical manipulator was verified.

2 Concept of a Master Slave Combined Manipulator for Laparoscopic Surgery

In laparoscopic surgery, the gripper's orientation of the forceps cannot be freely changed during the operation. However, it is highly desirable that the surgeon should be able to move the tip of the forceps as if it were his/her own hand. For that purpose, a technique employed for tele-operated robots that is analogous to the master slave manipulator is applicable. Surgical robots developed so far [1]-[6] are based on the same concept as that of the conventional master slave manipulator; that is, the slave arm is controlled from the master arm at an operational console separated from the patient. In this concept, the master arm and the slave arm can be designed independently, resulting in a more suitable design of the master arm for the surgeon in terms of operability, respecting such items as joint alignment and arm size. However, such a master slave manipulator makes a system mechanically and electrically complicated from the viewpoints of safety and maintenance. On the other hand, human/robot cooperative systems and advanced instruments have been variously developed [7]-[11]. Our approach is to develop a robotic tool, applying a master slave manipulator for an intuitive operation, which is able to be used near to a patient in combination with conventional surgical tools. Thus, a master slave combined manipulator is proposed for the robot forceps application [12] as shown in Fig.1. The manipulator should be a simple structure, highly reliable, and safe, and the surgeon should perform the operation near to the patient so as to be able to cope with any emergency, such as a sudden hemorrhage. Furthermore, the manipulator will be used for applications in general surgery rather than in cardiac surgery.

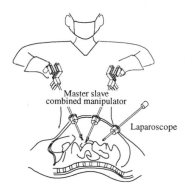

Fig.1. Image of laparoscopic surgey using master slave combined manipulators

3 Design of the Functional Model of a Master Slave Combined Manipulator

Fig.2 shows the structure of the developed surgical manipulator for laparoscopic surgery. The wrist joints are added to the forceps and they are operated from the grip in the same way as for a master slave operation. Since the master grip (control device) and the slave hand (operation device) are combined through the manipulator body, it is called a master slave combined manipulator (MCM). According to this concept, a surgeon will acquire greater skill in use of the MCM with practice, because it is a tool. In the previous paper [12], the support mechanism was proposed to hold the MCM in any position and compensate for its deadweight. Here, the functional model of the MCM without the support mechanism has been developed.

3.1   Structure of the Manipulator

A manipulator needs six degrees of freedom (DOF) in order to be deployed in a desired position and orientation in space. Since the tip position and the roll movement of the forceps are operated by the surgeon directly, the forceps needs more two DOF as a manipulator. Thus, two DOF are to be added to the forceps. Here, these two DOF are considered for performing the suturing task. In suturing, a semicircular needle is used generally. The needle has to be moved along a circular trajectory as shown in Fig.3. In the case that the tip joint of the MCM is roll axis, it is very easy to realize such a trajectory for any posture. However, if the tip joint is yaw axis or pitch axis, coordinated operation for orientational axes is required to operate along the circular trajectory. In the case of the MCM, such an operation is very difficult because of the structure. Therefore, the joint alignment of yaw axis (or pitch axis), roll axis, and a gripper is designed shown in Fig.2.

3.2   Slave Hand Mechanism

The slave hand consists of a gripper, roll and yaw axes. These axes are cable-driven by the DC servomotors mounted near the master grip. In order to reduce the number of DOF and decrease the weight of the manipulator, the roll axis around the manipulator body is commonly used for both the master grip and the slave hand. Additionally, the hand open/close motion is realized by the pinching mechanism of the master fingers.

3.3   Master Grip Mechanism

The master grip has yaw and roll axes and a gripper in the same order as the slave hand. The three axes of the master grip which roll, yaw and roll axes intersect at a point. In this structure, the operability of the MCM is found to be better in the case that the orientation is separated from the translation mechanically, because tip position does not move when the master grip orientation is changed. If the operation of the master grip orientation had an effect on the position of the slave gripper, precise surgical operation would be difficult. For the same reason, a gimbal mechanism has been widely adopted in previous master manipulators [13]. The master grip and the motor unit are to be separated from the body for the sterilization.

3.4   Control Method

The tip position of the MCM is controlled by the surgeon's direct motion and the orientation is determined by electrical signals generated by the master grip. The surgeon is responsible for the large and quick motion of the MCM. This is desirable from the viewpoint of safety. Fig.4 shows the control block diagram. The slave hand is controlled by the unilateral servo control method, i.e., each joint angle of the master grip is detected by the potentiometer and the slave hand is controlled to follow the joint angles by the encoders mounted on the servomotors. A notebook computer with an interface unit is used for the controller. By using motors, it would be possible to shift the motion area of the slave hand and change the motion ratio from the master to the slave hand for the improvement of the operability. Basic specifications and photograph of the developed MCM are shown in Table1 and Fig.5, respectively. In particular, the diameter of the manipulator is 12 mm, which is sufficient for conventional laparoscopic surgery.

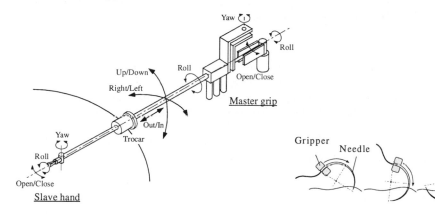

Fig. 2. Structure of the MCM

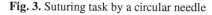

Fig. 3. Suturing task by a circular needle

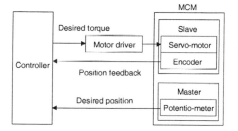

Fig. 4. Control block diagram

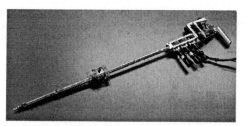

Fig. 5. Photograph of the developed MCM

Table 1. Specifications of the developed MCM

Items	Specification	
Size	Total Length	700 [mm]
	Pipe diameter	12 [mm]
Weght	0.6 [kg]	
Motion range	Yaw	±90 [°]
	Roll	±90 [°]
	Gripper	±30 [°] (10 [mm])
Control	Unilateral control	
Sensor	Master	Potentiometer
	Slave	Encoder

4   Basic Evaluation Experiments for the Functional Model of the MCM

Basic evaluation tests were performed for the MCM using a phantom model as shown in Fig.6. Here, the phantom model is made of a sponge for a stomach. Suturing and ligaturing tasks were performed to evaluate the position accuracy and operability of the MCM measured by the operation time and position errors. These tasks require dexterous manipulation in laparoscopic surgery.

4.1   Evaluation Task

Suturing and ligaturing tasks for evaluation were performed by operators who held the MCM in their right hands and the conventional forceps in their left hands, watching through the image of the laparoscope. The operators were three engineers who developed the MCM. Circular needles with 22 mm and 25 mm length were used for the evaluation task.

4.2   Operation Time for Suturing and Ligaturing

The operation time was measured from the insertion of the needle at any point to the completion of the ligature, four times per operator. In the ligaturing task, a surgical knot was used such as three single knots including double loop at the first knot. The result is shown in Fig.7 by box plots. The operation times shown is for suturing, knot-1, knot-2, knot-3, and total time, respectively. The average time is about 155 sec for the task. It was almost equal to the time using a conventional forceps instead of the MCM.

4.3   Operation Time for Continuous Suturing

Five continuous suturing tasks for horizontal and vertical directions were performed twice for three operators in Fig.8. The operation time and position accuracy of the continuous suturing task is shown in Fig.9. Fig.11 (1) shows the results. The phantom has marked points for insertion and penetration at suturing. The operation time contains changing time of the needle's posture for a suture. The error shows the position error between the marked point and actual insertion point. The average error was within 1 mm and one suturing time was about 65 sec in the continuous suturing in Fig.9. Angles of yaw and roll axes during the operation are shown in Fig.10. Note that roll axis was used effectively rather than the yaw axis in the suturing. Thus, the roll axis worked well for suturing.

4.4   360-Degree Suturing

One feature of the MCM is that suturing can be executed from any direction. This is impossible using a conventional forceps. To verify this feature clearly, 360-degree suturing was performed as shown in Fig.11 (2). In the horizontal plane, the task was almost realized. Although conventional forceps can move only around the axis of the forceps' body, the MCM can suture within the +-90 directions using the yaw axis. Rotating the tip roll axis of the slave hand, the needle is moved along the circular trajectory smoothly. The MCM was verified to be useful for suturing tasks.

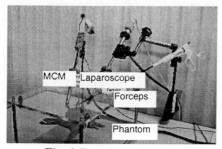

Fig. 6. Experimental setup

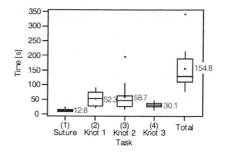

Fig. 7. Suturing and ligaturing time

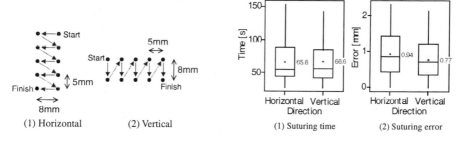

(1) Horizontal   (2) Vertical

Fig. 8. Continuous suturing task

(1) Suturing time   (2) Suturing error

Fig. 9. Continuous suturing time and position error

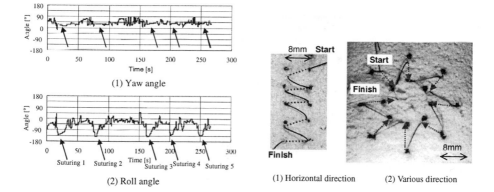

(1) Yaw angle

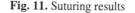

(2) Roll angle

Fig. 10. Joint angles of continuous suturing task

(1) Horizontal direction   (2) Various direction

Fig. 11. Suturing results

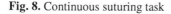

5   Preliminary Animal Experiment

The preliminary animal experiment was performed before the basic evaluation tests in Chapter 4. The purpose of the animal experiment is to identify any problems concerning the MCM. After the following experiments, gripping force and working area of the MCM were improved. The MCM was partially applied for the Nissen surgery involving suturing and ligaturing tasks. The surgeon practiced for an hour before the operation. In the surgical operation, the surgeon manipulated the MCM using his right hand and the conventional forceps using his left hand, watching the monitor from the laparoscope as shown in Fig.12.

5.1 Suturing Task

Fig.13 (1)-(4) show the suturing task performed using the MCM. During the penetration, it was confirmed that the yaw axis was not so moved and the roll axis of the slave hand was mainly used.

5.2 Ligaturing Task

Fig.13 (5)-(8) show the ligature task performed using the MCM. The ligature task consists of four knots; the MCM winds the thread twice around the conventional forceps, the forceps winds around the MCM once, and MCM winds around the forceps once. The MCM changes the posture of the slave hand depending on the conditions, such as, the case that the MCM winds the thread around the forceps, the case that the forceps winds around the MCM, and the case that the needle is passed between the MCM and forceps. In the operation, there are many requirements to change the posture of the MCM.

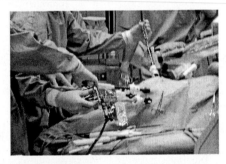

Fig. 12. Overview of the animal experiment

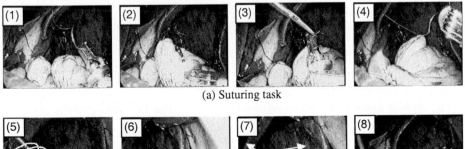

(a) Suturing task

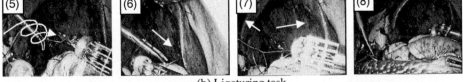

(b) Ligaturing task

Fig. 13. Suturing and ligaturing task performed using the MCM

6   Conclusion

The functional model of the master slave combined manipulator (MCM), a robotic forceps for laparoscopic surgery, has been developed. The validity of the MCM was confirmed by the basic evaluation experiments and the animal experiment as follows.

– Suturing from any direction that conventional forceps cannot perform is possible
– Suturing error is about 1 mm towards marked points

Next, with a view to proceeding to clinical tests, the operability and the reliability of the MCM should be improved, taking sterilization into consideration.

This development is carried out as part of a project concerning an advanced support system for endoscopic and other minimally invasive surgery by the New Energy and Industrial Technology Development Organization (NEDO) for 2000-2004.

References

1. http://www.computermotion.com
2. http://www.intuitivesurgical.com
3. A.J.Madhani, G.Niemeyer, J.K.Salisbury: The Black Falcon: A Teleoperated Surgical Instrument for Minimally Invasive Surgery, Proc. 1998 IEEE/RSJ Int. Conf. IROS (1998) 936-944
4. K.Ikuta, M.Nokata, S.Aritomi: Hyper Redundant Active Endoscope for Minimally Invasive Surgery, Journal of Robotics Society of Japan, Vol.16, no.4 (1998) 569-575 (in Japanese)
5. M.C.Cavusoglu, F.Tendick, M.Cohn, S.S.Sastry: A Laparoscopic Telesurgical Workstation, IEEE Trans. Robotics and Automation, Vol.15, No.4 (1999) 728-739
6. M.Mitsuishi, S.Tomisaki, T.Yoshidome, H.Hashizume, K.Fujiwara: Tele-micro-surgery system with intelligent user interface, Proc. IEEE Int. Conf. on Robotics and Automation, vol.2 (2000) 1607-1614
7. H.Kazerooni, Human/robot interaction via transfer of power and information signals Part I: Dynamics and Control analysis, Proc. IEEE Int. Conf on Robotics and Automation (1989) 1632-1640
8. M.O.Schurr: Robotic Devices for Advanced Endoscopic Surgical Procedures: An Overview, Journal of Robotics Society of Japan, Vol.18, No.1 (2000) 16-19
9. R.Kumar, P.Berkelman, P.Gupta, A.Barnes, P.Jensen, L.L.Whitcomb, R.H.Taylor: Preliminary Experiments in Cooperative Human/Robot Force Control for Robot Assisted Microsurgical Manipulation, Proc. IEEE Int. Conf. on Robotics and Automation (2000) 610-617
10. R.Nakamura, T.Oura, E.Kobayashi, I.Sakuma, T.Dohi, N.Yahagi, T.Tsuji, D.Hashimoto, M.Shimada, M.Hashizume: Multi-DOF Forceps Manipulator System for Laparoscopic Surgery - Mechanismminiaturized & Evaluation of New Interface -, Proc. 4th MICCAI2001 (2001) 606-613
11. S.Shimachi, Y.Hakozaki, A.Oguni, A.Hashimato: Weld Knotting and Contact Force Sensing for Laparoscoppic Surgery, Proc. 18th Annual Conf. of the Robotics Society of Japan (2000) 849-850 (in Japanese)
12. N.Matsuhira, H.Hashimoto, M.Jinno, T.Miyagawa, K.Nambu, Y.Morikawa, T.Furukawa, M.Kitajima, K.Nakazawa: Development of a Manipulator for Laparoscopic Surgery – Conceptual model of master slave combined manipulator and its evaluation -, Proc. 32nd ISR (2001) 630-635
13. N.Matsuhira, H.Bamba and M.Asakura: The development of a general master arm for teleoperation considering its role as a man-machine interface, Advanced Robotics, Vol.8, No.4 (1994) 443-457

Development of Three-Dimensional Endoscopic Ultrasound System with Optical Tracking

Naoshi Koizumi[1], Kazuki Sumiyama[2,3], Naoki Suzuki[2],
Asaki Hattori[2], Hisao Tajiri[4], and Akihiko Uchiyama[1]

[1] Sch. of Sci. & Eng., Waseda University
3-4-1 Okubo Shinjuku-ku, Tokyo, Japan
{koizumi,prof}@uchiyama.comm.waseda.ac.jp
[2] Institute for High Dimensional Medical Imaging, Jikei Univ. Sch. of Medicine
4-11-1 Izumihoncho Komae-shi, Tokyo, Japan
{nsuzuki,hat,kaz_sum}@jikei.ac.jp
[3] Dept. of Surg, Jikei Univ. Sch. of Medicine
3-25-8 Nishi-Shinbashi Minato-ku, Tokyo, Japan
[4] Dept. of Endoscopy, Jikei Univ. Sch. of Medicine
3-25-8 Nishi-Shinbashi Minato-ku, Tokyo, Japan
tajiri@jikei.ac.jp

Abstract. We have developed a new three-dimensional (3D) endoscopic ultra-sound system (EUS) with convex scanning echoendoscope to diagnose and navigate by using 3D image. We use an optical tracking system which is shaped like a ribbon to detect the position of the probe and to monitor the shape of the scope inside the body. The optical tracking system can measure bends and twists at each position along with the echoendoscope. Then, the position of the tip of the echoendoscope is allotted to a 2D image, and the system can reconstruct and visualize a 3D image in real-time. We have reported results of our experimental studies using phantom and 3D images of vessels in animal studies.

1 Introduction

3D-EUS system with spiral scanning has been used as one of the diagnostic imaging modalities in Gastroenterology [1-2]. But it is difficult to use 3D images effectively in real-time and it is impossible to navigate various therapeutic and diagnostic procedures with EUS [3]. As the technological advances in EUS have expanded its applications, a new way of diagnosis using the 3D image and navigation system of endoscopic puncture would be needed. Thus, we have been developing a new 3D-EUS system with a convex scanning echoendoscope to perform various procedures with 3D image.

2 Methods

2.1 Instruments

EUS was performed with a convex scanning echoendoscope (FG32UA PENTAX) equipped with transducers ranging 5 to 7 MHz and a display unit (EUB525

T. Dohi and R. Kikinis (Eds.): MICCAI 2002, LNCS 2488, pp. 60–65, 2002.
© Springer-Verlag Berlin Heidelberg 2002

HITACHI). Gray-scale and color Doppler video image data are fed into a personal computer (PC) (Precision 420 DELL) equipped with a video capture board (GV-VCP2M/PCI IO-DATA). To detect the position of the probe inside the body, we used an optical tracking system (Shapetape Measurand) and electromagnetic tracking system (Fastrak Polhemus). Shapetape whose shape was like a ribbon was attached along with the echoendoscope form controlling head side to the tip of the echoendoscope (Figure 1). The tip of the ribbon was fixed to the tip of the echoendoscope, and the ribbon could move smoothly between echoendoscope and surrounding tube. And Fastrak was fixed to the controlling head side. 3D reconstruction and visualization are performed with the above-mentioned PC.

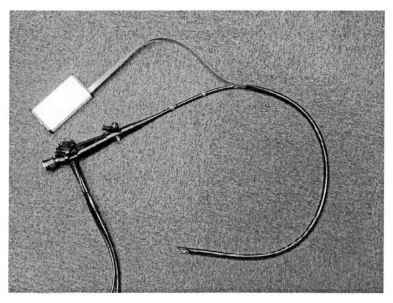

Fig. 1. Convex scanning echoendoscope with optical tracking system

2.2   3D Reconstruction and Visualization in Real-Time

In this system, the whole shape and relative position from the controlling head side to the tip of the echoendoscope are acquired by optical tracking system. The optical tracking system is composed of an array of fiber optic sensors (Figure 2), and can measure bends and twists at each position of the ribbon (Figure 3).

To calculate the twist and bend of each position from controlling head side to the tip, the whole shape of the ribbon is detected. In each position of the optical tracking system, there are three situations of coordinate systems. One is the original coordinate system before twist and bend (Σ_o). Next is the coordinate system after rotating twist (t), (Σ_t). Finally there is the coordinate system after rotating twist and bend (b), (Σ_b). Then the rotation matrix from Σ_o to Σ_t, (^oR_t), is defined as follows:

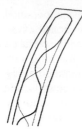 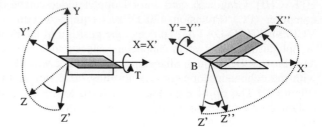

Fig. 2. Inner structure of the ribbon

Fig. 3. The definition of the twist and bend

$$
{}^{O}R_T = \begin{pmatrix} 1 & 0 & 0 \\ 0 & \cos t & -\sin t \\ 0 & \sin t & \cos t \end{pmatrix} \tag{1}
$$

In the same way, the rotation matrix from Σ_t to Σ_b, (${}^tR_b$), is defined as follows:

$$
{}^{T}R_B = \begin{pmatrix} \cos b & 0 & \sin b \\ 0 & 1 & 0 \\ -\sin b & 0 & \cos b \end{pmatrix} \tag{2}
$$

Then the rotation matrix from Σ_o to Σ_b, (${}^oR_b$), is defined as follows:

$$
{}^{O}R_B = {}^{O}R_T\,{}^{T}R_B = \begin{pmatrix} 1 & 0 & 0 \\ 0 & \cos t & -\sin t \\ 0 & \sin t & \cos t \end{pmatrix} \begin{pmatrix} \cos b & 0 & \sin b \\ 0 & 1 & 0 \\ -\sin b & 0 & \cos b \end{pmatrix} \tag{3}
$$

$$
= \begin{pmatrix} \cos b & 0 & -\sin b \\ \sin t \sin b & \cos t & \sin t \cos b \\ \sin b \cos t & -\sin t & \cos t \cos b \end{pmatrix}
$$

To use this rotation matrix, positions of each position of the ribbon are calculated. This rotation matrix calculates the number $(n, 1 \sim N)$ of twists and bends (${}^oR_b[n]$). The position of the number n from origin of the ribbon $(X[n], Y[n], Z[n])$ is calculated as follows:

$$
\begin{pmatrix} X[k] \\ Y[k] \\ Z[k] \end{pmatrix} = (\prod_{k=1}^{n} {}^{O}R_B[k]) \begin{pmatrix} x \\ y \\ z \end{pmatrix} + \begin{pmatrix} X[k-1] \\ Y[k-1] \\ Z[k-1] \end{pmatrix} \tag{4}
$$

In above-mentioned equation, (x, y, z) represented the position of the ribbon in Σ_o of number n=1. In addition to this relative position acquired by the optical tracking system, in measuring the original position of the ribbon with the electromagnetic tracking system can detect the position of the probe in world space coordinate system. These positions which are calculated are allotted to 2D image, and 3D image is reconstructed and visualized in real-time. Also, the display of our system can show the 2D image which is being scanned and the shape of the echoendoscope which is being monitored by optical tracking system and 3D image. A block diagram of the key components is shown in Figure 4.

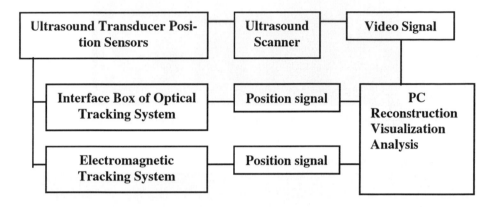

Fig. 4. A block diagram of the key components of the system

3   Results

Our system applied to experimental and animal studies. In experimental studies using a phantom of spherical shape, our system could reconstruct and visualize it in real-time and to observe the reconstructed 3D image, the shape of it could be confirmed as a sphere. (Figure 5). And to display the position of the 2D image that is scanning inside 3D image, the user could observe the 2D image with its surrounding information. Since our system can confirmed the updated 3D image as scanning 2D image, in the case of fail in scanning, the user could scan again speedy. In experimental studies, the characteristic of the optical tracking system and procedures in scanning were examined and confirmed. In animal studies, our system could reconstruct and visualize the portal vein of the hepatic hilum of the pig in real-time (Figure 6). In Figure.6, the upper left sub window shows 2D images which is scanning, and the frame that is composed of green and red lines show the region of interest (ROI). In Figure.6, the right window shows 3D image reconstructed by using ROI in 2D image. In Figure.6, lower left window shows the shape of the echoendoscope constructed by the data from optical tracking system, and to monitor and display the shape of echoendoscope inside body of animal, the operator could recognize the areas which were scanned intuitively.

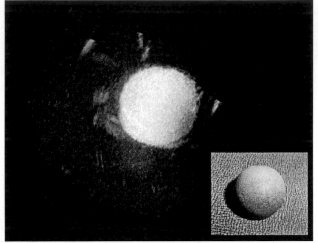

Fig. 5. Phantom and reconstructed 3D image in experimental studies

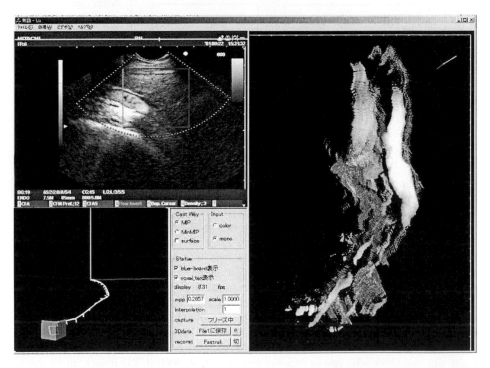

Fig. 6. Display of the system in animal studies. Upper left sub window shows Power Doppler sonography, and lower left shows the shape of echoendoscope inside body. The right window shows a real-time 3D image that was reconstructed

4   Discussion

According to the improvement of various medical imaging modalities, 3D images have been used in diagnosis and navigation field. In ultrasound, 3D images have been used in the obstetrics and gynecology field and the navigation system in open surgery of the liver and so on [4-6]. However in EUS, because of the difficulty in detecting the position of the probe inside the body, it is difficult to develop a system which makes good use of 3D images. In this study, our system established a foundation of 3D reconstruction and visualization in real-time using a convex scanning echoendoscope, and suggested the possibility of a navigation system of endoscopic punctures. Now, the problems of our system are ones of accuracy and ways of attaching to the optical tracking system. These kind of problems will be solved by combining it with our system and burying the optical fiber structure into the echoendoscope.

In summary, we developed new 3D-EUS system using a convex scanning echoendoscope with an optical tracking system. This system can reconstruct and visualize 3D image in real-time and monitor the shape of the echoendoscope inside the body. Experimental and animal studies demonstrated the technical feasibility of this system. We believe that further improvement of this system will be able to expand applications of 3D-EUS.

Reference

1.   Yoshino J, Nakazawa S, Inui K, Katoh Y, Wakabayshi T, Okushima T, Kobayashi T and Watanabe S: Surface-rendering imaging of gastrointestinal lesions by three dimensional endoscopic ultrasonography. Endoscopy 1999 Sep;31(7):541-5
2.   Kida M, Watanabe M, Sugeno S, et al: 3-Dimensional Endoscopic Ultrasonography for Upper Gastrointestinal Diseases. Endoscopy, 28(suppl): S38, 1996.
3.   Kazuya Y, Shunichi N, Shunichiro I, Tadayoshi K, Yoshihiro S: Imaging of the colorectal cancer using 3D-EUS system. Early Colorectal Cancer vol.3, number 3, 1999
4.   Baba K: Development of three-dimensional ultrasound in obsterics and gynecology: Technical aspects and possibilities. In 3-D Ultrasound in Obstetrics and Gynecology. Merz E ed., Lippincott Williams & Wilkins, Philadelphia, USA, 3-8, 1998.
5.   Nelson TR, Pretorius DH, Hagan-Ansert S: Fetal heart assessment using three-dimensional ultrasound. J Ultrasound Med, 14(suppl): S30 1995
6.   Steven c. Rose, Dolores H. Pretorius, Thomas B. Kinney, Thomas R. Nelson, Karim Valji, Horacio R. D'Agostino, Nannette M. Forsythe, Anne C. Roberts, Michael L. Manco-Johnson: Three-dimensional Sonographic Guidance for Transvenous Intrahepatic Invesive Procedures. Feasibility of a New Technique. JVIR 1999; 10:189-198

Real-Time Haptic Feedback in Laparoscopic Tools for Use in Gastro-Intestinal Surgery*

Tie Hu[1], Andres E. Castellanos[1,2],
Gregory Tholey[1], and Jaydev P. Desai[1]

[1] Program for Robotics, Intelligent Sensing, and Mechatronics (PRISM) Laboratory
3141 Chestnut Street, MEM Department, Room 2-115
Drexel University, Philadelphia, PA 19104, USA
{tie,gtholey,desai}@coe.drexel.edu
[2] Medical College of Pennsylvania, Hahnemann University
Andres.E.Castellanos@drexel.edu

Abstract. One of the limitations of current surgical robots used in
surgery is the lack of haptic feedback. While current surgical robots improve surgeon dexterity, decrease tremor, and improve visualization, they
lack the necessary fidelity to help a surgeon characterize tissue properties for improving diagnostic capabilities. Our work focuses on the development of tools and software that will allow haptic feedback to be
integrated in a robot-assisted gastrointestinal surgical procedure. In this
paper, we have developed several tissue samples in our laboratory with
varying hardness to replicate real-tissues palpated by a surgeon in gastrointestinal procedures. Using this tissue, we have developed a novel setup
whereby the tactile feedback from the laparoscopic tool is displayed on
the PHANToM haptic interface device in real-time. This is used for tissue
characterization and classification. Several experiments were performed
with different users and they were asked to identify the tissues. The
results demonstrate the feasibility of our approach.

1 Introduction

Surgeons rely primarily on their senses for the diagnosis and treatment of multiple surgical pathologies. Special attention has been paid to the development
of their visual and tactile perceptive abilites through surgical training. Surgeons have traditionally used palpation as the primary feedback for determining
whether a tissue is normal or abnormal [1]. The development of minimally invasive surgery has led to a better patient outcome at the expense of these visual
and tactile faculties. Through small incisions in the abdominal wall, the surgeon
introduces long instruments and camera to perform complicated abdominal procedures. The normal three-dimensional vision becomes two-dimensional and the
only advantages are that the new cameras allow the surgeon to have a better visualization of the operative field through increased magnification. Due to

---

* We greatfully acknowledge the support of National Science Foundation grant: EIA-
0079830 for this work.

T. Dohi and R. Kikinis (Eds.): MICCAI 2002, LNCS 2488, pp. 66–74, 2002.
© Springer-Verlag Berlin Heidelberg 2002

monocular vision feedback rendered on a two dimensional display, depth perception is lost and a surgeon adapts to this image over time. Haptic feedback is almost completely lost and in most cases limited to gross information. The learning curve becomes a prolonged process of adjustment to these conditions. While this has become an area of increasing interest, some preliminary laparoscopic forceps with force feedback have been tested with good results [2, 3].

The real role of haptic feedback in minimally invasive surgery and robotically assisted surgery has yet to be determined. Research seems to suggest that the introduction of haptic feedback can add substantial benefits to robotic systems and facilitate tissue recognition but there are still several hurdles to be resolved such as achieving at least half as much palpation capability through a robotic device [4–7]. Interaction with the laparoscopic tool remotely in a telesurgical framework poses additional challenges such as sufficiently high network bandwidth and latency issues in communicating over the network [8–12]. Several studies have been done in evaluating the ease of laparoscopic tools through remote manipulation. These studies (though limited to knot tying and suturing) have demonstrated that instrument based mapping gives a more realistic feel of the operative site compared to screen based mapping [13].

The primary goal of this paper is to provide a surgeon with haptic feedback through the PHANToM, a haptic feedback device (manufactured by Sensable Technologies, Inc.) for carrying out robotically-assisted, minimally invasive surgery. One of the chief applications of this research will be the localization of gastrointestinal polyps within the bowel lumen, a task almost impossible to perform with current laparoscopic and robotic devices. It will also enhance the resection of solid organs, allowing the surgeon to differentiate between tumor and normal tissue and between normal and abnormal lymph nodes. Even simple tasks like knot-suture tying can be improved by adding tactile feedback, especially with small sutures.

2   System Description

We have developed an interface to allow the surgeon to manipulate and characterize different tissue samples using the haptic feedback device. We have incorporated tactile sensing capability on conventional laparoscopic tools used in minimally invasive surgery without affecting the ergonomics of the current tool design. This is particularly important since we do not want the surgeon to get used to newer tools than what they currently use. Figure 1 shows the schematic of the overall system that we envision building. Currently, we are interested in solving the force feedback problem through the PHANToM and tool loop.

Our experimental testbed consists of a force sensing laparoscopic tool designed in our laboratory, a PHANToM haptic interface device (manufactured by Sensable Technologies, Inc.), DSpace DS1103 controller board, and tissue samples that we have developed in the laboratory of varying mechanical properties to simulate tissue palpated by a surgeon in gastrointestinal procedures. The experimental test-bed allows us to examine different tissue samples using the

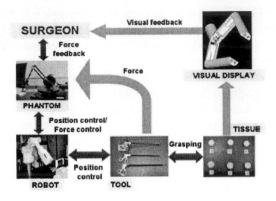

Fig. 1. Block diagram of the tissue characterization using haptic feedback.

force sensing forceps. The forceps are currently manipulated by the surgeon, but our eventual goal is to mount this on the robot arm and control the movement through the PHANToM. The force obtained by the forceps is displayed by the haptic interface device. In our setup, a user grasps the tool on one hand and closes the grasper (analogous to an automated laparoscopic grasper) while the surgeon interacts with the Phantom and feels the grasping force. Real-time force information is measured through appropriate calibration of the strain gages and recording of the signals by the DS1103 controller board.

3   Modeling

We have created our initial prototypes of the force sensing tool using disposable laparoscopic tools for minimally invasive surgery (manufactured by Ethicon, Inc). A laparoscopic grasper, scissor and dissector were modified for testing purposes by attaching strain gages. While these modifications to the tools created sensing capabilities that previously didn't exist, the overall functionality of the tools was preserved as used in practice. The standard laparoscopic tool consists of a 38 cm rod with a jaw mechanism at one end and a handle in the other end. Through an internal pole, the handle controls the opening and the closing of the jaws. These instruments are used to grasp, mobilize and cut the different tissues within the body. Two precision strain gages, manufactured by Measurements group, Inc, were attached to each side of the active handle of the instrument, opposite to each other, using a Wheatstone bridge configuration (see Figure 2). This allows for a deformation measurement of the instrument handle in response to the force applied, therefore producing force feedback correlating to a selected sample of tissue. A position sensor, manufactured by Midori Precision Co, Ltd, was attached to the pivot of the active handle (Figure 3) allowing accurate recording of the angular rotation of the handle. This further establishes a correlation between the deformation of the tissue and the exerted force. In order to increase sensing resolution, the sensors were connected to a transducer amplifier.

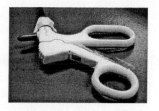

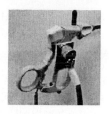

Fig. 2. Strain gage attached to the laparoscopic grasper handle.

Fig. 3. Position sensor attached to the laparoscopic tool.

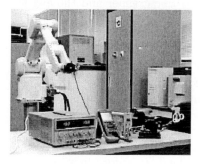

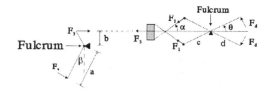

Fig. 4. Calibration setup for the strain gages on the force sensing forceps.

Fig. 5. Force diagram for analysis of the grasping force in relation to the exerted force on the laparoscopic tool.

Calibrating the strain gage and position sensor: In order to obtain valid results, a precise method of measuring the force applied to the active handle is required. For this, a mechanical setup for the laparoscopic tools was necessary. The setup was designed to securely hold the tool in place while incorporating a controlled motion to operate the handle. The force calibration for the laparoscopic tool was done by closing the grasper through the handle and placing an obstruction in the jaw of the grasper which was attached to the force sensor. Figure 4 shows the experimental setup for calibrating the strain gages on the laparoscopic tool. The detailed analysis for the calibration process is given below. Figure 5 shows the kinematic description of the laparoscopic grasper.

Based on Figure 5, we conclude that:

$$F_3 = 2F_1 cos\alpha, \quad F_1 sin(\alpha + \theta)c = F_d d, \quad F_v a = F_3 b$$

Finally, we get after simplification:

$$F_d = \frac{ac}{2bd} \left(\frac{sin(\alpha + \theta)}{cos\alpha} \right) Kv \qquad (3.1)$$

where F_d is the reaction force exerted on the grasper while grasping the tissue, F_1 and F_3 are the forces in the mechanism internal to the laparoscopic tool, and $F_v = Kv$ is the force exerted by the operator on the laparoscopic handle. The calibration process involved finding the value of K assuming a linear relationship of the applied load to the voltage generated by the strain gages. The experimental value of K was 3.9.

In another experiment, we calibrated the position sensor to measure the grasper movement for a given movement of the position sensor. The handle of the grasper was fixed for different positions of the jaws, which included full open, full close, and a few positions in between these extremes. Using the voltage feedback from the position sensor and the measured angle of the jaws with respect to a reference axis, the following relationship was experimentally determined between the angular movement (θ) of the laparoscopic grasper and the angular movement (β) of the handle:

$$\theta = -12.55\beta + 41.70 \tag{3.2}$$

Tissue modeling and characterization: To perform our testing we created several samples of Hydrogel material with varying consistency. The Hydrogel is created using a combination of polyvinyl alcohol (PVA) and polyvinyl pyrrolidone (PVP). A polymer blend of 90% PVA and 10% PVP was created. The solution was caste into cylindrical molds and subjected to subsequent cycles of freezing and thawing to crosslink the polymer blend, therefore increasing the Hydrogel consistency. A total of six cycles were performed and after each cycle a sample was removed. For the purpose of further discussion the samples were labeled from 1 to 6 based on their stiffness, where 1 was the softest and 6 was the hardest.

4   Experiments

We have conducted two experiments for tissue characterization, the first through force measurement while grasping the tissues without any haptic feedback and the second using haptic feedback.

4.1   Experiment 1

The principle objective of the tissue characterization experiment is to determine the property of the different tissues using a laparoscopic tool. For a given load applied through the grasper, we observed different angular movements of the grasper. In other words, for a given angular movement of the grasper, a stiffer tissue required higher force than a softer tissue. In this experiment, six artificial tissues with different stiffnesses were used (see Figure 6).

The sample tissues were numbered 1 through 6 in increasing hardness (see Figure 6). The operator grasped the samples and the DS1103 board records the real-time force and position signal. The sampling time was 0.4 ms. Figure 7 is the tissue characterization graph which shows the correlation between the deformation of the sample and the force exerted on the sample. The softer the tissue, the more degree of deformation with a lesser force; and the harder the

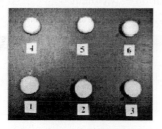

Fig. 6. Tissue Samples.

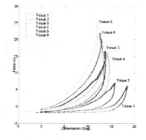

Fig. 7. Force vs. angular displacement plots for various tissue samples.

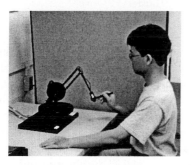

Fig. 8. Subject interaction with haptic interface.

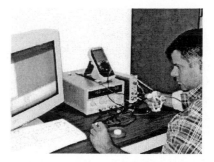

Fig. 9. Grasping of the tissue samples.

tissue, the less degree of deformation with higher force. This assumption made the Hydrogels a good model to represent simulated tissue samples with different consistency. It is clear from the figure that we were able to obtain quantitative estimate of the force-displacement relationship for the sampled tissues.

4.2 Experiment 2

In the second experiment (see Figures 8 and 9), we displayed the forces exerted on the laparoscopic tool to the PHANToM. The subjects were asked to rank three different Hydrogel samples, from softest to hardest, through pure haptic feedback using the PHANToM. They did not have visual or contact feedback of the different samples outside of the PHANToM. The angular displacement obtained with the laparoscopic tool was kept constant and monitored through the computer screen in order to repeat the same displacement for all the tissue samples. Therefore, as the samples increased in hardness, we can expect an increase in the amount of grasping force necessary to achieve the same angular displacement of the grasper.

The objective of the experiment is to use the PHANToM to differentiate between tissue samples when the displacement of these samples is more or less the same. According to the result of the tissue characterization experiment, we con-

Table 1. Tissue stiffness identification experiment

Subjects	Sample 2	Sample 3	Sample 6
S1	Soft	Hard	Harder
S2	Soft	Hard	Harder
S3	Soft	Hard	Harder
S4	Soft	Harder	Hard
S5	Soft	Hard	Harder
S6	Soft	Hard	Harder
S7	Soft	Hard	Harder
S8	Soft	Harder	Hard
S9	Soft	Hard	Harder
S10	Soft	Hard	Harder

cluded that we can use the laparoscopic tool to get different force/displacement characterization graphs of the 6 groups of tissues. When the displacement of the tissue is the same, the force applied on the tissues should be inversely proportional to the stiffness of the tissue. In this experiment, we chose Hydrogel samples 2, 3, and 6 as reference tissues. Sample 2 was the softest and sample 6 was the hardest. Ten subjects were tested, including several non-surgeons, surgeons and surgical residents with expertise in minimally invasive gastrointestinal surgery. When the subjects performed the experiment, the tissue samples were randomly arrayed and the subject did not know which sample they were testing. They were only in contact with the PHANToM while a second operator performed the grasping of the tissues using the laparoscopic tool. When the operator applied the force on the tissue with the laparoscopic tool, up to a constant angular displacement; the subjects were asked to rank those tissues based on the forces reflected in the PHANToM.

The results of the operator analysis after feeling all three tissues is tabulated in Table 1. As seen from the table, eight out of the ten subjects correctly identified the tissue samples qualitatively in terms of their stiffness. Only two subjects (non-surgeons) were unable to differentiate between samples 3 and 6 even though they were able to differentiate sample 2 as the softest when compared with the other two samples.

5   Discussion

We have developed an apparatus for use in laparoscopic surgery for tissue characterization. In our setup, the operator feels the force in real-time while squeezing the tissue. Our experimental work indicates that even non-surgeons can easily identify the tissue samples being grasped. We performed two experiments, one of which was to record the tissue grasping forces as a function of the angular displacement of the grasper and the other was to identify the stiffness of the tissue sample based on a randomly selected presentation of the samples for the operator to grasp.

We intend to extend this work to automated grasping of the tool through a motorized assembly. The laparoscopic tool would then be attached to the end of the robot arm which would be controlled by the PHANToM. One of the chief applications of this work would be provide haptic feedback to the surgeon in gastrointestinal surgery. By adding haptic feedback to robotic systems, the surgeon should be able to characterize tissue as normal or abnormal and titrate his dissection in order to spare normal tissue while completely removing the abnormal one. The best example is the removal of solid organ tumors, particularly liver tumors, where the surgeons use tactile feedback and intraoperative imaging to localize these tumors and perform an adequate resection with adequate margin. We will create liver models using different stiffness hydrogels in order to simulate liver tumors and perform surgical resection using the laparoscopic tools with force feedback using a robotic arm controlled by the surgeon using the PHANToM device. Our aim is to resect the tumor without disrupting the tumor surface while at the same time preserving the normal tissue.

While this paper addresses the first steps in this direction, there are several issues that need to be resolved. This includes the incorporation of visual feedback of the operative site with haptics and how it relates to operator performance. Also, an understanding of better tactile sensors for achieving palpation in real-time for exploratory tasks over an organ surface as is performed by a surgeon would be helpful. The results presented in this paper represent an important first step in that direction.

References

1. H. S. Chen and Sheen-Chenn, "Synchronous and early metachronous colorectal adenocarcinoma:analysis of prognosis and current trends," *Diseases of the Colon and Rectum*, vol. 43, pp. 1093–9, August 2000.
2. V. V. H. tot Dingshoft, M. Lazeroms, A. van der Ham, W. Jongkind, and G. Hondred, "Force reflection for a laparoscopic forceps," in *18th Annual International Conference of the IEEE Engineering in Medicine and Biology Society*, 1996.
3. J. Rosen, B. Hannaford, M. P. MacFarlane, and M. N. Sinanan, "Force controlled and teleoperated endoscopic grasper for minimally invasive surgery-experimental performance evaluation," *IEEE Transactions on Biomedical Engineering*, vol. 46, no. 10, pp. 1212–1221, 1999.
4. D. Salle, F. Gosselin, P. Bidaud, and P. Gravez, "Analysis of haptic feedback performances in telesurgery robotic systems," in *IEEE International workshop on Robot and Human Interactive Communication*, 2001.
5. A. Menciassi, A. Eisinberg, G. Scalari, C. Anticoli, M. Carroza, and P. Dario, "Force feedback-based micro instruments for measuring tissue properties and pulse in microsurgery," in *IEEE International Conference on Robotics and Automation*, May 2001.
6. P. Dario and M. Bergamasco, "An advance robot system for automated diagnostic task through palpation," *IEEE Transations on Biomedical Engineering*, vol. 35, February 1998.
7. E. P. Scilingo, A. Bicchi, D. D. Rossi, and P. Iacconi, "Haptic display able to replicate the rheological behavior of surgical tissues," in *IEEE 20th Annual International Conference*, 1998.

8. P. S. Green, R. E. Williams, and B. Hamel, "Telepresence: Dextrous procedures in a virtual operating field (abstract)," *Surgical Endoscopy*, vol. 57, p. 192, 1991.

9. A. Guerrouad and P. Vidal, "Stereotaxical microtelemanipulator for ocular surgery," in *Proc. of the Annual Intl. Conf. of the IEEE Engineering in Medicine and Biology Soc.*, vol. 11, (Los Alamitos, CA), pp. 879–880, 1989.

10. J. W. Hill and J. F. Jensen, "Telepresence technology in medicine: Principles and applications," *Proc. IEEE*, vol. 86, no. 3, pp. 569–580, 1998.

11. T. B. Sheridan, "Teleoperation, telerobotics, and telepresence: A progress report," *Control Eng. Practice*, vol. 3, no. 2, pp. 205–214, 1995.

12. S. E. Salcudean, S. Ku, and G. Bell, "Performance measurement in scaled teleoperation for microsurgery," in *First joint conference Computer vision, Virtual reality and Robotics in Medicine and Medical Robotics and Computer-Assisted Surgery* (J. Troccaz, E. Grimson, and R. Mösges, eds.), (Grenoble, France), pp. 789–798, Springer, March 1997.

13. F. Lai and R. D. Howe, "Evaluating control modes for constrained robotic surgery," in *2000 IEEE International Conference on Robotics and Automation*, (San francisco, CA), April 2000.

Small Occupancy Robotic Mechanisms
for Endoscopic Surgery

Yuki Kobayashi, Shingo Chiyoda, Kouichi Watabe,
Masafumi Okada, and Yoshihiko Nakamura

Department of Mechano-Informatics,
The University of Tokyo,
7-3-1, Hongo, Bunkyoku, Tokyo 113-8656 Japan,
nakamura@ynl.t.u-tokyo.ac.jp
http://www.ynl.t.u-tokyo.ac.jp/index.html

Abstract. To make the endoscopic surgery more precise and more accessible, computer-enhanced surgical robot systems are introduced and accepted in the surgical community. Present surgical robot systems unfortunately occupy a significant amount of space in operating rooms. It sometimes prohibits surgeons from emergency access to the patient. In this paper, we propose a design of small occupancy robots for endoscopic surgery. The design concept consists of three components. Namely, the Active Forceps, the Active Trocar, and the passive positioner. The detailed design of the Active Forceps and the Active Trocar presented, and the performance of prototypes are also reported.

1   Introduction

With the developments of robot assisted surgery system, various new procedures of minimally invasive surgery become possible [1][2][3][4]. It enables surgeons to perform surgery with high precision and smaller incisions so that the patient's trauma is reduced, scarring is minimized, and recovery is accelerated. Although several surgical robots are currently in use, they unfortunately occupy a significant amount of space in operating rooms. The manipulators stretched over patients sometimes prohibit surgeons from accessing patients in an emergency. This is due to the fact that the efforts of miniaturization are focused only on the forceps and hardly made for robotic mechanisms so far. The long arm needs high stiffness to move precisely, and the high stiffness makes the mechanism large and heavy. Therefore the robotic system for endoscopic surgery occupy a large space in operating rooms. In this paper, we propose design concepts of small occupancy robots for endoscopic surgery which has six degree-of-freedom. The efforts to make the surgical robot system small also realize mechanical stiffness and response.

2   Small Occupancy Robotic System

2.1   Design Specification

During endoscopic surgery, surgical instruments move focusing on the trocar port. As a way surgeon holds a surgical instrument in the endoscopic surgery,

T. Dohi and R. Kikinis (Eds.): MICCAI 2002, LNCS 2488, pp. 75–82, 2002.
© Springer-Verlag Berlin Heidelberg 2002

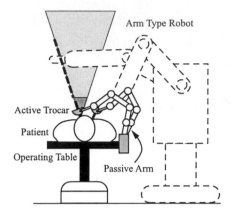

Fig. 1. Area Occupancy of the Surgical Robots

the surgical robot with arm shown on the right of Figure 1 with the dashed lines holds the back end of an surgical instrument. With this mechanism, a surgical robot moves, occupying large amount of space above of the patient. To miniaturize the area occupancy of the surgical robot, we propose a concept of surgical robot shown in Figure 1 with solid lines. The robot does not hold the back end of the surgical instrument but holds it right above of the trocar port so that it has the same operation range of the tip of the instrument as an arm type robot by smaller motion. In Figure 1, the portion of light gray expresses the space occupied with an arm type robot, and the portion of deep gray expresses that of the small surgical robot. The smaller space occupancy of surgical robot is, the larger the surgeon and the assistants can move in the operationg room. We call these small surgical robot which move right above of the trocar port, Active Trocar. The Active Trocar is installed in arbitrarily positions with a passive positioner which has six degree-of-freedom. It enables to use the range of operation of the Active Trocar effectively by making the initial position of it adapted for each operation method. On the basis of the above-mentioned concept, we designed a surgical robotic device. The designed robotic device consists of two parts. One is the High Stiffness Multi Degree-of-Freedom Active Forceps that has three degree-of-freedom which determines the posture at the tip of an surgical instrument, and the other is the Active Trocar that has three degree-of-freedom which determines the position of the end-effector in the abdominal cavity. To miniaturize a surgical robot system, we set the specification for the slave robot as follows:

Degree-of-Freedom: A slave robotic device for the endoscopic surgery is required to have at least six degree-of-freedom for dexterity and ease of use for surgeons. We designed the robot with a simple six degree-of-freedom mechanism as shown in Figure 2. One additional degree-of-freedom is for the function of end-effectors on the tip of the surgical instrument(e.g. grasping, scissoring etc.).

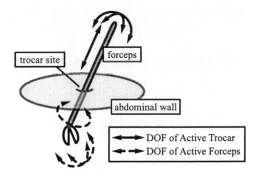

Fig. 2. Degree-of-Freedom of the Surgical Robic System

Field of Activity: The robot shall have the range of operation of 45 [degree] or more from its initial position to all the directions. If the initial position of the robot can be set up arbitrarily, it is considered that it is enough for the space where an endoscopic surgery is performed.

Size of the Robot System: The Active Trocar needs the small amount of motion compared with an arm type robot because of its concepts, and it can be turned into a small robotic system by intensive arrangement of actuators and mechanical composition parts. The size of the Active Trocar must be small enough to be arranged at least 3 bodies on the abdominal wall.

Sterilizability: Surgical instruments should be sterilizable or disposable so that they may not become the infection route. Since the actuator section, including motors, ball screws, and linear guides, is unsterilizable, the contact of the actuator section and surgical instruments which is set on the robot should be avoided. The portion of the robotic system which contact the patient's body is sterilizable, and the whole system is isolated with the patient's body with a drape.

2.2   Active Trocar

Figure 3 shows the Active Trocar. The mechanism is based upon the mechanism of the Additional Wrist Mechanism[5]. It consists of two actuated rotational joints with DC-servo motors and the Harmonic Drives which has 1/100 reduction ratio and one linear motion mechanism with DC-servo motor, a ball screw and a linear guide to realize three degree-of-freedom of position of the tip of a surgical instrument in the abdominal cabity. Figure 4 shows the mechanism of the Active Trocar. The closed kinematic chain which consists of Link A, Link B, Link E and Link F in Figure 4 restricts the sergical instrument on the Active Trocar to rotate around a certain point shown as point P in Figure 4. The kinematic chain is actuated with the rotational joint 2, and it has the flexibility of two degree-of-freedom centering on the point P by having a rotation mechanism expressed rotational joint 1 in Figure 4. Arranging the Active Trocar so that the point to be the trocar port, it does not damage the abdominal wall with excessive forces.

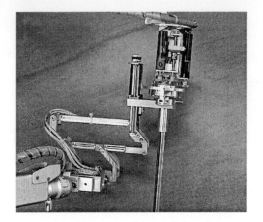

Fig. 3. The Active Trocar with Closed Kinematic Chain

In addition to these rotation mechanisms, three degree-of-freedom of position at the tip of the surgical instrument is decided according to the linear motion mechanism by which the insertion length of the instrument to the abdominal cabity is decided.

The size of designed Active Trocar is miniaturized with the concept of intensive arrangement of the actuators and mechanical parts, and the weight of the robotic device is also light and is approximately 630[g]. Figure 5 shows the size of Active Trocar.

2.3 Multi-degree-of-freedom Active Forceps

Most of the typical active forceps adopt wire driven mechanisms. Wire drive active forceps realize a compact and lightweight mechanism, while the elasticity of the wire causes low stiffness of the end-effector, the stretching and friction of the wire cause the low reliability of the system. Therefore we adopt link driven mechanisms, which realizes high stiffness, reliability and responsiveness. Figure 6 shows the mechanism of the active forceps shown as one degree-of-freedom of bending model. There are two links, one is fixed and the other slides along the axis of forceps. The model can be extended to the two degree-of-freedom of bending in the three dimensional space. We adopt it to the mechanism of the active forceps. In addition to these two degree-of-freedom, the active forceps has one degree-of-freedom of rotation, so that it determines the posture at the tip of an surgical instrument. As is mentioned in the section 2.1, the active forceps which contacts the patient's body should be sterilizable. Therefore the forceps section is designed detachable from the actuator section, and the actuator section should be covered with a clean drape.

Figure 7 shows the forceps section and the slide block on the tip and the bottom of the Active Forceps. It consists of three blocks, each of them is the devided part of a cylinder. The cut of each block has hooks so that they do not come apart, we call this mechanism "Jigsaw Block Slide". To decrease the

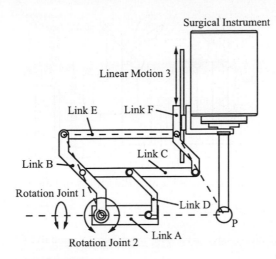

Fig. 4. Mechanism of Active Trocar with Closed Kinematic Chain

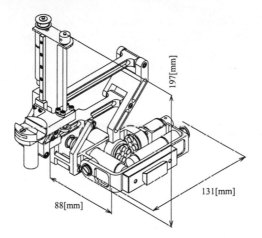

Fig. 5. Size of Active Trocar with Closed Kinematic Chain

friction between each block, Jigsaw Block Slide is made of Silicolloy™(Japan Silicolloy Industry Co., Ltd.) which is a kind of stainless steel includes as much as 4% silicon and has small friction for sliding. The diameter of forceps part is currently 10[mm] which is the standard size of endoscopes. The links are driven by linear motion mechanisms consist of 2.5[W] DC-servo motors, ball screws and linear guides. The length of the active forceps is currently 300[mm].

Although the power of actuators was efficiently transmitted with the Jigsaw Block Slide, the stiffness and strength of the mechanism were not satisfactory. The diameter of the endeffector which is shown in Figure 7 is 0.2[mm] although the diameter of the forceps is 10[mm]. By modifying the structure of the platform and reducing the number of mechanical elements, we designed another active forceps as shown on the left in Figure 8 compared with the present one on the

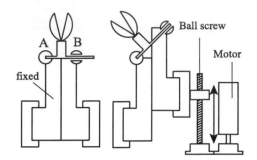

Fig. 6. The Mechanism of Active Forceps Illustrated in One Degree-of-Freedom

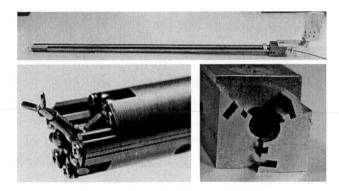

Fig. 7. The whole forceps part (above), The Tip (left) and the Bottom (right) Blocks of the Active Forceps with Biopsy Forceps

right. It uses Jigsaw Block Slide too, while its endeffctor is larger and has higher rigidity. The tip mechanism is changed so that the end plate might be larger. We call the mechanism the Triped Platform. Figure 9 shows the outline of it. The volume of the drive part of the second prototype is 60% of that of the first prototype.

3   Experiments of Master-Slave Control

We set up a master-slave control surgical robotic system for endoscopic surgery. It consists of a master device and a slave robot. We adopt PHANToM DESKTOP™(SensAble Technologies Inc.) as the master device which has six axes of measurable joints and three axes of haptic force feedback. The haptic sensation could be used to feedback the force interaction at the end-effector of the slace robot, or to establish haptic communication between the surgeon and the surgical navigation system. However, the current system has no force sensing device. The slave robot consists of the Active Trocar and the Multi Degree-of-Freedom Actuive Forceps, so that it has six degree-of-freedom at the endeffector. We evaluated the operativity of the system by *in vivo* experiments as shown in

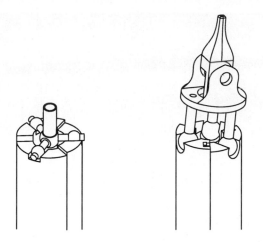

Fig. 8. The Active Forceps with Triped Platform

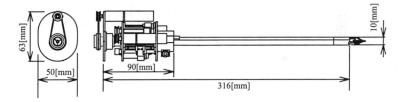

Fig. 9. Outline of the Second Prototype

Figure 10. The result of the experiment is shown in Figure 11. Three upper graphs express the response to the reference data from master device in each axes, and the lower graphs express the error. Although some big errors are seen in each axes, these are because the speed of the linear motion mechanism on the Active Trocar, and it is solvable by changing the pitch of the ball screw.

4   Conclusions

The result of this paper is summarized in the following points:

1. We introduced the concept of the Active Trocar that realizes miniaturization of the surgical robotic device.
2. We developed the surgical robot system including Active Trocar and the Multi Degree-of-Freedom Active Forceps.

Acknowledgements: This work was supported through "Development of Surgical Robotic System" (PI: Prof. Ichiro SAKUMA) under the Research for the Future Program, the Japan Society for the Promotion of Science, and through "Improving Manipulatability by Enhansment of Harmonic Scalpel for Laparoscopic Surgery" (PI: Prof. Minoru HASHIMOTO) under the grant-in-aid for scientific research (B).

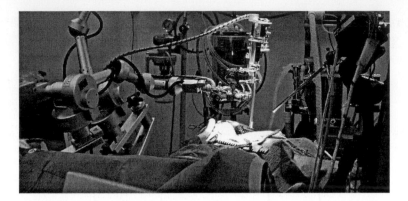

Fig. 10. *In vivo* Experiment on the Pig

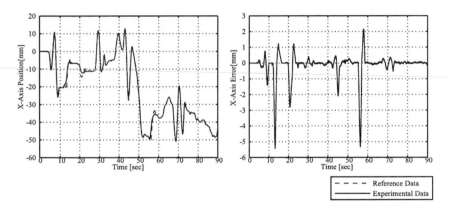

Fig. 11. The Response of the Slave Robot in the *in vivo* Experiment

References

1. Guthart G.S. and salisbury J.K. "The Intuitive™ Telsurgery System: Overview and application". *Proc. of the 2000 IEEE International Conference on Robotics & Automation*, Vol. 1, PP. 618–621, 2000.
2. Reichenspurner H. Damiano R.J., Mack M., Boehm D.H., and Detter C. Gulbins H. "Use of the voice-controlled and computer assisted surgical system ZEUS for endoscopic coronary artery bypass grafting". *J. Thorac Cardiovasc Surg.*, Vol. 118, No. 1, 1999.
3. Nakamura Y., Kishi K. and Kawakami H. "Heartbeat synchronization for robotic cardiac surgery". *Proc. of the 2001 IEEE International Conference on Robotics & Automation*, pp. 2014–2019, 2001.
4. Mitsuhiro H. and Nakamura Y. "Heartbeat syncronization for robotic cardiac surgery". *Proc. of the 2001 IEEE International Conference on Robotics & Automation*, pp. 1543–1548, 2001.
5. Hanafusa H. and nakamura Y. "Autonomous Trajectory Control of Robot Manipulators". *Robotics Research: The First International Symposium*, pp. 863–882, 1984.

Development of MR Compatible Surgical Manipulator toward a Unified Support System for Diagnosis and Treatment of Heart Disease

Fujio Tajima[1], Kousuke Kishi[1], Kouji Nishizawa[1], Kazutoshi Kan[1],
Yasuhiro Nemoto[1], Haruo Takeda[2], Shin-ichiro Umemura[3], Hiroshi Takeuchi[4],
Masakatsu G. Fujie[5], Takeyoshi Dohi[6], Ken-ichi Sudo[7], and Shin-ichi Takamoto[8]

[1] Mechanical Engineering Research Laboratory, Hitachi, Ltd.
502 Kandatsu, Tsuchiura-shi, Ibaraki 300-0013 Japan
{tajima,kishi,kouji,kan018,yas}@merl.hitachi.co.jp
[2] Systems Development Laboratory, Hitachi, Ltd.
1099 Ozenji, Asao, Kawasaki-shi, Kanagawa 215-0013 Japan
takeda@sdl.hitachi.co.jp
[3] Central Research Laboratory, Hitachi, Ltd.
1-280 Higashi-Koigakubo, Kokubunji-shi, Tokyo, 185-8601 Japan
sumemura@crl.hitachi.co.jp
[4] Medical Systems Division, Hitachi, Ltd.
1-5-1 Marunouchi, Chiyoda-ku, Tokyo, 100-8220 Japan
hi-takeuchi@med.hitachi.co.jp
[5] Department of Mechanical Engineering, Waseda University
3-4-1 Okubo, Shinjuku-ku, Tokyo, 169-8555 Japan
mgfujie@mn.waseda.ac.jp
[6] Graduate School, Institute of Information Science and Engineering, Tokyo University
7-3-1 Hongo, Bunkyo-ku, Tokyo, 113-8656 Japan
dohi@miki.pe.u-tokyo.ac.jp
[7] School of Medicine, Kyorin University
6-20-2 Shinkawa, Mitaka-shi, Tokyo, 181-8611 Japan
sudok@kyorin-u.ac.jp
[8] School of Medicine, Tokyo University
7-3-1 Hongo, Bunkyo-ku, Tokyo, 113-8656 Japan
takamoto-tho@h.u-tokyo.ac.jp

Abstract. We propose a new concept of a unified system for supporting both surgical treatment and intrasurgical diagnosis of heart diseases, especially ischemic heart disease like myocardial infarction, under a magnetic-resonance-imaging (MRI) environment. In developing the system, we first designed and built a prototype of maneuverable manipulator as a subsystem. We then evaluated MR compatibility of the manipulator by moving its arm tip close to a phantom in the field of view of an open-configuration MR imager. No noticeable deformation, but some signal-to-noise ratio (SNR) deterioration, was observed in the MR images taken during evaluation. It is planned to combine the manipulator with other subsystems and function modules in order to construct an easy-to-use unified support system. This system will then be applied to treat a variety of diseases of organs and tissues in the human body.

T. Dohi and R. Kikinis (Eds.): MICCAI 2002, LNCS 2488, pp. 83–90, 2002.

1   Introduction

Cardiovascular disease is the one of several major causes of death. Especially in Japan, it is said that one death out of four is caused by it, and ischemic heart disease like myocardial infarction accounts for some 50 percent of all cases of cardiovascular disease. This percentage is predicted to increase in the near future. Meanwhile, since the performance of various medical diagnosis devices, such as the magnetic resonance imager (MRI), has been making rapid progress over the last few years, it is no longer a dream that a surgeon can perform an operation while simultaneously watching images of multiple modalities acquired intrasurgically. To help make this dream a reality, we propose a unified system that supports intrasurgical diagnosis and minimally invasive surgery, mainly for ischemic heart disease, under MRI monitoring.

MRI has some advantages compared to conventional imaging devices like X-ray CT (computed tomography). Namely, it involves no exposure to radioactivity and can acquire tomographic images of a patient at any position from arbitrary orientation, and these imaging sequences provide many kinds of diagnostic information. Magnetic-resonance (MR)-compatible mechanisms for intervention and maneuverable surgical manipulator systems have been developed. Masamune [1] developed a needle-insertion manipulator for stereotactic neurosurgery in a conventional (i.e., not open-configured) MRI environment. It is a kind of stereotactic frame mechanism with motorized joints, and is composed of magnetic-insensitive materials like engineering plastics and metals like aluminum. In a collaborative research on an MR-compatible surgical robot system with an intraoperative MRI [2], Chinzei built a five-degree-of-freedom (5DOF) tool-positioning manipulator. This system used a "double-donuts"-type horizontal-magnetic-field open MRI, with a magnetic-field strength of 0.5 Tesla, manufactured by General Electric. The manipulator was maneuverable enough to hold surgical tools in a certain position and orientation.

Over the last several year research on manipulators that can perform surgical operations in the same way as a human hand has progressed considerably. Even commercial products have been clinically applied in many places in the world. The most popular one is called da Vinci (Intuitive Surgical) [3], which had FDA clearance for urology in June 2001 and clinical tests on cardiovascular surgery have been performed. Another is ZEUS (Computer Motion Inc.) [4]. These two products are so-called master-slave manipulator systems and they can perform very dexterous motion as an extention of a surgeon's hands. We have also been developing a multiple micromanipulator system that extends conventional stereotactic neurosurgery [5-7]. It enables an operator to make sub-millimeter manipulations that a surgeon's hand cannot do directly. We performed in-vivo operation experiments to improve the prototype system step by step. And it will be clinically tested in the near future. However, none of these manipulators referred to above are compatible with an MR environment (strong magnetic field and high-power radio-frequency waves).

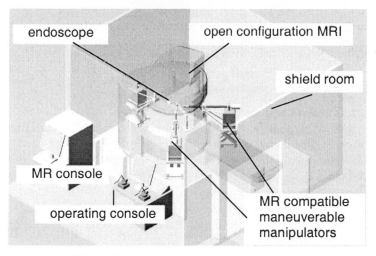

Fig. 1. Conceptual drawing of completed system

2   Conceptual Design

System Design

Figure 1 shows a conceptual drawing of the completed system. The system supports both diagnosis and treatment of cardiovascular disease under MR monitoring. It unifies image information from an optical endoscope, open MRI, an ultrasonic scanner, and conventional vital-sign detectors. Unified image information is updated periodically while surgery is being carried out. The updating period ranges from several tens of milliseconds to ten seconds, depending on the type of modalities. It helps and guides the surgeon and other medical staffs so they can make the right decisions. Moreover, the high-performance maneuverable manipulator can mimic the movement of the surgeon's hand precisely. The system uses a so-called master-slave control method in which an operation command through a master device is inputted and a slave manipulator moves according to the command almost instantly. The system also detects intrasurgical time-variant deformation of target organs by processing endoscopic images and information from a gap sensor attached at the distal end of the manipulator. The manipulator is then controlled so that the configuration of the arm tip in relation to the target point becomes appropriate for the operation. The manipulator mechanism is made of an insulator like ceramics or engineering plastics, or at least materials of low susceptibility to magnetism. This means that the MRI images do not suffer noise or distortion and that the manipulator is not affected by interference due to electromagnetic interaction. The actuators should not be electromagnetic-force driven for the same reason, so ultrasonic motors are used instead.

An example of the system operation is explained as follows. The manipulators are located at the side of the bed under open MRI. Before the surgery, the medical staffs perform preparation procedures like anesthetization, sterilization, and skin cleaning on the patient. After that, the bed moves so that the target organ or tissue is within the field of view of the open MR imager. Surgeons carry out the operation by using the maneuverable manipulators with the support of the image-information system, which gives them multi-modal images from the endoscope, ultrasonic scanners, and the open MRI. The configuration of the endoscope and operation viewpoints are controlled, and the images presented are changed and arranged by user interfaces like foot pedals and a voice recognition unit.

System Configuration and the Functions

The conceptual image in Fig. 1 is translated into a schematic diagram shown in Fig. 2, which shows how the total system works by presenting the subsystems and functional modules and the data flow among them. The system consists of three main parts: multimodal diagnostic devices, an intrasurgical information support system, and a maneuverable manipulator system. The functions of the developed subsystems are enclosed in bold-line rectangles and are summarized below:

(1) Surgical treatment using maneuverable manipulators compatible with MR;
(2) Shape-change compensation for surgical treatment without cardioplegia and cardio-pulmonary support;
(3) MR-compatible fast 3D ultrasonic scanning;
(4) Image processing for various modalities into understandable forms;
(5) Image presentation of surgical guidance information, endoscopic images, and various information from multimodal diagnostic devices and vital-sign detectors in a manageable manner;
(6) Fine operation such as anastomosis.

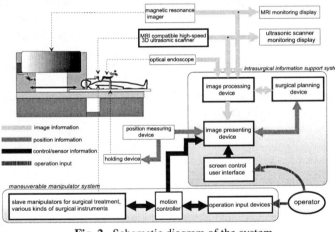

Fig. 2. Schematic diagram of the system

Design of Manipulator Mechanism

The maneuverable manipulator was designed so that a surgeon can perform MIDCAB (minimally-invasive direct coronary artery bypass), especially LITA (left internal thoracic artery)-LAD (left anterior descending branch) anastomosis. Before the manipulator mechanism was designed, preliminary studies were done on the motion of the surgeon during the operation.

First, motion and operation of a surgeon were analyzed. To do so, MIDCAB was decomposed into a series of operations, and it was found that anastomosis is usually required and can be done by a certain mechanical entity, namely, a maneuverable manipulator.

Then, the anastomosis operation was split into a series of single motions and measured the approximate distance of movement and the volume of workspace during each motion. Next, the transition of the manipulator configuration at the distal end of the surgical tools was investigated in order to find how many degrees of freedom are needed in each single motion (further explanation is not given here.)

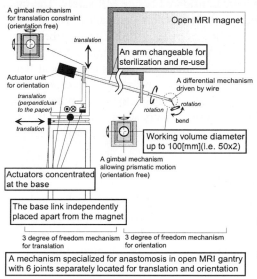

The above investigation was led to the following guiding principles for the manipulator design in Fig. 3:

(1) The manipulator mechanism should be specialized for anastomosis (light-loaded, small workspace, dexterous);

(2) The base link should be placed apart from the open MRI magnet so as not to interfere with the MRI image, and the long arm (made of magnetically insusceptible materials) should cover the whole field of view;

(3) Number of degrees of freedom should be at least six;

(4) Working distance at the arm tip should be at most 40 to 50 mm for all kinds of single motion;

(5) Actuators must be concentrated at the proximal end (i.e., as far from the magnetic field as possible)

Fig. 3. Basic concept of manipulator mechanism

(6) Joints for translation and orientation should be located separately (former concentrated around the base, latter around the distal end);

(7) The arm should be exchangeable for sterilization and re-use.

3   Implementation

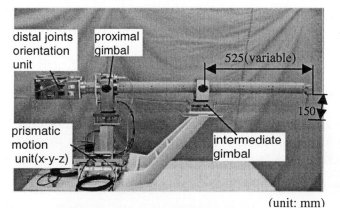

Fig. 4. Prototype of manipulator system

(unit: mm)

Figure 4 shows a view of the prototype of the manipulator. This manipulator has six degrees of freedom so that it can assume any configuration at its arm tip. Three prismatic motion units are fixed at its base. A motor at the proximal gimbal rotates the arm. The arm is supported and constrained by the intermediate gimbal to lessen deflection and vibration of the arm. The distal joints form a pair of differential gears, and the orientation of the arm tip is controlled by driving the gears with actuators at the proximal end through high-molecular-weight wires. Materials and components were selected according to preliminary examination under a 1.5 T MR environment. Especially at the arm tip, no damage to human tissue and the ability to withstand sterilization were considered beside MR safety. The main material of the prismatic motion units and gimbals was aluminum alloy. The arm and its distal joints were made of engineering plastics, mainly PEEK (poly-ether-ether-ketone). Two types of actuators were incorporated: an ultrasonic motor and a ceramic linear actuator. Position sensors were optical fiber rotary encoders and optical linear scales. These actuators and sensors were located a meter away from the center of the field of view, and no materials that are susceptible to magnetism incorporated were used. Light source and receiver of those position sensors were kept apart through optical fibers so that high power RF pulse emitted from the MRI does not affect sensor signals.

4   Evaluation of MR Compatibility

The manipulator was set up as shown in Fig. 5 to evaluate its effects on MR images. Preliminary studies were done under 1.5 T-MR environment (no details given here for want of space). A 0.3-T open configuration MRI (AIRIS II comfort, manufactured by Hitachi Medical Corporation, Japan) was used for imaging. Imaging sequences were spin echo (SE) and gradient field echo (GE). Imaging conditions are listed in the table 1.

Table 1. Imaging conditions

item	TR	TE	flip angle	number of pixels	FOV	slice thickness	band width
unit	[ms]	[ms]	[deg]	WxH	[mm]	[mm]	[KHz]
SE	200	27	-	256x256	220	10	15.0
GE	50	22.6	70	256x256	220	10	15.0

A phantom was used in the tests. It is a polyethylene cylindrical vessel filled with $CuSO_4$ solution (diameter: 150 mm, height: 300 mm). Images were taken while the manipulator was in motion. The manipulator repeatedly traced a rectangular trajectory at its arm tip between the narrow gap in the head coil.

Figure 6 shows MR images of the cylindrical phantom taken by SE and GE sequences. No severe artifacts were observed in the images, although the contrast in the image taken with GE sequence is deteriorated. These images were printed onto films usually used for diagnosis with the original data, and they were examined by clinicians. Their opinion was that they did not recognize any significant deformation even between the images taken with GE, and they are acceptable as long as they are used for intrasurgical survey, position tracking and the like, not for close diagnosis.

A quantitative comparison of contrast deterioration was done with signal-to-noise ratio (SNR) of each image, which is given by the definition:

$$SNR = Smean/SD, \tag{1}$$

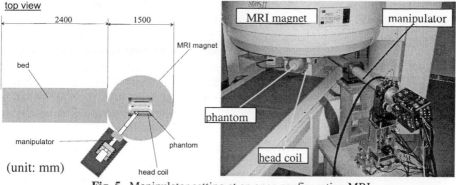

Fig. 5. Manipulator setting at an open configuration MRI

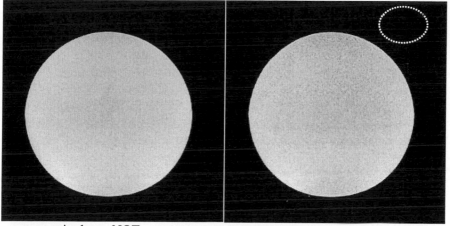

manipulator: NOT present   manipulator: in motion
(a) imaging sequence: spin echo

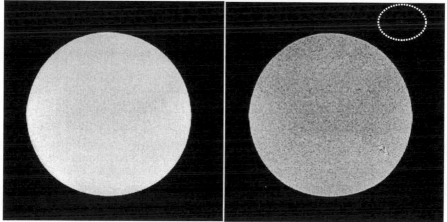

manipulator: NOT present   manipulator: in motion
(b) imaging sequence: gradient field echo

Fig. 6. MR images of a cylindrical phantom taken in two sequences. Dotted ellipses show the area where the tip of the manipulator moved.

where *Smean* is the average intensity value of 240 pixels in a circle at the center of the image, and *SD* is the average value of *SDn* (*n*=1–4), which is the standard deviation of 60 pixels in a circle at each corner of the image. Figure 7 compares *SNR* under several conditions. As a conventional method for comparing signal power, *SNR* values are plotted on a logarithmic scale, that is, a decibel ($20log_{10}SNR$) expression. As shown in Fig.6, *SNR* values were 38.3 dB (SE) and 33.4 dB (GE) when the manipulator was not present. They decreased to 33.6 dB (SE) and 27.0 dB (GE) when the manipulator was in motion.

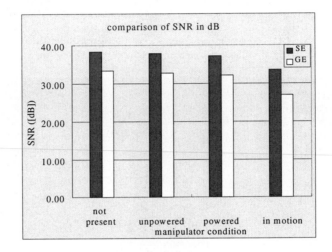

Fig. 7. Comparison of SNR in dB under 0.3-T open-configuration MRI

References

[1] Masamune, et al., *"Development of a MRI Compatible Needle Insertion Manipulator for Stereotactic Neurosurgery"*, Proc. MRCAS, pp. 165-172 (1995)

[2] http://www.aist.go.jp/MEL/soshiki/kiso/biomech/chin/MMM/mrmani0-e.htm

[3] http://www.intuitivesurgical.com/html/daindex.html

[4] http://www.computermotion.com/zeus.html

[5] Kan, K. et al., *"Microscopic Manipulator System for Minimally Invasive Neurosurgery"*, Proc. on the 12th International Symposium and Exhibition of Computer Assisted Radiology and Surgery (CAR'98), pp. 594-598 (1998)

[6] Kan, K. et al., *"Development of HUMAN System with Three Micro Manipulators for Minimally Invasive Neurosurgery"*, Proc. on the 15th International Symposium and Exhibition of Computer Assisted Radiology and Surgery (CARS 2001), pp. 144-149 (2001)

[7] Hongo, K. et al., *"Microscopic-manipulator system for minimally invasive neurosurgery Preliminary study for clinical application"*, Proc. on the 15th International Symposium and Exhibition of Computer Assisted Radiology and Surgery (CARS 2001), pp. 265-269 (2001)

Transrectal Prostate Biopsy Inside Closed MRI Scanner with Remote Actuation, under Real-Time Image Guidance

Gabor Fichtinger[1,2], Axel Krieger[1], Robert C. Susil[2,3], Attila Tanacs[1], Louis L. Whitcomb[4], and Ergin Atalar[2]

[1] Engineering Research Center, Johns Hopkins University, Baltimore, MD, USA
gabor@cs.jhu.edu
[2] Department of Radiology, Johns Hopkins University, Baltimore, MD, USA
[3] Dept. of Biomedical Engineering, Johns Hopkins University, Baltimore, MD, USA
[4] Department of Mechanical Engineering, Johns Hopkins Univ., Baltimore, MD, USA

Abstract. We present the proof-of-concept prototype of a prostate biopsy robot to be used inside a conventional high-field MRI scanner. A three degree-of-freedom (DOF) mechanical device translates and rotates inside the rectum and enters a needle into the body, and steers the needle to a target point pre-selected by the user. The device is guided by real-time images from the scanner. Networked computers process the medical images and enable the clinician to control the motion of the mechanical device that is operated remotely from outside the imager. The system is also applicable to localized prostate therapy and also demonstrates potential in other intra-cavitary procedures.

Introduction

Prostate diseases represent a significant health problem in the United States. After cardiac diseases and lung cancer, metastatic prostate cancer is the third leading cause of death among the American men over fifty years, resulting in approximately 31,000 deaths annually. The definitive diagnostic method of prostate cancer is core needle biopsy. Annually in the U.S., approximately 1 million prostate biopsies are performed revealing around 200,000 new cases. Currently, transrectal ultrasound (TRUS) guided needle biopsy is the gold standard for the diagnosis of prostate cancer [1] and contemporary intraprostatic delivery of therapeutics is also primarily performed under TRUS guidance. This technique has been overwhelmingly popular due to its excellent specificity, real-time nature, low cost, and apparent simplicity. At the same time, however, TRUS-guided biopsy fails to correctly detect the presence of prostate cancer in approximately 20% of cases [2,3]. Also importantly, the transrectal ultrasound probe implies variable normal force on the prostate through the rectal wall, causing dynamically changing deformation and dislocation of the prostate and surrounding tissue during imaging and needle insertion, an issue that has to be eliminated in order to achieve accurate and predictable needle placement. MRI imaging has a high sensitivity for detecting prostate tumors [3,4]. Unfortunately, MR imaging alone, without concurrent biopsy, suffers from low diagnostic specificity. Therefore, our primary objective was to develop a prostate biopsy system that couples superior imaging quality with accurate delivery hardware, inside a conventional MRI scanner. The

T. Dohi and R. Kikinis (Eds.): MICCAI 2002, LNCS 2488, pp. 91–98, 2002.

challenge was three-fold: (1) Conventional high-field MRI scanners apply whole-body magnets that surround the patient completely and do not allow access to the patients during imaging. The workspace inside the magnet is extremely limited, so conventional medical robots and mechanical linkages do not fit in the magnet. (2) Due to the strong magnetic field, ferromagnetic materials and electronic devices are not allowed to be in the magnet, which excludes the use of traditional electro-mechanical robots and mechanical linkages. (3) A real-time in-scanner guidance method is needed to operate the device.

Cormack, Tempany, Hata, D'Amico, et al. at the Brigham and Women's Hospital in Boston [5,6] proposed to use open MRI configuration in order to overcome spatial limitations of the scanner. This magnet configuration allows the physician to step inside the magnet and access the patient. The Brigham group proved the ability of MRI to detect cancer previously missed by TRUS biopsy and they performed success-ful targeted biopsy and brachytherapy inside the open MRI scanner. While this ap-proach has opened up a new chapter in managing prostate cancer, the open MRI scan-ner limits its potentials. Compared to closed magnets, open magnets tend to have lower signal-to-noise ratio, so the images also tend to be of lower quality. The in-curred cost and complexity of open MRI imaging are also substantial. The Brigham group applies transperineal access in biopsy, which it is significantly more invasive than the conventional transrectal approach.

Relevant work in robot assisted needle placement is also found in the literature. Recently, Fichtinger et al. [7] presented a 3-DOF remote center of motion robot for transperineal prostate access, the kinematic concept of which is not applicable to transrectal procedures. Rovetta et al. [8] applied an industrial robot to assist TRUS-guided prostate biopsy with the use of a conventional end-shooting probe. The robot mimicked manual handling of TRUS biopsy device in the patient's rectum, in a tele-surgery scenario. This system did not gain popularity, because the benefits of telesur-gery did not compensate for the added cost and complexity of the robot and many problems of TRUS-guided free-hand biopsy still remained unaddressed. The Brigham group, Chinzei, Hata et al. [9] reported a robotic assistant for transperineal needle placement in open MRI. In this design, the MR-compatible motors are situated outside the high field zone and two manipulator arms reach into the scanner. The arms are encoded and tracked by a FlashPoint tracker simultaneously. Unfortunately, these geometric and kinematic concepts are incompatible with our application. Cus-tom designed robots for use inside conventional closed MRI have also been investi-gated: Kaiser et al. [10] developed a system for breast biopsy and Masamune et al. published another one for brain surgery [11]. The kinematics and design concepts of these are also not applicable in transrectal prostate biopsy.

Multiple investigators, including our group at the Johns Hopkins University have studied intra-operative CT and X-ray guidance of surgical robots using passive fidu-cials attached to the interventional device. MRI imaging, however, is unique by of-fering the opportunity to apply micro-coil antennas as active fiducials [12]. In this scenario the signal processing software "listens" to a prominently present "signature" from the fiducial coils, allowing for true accurate real-time calculation of the coil positions, then using the these positions as rigid body markers on the device.

Our approach to image-guided prostate biopsy differs from other all the above so-lutions, in several aspects. Our objectives were to employ high resolution MRI imag-ing inside a closed MRI scanner, maintain the safe transrectal access, while replacing the manual technique with a remotely controlled needle insertion system, in order to maximize needle placement accuracy and also minimize dynamic tissue deformation. We also developed real-time tracking and guidance for the device, using solely the MRI scanner, without external tracking instruments.

Materials and Methods

Systems Design

The systems concept is shown in Figure 1. The device is secured to the table of the scanner with an adjustable mount that allows for flexible initial positioning. The patient is positioned comfortably on the scanner's couch in prone position with slightly elevated pelvis and the device is introduced to the rectum. A thin rigid sheath attached around a tubular obturator makes contact with the rectum, while the obturator can slide smoothly inside the sheath. The sheath prevents the obturator from causing mechanical distortion to the rectum wall and prostate while it is moving inside the rectum. After a satisfactory initial position is achieved, the mount is secured to hold this position. Using the sliding table of the scanner, the patient and device are moved into the scanner's magnet. The MRI scanner produces signal with the patient and device in the field, at the same time. Using signal-processing tools, we

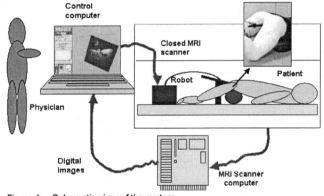

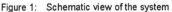

Figure 1:   Schematic view of the system

determine the spatial relationship between the device and the coordinate system of the MRI scanner. The images are transferred to a computer that produces a 3D representation of the device superimposed on the anatomic images. The physician interacts with the display and selects the target point for the needle. The computer calculates the kinematic sequence to bring the needle to the selected target position. The device realizes 3-DOF motion: translation of the end-effector inside the rectum, rotation of the end-effector around the axis of translation, and the depth of needle insertion. The order of translation and rotation are interchangeable, but both must be completed before the needle is inserted. The computer can also simulate the sequence of motion by moving a 3D model of the device, so that the physician could verify that the calculated sequence of motion would indeed take the needle from its current position to the pre-selected target position. The computer displays the three motion parameters to the operator. In the current embodiment of the system, the motion stages are powered manually, because motorized actuation was not considered to be a critical element in our proof of feasibility prototype. While the actuation of the device is in progress, the MRI scanner is collecting images in continuous mode and sends them immediately to treatment monitoring computer.   The computer processes the image data and

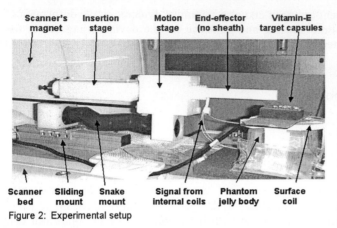

Figure 2: Experimental setup

visualizes the current image, with the model of the device superimposed in the scene, allowing the physician to monitor the motion of the device toward its target. The three parameters of motion (translation, rotation, insertion depth) are recalculated in each imaging cycle, enabling real-time dynamic control of the device. When the motion is motorized, we will have achieved the ideal of "point-and-click" surgery, when the surgeon points and clicks on a target in a computer screen, then a robot moves the needle and inserts it into the target, under real-time imaging surveillance but without manual intervention. An experimental setup with phantom is shown in Figure 2.

Description of the Device

The assembly of the needle insertion device is shown in Figure 3. The device consists of the following main components: (1) end-effector that is introduced into the patient's rectum, (2) motion stage to provide translation and rotation for the end-effector, (3) in-

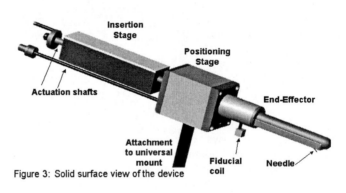

Figure 3: Solid surface view of the device

sertion stage to enter the needle into the prostate and retract it, (4) adjustable mount to bring and secure device in optimal initial position, (5) actuation shafts for remote operation from outside the scanner. In order to maintain material compatibility with MRI, the device was manufactured entirely from plastic, except the antennas, the needle, and two aluminum parts: the trigger of the biopsy needle and a sliding rail under the universal mount, but these two are situated far away from the field of imaging and produce no measurable artifact.

The end-effector is composed of a tubular obturator that translates and rotates in a thin rigid sheath. The sheath minimizes the deformation and displacement of the organ during positioning of the probe and it maintains a stationary position in reference to the organ of interest. The sheath also contains an MRI imaging loop antenna that produces real-time anatomic images stationary with respect to the subject anatomy. A small window is cut on the sheath through which the needle enters the body. A curved guiding channel is formed inside an obturator for a flexible standard MRI-compatible 18G biopsy needle. The needle exits on the side of the obturator and enters into the body through the rectum wall. Upon exiting the channel, the needle follows a straight trajectory. The obturator also holds three registration coils as active fiducials providing the spatial position of the probe in the MRI coordinate system.

The positioning stage transforms rotation of two concentric shafts into translation and rotation of a main shaft that serves as transmission to the end-effector. The concentric shafts are actuated from outside the scanner. The needle insertion stage transforms rotation of a knob into a well-defined insertion of the needle to a pre-determined target depth and actuates the shooting mechanism of a biopsy gun. In the current prototype, we adapted an 18G standard prostate biopsy needle (Daum GmbH, Schwerin, Germany). The insertion stage can also rotate the needle while it is being translated, thus achieving straight needle path when the needle needs to come out in a steeper angle from the end-effector.

Image Guidance

We apply computational image guidance, based on real-time collected MRI images. In this scenario, fiducial markers in a known geometric distribution are rigidly incorporated with the end-effector. Images are acquired with the device and patient together in the field of view. We use active MRI imaging antennas instead of traditional passive fiducial markers. Three imaging coils are situated in the end-effector of the device. Each coil winds around a small capsule containing gadolinium solvent, in order to provide strong signal in the vicinity of the coil. Two coils are located in the central axis of the end-effector to encode trans-

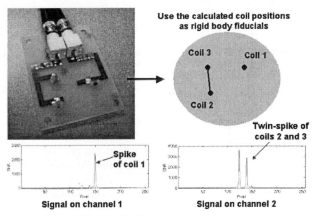

Figure 4: Dynamic Tracking Method

lation and the third coil is located off-axis to encode rotation. (More coils could provide redundancy to increase accuracy, but would also leave less channel capacity for anatomical imaging.) Figure 4 shows an early prototype of the tracking hardware. Each of these coils produces a single spike in the MR signal. Unlike other imaging modalities, MR gives us the ability to take direct, 1D projections. We acquire ten 1D projections of these fiducials along different orientations. This yields an overdetermined linear system for the positions of the points, which we can then solve for the coil locations. This yields enough information to define the scan plane. All together, the tracking sequence takes 50 ms, 5 ms for each 1D projection.

Calibration

The registration coils were fabricated manually, so the location of their signal centers with respect to the end-effector cannot be not be known without prior calibration. This information is constant for the entire lifetime of the device, assuming always the same image acquisition and processing parameters. We apply two tubes filled with gadolinium solvent. The first tube is placed inside the end-effector, while the other was attached around the needle. In a volumetric image of the device, the two tubes fully define the end-effector, while we also have readings on the coil positions. We repeat the calibration several times, in order to reduce the effects of measurement errors by simple averaging.

Results

The mechanical components of the device were analyzed separately, in laboratory environment. The accuracies of the translational and rotational mechanisms were found to be 1/100 mm, while the accuracy of the needle insertion stage is 0.1 mm. The computer software developed for calculation of targeting sequence, inverse and forward kinematics was tested on synthetic and real measurement and was found to be significantly more accurate than the mechanical components themselves. The appli-

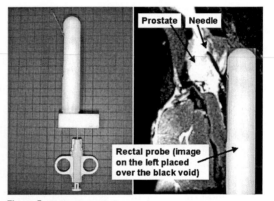

Figure 5: End-effector in live canine

cation and anatomical; feasibility of the end-effector was tested in vivo, when we performed transrectal needle biopsy of the prostate in a dog. Figure 5 shows the rectal sheath (left) and an 18 G biopsy needle entered through this end-effector (right). These experiments revealed that the combined system error has only one significant component and that originates from signal processing. The premise of our registration technique is that the readings on the positions of the fiducial coils define a rigid triangle at all times. We have performed extensive experiments that proved the feasibility of this concept. We used a mechanical frame that allowed for controlled translations and rotations of a board holding three fiducial coils in the same constellation as they are built in the end-effector. The three coils always define a triangle. We calculated the difference between the expected and measured centroids of the triangle and the difference between the expected and measured plane normal vectors of the triangle, which were 0.41 mm and 1.1 degree, respectively. Experiments were directed toward determining the effect of these errors on actual targeting accuracy. Total systemic accuracy has been tested in phantoms (Figure 6). Needle placement was found to be consistent throughout the field of imaging. The accuracy of needle placement was determined visually and it was below 2 mm in all trials. We expect to achieve similar accuracy in in-vivo, however, effects of possible displacement of the prostate during insertion is an important factor to be explored.

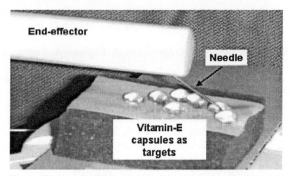

End-effector

Needle

Vitamin-E capsules as targets

Figure 6: Needle hitting a target in phantom experiment

Conclusion

We successfully demonstrated a proof-of-concept prototype for in-MRI biopsy of the prostate, under real-time image guidance, with remote actuation. We performed phantom and initial in-vivo canine studies. Determination of the combined systemic needle placement accuracy (considering errors from calibration, imaging, signal processing, target calculation, and mechanical actuation) is a work in progress. Our results so far justify the development of an advanced prototype suitable for human trials.

Acknowledgements

The authors acknowledge the support of the National Science Foundation under the Engineering Research Center grant #EEC-9731478. We are grateful to Theodore DeWeese, MD (Johns Hopkins University) for his guidance in clinical matters and to Dan Stoianovici, PhD (Johns Hopkins University) for contributing the universal snake mount (Figure 2) to our experiments.

References

1. Presti JC Jr. Prostate cancer: assessment of risk using digital rectal examination, tumor grade, prostate-specific antigen, and systematic biopsy. Radiol Clin North Am. 2000 Jan;38(1):49-58. Review
2. Norberg M, Egevad L, Holmberg L, Sparen P, Norlen BJ, Busch C. The sextant protocol for ultrasound-guided core biopsies of the prostate underestimates the presence of cancer. Urology. 1997 Oct;50(4):562-6.
3. Wefer AE, Hricak H, Vigneron DB, Coakley FV, Lu Y, Wefer J, Mueller-Lisse U, Carroll PR, Kurhanewicz J. Sextant localization of prostate cancer: comparison of sextant biopsy, magnetic resonance imaging and magnetic resonance spectroscopic imaging with step section histology. J Urol. 2000 Aug;164(2):400-4.
4. Yu KK, Hricak H. Imaging prostate cancer. Radiol Clin North Am. 2000 Jan;38(1):59-85, viii. Review.
5. Cormack RA, D'Amico AV, Hata N, Silverman S, Weinstein M, Tempany CM. Feasibility of transperineal prostate biopsy under interventional magnetic resonance guidance. Urology. 2000 Oct 1;56(4):663-4.

6. D'Amico AV, Tempany CM, Cormack R, Hata N, Jinzaki M, Tuncali K, Weinstein M, Richie JP. Transperineal magnetic resonance image guided prostate biopsy. J Urol. 2000 Aug;164(2):385-7.
7. G. Fichtinger, T. L DeWeese, A. Patriciu, A. Tanacs, D. Mazilu, J. H. Anderson, K. Masamune, R H. Taylor, D. Stoianovici: Robotically Assisted Prostate Biopsy And Therapy With Intra-Operative CT Guidance: Journal of Academic Radiology, Vol 9, No 1, pp. 60-74
8. Rovetta A, Sala R: Execution of robot-assisted biopsies within the clinical context., Journal of Image Guided Surgery. 1995;1(5):280-287
9. Chinzei K, Hata N, Jolesz FA, Kikinis R, MR Compatible Surgical Robot: System Integration and Preliminary feasibility study, Medical Image Computing and Computer-assisted Intervention 2000, Pittsburgh, PA. Lecture Notes in Computer Science, MICCAI 2000, Springer-Verlag, Vol. 1935, pp. 921-930
10. Kaiser WA, Fischer H, Vagner J, Selig M. Robotic system for biopsy and therapy of breast lesions in a high-field whole-body magnetic resonance tomography unit. Invest Radiol. 2000 Aug;35(8):513-9.
11. Masamune et. al., Development of an MRI-compatible needle insertion manipulator for stereotactic neurosurgery. Journal of Image Guided Surgery, 1995, 1 (4), pp. 242-248
12. Derbyshire JA, Wright GA, Henkelman RM, Hinks RS. Dynamic scan-plane tracking using MR position monitoring. J Magn Reson Imaging. 1998 Jul-Aug;8(4):924-32.

A New, Compact MR-Compatible Surgical Manipulator for Minimally Invasive Liver Surgery

Daeyoung Kim[1], Etsuko Kobayashi[2],
Takeyoshi Dohi[1], and Ichiro Sakuma[2]

[1] Department of Mechano-Informatics, Graduate School of Information Science
{young,etsuko}@miki.pe.u-tokyo.ac.jp
[2] Institute of Environment Studies, Graduate School of Frontier Sciences,
The University of Tokyo, 7-3-1 Hongo Bunkyo-Ku, Tokyo, 113-8656, Japan
{dohi,sakuma}@miki.pe.u-tokyo.ac.jp

Abstract. Recently, intra-operative magnetic resonance imaging (IO-MRI) has become an important clinical procedure. To perform this work, MR-compatible surgical equipment is necessary. In this study, our research team developed the technology for a MR-compatible manipulator for minimally invasive liver surgery that can operate in an MRI-scanner without any significant influence on MR imaging. The developed system that allows for 6 Degrees of Freedom (D.O.F) and a new RCM mechanism and bending forceps actuated by a motor-hydraulic actuation system. This manipulator provides enough power for liver surgery and is small enough to be operated within 45cm-high space in an Open-MRI. The image distortion within the MRI is minimal considering the effect of materials used in the system. These results demonstrate that it is feasible to operate the manipulator during MR operation and scanning.

1   Introduction

Recently, Intra-operative Magnetic Resonance Imaging (IO-MRI) has become a significant clinical procedure for minimally invasive surgery [1]-[4]. MR imaging is especially suitable for the intra-operative use because it does not require X-ray irradiation, allows for high soft-tissue contrast, and it can provide an arbitrary cross sectional image required for surgical planning. 3D-MR Angiograghy (3D-MRA) also provides information about blood vessel location. Surgeons can prevent unexpected bleeding during operation using this information.

However, space for the surgical operation within the MRI is still too limited for surgeons to perform conventional surgical work. Thus a mechanical manipulator that can perform precise surgical procedures in the limited space in open MRI is highly desirable. Furthermore, a MR image guided control of the manipulator can realize a new safer surgical procedure.

When we consider the application of an intra-operative MRI on minimally invasive liver surgery, the manipulator must be able to generate a large amount of power required for surgery. The simultaneous uses of multiple manipulators are often required, as demonstrated in the da Vinci system. In addition, since the liver is a soft organ, it is also necessary to conduct MR images during manipulator operation.

T. Dohi and R. Kikinis (Eds.): MICCAI 2002, LNCS 2488, pp. 99–106, 2002.

Non-ferromagnetic materials and ultrasonic motors are widely used today to realize MR-compatible manipulators. However, noise from ultrasonic motors will cause significant influence on MR imaging when such motors are placed near the Field of View (FOV). When the actuator was placed far from the FOV, the resulting mechanical system would be overly large. Thus, it would be difficult to install in the limited space such as an open MRI system.

In this study, we outline a newly developed MR-compatible manipulator for minimally invasive liver surgery. New materials, a new actuation system, and a manipulator mechanism were developed and incorporated in the design of this MR-compatible manipulator. The result is a tool that allows for minimally invasive liver surgery that can be operated in an MRI-scanner without any significant influence on MR imaging. We evaluated image distortion by several non-ferromagnetic materials and optimized their usage and propose a new hydraulic actuation system that provides enough power for actuation while the ultrasonic motor-based power generators are placed away from the FOV of the MRI scanner. A new remote center of motion (RCM) mechanism is also proposed to miniaturize the manipulator system. In numerous tests and experiments, we could evaluate the MR-compatibility of the system.

2   Manipulator Design

2.1   Material Selection

Special materials are required for the making of the MR-compatible device. For the material's MR-compatibility, Chinzei [3] evaluated the material's effect on the MRI by testing with 2cm Cubic metals, and Osada [5] analyzed the effect using the Finite Element Method (FEM). However, there is little data on the influence of material for practical mechanical structures used as surgical tools and manipulators. There is only a limited amount of quantitative data regarding the influenced area. In evaluating the effect of material on the MRI we used test pieces in the shape of pipe and rod that simulated the mechanical structure used in forceps.

For rods with a diameter of 10mm, the differences between observed MR images and the actual diameter was 10% of the actual diameter for Be-Cu and copper, 300% for titanium, and more than 1900% for SUS304, and SUS316 respectively. For titanium pipe with diameter of 10mm, the differences between observed MR images and the actual diameter was 70% of the actual diameter. SUS304, and SUS316 pipe showed much larger distortion (more than 400%). As for the test pieces with diameter of 3 mm (both for pipes and rods), there is very little distortion for Be-Cu, copper and titanium. There was significant distortion for SUS304, and SUS316 pipes. For 10 mm rods, range of influenced area was 10mm from the test piece for Be-Cu and copper, 30mm for titanium, and 300mm for SUS304 and SUS316. Therefore, it is appropriate to use Be-Cu for forceps that is placed near the center of FOV. Titanium pipe can be used for mechanical structure placed far from FOV by 30mm.

Since another mechanical part, such as a spring, might be used in manipulator mechanism, we also conducted the same evaluation on spring made of SUS 306, Be-Cu and NAS106N. The results are shown in Table 1.

Table 1. Evaluation of springs

Material of spring	SUS306	Be-Cu	NAS106N
Diameter of wire (mm)	0.3	0.3	0.3
Inner diameter of spring (mm)	0.9	0.9	1.3
Outside diameter of spring (mm)	1.5	1.5	1.9
Spring constant (gf/mm)	30	7	500
Observed image size evaluated two perpendicular diameter (mm)	58.5×94.5	1.8×1.8	7.0×11.0
Range of influenced area (mm)	100	≤10	≤10

As a result of these studies, Be-Cu was selected for the tip, and aluminum, brass, titanium for the structure. Only NAS106 N used in the metal of stainless for the pin, the spring, etc. considering hardness.

2.2   Actuation System

We used a hydraulic driving system both for forceps and forceps positioning manipulator to remove influence of the system on MR imaging even when the manipulator system was being driven during scanning. Ultrasonic motors placed far from RF coils of the MR scanner generated hydraulic power. It was transmitted with small tubes filled with sterilized saline. Thus the sterilization of the actuators is possible.

In a conventional hydraulic system, various mechanical elements, such as pressure source, accumulator, and valves are requiring leading to an increase in system size. We used hydraulic bilateral cylinder to improve the controllability and to reduce the size of the actuator [8].

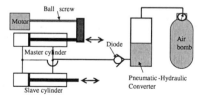

Fig. 1. Motor-hydraulic system

The system configuration of actuation system is shown in Fig.1. The torque of an ultrasonic motor controls the level of water pressure using a ball screw mechanism. Linear motion of the master cylinder is transmitted to the slave cylinder as shown in Fig.1. Leakage of fluid and immixture of air are two inherent problems in this system. To solve them, we added a fluid leakage compensation mechanism consisting of a compact air bomb, a pneumatic-hydraulic converter, and a hydraulic diode. This mechanism refills fluid when fluid pressure in the actuator cylinder is lower than a

certain level as shown in Figure 1. We can reduce the effect of air bubbles by setting the fluid pressure in the cylinder to high.

2.3   System Requirement

The mechanism of the manipulator was designed to consider the use of the system in a commercially available Open-MRI scanner (AIRIS2000, Hitachi Medical Co.). Detailed requirements for the manipulator system is summarized as follows:

- The system should have 6 degrees of freedom for ×15cm×6cm size under 10cm of abdominal wall considering the positioning and orientation of forceps in the abdominal space.
- The Range of motion of the forceps in the abdominal cavity is 25cm size of liver and working space created under pneumoperitoneum.
- The system should be placed inside the 45 cm high opening space of open MRI scanner.
- The system should generate 4kgf-cm torque around insertion port placed on the abdominal wall. This value was obtained by animal experiment with a pig that has 3cm-thickness abdominal wall.

The forceps should be able to bear 600gf considering the weight of liver tissue.

2.4   System Design

Since there was a restriction in height, the forceps should be inserted to the abdominal cavity from horizontal direction and should approach to the liver from vertical direction. Thus the bending of the forceps is indispensable.

In this system, bending was realized using a linkage mechanism. The length of the forceps tip (gripper) was 82mm and the remote center of motion was set at the point of 22cm from the tip of the forceps using the forceps positioning mechanism as described in section 2.5. The rotation of the gripper was achieved by cam mechanism. This mechanism enables the gripper to handle tissues such as a tubular blood vessel from any direction. Slave cylinders placed at the base of the forceps actuated the linkage mechanism and cam. Master cylinders were actuated by ball screw (lead: 2mm) driven by ultrasonic motors USR30-S4 (SHINSEI, Torque: 0.05Nm). Lengths of tubes connecting master and slave cylinder was 150cm and its inner diameter was 1.5mm.

In minimally invasive abdominal surgery, the Remote Center of Motion (RCM) of forceps is desirable where the forceps rotates around the insertion point on the abdominal wall [9]. We have developed a new RCM mechanism as shown in Figure 2.

To make RCM in this system, a ratio of d_t/d_b must be fixed during entire motion of the mechanism. This is obtained by fixing the ratio of two linkages' linear motion S_t/S_b. Since the motion of two master cylinders determines St/Sb, the distance between the lower linkage and remote center d_b was 5 cm.

The total movement of the RCM can be achieved by setting the gear ratio in ball screw driving mechanism. Ball screws (lead: 10mm) were driven by an ultrasonic motor USR60-S4 (SHINSEI. torque: 0.5Nm). Lengths of tubes connecting master and

slave cylinder was 150cm and its inner diameter was 1.5mm. This RCM has sufficient power (4kgf-cm at least), while the system is compact enough to install in the narrow space in open MRI scanner (9cm×14cm×45cm in height). The total system is shown in Fig.3.

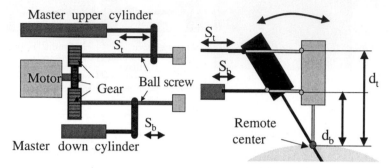

Fig. 2. RCM with linear actuators

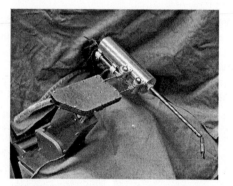

Fig. 3. MR-compatible Surgical Robot

3   Evaluation Experiments and Results

We evaluated the MR-compatibility of the system by placing and operating it in a conventional MR scanner (MRH-500 HITACHI Medical Co.). MR images were obtained and their distortions evaluated.

3.1   MR-Compatibility of Forceps' Material

Water and forceps were placed into acrylic plastic pipes of different diameters (ϕ22mm, ϕ58mm, ϕ107mm). The range of influenced area by the forceps was measured (Fig. 4). Sequence was SE, TE/TR: 30/300, FOV: 256mm×256mm, slice thickness: 10mm, and flip angle is 90 degrees. The results are summarized in Fig.4. We found that t distortions were small and limited in the area with a 10mm radius.

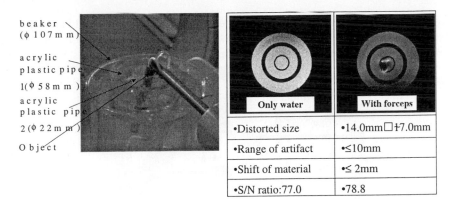

	Only water	With forceps
•Distorted size		•14.0mm□±7.0mm
•Range of artifact		•≤10mm
•Shift of material		•≤ 2mm
•S/N ratio:77.0		•78.8

Fig. 4. Evaluation :MR-compatibility of forceps' material

3.2   MR-Compatibility of Motor-Hydraulic Driving

We evaluated MR-compatibility of motor-hydraulic driving systems in the following four steps:
1. The manipulator was placed outside of RF coil, and electric power was unplugged.
2. The manipulator was placed inside of RF coil, and electric power was unplugged.
3. The manipulator was placed inside of RF coil, and electric power was plugged but did not drive the manipulator.
4. The manipulator was placed inside of RF coil, and electric power was plugged and drove the manipulator.

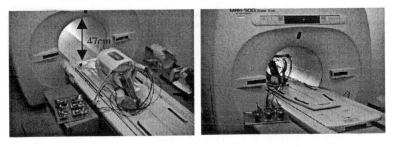

Fig. 5. Setting for evaluation: MR-compatibility of motor-hydraulic driving

Table 2. MR-compatibility of motor-hydraulic driving

Condition	Outside of RF coil Unplugged	Inside of RF coil Unplugged	Inside of RF coil Plugged	Inside of RF coil Being driven
Image				
S/N ratio	283.7	275.6	261.1	174.8

4.3   MR-Compatibility of the Total System

This evaluation was completed through two steps with a phantom used in 5.1 evaluations.

1. The manipulator was placed in the phantom unit to measure the distortion of the shape of the mechanism in the MRI, but was not actuated. Electric power was supplied.
2. The manipulator was placed in the phantom unit and was actuated.

The 8cm long tip of the forceps (gripper) was placed in the phantom. In step 2, bending mechanism was actuated. Results are shown in Table 3. Actuation of the manipulator slightly deteriorates image distortion and S/N ratio.

Table 3. MR-compatibility of total system

	Just plugged	With actuation
Forceps were put Into the phantom		
Distorted size	14×17(mm)	15×19.5(mm)
Range of artifact	≤10mm	≤10mm
S/N ratio	77.3	45.1

5   Discussion, Conclusion and Future Work

We developed a MR-compatible Surgical Manipulator System with Hydraulic Actuators. The driving method using bilateral cylinders was powerful effective enough to realize MR-compatibility, making it possible to produce a compact surgical manipulator. No significant influence on MR imaging was observed even when the mechanism was actuated during scanning. By adding a leakage compensation mechanism, stability and controllability of the system were improved.

As for manipulator design, we developed a bending forceps system that can be inserted into the abdominal cavity from a horizontal direction that allows liver to be approached from a vertical direction. The bending and rotation were realized by a linkage and cam mechanism driven by hydraulic actuators. A new RCM using linear actuators was also proposed. The developed system has 6 D.O.Fs. It is compact in size to be installed in narrow space in the scanner (45cm-high) and to be operated freely. The system has enough power (at least 4kgf-cm), and 600gf for holding the tissue while maintaining its compacted ness. It has the possibilities for enhanced safety [10] during usage as a medical robot.

Although the average S/N ratio of MR images deteriorated when the total manipulator system was actuated, the range of influenced area was limited to 10 mm in radius and there no significant noise on image was obtained. The image distortion was minimal considering the effect of materials used in the system. These results demonstrated that it is feasible to operate the manipulator during MR scanning.

Control of the surgical manipulator using real time image data of the important anatomical structure such as blood vessel's location will further advance minimally invasive liver surgery. Future research should focus on combining and overlapping the MRI and the laparoscope for more effective surgical procedures

To shorten setting time as can as possible, new type cylinder and new set method is advisable.

This study was partly supported by the Research for the Future Program (JSPS-RFTF 99I00904) Grant-in-Aid for Scientific Research (A) (14702070). NH was supported by Toyota Phsical&Chemical Research Institute, Suzuken Memorial Foundation, Kurata Grants.

References

1. Masamune K., Kobayashi E., et al.: Development of an MRI compatible Needle Insertion Manipulator for Stereotactic Neurosurgery, J image Guided Surgery,1pp.242-248(1995)
2. Chinzei K., et al.: Surgical Assist Robot for the Active Navigation in the intraoperative MRI, MICCAI Proc.pp.921-930(2000)
3. Chinzei K., Hata N., et al.: MRcompatible Surgical Assist Robot: System Integration and Preliminary Feasibility Study, IEEE/RSJ IROS2000,Proc. 727-732(2000)
4. Robert B.Lufkin: Interventional MRI, pp.55-69, Mosby, (1999)
5. Osada A. et al.: The fundamental Investigation for the designing of MRI compatible instruments, JSCAS Proc.pp107-108 (2000)
6. Ikuda K., Ichikawa H., et al.: Study on Micro Pneumatic Drive for Safety Active Catheter, JSCAS Proc.pp99-100 (2001)
7. M.laseroms al.: A Hydraulic Forceps with Force-feedback for Use in Minimally Invasive Surgery, Mechatronics Vol.6, No 4, pp.437-446 (1996)
8. Saitou Y.,Sunagawa Y.; A study of Hydraulic Bilateral Servo Actuator for welfare Robots, Life Support Proc.pp100 (1998)
9. Bishoff, J.T., Stoianovici, D., Lee, B.R., Bauer, J., Taylor, R.H., Whitcomb, L.L., Cadeddu, J.A., Chan, D., Kavoussi, L.R., RCM-PAKY: Clinical Application of a New Robotic System for Precise Needle Placement, Journal of Endourology, Vol. 12, pp. S82 (1998)
10. Davies BL.: A Discussion of safety issues of medical robots, Computer integrated Surgery: Technology and Clinical Applications. Cambridge, MA: The MIT press, pp287-296 (1995)

Micro-grasping Forceps Manipulator
for MR-Guided Neurosurgery

Nobuhiko Miyata[1], Etsuko Kobayashi[1], Daeyoung Kim[1], Ken Masamune[5],
Ichiro Sakuma[1], Naoki Yahagi[1], Takayuki Tsuji[1], Hiroshi Inada[2],
Takeyoshi Dohi[3], Hiroshi Iseki[4], and Kintomo Takakura[4]

[1] Graduate School of Frontier Scineces, the University of Tokyo,
7-3-1Hongo Bunkyo-ku Tokyo, 113-8656, Japan
{miyata,etsuko,young,sakuma}@miki.pe.u-tokyo.ac.jp
[2] Graduate school of Information, the University of Tokyo,
[3] Graduate School of Engineering, the University of Tokyo,
[4] Department of Neurosurgery, Tokyo Women's Medical University,
[5] Collage of Science & Engineering, Tokyo Denki University

Abstract. Mechanical support system is needed for minimally invasive surgery, since it enables precise manipulation of surgical instruments beyond human ability in a small operation space. Furthermore, a robot available for intra-operative MRI guided neurosurgical procedures could allow less invasive and more accurate image guided surgery. By combination of precise positioning to the target by intra-operative MRI guided surgery and dexterity by the multi function micromanipulator, safe and smooth operation is expected to be performed. In this approach, we have developed MR-compatible micro-forceps manipulator of the multi-function micromanipulator system for neurosurgery. By a new cam mechanism for two degrees of bending freedom, we achieved these excellent characteristics for the micro forceps. 1) Simple mechanism suitable for a micromanipulator, 2) Precise positioning, 3) Suitable mechanism for MR compatible manipulator. By evaluation experiments, we confirmed precise positioning of the manipulator and MR compatibility of the manipulator.

1   Introduction

Minimally invasive surgery is currently a hot topic because it can reduce a patient's post-operative discomfort and length of rehabilitation period, thus improving the patient's Quality of Life. Minimally invasive surgery has many advantages to the patient; on the contrary, it reduces the surgeon's dexterity. Precise manipulation of surgical forceps is indispensable for safe surgery, however, in minimally invasive neurosurgery, the precise manipulation of forceps through a small burr hole is particularly difficult. This difficulty is caused by, for example, hand trebling and insufficient degrees of freedom (D.O.F.) of the forceps. This has restricted the number of applicable clinical cases.

To achieve precise manipulation and enhance the surgeon's dexterity, mechanical operation support is useful. In this approach, various kinds of such surgical support systems have been developed [1][2]. In the neurosurgery, also, a mulch function micromanipulator system has been reported [3]. We have also developed a multi-function micromanipulator system (Fig.1) [4]. It consists of two micro grasping forceps manipulators (ϕ3.2mm), a rigid neuro-endoscope (ϕ4mm), a suction tube (ϕ3mm), and an irrigation tube (ϕ1.4mm). The components are inserted into a rigid tube (ϕ10mm). The micromanipulator is inserted into the burr hole with an insertion manipulator [5] that can determine the direction and position of the manipulator by reference to pre-operative images such as CT and Magnetic Resonance Imaging (MRI). The micro grasping forceps manipulator system has two degrees of bending freedom by a wire and a ball joint mechanism. However, the problem of the manipulator was stick-slip caused by wire mechanism and friction.

MRI techniques, including MRI angiography and functional MRI, are attractive for the development of interventional MRI therapies and operations [6][7][8]. A robot available for these neurosurgical procedures could allow less invasive and more accurate image guided surgery. From this background, we have developed MR-compatible stereo-tactic insertion manipulator [9].

From these backgrounds, by combination of precise positioning to the target by intra-operative MRI guided surgery and dexterity by the multi-function micromanipulator, safe, certain and smooth operation is expected to be performed.

Therefore, the goal of this research is achieve a micro grasping forceps manipulator of the multi-function micromanipulator. And the system has these characteristics; 1) two degrees of bending freedom, 2) precise positioning, and 3) MR-compatibility.

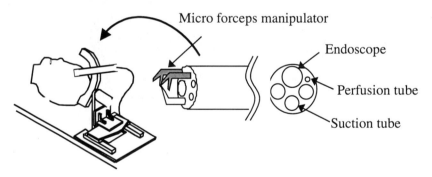

Fig. 1. Multi-function micromanipulator system for neurosurgery

2   Micro-grasping Forceps Manipulator

2.1   Requirements

Requirements of the micro grasping forceps are as follows;
1) MR-compatibility
2) Size; 3mm in diameter. As shows in Figure 1, the micro grasping forceps is inserted into a 10mm rigid tube. The size must be small.
3) Moving degrees of freedom (D.O.F.): It must have at least five D.O.F. Two degrees of bending, rotation around the axis, back and forth movement and grasping.

4) Precision positioning; Because the target is small tissue, the precise positioning is required.

Furthermore, because the manipulator requires small size with multi degrees of freedom, its mechanism must be simple.

2.2   MR Compatibility

MR-compatible material is the material that does not effect MR images and is not effected from strong magnetic field [10]. We validated MR-compatibility of materials and selected adequate material for the manipulator. ϕ3mm shaft was inserted into the beaker of 107mm in diameter and measured the range of artifact caused by the shaft.

Figure 2 shows the MR image and the range of artifact. We used MRI with 0.5T static magnetic field (MRH-500 Hitachi Medical corp., Japan) and the protocols of the image were T1 enhanced image, spin echo, 256x256mm FOV, 1mm image resolution, TR/TE 1500/35 and 2.0mm slice thickness. The image was taken in coronal plane. The range of the artifact caused by a stainless steel was almost same with a circle of 60mm in diameter. Aluminum and titan effected about the range of the circle of 15mm in diameter. Therefore, we used mainly titan and aluminum for the micro grasping forceps and used stainless steel for the part set far from the target.

Direction of a magnetic field   Area of artifact

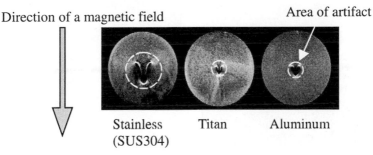

Stainless   Titan   Aluminum
(SUS304)

Fig. 2. MR image of the water with shafts of 3mm in diameter

2.3   New Cam Mechanism for a Micro-grasping Forceps Manipulator

To realize these requirements such as small size and precision positioning, we proposed a new cam mechanism for two degrees of bending freedom (Fig.3). A torsion spring is attached to a grasping forceps part and a cylinder cut aslant (named a cam cylinder) is set around the spring. The base of the grasping forceps part is push to an outer cylinder around the cam cylinder. Then by pushing the base of the grasping forceps part by the cam cylinder, the forceps manipulator is bend and by rotating the cam cylinder, bending direction can be changed. Rotation of the forceps is determined by the rotating the spring. Back and forth movement is achieved by a rack and pinion and grasping is by a wire. As we mentioned in chpt.2.2 we mainly used Aluminum and Titan for the manipulator. For the spring, we used Be-Cu. Ultrasonic motors drive all mechanisms.

Figure 4 shows a tip of the micro forceps manipulator. The diameter of the forceps was 3.2 mm. Figure 5 shows overview of the multi-function micromanipulator system.

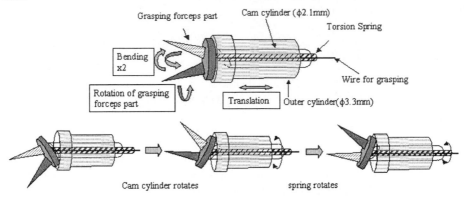

Fig. 3. Mechanism of the micro grasping forceps

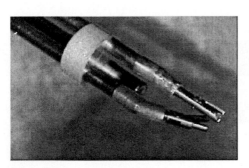

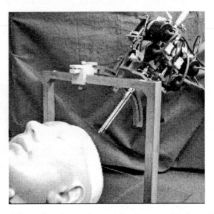

Fig. 4. Micro grasping forceps manipulator

Fig. 5. Overview of the multi-function micromanipulator system

3　Experiment

3.1　Positioning Accuracy

We evaluated the positioning accuracy of the bending when we put the command to move 1.0 degree. We set the high-definition digital micro scope (VH-6300, Keyence co. ltd., Japan) to observe the bending angle and measured the bending angle using the microscopic image (image resolution 0.015[mm/pixel]).

Figure 6 shows the relationship between the pushing distance of the cam cylinder and the measured bending angle. Average of the bending angle was 0.98 degree and standard deviation of the error was 0.68 degree. In bending movement, we achieved precise positioning without stick-slip movement. However, when the bending angle was more than 30 degree, the error was big, because the spring was extended rather than bending.

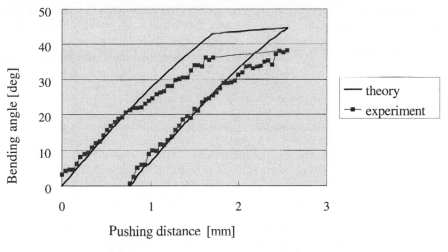

Fig. 6. Positioning accuracy of the bending

3.2   Evaluation of MR Image

We performed an evaluation of the MR image distortion. We put a sphere of 63mm in diameter into water and put the forceps on the surface of the sphere. We used a same MRI devices with the MR-compatible material evaluation (0.5T static magnetic field, MRH-500 Hitachi Medical corp.) The protocols of the image were T2 enhanced image, spin echo, 256x256mm FOV, 1mm image resolution, TR/TE 2500/100 and 2.0mm slice thickness. The image was taken in sagittal plane. For contrast, the non MR-compatible forceps manipulator was evaluated.

Micro grasping forceps manipulator

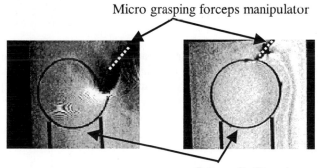

Sphere (ϕ 63mm)

Fig. 7. MR Image of a sphere with the micro forceps manipulator. Left: Image with non MR-compatible forceps. Right: Image with MR-compatible forceps

Figure 7 shows MR Images of the ϕ63mm sphere with the non MR-compatible and MR-compatible micro forceps manipulator. We measured the radius of the sphere from both images. In non MR-compatible forceps, maximum error of the radius was

5.3 mm. On the contrary, maximum error of the MR-compatible forceps was 1.5mm. From this result, the micro grasping forceps manipulator has enough MR compatibility to be used for intra-operative MRI guide surgery.

4   Discussion

Because the cam mechanism we have developed is simple and it has certain transmission of the positioning compare to wire mechanism, the manipulator has excellent characteristics as the micro forceps manipulator.

1) It consists of only simple parts. Therefore manufacturing and assembling is easily completed even if small parts are required.
2) Compare to the wire mechanism, precise positioning is possible.
3) It is also suitable for MR compatible manipulator.

In the experiment, we confirmed the precise positioning of 0.68 mm error.

In the image distortion evaluation, we confirmed little image distortion (maximum 1.5mm) caused by the manipulator. Because image resolution was 1.0 mm, the distortion was small enough to the positioning.

For MR-compatible materials, we used Be-Cu spring. The spring constant was 12.6gf/mm and it was not enough strength for the mechanism. We have to reselect the MR-compatible spring for more precise positioning and high torque occurrence.

Kan [3] achieved neurosurgery assist robotic system (HUMAN). In this system, however, forceps manipulator has only one degree of bending freedom. For dexterous operation, it is preferable to have the same degrees of freedom with the human wrist for the movement of the forceps. From this point of view, we have developed the forceps with two degrees of bending freedom and our system provide sufficient dexterity.

5   Conclusion

We have developed MR-compatible forceps manipulator for the multi-function micromanipulator system. For the bending mechanism we proposed new simple cam mechanism. By this forceps manipulator, we achieved precise bending positioning (0.68 degree) and MR compatibility (Maximum 1.5mm image distortion).

For future work, we combine the forceps and the MR-compatible insertion manipulator [9], and image distortion evaluation and positioning accuracy evaluation is performed.

Reference

1. Salisbury J. K.: The heart of microsurgery, Mechanical Engineering, v.120 n.12 Dec p46-51 (1998)
2. Mitsuishi M. et al, :A tele-micro-surgery system with co-located view and operation points and a rotational-foce-feedback-free master manipulator, Proc. of MRCAS '95, pp.111-118, (1995)

3. Berkelman P. J. et al :A Miniture instrument tip force sensor for robot/human cooperative microsurgical manipulator with enhanced force feedback, MICCAI2000, Proc. pp. 897-906 (2000)
4. Schurr M.O. et al.: Robotics and telemanipulation technologies for endoscopic surgery, Surgical endoscopy, 14, pp.375-381, (2000)
5. Kan K., et al. : Microscopic-manipulator system for minimally invasive neurosurgery, Proc. of CARS 98, pp.594-598, (1998)
6. Harada K. et al.: Development of a micro manipulator for minimally invasive neurosurgery, Proc. of CARS 2000, pp.116-120, (2000)
7. K Masamune, M Sonderegger, H Iseki, K Takakura, M Suzuki, T Dohi, Robots for Stereo-tactic neurosurgery, Advanced Robotics, Vol.10, No.3, pp.391-401 (1996)
8. Hwa-shain Y, et al.: Implantation of intracerebral depth delectrodes for monitoring seizures using the Pelorus stereotactic system guided by magnetic resonance imaging, J Neurosurg 78:138-141, (1993)
9. Robert B.Lufkin: Interventional MRI, pp.55-69, Mosby, (1999)
10. Chinzei K., Hata N., et al.: MR-compatible surgical assist robot: system integration and preliminary feasibility Study, IEEE/RSJ IROS2000, Proc. 727-732 (2000)
11. Masamune K., Kobayashi E., et al.: Development of an MRI compatible needle insertion manipulator for stereotactic neurosurgery, J Image Guided Surgery, 1 pp.242-248 (1995)
12. Chinzei K., et al.: Surgical assist robot for the active navigation in the intraoperative MRI, MICCAI2000, Proc. pp.921-930 2000

Endoscope Manipulator
for Trans-nasal Neurosurgery, Optimized
for and Compatible to Vertical Field Open MRI

Yoshihiko Koseki[1], Toshikatsu Washio[1],
Kiyoyuki Chinzei[1,2], and Hiroshi Iseki[2,3]

[1] National Institute of Advanced Industrial Science and Technology, 1-2 Namiki,
Tsukuba, Ibaraki 305-8564, Japan
koseki@ni.aist.go.jp
http://unit.aist.go.jp/humanbiomed/surgical/
[2] Dept. of Neurosurgery, Neurological Institute, Tokyo Women's Medical University,
[3] Field of Advanced Techno-surgery, Graduate School of Medicine,
Tokyo Women's Medical University

Abstract. This paper preliminarily reports the robotic system working
inside the gantry of vertical field Open MRI. This manipulator is new in
terms of the application to vertical field Open MRI, cost effectiveness,
accuracy and stiffness sufficient for endoscope manipulation. The endoscope manipulation for trans-nasal neurosurgery under MR-guidance
was selected as the sample task. The endoscope operation in MR-gantry
might provide the surgeon(s) with real-time feedback of MR image to
endoscopic image and the reverse. This facilitates the comprehensive understanding, because MRI compensates the vision lost through narrow
opening of keyhole surgery with global view. So this surgery is a good
motivation for combination of MRI and robotic systems. In this paper,
the design and implementation are presented and preliminary test shows
good MR-compatibility, accuracy and stiffness.

1 Introduction

The merits of MRI (Magnetic Resonance Imaging) are not limited to visualization behind the surface anatomy but also excellent soft tissue discrimination,
functional imaging, and non X-ray exposure. Its intra-operative usage can make
so-called keyhole surgery safer and effective[1]. Because MRI can compensate the
limited view from the narrow opening, and can distinguish the residual tumor
from normal tissues. For such usage, some types of widely open MRI have been
provided recently.

Many researchers have proposed that the combination of tomography and
numerically controlled robot potentially improves the performance of keyhole
surgery[2, 3]. The robot can position tools and devices referring to precise 3D
coordinate of tomography. The technical drawbacks of MRI are that the most
conventional materials and devices affect and are affected by the strong and

T. Dohi and R. Kikinis (Eds.): MICCAI 2002, LNCS 2488, pp. 114–121, 2002.
© Springer-Verlag Berlin Heidelberg 2002

precise magnet[4]. Because of clinical advantages, an MR-compatible robotics has been requested however.

An MR-compatible manipulator was firstly proposed by Masamune to assist needle insertion for stereo-tactic neurosurgery under closed gantry MRI[5]. Kaiser also proposed one for breast cancer[6]. The closed gantry MR scanners generally have better magnetic field properties and are widely used, but have less accessibility to patient. The accessibility to patient must be secured for emergencies during scanning, so the operation inside gantry must be as simple as needle insertion.

We have also investigated the MR-compatibility of mechanical parts and have summarized MR-compatible techniques[7]. Firstly, we developed one prototype for horizontal field Open MRI[8]. This type of MRI is vertically open enough for the surgeon to stand by the patient and to perform the operation inside gantry. In this case, the manipulator is requested not to occupy the surgeon's space nearby the patient.

On the other hand, the vertical field Open MRI is vertically so narrow that the surgeon(s) doesn't stand by the patient while the patient is inside gantry. The hand-works must be done outside and on demand of MR imaging the patient is carried in. This method is clinically and commercially reasonable because a lot of conventional apparatus can be available in many situations. However, a manipulator needs work inside the gantry instead of surgeon.

In case of vertical field Open MRI, the space around the patient remains unoccupied and a manipulator can be closed to the deep inside gantry. This is advantageous in terms of stiffness and precision of the manipulator but disadvantageous in terms of MR-compatibility.

Accordingly, the vertically small shaped prototype was newly designed and implemented for vertical field Open MRI. The prototype is installed to imaging area and has good performance of precision and stiffness. Our continuing studies have revealed that magnetically not ideal parts can be used according to the distance from the imaging area. The cutback of excessively fine MR-compatibility can reduce the cost.

To determine the detailed specifications, an endoscope manipulation of trans-nasal neurosurgery was selected as a sample application. Because the importance of intra-operative MRI is high but almost hand-works have to be performed outside gantry and imaging is not frequent.

2　Design and Implementation

2.1　Scenario

The trans-nasal neurosurgery is one of the most typical keyhole surgeries, where the surgeon(s) approach the pituitary tumor behind sphenoid through the narrow nasal cavity[9]. The surgeon spends the most time on making an approach through sphenoid and resection of the tumor.

The global view and good contrast of soft tissue of MRI are helpful to avoid trauma to critical structures of brain and remove the residual tumor. The real-time feedback of MRI to endoscopic image and the reverse will enhance the performance and safety of trans-nasal neurosurgery. Although the surgeon cannot hold, pan, or tilt the endoscope stably in vertically narrow MR-gantry, a robotic system can do.

The greater part of this surgery is done in the fringe field and the patient and bed are carried into the gantry on demand of intra-operative MRI. The manipulator should be embedded on the bed for easy carrying in/out. The endoscope should be inserted and removed outside of gantry because the back of endoscope is blocked by the upper magnet while the patient is inside.

2.2   System Requirements

The prototype was designed for Hitachi's AIRIS-II (Hitachi Medical Corp., Tokyo, Japan), whose magnets are 1400[mm] in diameter and are 430[mm] open vertically.

2 DOF (Degree of Freedom) of rotational motions are required for pan and tilt. 2 DOF of translational motions are required for positioning. One DOF around endoscope might be required for potential future usage of angled endoscope but currently not installed.

2.3   Implementation

Previously, MR-compatibility has been applied uniformly. The materials such as titanium and MC Nylon, which are highly compatible, but expensive and weak. Our pretests led that the magnetic effect is inverse proportional to the distance and proportional to the volume. This time incompatible materials and parts were used according to their distance from imaging area and their amount. This enables the stiffness to be improved and the cost to be reduced. The guidelines was set as shown in Table 1.

Fig. 1 shows the mechanism and coordinate system. A rotational 5-bar linkage mechanism was adopted for 2 DOF of translational motions. The reasons are that the actuators are set on distant and immobile points, and the planar parallel mechanism is vertically small compared to a serial mechanism because driving units are arranged in the same plane in parallel. The endoscope is panned around an axis away from the actuator with a parallelogram. This mechanism enabled the actuator distant from imaging area. The endoscope is tilted with the rotation of the parallelogram.

All axes were driven by non-magnetic ultrasonic motors, USR60-S3N (Shinsei Kogyo Corp., Tokyo, Japan) via strain wave gears and hand clutches. Normal strain wave gears, CSF-17 (Harmonic Drive Systems Inc., Tokyo Japan) were used for axis 1 & 2 and low-magnetic ones (custom-made by Harmonic Drive Systems) are used for axis 3 & 4. The strain wave gears reduce the velocity of motors to safe level. The hand clutches can switch from motor drive to manual operation for emergency.

Rotary encoder units, VR-050M&SR-050M (5000P/R, Canon Inc., Tokyo Japan) and potentiometers, JC22E (Nidec Copal Electronics Corp., Tokyo,

Table 1. Zone control of MR-compatibility

	Zone	Guideline	Compatible Materials & Devices
I	Neighborhood of Imaging Area (Within a radius of 300[mm])	Non-magnetic Materials, No Electrical Components	Ti, MC-Nylon, Ceramic Bearing
II	Fringe of Imaging Area (Without a radius of 300[mm])	A Small Amount of Low-Magnetic Materials Electrical Components	Al, SUS304, Low-Magnetic Harmonic Drive, Ultrasonic Motor, Potentio-meter, Rotary Encoder
III	Fringe of Magnet (Without a radius of 700[mm])	A Small Amount of Ferro-magnetic	Harmonic Drive, Normal Bearing

The guideline of outer zone includes those of inner zones.

Japan) were installed for precise incremental measurement and absolute measurement of axes respectively. The motor unit and sensors are connected in parallel to axis via parallelogram so the sensors follow the axial motion while the clutch is open. The electrical signals of rotary encoder are optically transmitted to the outside of operation room. Fig. 2 shows the prototype deployed in a dummy of Hitachi's AIRIS-II with a human phantom.

3 Experiments

3.1 Accuracy Test

The accuracy and repeatability of this prototype were tested. Five, 3, and 3 points were selected for X-Y coordinate, axis 3 and 4, respectively. The manipulator moved to each point 20 times on random path. The displacement was measured with two CCD laser micrometers (VG-035/300, KEYENCE, Osaka, Japan). The rotational displacements were indirectly measured by measuring translational displacement of different two points. Table 2 shows ideal positions calculated by kinematics, averages, and standard deviation of measured position.

The accuracy and repeatability were totally good for endoscope positioning. The calibration of mechanical parameters of 5-bar linkage mechanism will improve the accuracy in X- and Y-axes. The error in axis-3 & 4 are relatively large considering of its effect on the tip of 100[mm] endoscope. The error is mainly due to backlash because the error of single path was very small. The pretests revealed that the frictions of these axes increased backlash. As is similar to stiffness, minor changes are necessary.

3.2 Stiffness Test

The major elasticity of this prototype was tested. Up to 20[N] (2.0[kgf]) force was applied on one point close to, and the other point distant from the origin

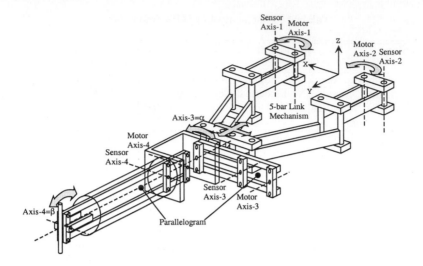

Fig. 1. Mechanism of MR-compatible endoscope manipulator prototype

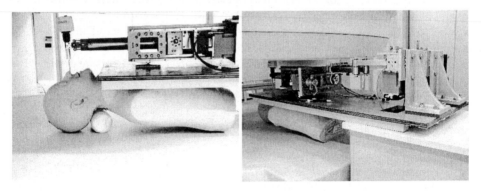

Fig. 2. Prototype of MR-compatible endoscope manipulator in dummy MR gantry

of end-plate, in each direction. The displacements were measured similarly as accuracy test. The coordinate and axes are shown in Fig. 1 and θ_x, θ_y, and θ_z are the rotation around X-, Y-, and Z-axis, respectively. Table 3 shows the elasticity and backlash in positive and negative direction of X, Y, Z θ_x, θ_y, and θ_z.

The elasticity in X-axis was large. The axis 4 was supported by open sided structure (See Fig. 1). The offset of θ_x was also large. Some weak parts were used for knockdown structure around the axis-4. A minor change in mechanism will improve these weaknesses. The stiffness in other directions were excellent.

3.3   MR-Compatibility Test

MRI's Effect to Manipulator. The MR-compatibility of this prototype was tested by real Hitachi's AIRIS-II in Intelligent Operating Room in Tokyo

Table 2. Accuracy & repeatability test

Direction	Ideal	Real Average	STDV
(X, Y)	(0.00, 0.00)	(-, -)	(0.03, 0.02)
([mm], [mm])	(0.00, 5.11)	(0.04, 5.13)	(0.03, 0.01)
	(0.00,-5.34)	(0.05,-5.40)	(0.03, 0.01)
	(7.43,-0.09)	(7.47,-0.03)	(0.02, 0.01)
	(-7.43,-0.09)	(-7.38,-0.20)	(0.02, 0.01)
Axis 3	0.00	-	0.01
[Deg]	5.40	5.40	0.02
	-5.40	-5.38	0.02
Axis 4	0.00	-	0.03
[Deg]	5.40	5.44	0.03
	-5.40	-5.41	0.03

STDV: standard deviation

Table 3. Major elasticity of the prototype

Direction	Pos. [m/N] ([mm/kgf])	Neg. [m/N] ([mm/kgf])	offset [m] ([mm])
x	1.28×10^{-4} (1.28)	1.33×10^{-4} (1.33)	$\pm 0.22 \times 10^{-3}$ ($\pm$0.22)
y	0.07×10^{-4} (0.07)	0.09×10^{-4} (0.09)	$\pm 0.05 \times 10^{-3}$ ($\pm$0.05)
z	0.19×10^{-4} (0.19)	0.24×10^{-4} (0.24])	$\pm 0.03 \times 10^{-3}$ ($\pm$0.03)

Direction	Pos. [Deg/N·m] ([Deg/kgf·cm])	Neg. [Deg/N·m] ([Deg/kgf·cm])	offset [Deg]
θ_x	0.73 (0.073)	0.75 (0.075)	$\pm$1.42
θ_y	0.46 (0.046)	0.54 (0.054)	$\pm$0.66
θ_z	0.25 (0.025)	0.25 (0.025)	$\pm$0.05

Women's Medical University. The manipulator was scanned with spin echo and gradient echo sequence. The followings were confirmed while the manipulator was hard-wired and set on regular position at a standstill.

1. The manipulator was not attracted by the magnet.
2. No heat or noise occurred.
3. The ultrasonic motors worked regularly.
4. The counts of rotary encoders did not change.
5. The noise of potentio-meters was slightly increased at the beginning of scanning.
6. The status of limit switches did not change.
7. The status of emergency switches did not change.

Manipulator's Effect to MRI. The prototype's effect to the images was examined. $1.0l$ aqueous solution of $_2$ 1.8×10^{-4} mol/l NiCl and 0.1% NaCl was imaged as a phantom. The intensity of magnetic field was 0.3 Tesla, and other parameters were TE/TR=20/100[ms], bandwidth=30kHz, Flip Angle=30.0[Deg]. The spin echo image, gradient image, and spectrum of MR on the following conditions were obtained. The 3rd condition is just an auxiliary experiment because the endoscope needs not be operated while MR scanning.

1. The prototype was not installed to the gantry. Only phantom.
2. The prototype was installed to the gantry and hard-wired.
3. The prototype was actuated with the repeat of acceleration and deceleration.

Fig. 3 shows gradient echo MR images on these 3 conditions. Fig. 3 also shows the difference image between condition 1 and 2. Table 4 shows the signal-to-noise ratio (S/N ratio) and half width of MR spectrum. The S/N ratio is the ratio of the mean value of the phantom to the standard deviation of the air. The half width of MR spectrum corresponds to the sharpness of magnetic resonance and indicates the distortion of image. If the magnetic field is distorted, the resonance will be dull.

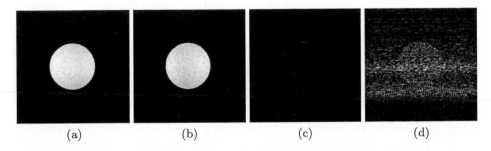

Fig. 3. Gradient echo MR images of phantom, (a)only a phantom, (b)the manipulator is deployed, (c)the difference image between (a) and (b), (d) the manipulator is actuated

Table 4. Signal to noise ratio and half width of phantom's MR spectrum

Condition	S/N Ratio		Half Width	
	SE	GRE	SE	GRE
Only Phantom	216.7	61.2	33.0	36.1
Manipulator Deployed	208.0	66.4	36.9	37.7
Manipulator Actuated	14.4	11.9	36.1	38.8

The difference images (Fig. 3(c)) led that the manipulator's effect on MRI was negligible. S/N ratio and half width also indicated that no noise or distortion was caused by manipulator as long as the motor was inactive. The actuator caused large noise on MR scanning, however. Assume that the endoscope focuses one area imaged by MRI, the endoscope manipulator needs not move while MR scanning. So this noise doesn't cause trouble.

4   Conclusion

The robotic system working inside the gantry of vertical field Open MRI was studied in this paper. The design and implementation were discussed and the pre-clinical evaluation of our first prototype like, accuracy test, stiffness and MR-compatibility were reported.

The technical significances of this paper are

1. A manipulator was specially designed for vertical field Open MRI, which is vertically narrow.
2. The zone control reduces the cost and improves the accuracy and stiffness remaining the MR-compatibility.

The clinical significances are

1. This manipulator system enables real-time feedback of MR image to endoscopic image and the reverse.
2. The combination of MRI and endoscope enhances the performance and safety of keyhole surgery.

The pre-clinical evaluations led that some minor modifications are necessary.

References

1. Pergolizzi R.S., et.al.: Intra-Operative MR Guidance During Trans-Sphenoidal Pituitary Resection: Preliminary Results. J. of Magnetic Resonance Imaging, **13** (2001) 136–141
2. Burckhardt C.W., Flury P., Glauser D.: Stereotactic Brain Surgery. IEEE Engineering in Medicine and Biology Magazine, **14(3)**, (1195) 314–317
3. Kwoh Y.S., Hou J., Jonckheere E., Hayati S.: A Robot with Improved Absolute Positioning Accuracy for CT Guided Stereotactic Brain Surgery. IEEE tran. on Biomedical Engineering, **35(2)**(1988), 153–160
4. Jolesz F.A, et. al.: Compatible instrumentation for intraoperative MRI: Expanding resources. JMRI, **8(1)** (1998) 8–11
5. Masamune K., Kobayashi E., Masutani Y., Suzuki M., Dohi T., Iseki H., Takakura K.: Development of an MRI-compatible needle insertion manipulator for stereotactic neurosurgery. Journal of Image Guided Surgery. **1(4)** (1995) 242–248
6. Kaiser W.A., Fischer H., Vagner J., Selig M.: Robotic system for Biopsy and Therapy in a high-field whole-body Magnetic-Resonance-Tomograph. Proc. Intl. Soc. Mag. Reson. Med. **8** (2000), 411
7. Chinzei K., Kikinis R., Jolesz F.A.: MR Compatibility of Mechatronic Devices: Design Criteria. Proc. of MICCAI'99, (1999) 1020–1031
8. Chinzei K., Hata N., Jolesz F.A., Kikinis R.: MR Compatible Surgical Assist Robot System Integration and Preliminary Feasibility Study. Proc. of MICCAI 2000 921–930
9. Griffith H.B., Veerapen R.: A direct transnasal approach to the sphenoid sinus. Technical note. J Neurosurgery **66** (1987) 140–142.

A Motion Adaptable Needle Placement Instrument Based on Tumor Specific Ultrasonic Image Segmentation

Jae-Sung Hong[1], Takeyoshi Dohi[2], Makoto Hasizume[3],
Kozo Konishi[3], and Nobuhiko Hata[2]

[1] Environmental Studies, Graduate School of Frontier Sciences,
The University of Tokyo, 7-3-1 Hongo, Bunkyo-ku, Tokyo 113-8654, Japan
hjsshep@atre.t.u-tokyo.ac.jp
[2] Mechano-informatics, Graduate School of Information Science and Technology,
The University of Tokyo, 7-3-1 Hongo, Bunkyo-ku, Tokyo 113-8654, Japan
{dohi@miki.pe,noby@atre.t}.u-tokyo.ac.jp
[3] Disaster and Emergency Medical, Graduate School of Medical Sciences,
Kyushu University, Maidashi 3-1-1, Higashi-ku, Fukuoka, 812-8582, Japan
{konizou@surg2,mhashi@dem}.med.kyushu-u.ac.jp

Abstract. This paper suggests an ultrasound guided needle insertion instrument which can track target motion in real-time. Under traditional ultrasound guided needle insertion therapies, surgeons have had much burden to find out the precise targeting position, particularly when the organ is moving due to the respiration or heartbeat. We developed a new needle insertion instrument which can track moving target based on visual servo control. In addition, this paper proposed a tumor specific active contour model which can conduct a fast and robust segmentation for tumor, and utilized Hough transform for needle recognition. In the experiment, the proposed system could track a moving phantom successfully at speed of 3 frames/sec processing.

1 Introduction

Interventional radiology (IR) has been widely accepted in that the therapy is performed with minimal invasiveness so that the period of hospital treatment is significantly reduced [1]. In IR therapy, percutaneous microwave coagulation therapy (PMCT) or percutaneous ethanol injection therapy (PEIT) is performed under ultrasonic image-guided environment without performing laparotomy [2]. However these type of operations require highly experienced techniques due to the limitation of visibility on the paths of needle insertion. This imposes a burden on the operator, thus leading to surgical complications such as a missing the target or inaccurate insertion which can cause hemorrhage.

Recently a number of researches on needle accessing instruments based on medical image processing were reported to be in process. Loser *et al.* proposed a prototypical robot for image-guided interventions optimized for usage inside

T. Dohi and R. Kikinis (Eds.): MICCAI 2002, LNCS 2488, pp. 122–129, 2002.
© Springer-Verlag Berlin Heidelberg 2002

a CT gantry [3]. Patriciu *et al.* proposed that the simple and precise targeting method under portable x-ray fluoroscopy [4], and the authors of this paper developed a manipulator to insert needle for brain tumor using CT images [5]. Nakamura *et al.* presented a surgical instrument which can track the motion of heartbeat. It can track the target in real-time based on efficient master-slave system, yet this work is performed under CCD camera, i.e. requiring abdominal operation [6].

Inspired by previous works [3–7] on visual-servoing in medical robotics, this paper introduces a novel method to drive a needle based on real-time ultrasonic image segmentation. The proposed method can compensate for a motion or unexpected trembling of the target caused by respiration or heartbeat and execute a reliable tumor specific segmentation on ultrasonic images to support real-time motion tracking. The image-guided visual servo configuration which is robust to calibration was utilized to achieve real-time tracking for the moving target, and by joining manipulator to ultrasound probe as one unit, eye in hand mechanical organization which is relatively stable to calibration was implemented. In the following sections, we will describe the details of tumor specific ultrasonic image segmentation method, and report about the tracking process with experimental results.

2   The Robot's Design

The proposed instrument comprises a five DOF passive arm which is to guide the manipulator to the desired position on the skin providing sufficient visibility and a two DOF active manipulator which is for the control of the access direction of the needle and the distance to the target. Currently we are processing in 2-D space on ultrasonic image. Although an approaching in 3-D space was considered, it turned out to be anatomically impossible because ultrasound probe has to be placed between the ribs in parallel for needle insertion inside liver in most cases. Therefore we assumed the movement of target can be observed on the 2-D image plane. For convenience, we would name the proposed instrument UMI which stands for Ultrasound guided Motion tracking Instrument in the rest part of this paper.

To describe the structure of UMI, the main feature of UMI is that the probe and needle are joined as one unit to be put on the same plane so that the needle position can be observed on the ultrasonic image always during insertion therapy, and this relationship is maintained in spite of any shock or alteration from outside. The needle was inserted by frictional power by motorized rollers of which structure enable the instrument to be made small-sized and the insertion length of needle to be freely adjustable. Inevitable slip of needle can be controlled according to visual feedback. The needle moves around describing imaginary circular arcs and the center of circle corresponds to the puncture point of patient's skin which is fixed as fulcrum of needle. This arc revolution is realized by moving along arc shape guide rail. The fixed guide rail assures the stillness of fulcrum so that the needle does not hurt around skin puncture point. This kind of phys-

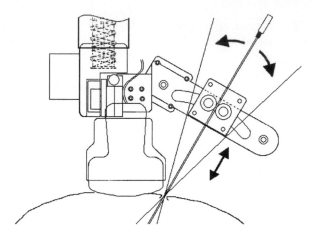

Fig. 1. The probe mounted instrument

ical guide rail often has demerits in burdensome size but UMI has one in small size because only ±15 degree give us enough space to move on high resolution ultrasonic images. Fig. 1 shows the front view of the proposed instrument UMI.

3   Real-Time Tracking Based on Visual Servo Control

The human body has inevitable internal movements due to respiration, heartbeat or unexpected patient action caused by needle insertion pain. Surgeons often perform needle insertion during the 15 seconds when the patient's respiration is stopped intentionally. Accordingly they have much burden to perform the precise insertion watching the ultrasonic image within a definite time limit, and this kind of therapy needs highly trained technique. UMI can assist the operator to perform accurately and without hastening based on image-guided tracking.

In robotic system, vision has been widely used due to its non-contact sensing and superior informative ability. In medical robotics, the visual servoing has been utilized in the field of minimally invasive surgery to control motion of a camera or medical instrument [8, 9]. In most cases, the calibration problem is cumbersome, which is even more difficult in the case of accessing a moving objective in the unstable human body. As compared to position-based image servoing, image-based visual servo control uses vision alone to stabilize the mechanism as shown in Fig. 2, therefore it is less sensitive to camera calibration [10]. In addition, the proposed manipulator uses the eye-in-hand configuration which has a constant relationship between the pose of the camera (probe) and that of the end-effector (needle)[11].

4   Image Segmentation for Region of Interest

In ultrasonic images, Regions of interest(ROIs) of our system are tumor and needle. The distance between tumor and needle, plus the status of collision be-

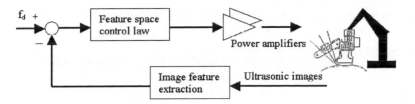

Fig. 2. Image-based visual servoing configuration

tween them are checked from image processing during the therapy. The specified techniques fit for ultrasonic images were utilized.

4.1   Target Recognition

The automatic segmentation of ultrasonic image is considerably difficult when using the traditional segmentation methods. Furthermore tumor is more vague than vessel because of its histology. The gradient operators such as sobel or canny detect only some parts of the tumor edge and extracts at once many undesirable edges irrelevant to the tumor.

Kass *et al.* presented the active contour model (snakes) which can yield a fully connected edge using not only image information but model's own feature [12]. The method defines energy function E_{snake} which consists of $E_{internal}$ and $E_{external}$. Given that there are N control points and (x_i, y_i) means the coordinate of the pixel of ith control point, active contour is expressed as follows,

$$E_{snakes} = \int_C E_{internal} + E_{external}\ ds \cong C(x_i, y_i, \ldots, x_N, y_N) + \sum_i^N G(x_i, y_i) \quad (1)$$

$C(x_i, y_i)$ denotes elastic energy and $G(x_i, y_i)$ means gradient of image in our system. Moving the contour to the direction to which the total energy decrease, the optimal contour is determined through the iteration process. This model is robust to the texture of image, so it was also employed as the edge detector for the CT or MRI images [13]. In addition because the contour is determined by control points, the contour can be altered easily by changing the position of the control points, that is, according to the processing for only the pixels around control points not the whole pixels in image plane or window, the edge moves and settles down at the final position. This operation is useful for real-time processing and the moving picture segmentation which needs reference to previous edge trail. However, active contour requires the designation of initial contour, and improper designation leads the contour astray or lengthens the time to search right path, therefore considerate inspection is required for initial contour setting.

We devised a method which can set an initial contour most closely to the final contour by using the partially extracted edge produced by a gradient operator and the anatomical prior knowledge. Unlike blood vessels, tumors have elliptical shapes in general [14]. Accordingly we presumed that the initial contour should be a circle that surrounds the tumor. The radius and coordinate of the center point of the circle can be calculated by referring to the partially extracted edge before, and a small intended enlargement of the calculated radius makes the fittest initial contour which encloses the tumor region. To extract partial, but connected edge of a tumor the edge following method [15] modified from the Delp's algorithm [16], was utilized. Fig. 3 shows the process of contour variation towards the optimal position. We can see the connected contour is extracted successfully which is virtually impossible by traditional edge detectors.

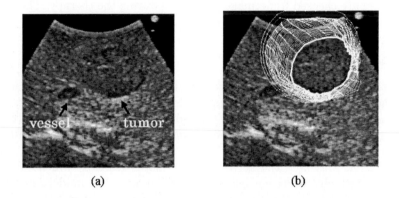

(a)   (b)

Fig. 3. Segmentation by Snakes. (a) Original image, (b) Approaching process for tumor contour

4.2   Needle Recognition

The needle equipped in UMI is a $20G$ PTC needle. It usually appears as a straight line on image, but there can be gaps in the line and also some line fragments of other objects irrelative to needle. Therefore, we first have to find out dominant line element on image which represents PTC needle, then locate the endpoint of needle referring to that line.

Hough transform [17] is useful in determination of line parameters such as slope and offset of line even though there are some gaps in line. According to the Hough transform, the pixels on the identical line in image gather into one point in transformed parameter space and the most concentrated point in parameter space is related to a dominant line in image plane which eventually stands for PTC needle. The gradient edge image is used as input for Hough transform. On the other hand in order to locate the endpoint of the needle, the previously acquired line is used as a guide line. Moving along the guide line the connection of edge is verified. When the unconnected point is detected we consider it as endpoint of needle. The small gaps less than a defined threshold are ignored during the check process. Fig. 4 shows the needle on ultrasonic image and the detected endpoint of the needle.

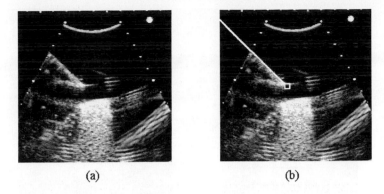

(a)   (b)

Fig. 4. Needle recognition using Hough transform, (a) original needle image, (b) detected endpoint of needle

5   Experiment

A tumor specific segmentation is tested with ultrasonic images taken under microwave coagulation therapy for liver cancer. On the other hand the tracking ability of the proposed instrument is tested using a phantom. A phantom made by spongy was used as a target. The PC used for image processing and visual servo control is equipped with a Pentium 3 processor, a frame grabber, and a motor control board. The software is programmed using C++ and Tcl/Tk language on a Linux platform. The ultrasound instrument used for this experiment is a 11MHz probe system. The phantom in a cistern was moved manually and the ultrasonic image was taken during the motion. The end-effector of the actuator was instructed to follow the center of the phantom in real-time. Fig. 5 shows the proposed instrument UMI.

6   Results and Discussion

The proposed algorithm could extract the connective contour of the tumor successfully as described previously while the traditional gradient operators in most cases fail to extract. The result images are presented in the previous chapter 4 (See the Fig. 3.) We can also see that the extracted contour is slightly different from the original tumor contour as expected because the computerized algorithm could not performed successfully at the place where the image is severely obscure.

In phantom test, UMI could process 3 frames per a second. Assuming target is moving with speed about 5cm/sec, the error distance between target and needle is about 1.7cm theoretically. We believe the error caused by time latency would decrease with the improvement of hardware such as use of Pentium 4 processor and software such as thread programming. In the future we will carry out an experiment with ultrasonic liver images using UMI and the results of which will be reported.

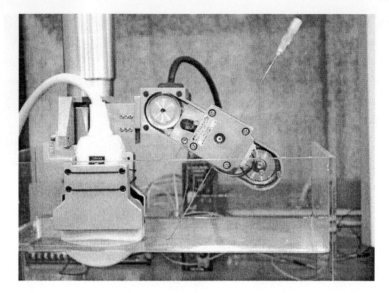

Fig. 5. UMI(Ultrasound guided Motion tracking Instrument)

7   Conclusion

This paper suggested an needle insertion instrument which can compensate the unpredictable motion of organs due to the patient respiration or sudden action during the therapy. The tumor specific active contour model based on anatomical knowledge was proposed to achieve the reliable and fast segmentation for relatively vague ultrasonic images. The proposed instrument used visual servo control to track the moving target in real-time, and it was designed as the probe mounted end-effector which ensures always the constant relationship between probe and needle on image. In the experiment, The fine contour for tumor was acquired and the tracking was accomplished for the moving phantom with a 3 frames/sec processing speed.

Acknowledgements

This work was supported by the Grant-in-Aid for Scientific Research (B13558103, A14702070) in Japan and NH was supported by Toyota Phsical & Chemical Research Institute, Suzuken Memorial Foundation, Kurata Grants.

References

1. M. Kudo : Percutaneous needle placement into hepatic tumors under ultrasound vascular image guidance. Journal of clinical surgery, Vol. 55. (2000) 1551–1555
2. M. Hiroda, T. Becpoo, S. Shimada, M. ogawa : Percutaneous ultrasound-guided microwave coagulation therapy for hepatic neoplasms. Journal of clinical surgery, Vol. 55. (2000) 1557–1560
3. M.H. Loser, N. Navab : A New Robotic System for visually Controlled Percutaneous Interventions under CT Fluoroscopy. MICCAI 2000, Lecture Notes in Computer Science, Vol. 1935. Springer-Verlag (2000) 887–896
4. A. Patriciu, D. Stoianovici, L.L. Whitcomb, T Jarrett, D. Mazilu, A. Stanimir, I. Iordachita, J. Anderson, R. Taylor, L.R. Kavoussi : Motion-Based Robotic Instrument Targeting Under C-Arm Fluoroscopy. MICCAI 2000, Lecture Notes in Computer Science, Vol. 1935. Springer-Verlag (2000) 988–998
5. T. Dohi, "Medical Imaging for Computer Aided Surgery : IEICE Trans. Inf. and Syst., Vol. J83-D-II. (2000) 27–33
6. Y. Nakamura, K. Kishi, H. Kawakami : Heartbeat Sysncronization for Robotic Cardiac Surgery. ICRA2001, IEEE International Conference on Robotics and Automation (2001) 2014–2019
7. S.E. Salcudean, G. Bell, S. Bachmann, et al. : Robot-assisted diagnostic ultrasound - design and feasibility experiments. Proc. MICCAI 1999, Lecture Notes in Computer Science, Vol.1679 (1999) 1062–1071
8. R. H. Taylor, J. Funda, B. Eldridge, D. Larose, M. Talamini, L. Kavoussi, J. Anderson : A telerobotic assistant for laparoscopic surgery. in Proc. Int. Conf. On Advanced Robots (1995) 33–36
9. G.Q. Wei, K. Arbter, G. Hirzinger : Real-Time Visual Servoing for Laparoscopic Surgery IEEE Eng. in Med. and Biol, Vol.16 (1997) 40–45
10. G.D. Hager, S. Hutchinson and P. Corke : A Tutorial on Visual Servo Control. IEEE Transactions on Robotics and Automation, Vol. 12 (1996) 651–670
11. R. Kelly, R. Carelli, O. Nasis, B. Kuchen, F. Reyes:Stable Visual Servoing of Camera-in-Hand Robotic Systems. IEEE Trans. Mechatoronics, Vol.5 (2000) 39–48
12. M. Kass, A.Witkin, and D. Terzopoulos : Snakes:Active Contour Models. Proceeding of First International Conference on Computer Vision (1987) 259–256
13. M. Mignotte, J.Meunier : A multiscale optimization approach for the dynamic contour-based boundary detection issue. Computerized Medical Imaging and Graphics, Vol 25. (2001) 265–275
14. J.S. Hong, T. Kaneko, R. Sekiguchi and K.H. Park : Automatic Liver Tumor Detection from CT. IEICE Trans. Inf. and Syst., Vol. E84-D. (2001) 741–748
15. C. Choi, S.M. Lee, N.C. Kim, and H. Son : Image segmentation and coding using edge tracing. J. KITE, Vol. 26. (1989) 105–112
16. E.J. Delp and C.H. Chu : Detecting edge segments. IEEE Trans. On Sys. Man and Cybern., Vol SMC-15 (1985) 144–152
17. Hough P.V.C. : A Method and Means for Recognizing Complex Patterns. U.S. Patent No. 3069654 (1962)

Experiment of Wireless Tele-echography System by Controlling Echographic Diagnosis Robot

Kohji Masuda, Norihiko Tateishi, Yasuyuki Suzuki,
Eizen Kimura, Ying Wie, and Ken Ishihara

Department of Medical Informatics, Ehime University Hospital,
Shigenobu-cho, Onsen-gun, Ehime 791-0295 Japan
masuda@vishnu.m.ehime-u.ac.jp
http://www.medinfo.m.ehime-u.ac.jp/

Abstract. We have developed a wireless tele-echography system for controlling an echographic diagnosis robot (EDR) that was developed in our laboratory. The examiner can control the robot at a distance from the patient and ob-
tains both an image of the patient's status and an echogram of the internal
organs. The locations of the examiner and the patient are connected by a wireless network. Remote control was realized by means of the Object Request
Broker technique. By this experiment, we have thus verified the usefulness of
our system for clinical practice. Remote diagnosis of an echogram with sufficient image quality was possible after a skilled examiner had become used to
controlling the robot. The adult patient never felt any discomfort or pain from
the robot. Since the maximum bandwidth required by this system was 1Mbps,
we have confirmed that wireless tele-echography can become a reality in telemedicine and telecare.

1 Introduction

We have developed an echographic diagnosis robot[1,2] to control an ultrasound
probe. The examiner captures echograms by placing the robot on the body surface of
a patient. The robot is designed to move the probe on the human abdomen in three
dimensions, has 6 degrees of freedom of movement, detects contact force on the body
and encompasses carefully considered safety measures. Although several groups have
previously developed mechanisms to handle an ultrasound probe, almost all of these
are of the manipulator type [3,4] and involve a large system [5]. In applying such manipulator robots to medical needs, position control is difficult to achieve when the
body motion of the patient has to be followed. Thus, we considered that the entire
mechanism for moving the ultrasound probe should be lightweight and be placed on
the body itself [6].

 We have already tried a preliminary experiment involving tele-echography via the
Internet and an ISDN network [1,2]. Just a few years ago, the bandwidth of a popular
ISDN network was mostly 128 kbps in Japan. Surprisingly, there has been rapid progress in line speed, and ADSL at 1Mbps became available to private users quite recently. Thus, we considered the feasibility of extending the tele-echography system
rather than adhering to line speed. In this paper, we describe a preliminary experiment

T. Dohi and R. Kikinis (Eds.): MICCAI 2002, LNCS 2488, pp. 130–137, 2002.

in wireless tele-echography involving the control of our echographic diagnosis robot in order to verify the possibility of clinical use.

2   Wireless Tele-echography System

2.1   Overview

Fig.1 shows the concept of our wireless tele-echography system. An examiner is located quite separate from the patient and controls the echographic diagnosis robot which has been placed on the abdomen of the patient. The ultrasound probe is held by the robot and it moves on the abdomen under the control of the examiner. The patient status images and echograms are transferred back to the examiner. The patient and examiner can communicate by seeing and talking to each other.

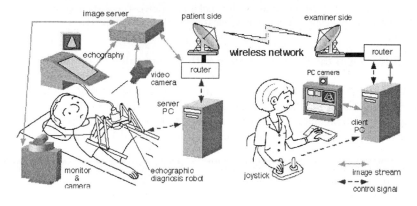

Fig. 1. Scheme of wireless tele-echography system

The most recent internet applications are moving towards wireless and mobile. Wireless network technology is very useful for telemedicine, especially in Ehime district, as there is no need to run wires and cables. Ehime prefecture includes both high mountains and isolated islands, which are typical Japanese geographical features. Although the present accessibility distance is several kilometers at most, international connection might be possible in the future. Wireless networks can be established quickly at low cost, which enables the possibility of setting up a temporary clinic in the case of a large-scale disaster.

We used two wireless LAN bridges SB-1100 (ICOM Co. Ltd.). One is included in the ordinary LAN in Ehime University which we usually use at 10Mbps. The other is used as a temporary network with a router and notebook PC in a temporary examination room located separately from Ehime University Hospital.

Fig. 2 shows the map of Shigenobu-cho(town) in Ehime prefecture, Japan. We selected a temporary examination room in the Twin Dome Shigenobu which is located 1.4 km from our hospital. There is no obstruction for wireless telegraphy between the Twin Dome and the hospital. In this experiment, we established the examiner site in the Twin Dome because the echographic diagnosis robot is complicated in wiring and power supply at present, and is difficult to remove from the hospital.

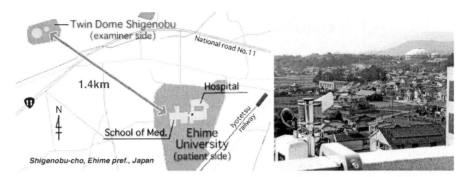

Fig. 2. Geographical situation. Map of Shigenobu-cho (left). The distant view of Twin Dome Shigenobu from Ehime University with wireless network antenna (right)

2.2   Situation at the Patient Location with Echographic Diagnosis Robot

Fig. 3 shows the situation at the patient site. The image streaming server (PCS-1600, Sony Co. Ltd.) is on the monitor beside the patient, as shown in Fig. 3 (a). It captures not only two patient status images from two video cameras, but also echograms captured by echography (EUB-565S, Hitachi Medical Co. Ltd.) and encodes this into the image stream. The examiner is able to switch among these images via the network.

The echographic diagnosis robot, which we have developed to realize 6 DOF motion of three-dimensional rotation and translation, moves according to the command from the examiner. Precise mechanism is shown in Fig. 3 (b). The echographic diagnosis robot is placed on the abdomen of the patient. Its total weight is 3.3 kg, which is insufficient for adults to feel heavy.

The robot consists of gimbal, pantograph and slide mechanisms. The gimbal mechanism tilts the probe by three independent motors. The probe is fixed in an acrylic resin column which has a brim where four miniature force sensors are located, to detect contact forces against the body surface as shown in Fig. 3 (c). The reason for using four sensors is as follows. Since a summation of output of four sensors reveals the total contact force on the body, the pantograph motion can be limited so that it will not push the body by strong force. Furthermore, the difference in output between two symmetrical sensors indicates the angle of the probe to the body surface. Thus, safety control is possible by computing the output of four sensors so that dangerous physical positions can be avoided [1].

Both the pantograph and the slide mechanisms effect translation of the probe on the abdomen. Parallel (x) and rectangular (y) translation of the probe are done by moving actuators located at the bottom of the pantograph. Two slide actuators are set on the abdomen to move the pantograph mechanism in the body axis direction. Each side of the slide effects linear motion by a linkage between two joints.

Since the bottom of the pantograph mechanism is put on the side of the abdomen, the arms of the pantograph never harm the patient's body. Fig. 3 (d) shows the geometry of the pantograph mechanism. Defining the positions of the slide actuators as

(0, 0) and $(d, 0)$ in rectangular coordinates and the intersection point of the gimbal axis as $P(x_p, y_p)$ shown in Fig. 3(d), while either of the angles of motors θ_1 and θ_2 do not exceed $\pi/2$, the coordinates of $P(x_p, y_p)$ can be expressed as follows.

$$x_p = \frac{a(\cos\theta_1 - \cos\theta_2) + d}{2} \tag{1}$$

$$y_p = a(\sin\theta_1 + \sin\theta_2)/2$$

$$-\frac{1}{2}\sqrt{4b^2 - (a-c)^2 + 2a(a-c)(\cos\theta_1 + \cos\theta_2) - 2a^2\{1 + \cos(\theta_1 + \theta_2)\}} \tag{2}$$

In these equations, a, b represent the arm lengths of the pantograph, c, the width of the gimbal and d, the distance between two slides, respectively.

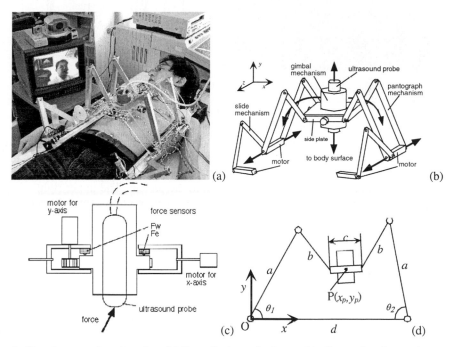

Fig. 3. Situation at patient location. (a) Overall view of echographic diagnosis robot on human abdomen. (b) Precise mechanism of the robot. (c) Cross-section of the gimbal mechanism. (d) Geometry of the pantograph mechanism

2.3   Situation at Examiner Location with Human Interface

Fig. 4 shows the scene at the examiner site. A skilled medical doctor controls the remote robot by a two-axis joystick (Compact analog stick, Hori Co. Ltd.). The control interface was designed for the examiner in the way of observing the patient from the direction of the feet. The method of control is shown to the right of Fig. 4. The angle of the right stick corresponds completely to the angle of the gimbal mechanism. Rotation of the probe axis is done by pushing two buttons with the right forefinger. The left stick is used for pantograph motion. After adjusting the initial position and gain, which depend on the body size of the patient, the angle of the left stick corresponds to the coordinates of the probe position $P(x_p, y_p)$. Slide motion in body axis is made by pushing two buttons with the left forefinger.

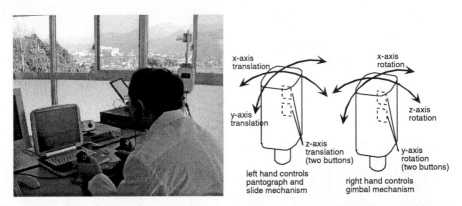

Fig. 4. Situation at examiner location. The examiner controls the remote robot by two-axis joystick while observing the patient status on a PC monitor. Ehime University Hospital can be seen out of the window (left). Method of controlling the robot by the joystick (right)

The examiner inspects the echogram and the patient status image simultaneously on the PC monitor, as shown in Fig. 5. The upper right window is the echogram, the upper middle is a robot image to confirm the position of the probe, and at the upper left is the examiner's own image which is sent to the patient. The upper right window can be changed regarding input source. The lower window is for input selection and the control of camera angle. Voice communication between the examiner and the patient is also possible.

2.4   Object Request Broker

To control the robot via a network, we applied the HORB [7] technique, which is derived from ORB (Object Request Broker) technique in distributed object systems. HORB satisfies higher speed transfer and better facility of development compared to CORBA [8]. We developed the software under the C++ and Java platforms [9].

3   Results of Experiment

We prepared to conduct the experiment over two days in February. The first day was rainy and it snowed intermittently. The next day was very fine. On both days, the line speed was sufficient to enable communication at up to 6Mbps bandwidth, confirming that the weather was not important for wireless communication. The robot followed the command from the examiner and touched closely on the surface of abdomen. We adopted ITU T.120 standard data protocols with ITU G.728 standard voice compression, which enabled high quality conference conditions with real-time moving echogram. The time delay was less than 1 sec when image size was CIF 352 x 288 pixels for the echogram at 512Kbps and QCIF 176 x 144 pixels for the patient status image at 100-200Kbps. This was much more comfortable than our previous experiment [1,2] where we used motion-JPEG encoding and the time delay was 4-5 sec, which was very stressful.

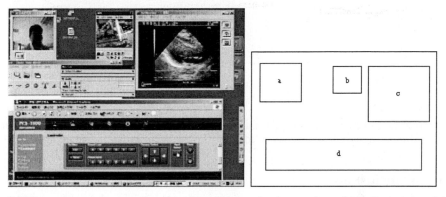

Fig. 5. PC monitor at the examiner location. (a) examiner's own face, (b) patient status, (c) echogram and (d) video camera control with input selection. The examiner's facial image is transferred to the patient location. Two kinds of patient status image and the echogram can be switched as desired by the examiner

The examiner got used to operating the controls after a few minutes of practice. The quality of the echogram was sufficient for diagnosis. Communication with the patient was as easily achieved as good-quality telephone link. When observing the heart, the examiner had no difficulty in instructing the patient to stop breathing and to resume.

The adult patient did not feel any discomfort after the robot had been put on the abdomen, and even after an experiment lasting more than one hour. Only the slide part touched to the body (after adjusting the width of the slide according to the body size). However, we do not know whether this design would be for a pregnant woman or an infant. Thus, for clinical use, several different types of robot construction should be prepared to suit different patients.

Before the experiment, we thought that one patient image would be enough on the examiner's monitor because the examiner can switch between echogram and patient status images as desired. However, if the examiner observed the echogram alone, the direction of ultrasound probe on the body surface became confused. To avoid stress, at least two kinds of image are necessary on the PC monitor at the same time.

Fig. 6 shows the variation in packet number and bit rate which passed through the wireless LAN bridge during the experiment. The horizontal line expresses time during the experiment. Coloured areas express packet number of image stream and control signal, respectively, which are designated on the left axis. The solid line expresses total bit rate, which is designated on the right axis. Total bit rate was at most 1Mbps, so that this system can be accepted into the infrastructure of recent fast digital networks.

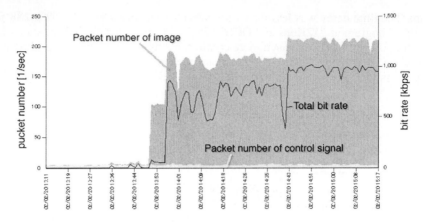

Fig. 6. Time variation of packet number and bit rate during the experiment. Total bit rate was at most 1Mbps, so that this system can be adopted using an ordinary fast digital network

4   Conclusions

We have experimented with a wireless tele-echography system to control our echographic diagnosis robot. The examiner could obtain an echogram of a patient at a remote location by control involving a two-axis joystick without any discomfort. The robot never subjected the patient to danger. We have thus confirmed the applicability of tele-echography to telemedicine. This system could be used for remote patients who are living in villages lacking appropriate medical care, or isolated islands far from a main hospital. Japan especially has many mountain areas and small islands, so that demand for telemedicine and telecare is high. Although this system required an assistant on the remote side to place the robot in position, we aim to develop a new system where no personnel are involved. We envisage that this system would be applicable to diagnosis in an emergency situation involving an ambulance or a helicopter, in order to gain time during critical patient transport. Since the advent of satellite systems, international telemedicine and telecare is no longer a dream. We trust that our system will be an effective demonstration of the importance of robotic telemedicine and telecare.

Acknowledgements

We wish to thank to third grade students of Ehime University, Mr. Sohei Takamori and Miss Toshiko Hidaka who assisted with this experiment. Part of this research was supported by Nakatani Electronic Measuring Technology Association, Japan.

References

1. K.Masuda, E.Kimura, N.Tateishi and K.Ishihara: "Three Dimensional Motion Mechanism of Ultrasound Probe and its Application for Tele-echography System," Proc. of International Conference of the IEEE Intelligent Robots and Systems (IROS), 2001, Maui, pp.1112-1116

2. K.Masuda, E.Kimura, N.Tateishi and K.Ishihara: "Construction of 3D Movable Echographic Diagnosis Robot and Remote Diagnosis via Fast Digital Network," Proc. of 23rd Annual International Conference of the IEEE Engineering in Medicine and Biology Society (EMBS), 2001, Istanbul, CD-ROM
3. P.Abolmaesumi, S.E.Salcudean, W.H.Zhu, S.P.DiMaio and M.R.Sirouspour: "A User Interface for Robot-Assisted Diagnostic Ultrasound," Proc. of IEEE Int'l Conf. on Robotics and Automation, pp.1549-1554, 2001, Seoul, CD-ROM
4. R.P.Goldberg, M.Dumitru, R.H.Taylor and D.Stoianovici: "A Modular Robotic System for Ultrasound Image Acquisition," Proc. of Medical Image Computing and Computer-Assisted Intervention (MICCAI), 2001, Utrecht, pp.1430-1432
5. M.Mitsuishi, S.Warisawa, T.Tsuda, T.Higuchi, N.Koizumi, et al.: "Remote Ultrasound Diagnostic System," Proc. of IEEE Int'l Conf. on Robotics and Automation, pp.1567-1574, 2001, Seoul, CD-ROM
6. A.V.Gonzales, P.Cinquin, J.Troccaz, A.Guerraz, B.Hennion, et al.:"TER: A System for Robotic Tele-Echography," Proc of Medical Image Computing and Computer-Assisted Intervention (MICCAI), 2001, Utrecht, pp.326-334
7. HORB http://horb.etl.go.jp/horb
8. S.Hirano, Y.Yasu, and H.Igarashi: "Performance Evaluation of Popular Distributed Object Technologies for Java," Proc. of ACM 1998 Workshop on Java for High-performance Network Computing, 1998
9. E.Kimura, K.Matsubara, K.Masuda, N.Tateishi and K.Ishihara: "Remote fetal cardiotocograph watching system with mobile telephone," Proc. of 10th World Congress on Medical Informatics, 2001, London, CD-ROM

Experiments with the TER Tele-echography Robot

Adriana Vilchis[1], Jocelyne Troccaz[1], Philippe Cinquin[1], Agnes Guerraz[2],
Franck Pellisier[2], Pierre Thorel[2], Bertrand Tondu[3], Fabien Courrèges[4],
Gérard Poisson[4], Marc Althuser[5], and Jean-Marc Ayoubi[5]

[1] TIMC/IMAG laboratory, Domaine de la Merci, F-38706 La Tronche cedex - France
{adriana.vilchis,jocelyne.troccaz}@imag.fr
[2] France Telecom R&D
[3] INSA Toulouse
[4] LVR Bourges
[5] CHU Grenoble

Abstract. This paper presents a master-slave system applied to the remote diagnosis from echographic data. The motion of the master manipulator is remotely controlled by a physician and reproduced by a slave robot carrying the echographic probe. The contact force between the probe and the patient is fed back to operator allowing him to have a haptic virtual environment. The innovation of this haptic control is to preserve medical expert proprioception and gesture feelings, which are necessary to synchronize the ultrasound images with the motion made by the medical doctor. The slave robot is a cable-driven manipulator using pneumatic artificial muscle actuators to control the motion of the ultrasound probe. In this paper we present the architecture and the performances of the slave robot and the first experiments of the master-slave remote echography system for examinations of pregnant women.

1   Introduction

Among many types of medical equipment, ultrasound diagnostic systems are widely used because of their convenience and innocuously. Performing an ultrasound examination involves good hand-eye coordination and the ability to integrate the acquired information over time and space; the physician has to be able to mentally build 3D information from both the 2D images and the gesture information and to put a diagnosis from this information. Some of these specialized skills may lack in some healthcare centers or for emergency situations. Tele-consultation is therefore an interesting alternative to conventional care. Development of a high performance remote diagnostic system, which enables an expert operator at the hospital to examine a patient at home, in an emergency vehicle or in a remote clinic, may have a very significant added value.

Some previous tele-echography and robot-based echography systems have been developed [1-8]. Some of these approaches are purely tele-medicine projects (see [5] for example). A second class of systems allows to automate an echographic examination using a robot [3,4]. Finally, a last category of robot-based systems enables the remote examination of patients by a distant expert with [3,6] or without [2, 8] force feedback. Many of the robot-based systems integrate conventional robot architectures

T. Dohi and R. Kikinis (Eds.): MICCAI 2002, LNCS 2488, pp. 138–146, 2002.
© Springer-Verlag Berlin Heidelberg 2002

and actuation. One objective of this research was to propose a new architecture of low weight, compliant and portable medical robots.

2   Overview of the TER System

2.1   Description of the TER System

The tele-operated TER system allows the expert physician to move by hand a virtual probe in a natural and unconstrained way and safely reproduces this motion on the distant robotic site where the patient is. For a global description of the TER project see [9]. Figure 1.a shows a schematic diagram of the TER system. The physician located in the master site moves the virtual probe placed on a haptic device to control the real echographic probe placed on the slave robot. The haptic control station in the master site is developed to give a realistic environment of what remotely occurs [10]. It integrates a PHANToM device (from SensAble Device Inc) which has 6 degrees of freedom (dof) and renders 3D-force information. Position and orientation tracking of the virtual probe is performed within a workspace of 16cmx13cmx13cm and with maximum a force of 6.4N. Real time force feedback information and a virtual geometric model of the patient (see [11]) are rendered to the expert operator. The obtained ultrasound image is continuously sent from the slave site to the operator that has to perform the examination and to provide a diagnosis. The precise position of the ultrasound probe is provided by an optical localizer and is sent to the master site where the position is represented as a visual information. A non-expert operator is located close to the patient and supervises the procedure that he can interrupt in an emergency case. The patient can at all times communicate with the operator or with the expert. Two IDSN 128kb/s connections are used; one is for the Visio-phonic data and echographic images and the other one is for the transmission of the control information for the slave-robot.

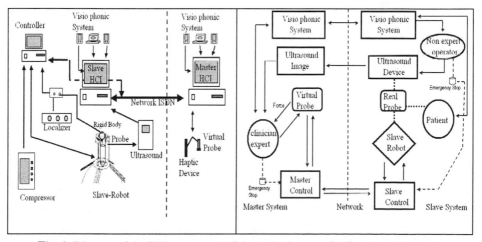

Fig. 1. Diagram of the TER system. (a) Schematic diagram. (b) Functional diagram

2.2   Procedure of Tele-echographic Robotic Examination

The procedure of the tele-echographic robotic examination is performed in three phases: initialization, echographic examination and end of the session. Table 1 shows the steps of a typical procedure with the TER system and figure 1.b gives its functional diagram. Medical experts who tested the system followed this procedure.

Table 1. Procedure of examination of TER system

Master site	Slave site
	- Position of the slave robot relatively to the patient body
	- Gel application
- Initialization of:	- Initialization of:
• Virtual Probe parameters	• Robot parameters
• Communication parameters	• Communication parameters
• Visio phonic parameters	• Visio phonic parameters
• Haptic Environment	• Initial Position of Robot
- Establishing communications	- Waiting for communications
- Examination (continuous loop until end of session):	- Examination (continuous loop until end of session):
• Motion of the Virtual Probe	• Motion of the slave robot
• Analysis of ultrasound images	• Sending ultrasound images
• Ask for the tuning of image parameters of the echographic system	• Tuning of image acquisition parameters by the non expert operator
• Communication with the patient or with the non expert operator	• Communication with the medical expert
- End of session:	- End of session:
• Disconnection with the slave robot	• Disconnection with the master haptic environment
	• Take the slave robot away from the patient's body
• Final discussion with the patient and with the non expert assistant	• Final discussion with the medical doctor
• Close the Visio phonic session	• Close the Visio phonic session

2.3   Analysis of the Echographic Probe Motions

To determine the motion and force range of the remote echography system, the executed motions and applied forces of a real echographic probe were analyzed while a physician was examining a patient with a conventional procedure. The observed motions and gestures zones were used to define the working surface used during the examination by the physician. In the application to the diagnosis of pregnant women, this surface depends on the stage of pregnancy. As the pregnancy evolves the working surface becomes larger and rounder. This surface is taken into account at the beginning of the examination.

The condition of permanent contact of the echographic probe with the patient's body must be satisfied at each moment to allow the formation of images. The measurements of the effort variation on the abdomen during the examination using a dynamometer are of three types: minimal pressures from 0.6 to 0.7dN, standard pressures from 0.8 to 1.1dN and maximum pressures from 1.3 to 1.5dN. These measurements determine a range of authorized efforts, which have to be considered for remote examination.

3   Ultrasound Slave-Robot Design

3.1   Slave Robot Mechanical Architecture

The robot architecture is rather different from classical existing ones. The application simulation (a), the translation component of the slave robot prototype (b) and a close up of the orientation component of our current slave robot prototype attached to an abdomen phantom (c) are pictured in figure 2. The slave robot is a parallel uncoupled one. It includes two independent parallel structures having two independent groups of pneumatic artificial muscle actuators (McKibben artificial muscles) [12]. Thin and flexible cables are used to position and orient the echographic probe. The cables are connected to the pneumatic artificial muscles.

The artificial muscle is made of a thin rubber tube covered with a shell braided according to helical weaving. The muscle is closed by two ends, one being the air input and the other the force attachment point. When the inner tube is pressurized to a given pressure, the textile shell converts circumferential pressure force into axial contraction force, which reduces the muscle length while its radius increases. This means of actuation is simple, lightweight and has the added benefit of passive compliance. Moreover compressed air sources can be very easily found in the clinical environment.

The translation movements are controlled by four identical antagonistic artificial muscles connected by cables to a metal ring supporting the second parallel structure (see figure 2.b). The second parallel structure enables 3D orientation and translation along the Z axis of the echographic probe (see figure 2.c). It is actuated by four artificial muscles: three of them are identical and they control two of the three orientations and the translation. The fourth muscle controls the rotation of the ultrasound around its vertical axis. Both subsystems can be controlled simultaneously.

4   Experimental Results

4.1   Performances of the Slave Robot

Several control modes [13] can be used for such a robot: closed-loop pressure control, open-loop position control, closed-loop position control and hybrid position/force control. The results presented in this work correspond to the position open-loop control (see picture 3).

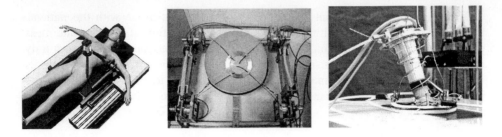

Fig. 2. Slave Robot. (a) Conception Design. (b) Translation Robot. (c) Orientation Robot

The data set of points (P_d) generated by the motion of the virtual probe held by the expert are sent every 500ms to the robot controller which converts this information to cable lengths (q^d) using an inverse model of the robot. These lengths are turned to pressure joint values (Pi) to be sent to the muscles. PIDA and PID regulators were respectively implemented for the closed-loop joint control of the translation and orientation structures of the robot [14]. As compared to a conventional robot, using only an open-loop position control is compensated here by the fact that the operator closes the loop from the image interpretation. However, the model allowing to compute cable lengths from Cartesian orders is not very precise because the working surface is a free-form surface and is not modeled perfectly for each patient.

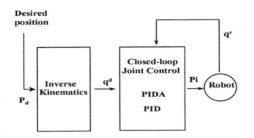

Fig. 3. Position Open-loop Control

The muscles have an intrinsic response time of 340ms due to friction and inertial effects. Figure 4 shows the joint errors for both structures of the slave robot for a single position. The error between 0 and 400ms in the figure 4 corresponds to the error resulting fromr the previous position. In figure 4.a we can see that the joint errors for the translation joints converge to zero after 600ms, which represents a good response time. Figure 4.b shows that the orientation joint errors correctly converge to zero after 1000ms.

Figure 5 shows the position error during a tracking task. The desired "trajectories" are a circle and a straight line that are defined by a sequence of points on the working surface. The robot does not perform a perfect tracking of the trajectory. The behavior in the lower part of figure 5.a can be explained by the imprecision with the two channels of the input board that read the values of the encoders associated with this part of the robot. In the example, the distance of the initial point to the trajectory also contributes to a tracking error since a new order is sent before the previous position is reached. Finally, the error is also due to the fact that the control is independent for each muscle. It could be reduced with a controller providing global and asymptotic error convergence for the closed-loop control. In Figure 5 we can see that the robot is more precisely in the straight-line trajectory that in the circle trajectory.

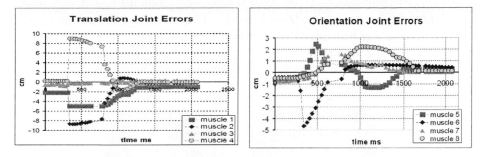

Fig. 4. Joints Errors. (a) Translation Joint Errors. (b) Orientation Joints Errors

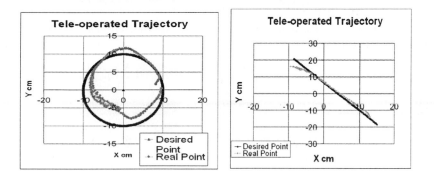

Fig. 5. Trajectory Errors. a) Circle Trajectory. b) Straight Line Trajectory

4.2 Tele-operation Experiments

After the integration of the system TER last january, some experiments have been performed using an echographic phantom (see figure 6.a) and one experiment in a voluntary patient. The objective of the test with the echographic phantom consisted in identifying the internal structures and in following them like in a real examination. The phantom was unknown to the medical experts. The objectives of the test performed with in a voluntary person belonging to the TER consortium patient consisted in identifying the internal organs and validating the ability of the robot TER to move on an unknown surface.

Three physicians (two obstetric gynecologists and one radiologist, all three being expert in echographic examinations) have carried out the examination with the echographic phantom and only one of the physicians has carried out the examination with the voluntary person. The medical experts handle the virtual probe fixed to the haptic system from the haptic information and from what that they see in the transmitted echographic images. Trajectory motions performed by the virtual probe are converted in a sequence of points, which are sent every 500ms to the slave site. The system converts these points into joint values for the slave robot. The master and slave sites where about 10 kilometers distant. After experimenting with the system each physicians had to fill a questionnaire. The general appreciation of the system is good. The experiment time was between 45 minutes and 60 minutes approximately. Figure 6.b shows one of the echographic images seen by the experts during the experiments. Figure 7 presents different steps of experiment with the echographic phantom and figure 8 presents the experiment with a volunter.

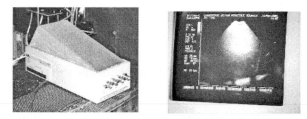

Fig. 6. (a) Echographic phantom used by the first experiments, (b) Echographic image of the internal structures of the phantom

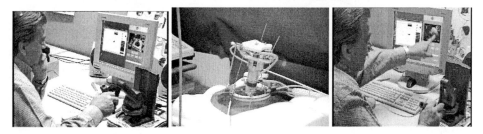

Fig. 7. (a) Doctor and haptic device (Master site), (b) Slave Robot on a medical phantom, (c) Doctor recognizing internal structures

5   Conclusion

In this paper, an original slave robot architecture was described and preliminary experiments with the TER system were presented. The system enables a medical expert to perform in real time, via ISDN communication links, an echographic examination on a patient remotely located. The first experiments realized with the TER system are very promising.

The TER system was developed for the realization of pregnancy echographic examination but the system can naturally be used for other types of echographic examination like heart, abdomen and others.

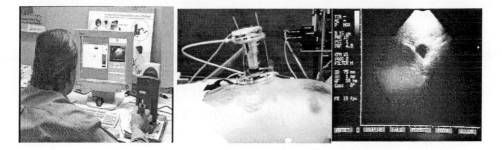

Fig. 8. (a) Doctor and the haptic device (Master site), (b) Slave Robot on voluntary patient, (c) Ultrasound Image seen by the doctor

Experiments demonstrated that the use of the TER system is very intuitive; there is a short adaptation time of 5 to 10 minutes necessary to the medical expert to feel comfortable with moving the virtual probe using the haptic device. The quality of images and robot controllability are considered as good. The medical experts were able to recognize the internal structures of the echographic phantom and to follow them. The position errors of the slave robot are not very important for the medical expert because he controls the probe motion in function of what he sees in the echographic image -internal structures- rather than in function of the position of the real probe.

Next developments will consist in experimenting other control schemes, in particular hybrid position/force control which should allow to keep a more constant contact force with the body of the patient. In parallel, clinical validation will be performed on a larger number voluntary persons and on patients.

Acknowledgments

This project is supported by the French Ministry of Research and Technology (action line "ACI Telemédecine"), by France Telecom R&D and by UAEM Mexico. We thank the clinicians, Dr Marc Althuser, Dr Jean Marc Ayoubi and M. Schneidern for testing the system. We also thanks PRAXIM, SINTERS, LVR and Pr Arbeille for their significant contribution to the project; and Dr. Kohji Masuda for lending us his vascular echographic phantom.

References

1. De Cunha, D., P. Gravez, C. Leroy, E. Maillard, J. Jouan, P. Varley, M. Jones, M. Halliwell, D. Hawkes, P.N.T. Wells and L. Angelini (1998). The midstep system for ultrasound guided remote telesurgery. *20th Annual International Conference of the IEEE Engineering in Medicine and Biology Society.* Vol. 20. pp. 1266-1269.

2. Gourdon, Ph. Poignet, G. Poisson, Y. Parmantier and P. Marché (1999)). Master-slave robotic system for ultrasound scanning. *European Medical and Biological Engineering Conference*. Vol. II. pp. 1116-1117.

3. S. Salcudean, G. Bell, S. Bachmann, W.H. Zhu, P Abolmaesumi and P.D. Lawrence (1999). Robot-assisted diagnostic ultrasound-design and feasibility experiments. *Lecture Notes in Computer Science. Medical Image Computing and Computer-Assisted Intervention* (MICCAI'99). pp. 1062-1071.

4. F. Pierrot, E. Dombre, E. Dégoulange, L. Urbain, P. Caron, S. Boudet, J. Gariépy and JL. Mégnien (1999). Hippocrate : a safe robot arm for medical applications with force feedback. *Medical Image Analysis*, Vol 3, pp 285-300.

5. on line http://www.crcg.edu/projects/teleinvivo.html.

6. M. Mitsuishi, S. Warisawa, T. Tsuda, T. Higuchi, N. Koizumi, H. Hashizume and K. Fujiwara. Remote Ultrasound Diagnostic System. *Proceedings of the IEEE International conference on Robotics & Automation*, Seoul, Korea May 21-26 2001, pp 1567-1574.

7. R. P. Goldberg, M Dumitru, R. H. Taylor and D. Stoianovici. A Modular Robotic System for Ultrasound Image Acquisition. *Fourth International Conference on Medical Image Computing and Computer Assisted Intervention,* Utrecht, the Netherlands 14-17 October 2001, pp 1430-1432.

8. K. Masuda, E. Kimura, N. Tateishi and K. Ishihara. Three dimensional motion mechanism of ultrasound probe and its application for tele-echography system. *Proceedings of the IEEE/RSJ International Conference on Intelligent Robots and Systems*. Maui, Hawaii, USA, Oct 29-Nov 03 2001. pp 1112-1116.

9. Vilchis, P. Cinquin, J. Troccaz, A. Guerraz, B. Hennion, Franck Pellisier, Pierre Thorel, F. Courreges, Alain Gourdon, G. Poisson, Pierre Vieyres, Pierre Caron, Olivier Mérigeaux, Loïc Urbain, Cédric Daimo, Stéphan Lavallée, Philippe Arbeille, Marc Althuser, Jean Marc Ayoubi, B. Tondu and Serge Ippolito, "TER: a system for Robotic Tele-echography". *Fourth International Conference on Medical Image Computing and Computer Assisted Intervention,* Utrecht, the Netherlands 14-17 October 2001, pp 326-334.

10. Guerraz, A. Vilchis, J. Troccaz, P. Cinquin, B. Hennion, Franck Pellisier and Pierre Thorel, "A Haptic Virtual Environment for tele-Echography". *10th Annual Medicine Meets Virtual Reality Conference*, Newport California January 23-26 2002.

11. Guerraz, B.Hennion, P. Thorel, F. Pellissier, A. Vienne and I. Belghit, "A haptic command station for remote ultrasound examinations", *Tenth Annual Symposium on Haptic Interfaces for Virtual Environment and Teleoperator Systems*, Orlando, FL, on March 24-25, 2002 in conjunction with the IEEE Virtual Reality 2002 Conference

12. Tondu and P. Lopez, "Modeling and control of Mckibben artificial muscle robot actuators", *IEEE Control Systems Magazine*, vol. 20, no. 2 pp 15-38, 2000.

13. Vlchis, J. Troccaz, P. Cinquin, F. Courrèges, G. Poisson and B. Tondu, "Robotic Tele-Ultrasound System (TER): Slave Robot Control", *1st IFAC Conference on Telematics Application in Automation and Robotics,* Weingarten, Alemania 24-26 2001, pp 95-100.

14. F. Courreges, G. Poisson, P. Vieyres, A. Vilchis, J. Troccaz and P. Cinquin, "Low level control of antagonist artificial pneumatic muscles for a tele-operated ultrasound robot: TER". *12th International Symposium on Measurement and Control in Robotics,* (Bourges June 20-22 2002).

The Effect of Visual and Haptic Feedback on Manual and Teleoperated Needle Insertion

Oleg Gerovichev[1,3], Panadda Marayong[2], and Allison M. Okamura[2,3]

[1] Department of Biomedical Engineering
[2] Department of Mechanical Engineering
[3] Engineering Research Center for Computer-Integrated Surgical Systems and Technology
Johns Hopkins University, Baltimore, MD
{oleg,panadda,aokamura}@jhu.edu

Abstract. In this paper, we present a study that evaluates the effect of visual and haptic feedbacks and their relevance to human performance in a needle insertion task. A virtual needle insertion simulator with a four-layer tissue model (skin, fat, muscle, and bone) and haptic feedback is used for perceptual experiments. The task was to detect the puncture of a particular layer using haptic and visual cues provided by the simulation. The results show that the addition of force feedback reduces error in detection of transitions between tissue layers by at least 55%. The addition of real-time visual feedback (image overlay) improved user performance by at least 87% in scenarios without force feedback. Presentation of both force and visual feedback improved performance by at least 43% in comparison to scenarios without feedback. These results suggest that real-time image overlay provides greater improvement in performance than force feedback.

1 Introduction

Current medical practice relies heavily on the manual dexterity of medical personnel. Cardiac bypass surgery, microsurgery, and percutaneous needle therapy are several examples of procedures where human abilities are exercised to the maximum. In addition, the target area is often occluded, particularly in percutaneous therapy. Robotic and imaging technologies have become important aids to assist medical personnel in these tasks. Fichtinger, *et al.* identify a need for increased precision in aiming and delivery of needles in nerve block and facet joint injection procedures, and propose robot-assisted mechanisms with CT guidance to alleviate the problem [4]. Chinzei, *et al.* suggest a surgical assist robot to be used with intraoperative MRI, which offers exceptional soft tissue discrimination, for instrument insertion in procedures like prostate tumor biopsy [2]. Masamune, *et al.* present a needle insertion system for use with MRI-guided neurosurgery [8]. There are also skill-enhancing systems, not targeted specifically at needle insertion tasks, such as the da Vinci™ Surgical System (Intuitive Surgical Inc., Mountain View, CA) and the ZEUS® Surgical Robotic System (Computer Motion, Inc., Goleta, CA). These robot-assisted surgical systems offer a novel approach to dexterous manipulation of surgical instruments for minimally invasive surgery. However, the systems above do not address the use of force feedback, which could improve performance of the surgeon.

T. Dohi and R. Kikinis (Eds.): MICCAI 2002, LNCS 2488, pp. 147–154, 2002.
© Springer-Verlag Berlin Heidelberg 2002

While visual information is used whenever possible, clinicians traditionally rely on manual force feedback in visually obscured areas. In this paper, we assess the value of visual and force feedback for improving medical tasks, specifically needle insertion. To our knowledge, no similar studies have been performed in the past, although Kontarinis and Howe [6] performed an experiment in which the user was asked to penetrate a thin membrane with a needle held by a slave manipulator while being given combinations of visual (manipulator exposed/hidden), filtered force, and vibratory feedback at the master manipulator. The result was that a combination of force feedback and vibration reduces reaction time in comparison to visually guided approach in puncture tasks. In addition, there are several needle insertion simulators that used the PHANToM™ haptic interface (SensAble Technologies, Inc., Woburn, MA) to provide 3-DOF force feedback, but no studies validated an improvement in subject performance [3, 7, 9]. In typical approaches, force models have been created from lumbar needle insertion procedure analysis and programmed into a virtual environment. Another approach used force data acquired during *ex vivo* needle insertions into a porcine specimen to create the force model [1]. A third approach used materials modeling of mechanical tissue properties and MRI imaging for layer anatomy determination [5].

We propose a needle insertion simulation that would assess the advantages of enhanced feedback to the user to improve performance in dexterous tasks. For the purpose of testing human abilities, we created a multi-layer tissue model that provides an illusion of puncture upon needle insertion. The Impulse Engine 2000 (IE2000™) (Immersion Corp., San Jose, CA) is a 2-DOF haptic interface that has sufficient capability to perform the task proposed.

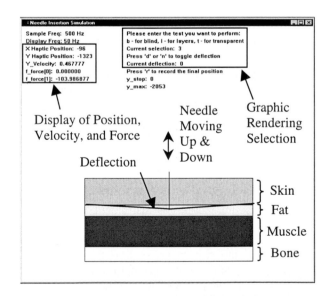

Fig. 1. Needle Insertion Simulation GUI showing layer deflection for visual feedback

2   System Design

2.1   Haptic Hardware and Software

The system uses one degree-of-freedom of the IE2000™. The simulation was created with Microsoft Visual C++ 6.0 and IE2000™ SDK 4.2 on a Pentium III-based system with a Windows NT operating system. The servo loop ran at 500 Hz. The graphics were updated at 50 Hz. The simulation provides the user with different graphical and haptic rendering of multi-layered tissues composed of skin, fat, muscle, and bone layers. We recorded position, velocity and force information during task execution. A screenshot of GUI is shown in Figure 1.

2.2   Force Model

Force feedback to the user was based on stiffness force before puncture and damping force during needle translation through the tissue layers. As the needle penetrates deeper into the layers, the user feels the total damping force accumulated from the above tissue layers. Each tissue has different stiffness and damping coefficients, as shown in Table 1. Nominal stiffness coefficients were assigned to reflect differences in tissue densities, and nominal damping coefficients were assigned to reflect the friction between the tissue and the needle shaft. We considered the bone as a solid structure that has a very high stiffness and no viscosity. We implemented the following force model:

Skin:	Upon puncture =>	$F = k_s y$	(1)
	After puncture =>	$F = b_s y\,v$	(2)
Fat:	Upon puncture =>	$F = k_f y + b_s y_s v$	(3)
	After puncture =>	$F = (b_s y_s + b_f y)v$	(4)
Muscle:	Upon puncture =>	$F = k_m y + (b_s y_s + b_f y_f)v$	(5)
	After puncture =>	$F = (b_s y_s + b_f y_f + b_m y)v$	(6)
Bone:	Upon puncture =>	$F = k_b y + (b_s y_s + b_f y_f + b_m y_m)v$	(7)

where k_s, k_f, k_m, and k_b are stiffness coefficients of skin, fat, muscle, and bone, respectively; b_s, b_f, and b_m are damping coefficients per unit thickness of skin, fat, and muscle, respectively; y_s, y_f, and y_m are thicknesses of each layer; y is the amount of needle penetration with respect to the current layer boundary; and v is needle velocity.

Table 1. Simulation Parameters

Tissue Type	Stiffness Coefficient (k), N/m	Damping Coefficient per unit length (b), N·s/m^2
Skin	331	3
Fat	83	1
Muscle	497	3
Bone	2483	0

Table 2. Test Conditions (L = Layers, N = Needle, D = Deflection, F = Force)

Test	Simulation	L	N	D	F
1	Real-time image overlay and needle tracking for tele-insertion	X	X	X	
2	Real-time needle tracking for tele-insertion with force feedback and pre-op image overlay (or manual insertion)	X	X		X
3	Real-time image overlay and needle tracking for tele-insertion with force feedback (or manual insertion)	X	X	X	X
4	Insertion based on anatomical knowledge with preoperative image overlay	X			
5	Tele-insertion based on anatomical knowledge with real-time image overlay	X		X	
6	Tele-insertion based on anatomical knowledge with pre-op image overlay and force feedback (or manual insertion)	X			X
7	Tele-insertion based on anatomical knowledge with real-time image overlay and force feedback (or manual insertion)	X		X	X
8	Tele-insertion based on anatomical knowledge with force feed-back				X
9	Manual insertion in inaccessible area with poor/no visibility				X

3   Experimental Procedure

Perceptual experiments were conducted with 10 volunteer subjects aged 21-31, 8 of them male and 2 female (Group I). On average, the subjects had medium exposure to haptic interfaces and virtual environments in the past and low exposure to real needle insertion. We also conducted experiments with 4 volunteer male subjects aged 26-40 that had extensive experience with real needle insertion through medical training or research, but no experience with haptic devices (Group II). We presented a training simulation to the subjects in the beginning of the experiment to get them familiar with the mechanics of IE2000^{TM}, introduce different insertion scenarios and allow them to find a comfortable position for joystick operation.

The actual experiments consisted of three trials of nine tests each. In each trial, the tests were presented in random order to minimize learning effects. The goal of each test was to successively detect the transition between the layers either due to haptic or visual cues. For each test, the subject was asked to insert the "virtual" needle into the skin, move from skin into fat, and from fat into muscle. After each transition the subject was to stop the movement of the joystick as soon as possible and allow the experimenter to record appropriate data, then extract the needle from the tissue completely. The data recorded was the penetration depth into the layer after puncture with respect to the layer boundary.

Each of nine presented tests simulated a different needle insertion environment. The conditions for each test are outlined in Table 2. "Deflection" refers to graphical deflection of layer boundary prior to puncture due to the needle. In test 8, subjects could only see the skin boundary, but none of the internal boundaries, whereas in test 9, the subjects were blindfolded and relied completely on force feedback. Tests 4, 5, 6, and 7 require some anatomical knowledge on the part of the user since they mimic situations where the imaging (a) provides real-time visual feedback, but does not capture the needle in the imaging plane, or (b) is not real time.

4   Results and Discussion

To evaluate subject performance, we calculated the error between the penetration depth and the layer boundary for skin, fat, and muscle in each test. We then averaged the error over three trials for each subject. Afterwards, we averaged the resulting errors over all subjects for skin, fat, and muscle in each test. Then, all values were converted from counts into millimeters. Finally, we grouped the results by the following criteria:

1. Group of tests where force feedback was always present and visual cues differed. This studies the effect of imaging on manual insertion or teleoperated tasks (with force feedback).
2. Group of tests where force feedback was always absent and visual cues differed. This studies the effect of imaging on teleoperated tasks.
3. Group of tests where visual feedback was limited and force feedback differed. This studies the effect of force feedback on insertion tasks with or without limited visual feedback.

4.1   Force Feedback with Varying Visual Feedback

Figure 2 shows the results of experiments where the subjects received force feedback, yet visual feedback was different in each test (tests 2, 3, and 6-9 in Table 2). As compared to experiment 8 (case "no visual" in Figure 2) when no visual feedback was present, we observed that subjects in Group I (regular subjects) had a 43% reduction in error (t_{18}=1.365, p<0.09) in tests with fat layer puncture when only the needle was rendered (cases "ND,WN," "WD,WN," and "WD,NN" in Figure 2), but a 67% reduction in error (t_{18}=2.586, p<0.01) when only the deflection was rendered. Group II (medical subjects) showed at least a 45% reduction in error (t_6=0.889, p<0.21) when only the needle was rendered and 75% reduction in error (t_{18}=1.671, p<0.08) when only the deflection was added. Skin and muscle trials did not show a significant reduction in error. This shows that in low-level force display scenarios (e.g. fat), users greatly benefit from presence of visual feedback based on real-time tissue boundary tracking, whereas in high-force displays (e.g. skin, muscle), force rendering is sufficient. We observed similar performance and error reduction from the two groups, indicating that performance with force feedback is independent of prior needle insertion experience.

4.2   No Force Feedback with Varying Visual Feedback

Figure 3 shows the effect of visual feedback on the performance of the subjects when force feedback is absent. For this set of tests (tests 1, 4, and 5 in Table 2), layer boundaries were rendered, which is equivalent to overlay of pre-operative image data.

When the deflection of the boundary layer and rendering of the needle were absent, the subjects performed badly for all tissue types. Clearly, without any force feedback and needle rendering, the subject has to guess about the location of the needle based on their abstract spatial representation of the needle with respect to the boundaries (anatomical knowledge). As compared to the experiment with needle and layer deflection absent, subjects in Group I showed a 91% reduction in error (t_{18} = 5.683, p<0.0001), and Group II showed a 96% reduction in error (t_6 = 3.9, p<0.004) with the addition of deflection rendering. With the addition of both deflection and needle rendering, subjects in Group I showed an 87% reduction in error (t_{18} = 6.061, p<0.0001), and Group II showed a 95% reduction in error (t_6=3.839, p<0.004) as compared to the experiment with needle and layer deflection absent. Therefore, boundary layer deflection is a sufficient aid to improve performance, possibly more important than the additional visibility of the needle. This result indicates that the use of real time image overlay will improve insertion depth accuracy.

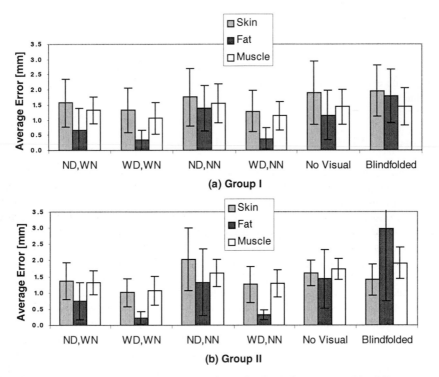

Fig. 2. Average error in millimeters when force feedback is present with different types of visual feedback where ND = No Deflection, WD = With Deflection, NN = No Needle, and WN = With Needle for a) Group I, b) Group II

4.3   Limited Visual Feedback with Varying Force Feedback

In Figure 4, visual feedback was limited to tissue boundaries (no deflection and no needle) in each experiment (tests 4, 6, and 8 in Table 2), and no visual feedback at all in one case (test 9 in Table 2). The addition of force feedback reduced the error in Group I by at least 62% (t_{18}=3.257, p<0.004) as compared to the no force feedback case, and Group II showed at least a 55% reduction in error (t_6=1.613, p<0.07). This shows that addition of force feedback to telesurgical systems could improve surgical performance in situations where vision is occluded. We also observe that the visibility of tissue boundaries has little effect on performance in this scenario because experiments in which tissue layers alone were visible showed little difference in error from experiments where the tissue layers were invisible.

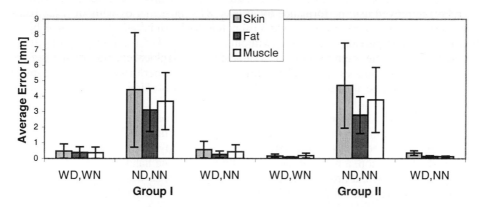

Fig. 3. Average error in millimeters when force feedback is absent with different types of visual feedback where ND = No Deflection, WD = With Deflection, NN = No Needle, and WN = With Needle.

The larger errors in tests with force feedback are due to overshoot after puncture. When the user pushes against a boundary that is suddenly removed, he or she is not able to stop immediately. To prevent this particular effect, a teleoperated robot with no force feedback may be most appropriate. In general, the results demonstrate that visual feedback alone is a more effective aid than haptic feedback alone. While a teleoperated procedure (where no force feedback is provided) could benefit from addition of force feedback, better performance can be obtained from real-time image overlay for manual or teleoperated needle insertions.

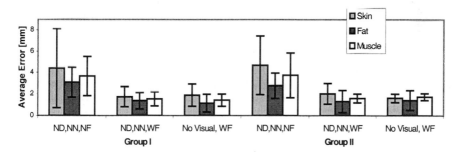

Fig. 4. Average error in millimeters when visual feedback is limited with/without force feedback where NN = No Needle, WN = With Needle, NF = No Force, and WF = With Force

5   Conclusion

We created a virtual needle insertion simulator with visual and force feedback, and performed a series of perceptual experiments to evaluate performance in a needle insertion task. Users experienced different combinations of visual and haptic feedback, mimicking manual or teleoperated scenarios with and without image overlay (real time or pre-operative). The results show that the addition of force feedback to systems that obstruct field of view reduces error in the detection of transitions between tissue layers by at least 55%. The addition of real-time visual feedback (image overlay) improved user performance by at least 87% in scenarios without force feedback. Presentation of both force and visual feedback improved performance by at least 43% in comparison to scenarios without any feedback. Even though haptic feedback provides some improvement, we conclude that graphical display of the deflection of tissue boundaries has a dominating influence on performance. This prompts the use of real-time imaging in medical procedures to provide the user with image overlay to assist in task visualization.

We plan to perform a set of experiments to obtain force profiles for real needle insertions and fit appropriate force models for more realistic simulations. It is also desirable to have experiments for different areas of the body to serve a variety of training needs. In addition, a haptic device that allows the same hand movement as in real needle insertion would provide more realistic simulation, as well as allow training of medical personnel without the use of cadavers or artificial materials.

References

1. Brett, P. N., Harrison, A. J., Thomas, T. A., "Schemes for the Identification of Tissue Types and Boundaries at the Tool Point for Surgical Needles," *IEEE Transactions on Information Technology in Biomedicine*, Vol. 4, No. 1, pp. 30-36, 2000.
2. Chinzei, K., Hata, N., Jolesz, A., Kikinis R., "Surgical Assist Robot for the Active Navigation in the Intraoperative MRI: Hardware Design Issues," *Proceedings of the IEEE/RSJ International Conference on Intelligent Robots*, Vol. 1, pp. 727-732, 2000.
3. Dang, T., Annaswamy, T.M., Srinivasan, M. A., "Development and Evaluation of an Epidural Injection Simulator with Force Feedback for Medical Training," *Studies in Health Technology and Informatics*, Vol. 29, pp. 564-579, 1996.
4. Fichtinger, G., Masamune, K., Patriciu, A., Tanacs, A., Anderson, J.H., DeWees, T.L., Taylor, R., Stoianovici, D., "Robotically Assisted Percutaneous Local Therapy and Biopsy," *The 10th International Conference on Advanced Robotics*, pp. 133-151, 2001.
5. Hiemenz Holton, Leslie L., "Force Models for Needle Insertion Created from Measured Needle Puncture Data," *Medicine Meets Virtual Reality*, pp. 180-186, 2001.
6. Kontarinis, D.A. and Howe, R.D., "Tactile display of vibratory information in teleoperation and virtual environments," *Presence*, Vol. 4, pp. 387-402, 1995.
7. Kwon, D. S., Kyung, K. U., Kwon, S.M., Ra, J. B., Park, H.W., Kang, H. S., Zeng, J., Cleary, K.R., "Realistic Force Reflection in a Spine Biopsy Simulator," *Proceedings of the IEEE International Conference on Robotics and Automation*, pp. 1358-1363, 2001.
8. Masamune, K., Kobayashi, E., Masutani, Y., Suzuki, M., Dohi, T., Iseki, H., Takakuro, K., "Development of an MRI-compatible needle insertion manipulator for stereotactic neurosurgery," *Journal of Image Guided Surgery*, Vol. 1, No. 4, pp. 242-248, 1995.
9. Ra, J. B., et al. A Visually Guided Spine Biopsy Simulator with Force Feedback, *SPIE International Conference on Medical Imaging*, pp. 36-45, 2001.

Analysis of Suture Manipulation Forces for Teleoperation with Force Feedback

Masaya Kitagawa[1], Allison M. Okamura[1], Brian T. Bethea[2],
Vincent L. Gott[2], and William A. Baumgartner[2]

[1] Johns Hopkins University, Department of Mechanical Engineering, 200 Latrobe Hall,
3400 N. Charles Street, Baltimore, MD 21218
{aokamura,mkitagawa}@jhu.edu
http://haptics.me.jhu.edu
[2] Johns Hopkins Medical Institutions, Division of Cardiac Surgery, 618 Blalock,
600 N. Wolfe Street, Baltimore, MD 21287
{bbethea,vgott,wbaumgar}@csurg.jhmi.jhu.edu

Abstract. Despite many successes with teleoperated robotic surgical systems, some surgeons feel that the lack of haptic (force or tactile) feedback is detrimental in applications requiring fine suture manipulation. In this paper, we study the difference between applied suture forces in three knot tying exercises: hand ties, instrument ties (using needle drivers), and robot ties (using the da Vinci™ Surgical System from Intuitive Surgical, Inc.). Both instrument and robot-assisted ties differ from hand ties in accuracy of applied force. However, only the robot ties differ from hand ties in repeatability of applied force. Furthermore, comparison between attendings and residents revealed statistically significant differences in the forces used during hand ties, although attendings and residents perform similarly when comparing instrument and robot ties to hand ties. These results indicate that resolved force feedback would improve robot-assisted performance during complex surgical tasks such as knot tying with fine suture.

1 Introduction

Robot-assisted surgical systems are enhancing the ability of surgeons to perform minimally invasive procedures by scaling down motions and adding additional degrees of freedom to instrument tips. Thousands of general surgeries and several hundred cardiac surgeries have been performed worldwide with teleoperated robotic surgical systems [1]. Moreover, both the ZEUS® Surgical Robotic System from Computer Motion (Goleta, CA) [2, 3] and the da Vinci™ Surgical System from Intuitive Surgical, Inc. (Mountain View, CA) [4-8] have been used in cardiac surgery to perform coronary artery bypass grafting and mitral valve repair [9]. Despite these successes, many surgeons claim that further progress in this field is limited by an unresolved problem: the lack of haptic (force and tactile) feedback to the user. This is especially detrimental in fields where force is applied to fine suture and delicate tissues, such as cardiac surgery. Appropriate applied forces are critical in creating knots that are firm enough to hold, but do not break sutures or damage tissue.

Until now, the problem of the lack of force feedback has only been described anecdotally. The goal of this work is to quantify the effect of force feedback on performance in a suture manipulation task. This will allow us to determine whether bilat-

T. Dohi and R. Kikinis (Eds.): MICCAI 2002, LNCS 2488, pp. 155–162, 2002.
© Springer-Verlag Berlin Heidelberg 2002

eral telemanipulation with force feedback would improve performance in applied force accuracy and repeatability. A bilateral telemanipulation system provides bilateral interaction between the robot and the user: the user specifies the robot motion using the master, and also feels resolved forces that are sensed by the robot.

It is important to distinguish between haptic, tactile, and force feedback. Haptic information is a broad term used to describe both cutaneous (tactile) and kinesthetic (force) information. Both types of information are necessary to form the typical sensations felt with the human hand. In this paper, we consider force feedback, where forces are resolved to a single point, and are displayed to the user through a tool. A haptic device such as the Phantom from SensAble Technologies (Woburn, MA) [10] can provide this type of feedback. The master of the da Vinci™ is also equipped to provide force feedback, although currently little to no feedback is provided. Tactile display devices are not yet commercially available, and are not likely to meet the size and weight constraints for multi-degree-of-freedom systems in the near future.

1.1   Previous Work

Although a significant effort has been put forth in motion analysis, e.g. [11], little work has focused on characterizing the forces resulting from surgical tasks. Force feedback in teleoperated systems is known to improve the performance of a user in some situations [12, 13]. Moreover, the "addition of kinesthetic force feedback is of substantial help in moving performance toward the extreme demonstrated by the barehanded human" in a force-reflecting teleoperated system [14]. In addition, Rosen, et al. showed that bilateral telemanipulation of an endoscopic instrument returned haptic information that was lost when a surgeon manipulated soft tissues using a traditional endoscopic tool/grasper. [15].

However, there exists some anecdotal evidence against the use of bilateral telemanipulation in a suturing task. In [16], the tip forces of the robot were indirectly sensed using actuator torques. Using this sensing method during robot-assisted suturing, it was found that force feedback "was more of an annoyance than a help." It is suspected that the tip forces were not appropriately sensed; without a comprehensive study, one cannot characterize the appropriate resolution and distribution of force sensors, or the change in performance when force feedback is provided.

2   Experiments

The experiments were designed to evaluate three claims:
1. *Accuracy*: The force magnitudes applied with the needle driver are indistinguishable from those applied solely by hand, while the forces applied with the robot are different from those applied by hand. This claim seeks to show that forces can be applied more accurately with resolved force feedback than without.
2. *Repeatability*: The normalized standard deviation of force (standard deviation as a percentage of the average force level) for instrument ties is indistinguishable from hand ties. However, the normalized standard deviation for robot ties is different from that of hand ties. This claim intends to demonstrate that forces can be applied with better repeatability with the instrument than with the robot.

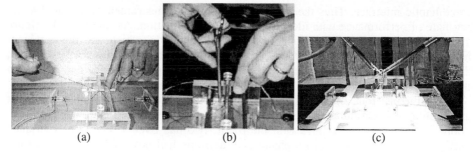

Fig. 1. A tension measurement device is used to measure the forces applied to sutures, (a) by hand, (b) by instrument, and (c) using the robot

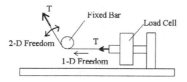

Fig. 2. Side view of the measurement device. The pulling force in two dimensions is resolved into the direction parallel to the axis of the load cell. This design allows users to perform the task in a natural way even though the measurement device has only one degree of freedom

3. *Skill Comparison*: Residents have higher normalized standard deviations than attendings for hand ties and instrument ties. With the robot, there will be a reduction in performance margin between the two groups.

2.1   Experiment Design

Complex surgical tasks, such as knot tying, require force feedback. In practice sessions with the robot, novice users occasionally broke fine polypropylene sutures during the first throw of a knot. In our experiments, we measured the tension applied to sutures during the first throw of a knot by the left and right hand using a tension measurement device (Figure 1). The device consists of two one-degree-of-freedom Entran® load cells tied to sutures, and bars used to orient the applied force in the direction parallel to the axes of the load cells. The device design made it possible for users to perform the task in a natural way and to record the tension in the suture (Figure 2). Separate sutures were used for the left and right hands, and each suture was replaced after 5 ties. While data was acquired for both hands, only the dominant hand (the right hand for all the subjects) was used in data analysis.

Three conditions were used, as shown in Figure 1. The first condition was a hand tie, representing the feedback received by a surgeon during traditional execution of a procedure. The second condition was an instrument tie, which is commonly used in procedures where it is difficult for the surgeon to access the suture by hand. The instrument tie mimics the type of feedback a surgeon would receive through a resolved-

158   M. Kitagawa et al.

force haptic interface. Thus the performance during an instrument tie is used as an estimate of performance with ideal bilateral telemanipulation. As shown in the figure 1 (b), the instrument was used only on the right hand side, which was the dominant hand for all subjects. The third condition used the da Vinci™. In this final condition, the surgeon observed a magnified, three-dimensional display from the endoscope. In the other conditions, the surgeon could directly observe the suture.

Six surgeons, four attendings, and two residents performed the hand, instrument and robotic ties. Of the attendings, one had performed over one hundred nissen fundoplications and splenectomies with the robot, two had over 5 hours of experience with the robot (tying sutures on phantoms), and one had not used the robot before. The two residents had less than 1 hour of previous experience with the robot. Six different sutures used in general and cardiac surgeries were employed in this experiment. The sutures, which varied by type and size, were: 2-0 Silk, 2-0 Ti-Cron, 4-0 Polypropylene, 5-0 Polypropylene, 6-0 Polypropylene, and 7-0 Polypropylene from various manufacturers (e.g., Ethicon, USSC and Sherwood-Davis & Geck). Five tension recordings were taken for each suture used by each surgeon. The data set for one subject, an attending, is provided in Figure 3.

A total of 30 throws were recorded for each surgeon under a single condition (hand, instrument, or robot). The testing for hand and instrument were performed together for four of the six subjects, and the other two subjects separated their hand and instrument ties by at least one day. The robot experiments were performed at least one week later for all subjects. The task was to perform a single throw of a knot in standard fashion around a circular rod in the middle of the tension measurement device. The subjects were instructed to aim for consistency and accuracy in applied force, rather than speed of completion. In addition, the subjects were asked to hold the throw for three seconds at the desired tension level.

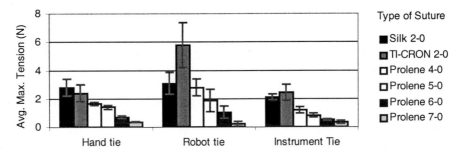

Fig. 3. Data summary for a single subject (attending surgeon). The forces applied to various sutures change with suture strength. For this subject, the instrument tie force levels and standard deviations of the hand tie and instrument tie are similar, while those of the robot tie are different

2.2   Data Segmentation

The data obtained was force applied to the suture for the left and right hands. The tension data was plotted against time for each run (one run is shown in Figure 4). The graph consists of 3 active regions: (a) increasing tension, (b) holding tension, and (c)

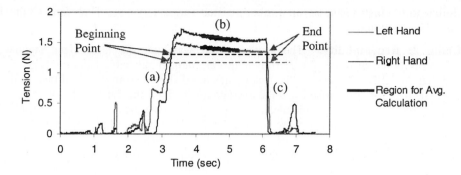

Fig. 4. Data recorded from a single throw. The data is segmented into three areas: (a) increasing tension, (b) holding tension, and (c) decreasing tension. The average of forces in the middle 40% of the holding region is used in data analysis

decreasing tension. The holding region was automatically segmented from the other two regions at points that were 90 percent of the maximum tension measured during each run. The middle 40 percent of the holding region was the only portion of the data included in the calculation of the average applied tension for each run. From Figure 4, it is clear that different forces are used for the two hands, which is possible because forces were measured on two separate sutures. In practice, the left and right hand forces in a single suture can also differ due to friction between the suture and the tissue, or the suture and itself. The tension measurement device was designed to minimize friction.

2.3   Results

For each of the three claims described previously, the Student's t-test was used for data analysis. We will now describe the results and implications of these three claims individually.

Claim 1: Accuracy.   The first claim was that the instrument ties would produce the same applied tension as the hand ties, whereas the robot-assisted ties would not. First, we compared the means of the forces applied during hand and instrument ties for each user and each suture (n= 30). The number of these comparisons with a p-value of greater than 0.1 was 19, meaning that 63.3% of the trials showed that there is a difference between the instrument tie and the hand tie. Second, we compared the means of the forces applied to hand and robot-assisted ties for each user and each suture (n=30). The number of these comparisons with a p-value greater than 0.1 was 22, meaning that 73.3% of the trials showed that there is a difference between the robot tie and the hand tie.

These results indicate that forces used for instrument ties are slightly better than robot ties, when the goal Is to apply the same force as for hand ties. However, this difference is not large enough to conclude that accuracy would be improved to the level of hand ties with the inclusion of resolved-force feedback (which would feel similar to the instrument tie) in a robot-assisted surgical system. Therefore, Claim 1 cannot be validated.

Claim 2: Repeatability.   The second claim was that the normalized standard deviation (NSD) of forces for instrument ties are indistinguishable from the hand ties, and that the NSD of forces for the robotic ties are different from the hand ties. In this case, the data for comparison was the average normalized standard deviation for each subject. First, we compared the mean hand ties NSD to the mean instrument ties NSD for each user. The number of these comparisons with a p-value of greater than 0.1 was 0 (n= 5), meaning that none of the subjects demonstrated a difference between instrument ties and the hand ties. Second, we compared the mean hand ties NSD to the mean robot ties NSD for each user. The number of these comparisons with a p-value of greater than 0.1 was 3 (n=5), meaning that 60.0% of the subjects demonstrated a difference between robot ties and hand ties.

These results indicate that instrument ties provide an NSD more similar to the hand ties than do the robot ties. The hand tie had the lowest NSD of all methods. We can conclude that this claim is satisfied; repeatability would be improved with the inclusion of resolved force feedback (which would feel similar to the use of an instrument) in a robot-assisted surgical system.

Claim 3: Skill Comparison.   The third claim was that, while residents have higher NSD than attendings for hand ties and instrument ties, the robot significantly mitigates this difference. In our group of subjects, the residents had significantly less surgical experience than the attendings, so one can also consider these groups to be "novice" and "expert." This experiment consists of three different tests comparing resident and attending by: (1) hand ties, (2) instrument ties, and (3) robot ties. Our results demonstrate a significant difference in hand ties (p=0.03), however, no statistically significant difference was demonstrated for instrument (p=0.40) or robotic (p=0.25) ties. Thus, this claim is not satisfied because both the instrument and the robot reduce the performance margin between expert and novice users.

3   Discussion

The goal of these experiments was to examine claims about the necessity of force feedback for robot-assisted surgical systems. All of the claims were partially satisfied in that user performance (both accuracy and repeatability) for robot ties was worse than user performance for hand ties. However, the claims also purported that the application of force feedback to the user would eliminate these differences, and this was not always found to be true.

There has been much discussion in the robotics and medical communities about the application of force feedback to robot-assisted surgical systems, and this work provides the first statistically significant data indicating that doing so may not enhance performance to the level of direct manual operation. When surgeons manipulate sutures by hand, some local tactile information is being used to sense suture tension, even when a surgical glove mediates the forces. It is possible that this tactile information is critical to maintaining accuracy and repeatability in the application of suture forces, since tactile sensation is very important in exploration and manipulation [17].

Unfortunately, practical application of such tactile feedback to teleoperated systems is not likely to happen in the near future.

Since current robot-assisted surgical systems continue to be limited by a lack of haptic feedback, a form of sensory substitution may be a short-term solution. By using data obtained from the hand ties as the standard, one could create a system where the current and desired amounts of tension applied to suture can be displayed to the surgeon. This would facilitate the accomplishment of complex surgical tasks such as knot tying. This study represents an initial step, and further research is needed before appropriate feedback can be relayed to the surgeon.

Acknowledgements

The authors acknowledge the encouragement and assistance of the Divisions of Cardiac Surgery and Surgery at the Johns Hopkins Medical Institutions, including Dr. Mark A. Talamini, Dr. Marc S. Sussman, Dr. David D. Yuh, and Dr. Stephen Cattaneo. This material is based upon work supported in part by the National Science Foundation under Grant No. EEC9731478, the Engineering Research Center for Computer-Integrated Surgical Systems and Technology.

References

1. Yoshino, M. Hashizume, M. Shimada, M. Tomikawa, M. Tomiyasu, R. Suemitsu, and K. Sugimachi, "Thoracoscopic Thymomectomy with the da Vinci Computer-Enhanced Surgical System," Journal of Thoracic and Cardiovascular Surgery, vol. 122, no. 4, pp. 783-785, 2001.
2. W. D. Boyd, R. Rayman, N. D. Desai, A. H. Menkis, W. Dobkowski, S. Ganapathy, B. Kiaii, G. Jablonsky, F. N. McKenzie, and R. J. Novick, "Closed-Chest Coronary Artery Bypass Grafting on the Beating Heart with the Use of a Computer-Enhanced Surgical Robotic System," The Journal of Thoracic and Cardiovascular Surgery, vol. 120, no. 4, pp. 807-809, 2000.
3. E. A. Grossi, A. LaPietra, R. M. Applebaum, G. H. Ribakove, A. C. Galloway, F. G. Baumann, P. Ursomanno, B. M. Steinberg, and S. B. Colvin, "Case Report of a Robotic Instrument-Enhanced Mitral Valve Surgery," The Journal of Thoracic and Cardiovascular Surgery, vol. 120, no. 6, pp. 1169-1171, 2000.
4. F. W. Mohr, V. Falk, A. Diegeler, T. Walther, J. F. Gummert, J. Bucerius, S. Jacobs, and R. Autschbach, "Computer-Enhanced "Robotic" Cardiac Surgery: Experience in 148 Patients," The Journal of Thoracic and Cardiovascular Surgery, vol. 121, no. 5, pp. 842-853, 2001.
5. U. Kappert, R. Cichon, J. Schneider, V. Gulielmos, S. M. Tugtekin, K. Matschke, I. Schramm, and S. Scheuler, "Closed-Chest Coronary Artery Surgery on the Beating Heart with the Use of a Robotic System," The Journal of Thoracic and Cardiovascular Surgery, vol. 120, no. 4, pp. 809-811, 2000.
6. W. R. Chitwood, L. W. Nifong, J. E. Elbeery, W. H. Chapman, R. Albrecht, V. Kim, and J. A. Young, "Robotic Mitral Valve Repair: Trapezoidal Resection and Prosthetic Annuloplasty with the da Vinci Surgical System," The Journal of Thoracic and Cardiovascular Surgery, vol. 120, no. 6, pp. 1171-1172, 2000.
7. Carpentier, D. Loulmet, B. Aupecle, A. Berrebi, and J. Relland, "Computer-assisted cardiac surgery," The Lancet, vol. 353, no. 9150, pp. 379-380, 1999.

8. H. Shennib, A. Bastawisy, M. J. Mack, and F. H. Moll, "Computer-assisted telemanipulation: an enabling technology for endoscopic coronary artery bypass.," Annals of Thoracic Surgery, vol. 66, no. 3, pp. 1060-1063, 1998.

9. R. J. Damiano, "Editorial: Endoscopic Coronary Artery Bypass Grafting - The First Steps on a Long Journey," The Journal of Thoracic and Cardiovascular Surgery, vol. 120, no. 4, pp. 806-807, 2000.

10. T. H. Massie and J. K. Salisbury, "The PHANTOM Haptic Interface: A Device for Probing Virtual Objects," Proceedings of the ASME Winter Annual Meeting, Symposium on Haptic Interfaces for Virtual Environment and Teleoperator Systems, vol. 55-1, pp. 295-299, 1994.

11. G. L. Cao, C. L. MacKenzie, and S. Payandeh, "Task and Motion Analyses in Endoscopic Surgery," Proceedings of the ASME Dynamic Systems and Control Division, Symposium on Haptic Interfaces for Virtual Environment and Teleoperator Systems, vol. 58, no. 583-590, 1996.

12. J. T. Dennerlein, D. B. Martin, and C. Hasser, "Force-feedback improves performance for steering and combined steering-targeting tasks," Proceedings of the Conference on Human Factors in Computing Systems, pp. 423-429, 2000.

13. J. T. Dennerlein and M. C. Yang, "Haptic force-feedback devices for the office computer: Performance and musculoskeletal loading issues," Human Factors, vol. 43, no. 2, pp. 278-286, 2001.

14. Hannaford, L. Wood, D. A. Douglas, and H. Zak, "Performance evaluation of a six-axis generalized force-reflecting teleoperator," IEEE Transactions on Systems, Man and Cybernetics, vol. 21, no. 3, pp. 620-633, 1991.

15. J. Rosen, B. Hannaford, M. P. MacFarlane, and M. N. Sinanan, "Force controlled and teleoperated endoscopic grasper for minimally invasive surgery - experimental performance evaluation," IEEE Transactions on Biomedical Engineering, vol. 46, no. 10, pp. 1212-1221, 1999.

16. J. Madhani, G. Niemeyer, and J. K. Salisbury, "The Black Falcon: A Teleoperated Surgical Instrument for Minimally Invasive Surgery," IEEE/RSJ International Conference on Intelligent Robotic Systems, vol. 2, pp. 936-944, 1998.

17. S. J. Lederman and R. L. Klatzky, "Feeling through a probe," Dynamic Systems and Control Division, Proceedings of the 1998 ASME International Mechanical Engineering Congress and Exposition, vol. 64, pp. 127-131, 1998.

Remote Microsurgery System for Deep and Narrow Space – Development of New Surgical Procedure and Micro-robotic Tool

Koji Ikuta, Keiji Sasaki, Keiichi Yamamoto, and Takayuki Shimada

Department of Micro System Engineering, Graduate School of Engineering,
Nagoya University, Furo-cho, Chikusa-ku, Nagoya, Aichi, 464-8603, Japan
Tel: +81 52-789-5024, Fax: +81 52-789-5027
ikuta@mech.nagoya-u.ac.jp

Abstract. We developed a new medical operation procedure and robotic tool of microsurgery in deep and narrow site. It enables us to operate a difficult microsurgery that conventional method can't be achieved. Our system consists of flexible slave micro manipulators which can enter deep site of human body like a flexible catheter and master manipulators. Owing to difference of their sizes, it enables to convert micro motion of slave into natural size motion of master. Finally, both feasibility and effectiveness of the total system were verified experimentally.

1   Introduction

The target of this study is microsurgery in deep, narrow sites of the body, which are currently the most difficult areas to perform minimally invasive surgery. Typical examples are neurosurgery, head and neck surgery in otolaryngology, and microsurgery on esophageal cancer in the outer wall of the esophagus, an area that is not accessible with an endoscope through the mouth. We proposed and developed both a new method of microsurgery and surgical tools. Through a two-step development, a system was successfully created in which a slave manipulator with seven degrees of freedom in movement is remotely controlled from outside the body. The driving system is the size of a notebook computer and weighs approximately 1 kg. It can be hung on a bedside stand when in use. Dramatic reductions in size and weight from the current surgical robot prototype were accomplished. Finally, the effectiveness of the system was verified in animal experimentation.

2   Sophisticated Medical Treatment and Cases in Which Microsurgery Is Impossible

The current method of microsurgery has the following problems:
1. It is not applicable to deep sites of the body or the nasal cavity, which are difficult to access
2. Microscopic manipulation cannot be done at a level beyond the skill of the surgeon.
3. It requires a large incision.

T. Dohi and R. Kikinis (Eds.): MICCAI 2002, LNCS 2488, pp. 163–172, 2002.
© Springer-Verlag Berlin Heidelberg 2002

In current medical treatment, there are other types of surgery that are very difficult or nearly impossible to perform, such as those on the esophagus and other digestive organs, those on the spleen and other organs located deep inside the body, and those on fetal organs. This is because there are critical organs, such as the lungs and the heart, that are in the approach path to the site to be operated.

Factors that prevent surgery are shown below:

1. Critical organs, such as the lungs and the heart, that are in the approach path must not be touched
2. Even when the site is accessible, a severely restricted space will not allow for any surgery in which forceps are inserted from the outside.
3. The surgery itself is very difficult because it is extremely microscopic.

There are also surgeries that are performed under X-ray exposure. In these cases, remote medical treatment will be necessary to protect surgeons from exposure to X-rays[1]. Among remote microscopic surgical systems, there are the Tele Microsurgery System by Mitsuishi et al.[2] and the HUMAN Manipulator System by Kan et al. [3].

Most of these systems are basically used in open surgery to perform microscopic manipulation remotely. In other words, they are the current remotely controlled surgical systems. Therefore, it is very difficult to apply them to the cases mentioned above.

3   Proposal of a New Method of Microsurgery

The new method of microsurgery we propose is shown in Fig. 1.

1. As in a catheter procedure, a guide tube is inserted following after insertion of a guide wire and is threaded through the space between organs to the site to be operated.
2. The guide wire is withdrawn, and the slave micromanipulator is inserted along the tube to the site to be operated. More slave manipulators and an endoscope may be inserted in the same way as necessary.
3. While monitoring the images from the endoscope, the master manipulator is used in the microsurgery performed by the slave manipulator in the restricted space.

To use the new method of microsurgery in deep sites of the body and in restricted space, we propose the remote microsurgery system as shown in Fig. 2. In this system, the microscopic procedure is performed by a slave manipulator controlled through a master manipulator, which is several times larger in scale than the slave manipulator, by the operator. Furthermore, the slave manipulator allows a winding approach to be taken, going around organs to reach the site to be operated in the patient's body.

The features of the system are shown below:

1. Flexible movement of the slave manipulator makes it possible for microsurgery to be performed at deep sites of the body.
2. Minimally invasive surgery can be performed since no incision is required.
3. The difference in size between the master and slave manipulators makes it possible to perform microsurgery at a level beyond the skill of the doctor.

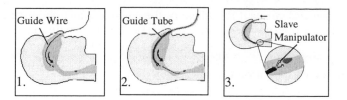

Fig. 1. New Method of Microsurgery in Deep and Narrow Site

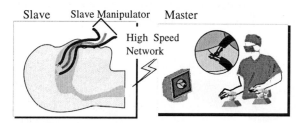

Fig. 2. Proposed Concept of Remote Microsurgery System

4   Preparation of the System

4.1   Requirements for the Slave Mechanism

Requirements for the slave mechanism are shown below:
1.   Miniaturized tip manipulator
2.   Able to follow a winding approach to the site
      To meet requirement 1, the degree of freedom in movement of the tip manipulator
was limited to five (the smallest number considered necessary to be useful as a microsurgical tool): (1) translation, (2) torsion, (3) grasping, (4) base joint, and (5) tip joint.
At the same time, the tip manipulator unit is to be separated from the driving member
unit. As for translation and torsion, the slave manipulator was devised so that it can
move its main body itself in such a way that translation and torsion is obtained at the
tip manipulator.
      To meet the requirement 2, a microwire transmission mechanism was adopted as a
transmission mechanism from the driving member to the tip manipulator so as to
make the intermediate portion of the slave manipulator flexible.
      In general, the wire system can cause the following problems, which have been
solved by adopting a noninterference microjoint mechanism and the S-Drive, which
will be explained later, to compensate for any slack:
1.   Redundant movement of multiple degrees of freedom is difficult
2.   Slack in the wire

4.2   Decoupled Microjoint Mechanism [4]

Fig.3 is a diagram of the "decoupled microjoint mechanism". Since the wire for driving the tip joint always passes through the axis of the base joint, the path length of the

driving wire remains constant regardless of the angle at which the base joint is bent. Therefore, there will be no interference of the base joint by the tip joint.

4.3   S-Drive for Elongation Compensation

Fig. 4 is a diagram of the S-Drive. The S-Drive compensates for any elongation in the wire to keep the wire's tension constant using a spring, which is based on Tendon-Drive Mechanisms by S.Hirose et al.[5] The drive also features the ability to apply the maximum amount of static friction between the wire and the pulley on the motor

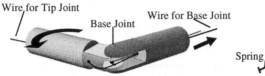
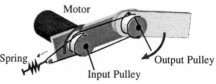
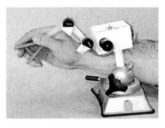

Fig. 3. Decoupled Microjoint Mechanism with 2D.O.F

Fig. 4. S-Drive Mechanism to compensate elongation after long term driving

Slave   Master

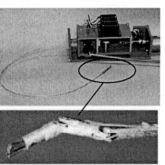

Fig. 5. First Prototype of Remote Microsurgery System (2000)

Slave   Master

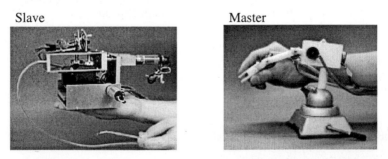

Fig. 6. Second Prototype of Remote Microsurgery System (2001)

side using the spring. Therefore, adjustments to the spring will determine the maximum torque to be transmitted to the tip, thus functioning as a torque limiter.

5   Development of Prototypes

In this study, the first prototype used in the verification of the basic principle was created in 2000.[6] In the model (Fig.5), the tip manipulator of 3 mm has five degrees of freedom in movement (a grasping mechanism, two joints, translation, and torsion), each of which was successfully driven independently. The first prototype, however, could not be operated steadily over long periods of time due to an insufficient driving capability resulting from a lack of rigidity.

To improve stability so that the manipulator could be used in long-term animal experimentation, a second prototype for animal experimentation was created in 2001 (Fig. 6).[7]

With the second prototype, animal experimentation on a chicken was conducted, and the following results were obtained:
1.   In the proposed method, deep sites of the body were accessed.
2.   The manipulator was inserted from the neck of the chicken to the abdominal cavity, where the manipulator's capability for surgical manipulation was verified.

Based on the results, it was verified that access to deep and narrow sites of the body was possible and that microscopic manipulation was also possible at such sites. Thus, the effectiveness of the prototype system was verified. However, before going onto the clinical application in the next step, the following had to be realized:
1.   Improvement in the driving properties and power
2.   Increase in the degree of freedom in movement of the slave manipulator tip
3.   Improvement in the operability of the master manipulator

Slave

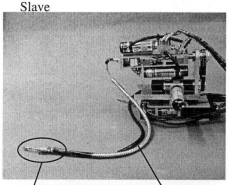

Micro Manipulator   Guide Tube

Master

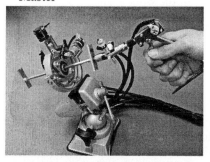

Fig. 7. Newly Developed Clinical Applicable Prototype of Remote Microsurgery System (2002)

6   The Third Prototype for Clinical Application

Fig. 7 shows an external view of the prototype created for clinical application in this study. Pitch and yaw are added to this prototype to increase the degree of freedom in movement of the tip. Thus, the tip of the guide tube is provided with a total of seven degrees of freedom in movement.

The prototype features the following:
1. Increase driving capability through an improvement in wire transmission properties
2. Increase in the degree of freedom in movement through the introduction of a tip driving guide tube (seven degrees of freedom in movement at the tip)
3. Increase operability through an improvement in the master manipulator
4. Reduction in size and weight of the entire system

Each of the items above is explained below:

6.1   Driving Member of the Slave Manipulator

The driving member of the slave manipulator is a unit into which the actuators of the tip manipulator are integrated. The changes made from the second prototype are shown below:

1. *A guide tube driving system is added*
An actuator is newly added to the guide tube, and the driving system for the guide tube is made to be interchangeable with the driving system for the tip manipulator so that it would be able to cope with changes in the tip manipulator.
2. *The amount of translation and torsion is increased*
The amount of translation and torsion is increased to 1.5 times the current amount so as to extend the work area.
3. *The size and weight of the system is reduced*
Due to an optimized motor arrangement and materials, the size and the weight of the entire system are greatly reduced despite an increase in the number of motors and the size of the work area.

The properties of the new slave mechanism are compared to those of the current one in Table 1.

6.2   Tip Micromanipulator

The tip manipulator is a microscopic manipulator that performs operations in deep and narrow sites of the body. It is 3mm in diameter, providing five degrees of freedom in movement: grasping, tip joint, base joint, translation, and torsion. The external view of the manipulator is shown in Fig. 8.

An improvement in the manipulator design and the use of an outer casing to increase the wire transmission capability greatly improve the driving property of the tip manipulator, providing sufficient power required for microscopic suturing in the body.

Table 1. Comparison of the Characteristic

	Clinical applicable prototype('02)	Previous Prototype('01)
D. O. F.	7	5
motor	Harmonic Drive (RH-5A 1/80) *4 DCmotor (maxon 4.5W 1/84) *2 DCmotor (COPAL LC20G 1/100) *1	DC servomotor (Futaba S9450)
Width(mm)	155	261
Extend(mm)	70	107
Height(mm)	130	120
Weight(g)	1064	1087
Thrust movement (mm)	40	25
movable angle(deg.)	±150	±90
Max speed Thrust(mm/s)	62	
Twist(rpm)	55	

6.3   Additional Degrees of Freedom on the Tip of Guide Tube

In the method proposed in this study, "guide tube" is defined as a tube used to secure the path of the slave manipulator. So that a tip manipulator could work in the target position, pitch and yaw are newly added to the guide tube. It is constructed so that a universal joint with a controllable tip is joined at the tip of a stainless steel flexible tube (Fig. 9).

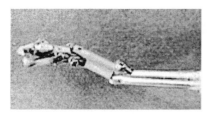

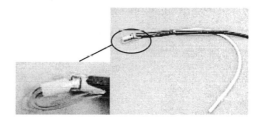

Fig. 8. Newly Developed Micromanipulator with 7D.O.F

Fig. 9. Decoupled microjoint with 2D.O.F on the tip of guide tube

The system features the following:

1. *Seven degrees of freedom in movement, including pitch and yaw, provided for the tip*

The two new degrees of freedom in movement provided for the tip of the guide tube increase the number of degrees of freedom in movement at the tip portion to seven (together with the five degrees of freedom in movement of the manipulator). This greatly contribute to an increase in operability.

2. *Flexible body trunk*

The entire flexible construction of the body trunk is similar to that of a catheter, allowing the manipulator to be inserted and operated without damage to the human body.

3.   *A driving source placed outside of the body*
The wire mechanism allows the driving source to be placed outside of the body. This makes it an excellent system in terms of safety because there is nothing in the body that is electrically run.

6.4   Master Mechanism Member

The master mechanism is a control stick with which a doctor operates the system. Because microsurgery requires microscopic manipulation, which is very difficult to do, it takes a lot of time. Therefore, the master mechanism must be easy for the doctor to operate, causing little fatigue even in a prolonged procedure.

The master mechanism previously reported had the following problems:
1.   Insufficient operability
2.   Limited work area

As to item 1, because the previous master mechanism was of the same pen-shaped structure as the slave mechanism, holding and operating the master mechanism was very difficult. Thus, the problem of operability remained.

As to item 2, because the master and slave manipulators were of the same structure, their work areas were identical. This allowed for intuitive operation, but there was the same restriction with the degree of freedom in movement on the master side as on the slave side, forcing the doctor to operate it in an unnatural position. The restricted degrees of freedom in movement may have been the cause of stress in doctors.

To solve these problems, a forceps-shaped master is created for this study.

Features of the master are shown below:

1.   *Increase in the degree of freedom in movement*
A tip driving guide tube is newly added to increase the number of degrees of freedom in movement to seven, and a corresponding change is made on the master side so as to control these seven degrees of freedom in movement.

2.   *Good operability, giving the doctor a sense of congruity*
A structure shaped like forceps, which is a familiar object to doctors, allows the doctor to perform microsurgery with the same feeling as in laparoscopic surgery, which is becoming increasingly popular. Furthermore, fewer restrictions on the degree of freedom in movement eliminate operative restrictions, successfully providing good operability.

3.   *Good control of the slave*
The degree of freedom in movement on the master side corresponds to that on the slave side, although the master has a different structure. This eliminates the need for coordinate transformation, thus creating a unique master that provides a feeling of intuitive operation, which is an advantage of masters of the same structure, as well as good operability, which is an advantage of masters of a different structure.

The corresponding degrees of freedom in movement on the slave side are shown in Fig. 10. The gimbals equipped with a locking mechanism senses the pitch and yaw of the guide tube and the forceps mechanism senses the grasping, two joints, translation, and torsion of the tip manipulator.

When operating the mechanism, the gimbals is used to control the pitch and yaw of the guide tube for the rough positioning of the tip. Then, the gimbals is locked and the rest of the forceps mechanism is used to drive the tip manipulator in five degrees of freedom in movement to perform microsurgery.

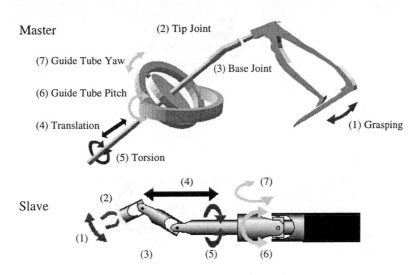

Master

(2) Tip Joint

(7) Guide Tube Yaw

(3) Base Joint

(6) Guide Tube Pitch

(4) Translation

(1) Grasping

(5) Torsion

(4)   (7)

(2)

Slave

(1)

(3)   (5)   (6)

Fig. 10. Correspondence of D.O.F between Master and Slave Micromanipulator

7   Verification Experiment

To verify the functions of this system, experiments were conducted on animals. Livers of chicken were used to perform suturing, which is the most difficult of the basic procedures in microsurgery (Fig. 11). A curved, semicircular needle was used.

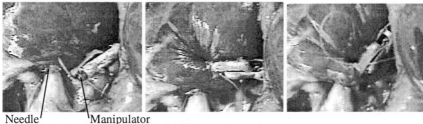

Needle   Manipulator

Fig. 11. Suture Experiment (from VCR image)

The results of the experiments showed that the series of operations performed-transferring a needle from the forceps, grasping the needle with the tip manipulator, moving it to a desired point, inserting the needle, and withdrawing the needle was successful. Thus, the effectiveness of the system was verified.

8   Conclusion

We developed a new medical operation procedure and robotic tool of microsurgery in deep and narrow site. It enables us to operate a difficult microsurgery that conventional method can't be achieved. Our system consists of flexible slave micro manipulators which can enter deep site of human body like a flexible catheter and master manipulators. A prototype for clinical application was created. By improving the driving property, degree of freedom in movement, and operability of the tip manipulator, a prototype of a total system with a dramatically improved performance was created.

Especially in the tip manipulator, work efficiency and multipurpose applicability were successfully improved by increasing the degrees of freedom in movement of the tip to seven while keeping the size the same as that of the current tip (3 mm in diameter). Furthermore, a verification experiment on a chicken verified that the basic procedures of microsurgery -ablation, partial excision, movement, fixing, and suturing- could be successfully performed.

Acknowledgment

The authors thank Dr. H.Iseki at Tokyo Woman's Medical University, Dr. D.Hashimoto and Dr. K.Shinohara at Saitama Medical School for their useful advice. We also acknowledge the assistance of all contributors.

References

1. K. Ikuta, T. Shimada, K. Ishizuka and Y. Nakayama, "Servo Forceps with Force Sensation for Remote Minimal Invasive Surgery", Proc. of 1999 JSME Conference on Robotics and Mechatronics (ROBOMEC 99), 1P2-10-004, 1999 (in Japanese).
2. M. Mitsuishi, et al "A Tele-Micro-Surgery System", Proc. of the 8th Annual Conference of the Japan Society of Computer Aided Surgery (JSCAS 99), pp.123-124, 1999 (in Japanese).
3. K. Kan, et al, "An Operation Experiment of HUMAN-Manipulator Prototype System for Neurosurgery", Proc. of the 8th Annual Conference of the Japan Society of Computer Aided Surgery (JSCAS 99), pp.105-106, 1999 (in Japanese).
4. K. Ikuta, F. Higashikawa and K. Shimoya, "Study on High Performance Hyper Endoscope", Proc. of 1998 JSME Conference on Robotics and Mechatronics (ROBOMEC 98), 1AIII2-5, 1998 (in Japanese).
5. Shigeo HIROSE, Yasuyuki UCHIDA, Richard CHUConsideration of New Tendon-driven Mechanisms, Proc. of 1998 JSME Conference on Robotics and Mechatronics (ROBOMEC 98), 1CI2-3, 1998 (in Japanese).
6. K. Ikuta, T. Shimada and K. Sasaki , "Study on Remote Microsurgery System", Proc. of 2000 JSME Conference on Robotics and Mechatronics (ROBOMEC 00), 2A1-13-017, 2000 (in Japanese).
7. K. Ikuta, K. Sasaki and T. Shimada, "Prototype and in vivo surgical experiment of Remote Microsurgery System", Proc. of 2001 JSME Conference on Robotics and Mechatronics (ROBOMEC 01), 2P1-D6, 2001 (in Japanese).

Hyper-finger for Remote Minimally Invasive Surgery in Deep Area

Koji Ikuta, Shinichi Daifu, Takahiko Hasegawa, and Humihiro Higashikawa

Department of Micro System Engineering, Graduate School of Engineering, Nagoya University
Furo-cho, Chikusa-ku, Nagoya, Aichi, 464-8603, Japan
Tel: +81 52-789-5024, Fax: +81 52-789-5027,
ikuta@mech.nagoya-u.ac.jp

Abstract. A new robotic system named Hyper Finger for minimally invasive surgery in deep organs has been developed. The finger size of the latest version is 10 mm and the entire system is much smaller and lighter, and can be set up on a camera tripod. This is one of the smallest master-slave robots in medicine. Each finger has nine degrees of freedom and several unique mechanisms are employed to solve the fundamental issues of conventional wire drive manipulators. The new concept and system were verified successfully by in-vivo remote minimally invasive surgery. Further improvements of the system toward a clinical version are now underway.

1 Introduction

A major focus of advanced medical technology development based on mechatronics is minimally invasive techniques in surgical operations, particularly the development of surgical instruments for laparoscopic surgery. We have been proposing and developing a Hyper Finger (hyper redundant multiple degrees of freedom active forceps) as a next-generation surgical instrument that enables more advanced and extensive laparoscopic surgery [1][2].

This study describes miniaturization of the arm to 10 mm diameter for clinical use, development of a compensation mechanism for drive wire elongation, and construction of a master-slave system with a pair of Hyper Fingers with this arm and mechanism.

Finally, further miniaturized prototype of Hyper Finger with nine degree of freedom was produced. The effectiveness of the system was also verified by in-vivo experiments.

2 Remote Laparoscopic Surgery Using Hyper Fingers

Different from standard open abdominal surgery, laparoscopic surgery is a minimally invasive operation technique, performed in the abdominal cavity with surgical instruments inserted through skin incisions of about 10 mm near the affected area. This

T. Dohi and R. Kikinis (Eds.): MICCAI 2002, LNCS 2488, pp. 173–181, 2002.

surgical method is performed in the abdominal cavity which is expanded like a dome by gas pressure, using inserted instruments such as an endoscope to look inside the cavity, working forceps, etc. Compared to open abdominal surgery, this surgical approach offers the advantage of less physical and mental stress for patients due to the smallness of the incisions. However, the approach is still under development and entails the following problems.

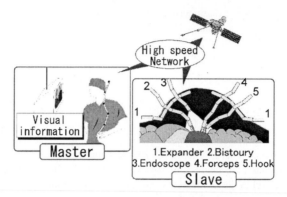

Fig. 1. Schematic diagram of remote laparoscopic surgery by using several type of Hyper Finger

1) Difficulty of observation and operation on a deep organ or on the backside of an organ

2) Limited operation area due to straight shaped forceps

3) Difficulty in cooperative work by many doctors

We have been developing the Hyper Finger (hyper redundant multiple degrees of freedom active forceps) surgical instrument to solve these problems [1].

As shown in Fig. 1, Hyper Fingers are active forceps with redundant degree-of-freedom multiple joints, and various functions can be attained by exchanging end-effectors. Independent or cooperative operation of two or more Hyper Fingers with high degrees of freedom enables advanced and extensive laparoscopic surgery to be performed.

This method can be developed for remote laparoscopic surgery with a master-slave system through high-speed communication of the endoscopic image, positional information and power sensor information of Hyper Fingers. A person at a remote location or under radiation exposure can thus receive advanced laparoscopic surgery.

3   Functional Verification Model

In our previous study, we developed a master-slave system with a pair of Hyper Fingers (Fig. 2) for feasibility check.

Although the system is wire driven, decoupled drive is possible in all degrees of freedom due to the use of two new mechanisms: an active universal joint and a decoupled link mechanism. The results showed good performance in position tracking and responsiveness of the master-slave system as well as enough force for surgery [2].

However, it was impossible to use this prototype for laparoscopic surgery because it was fabricated as a functional verification model of twice the size of devices used for surgery, as well as the following problems in clinical application:

1) Model of twice the size of devices used for surgery
2) Wire elongation
3) Friction between wire and wire path
4) Development of surgical end-effectors

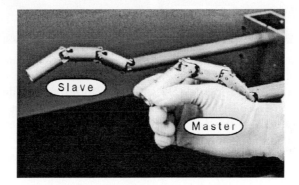

Fig. 2. First prototype of Master-Slave Hyper Finger (Mark-1 with 6 D.O.F.) [2]

4   Development of a Surgically Applicable Prototype

Figure 3 shows the developed miniaturized prototype of Hyper Finger (Mark-2) which is applicable to laparoscopic surgery. This model is not only smaller with an outer diameter of just 10 mm, but also has new movement and arm mechanisms to solve the above problems. Better position tracking, stability and expandability were thus achieved compared with the previous functional verification model. The new mechanisms are as follows:

1) Decoupled ring joint
2) Compensation mechanism for wire elongation
3) Unit-type regular hexagonal pyramid structure
4) Detachable gripper mechanism

4.1   Decoupled Ring Joint

The decoupled ring joint consists of a pair of arms connected to each other with a joint ring, and allows two degrees of freedom (horizontal/vertical) rotation manipulated by two wires each (Fig. 4). Since each axis and the corresponding wire-connecting points are located in the same plane, one rotational drive system has no effect on the other. Thus, each joint can be driven independently with two degrees of freedom.

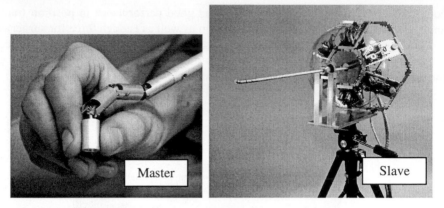

Fig. 3. Miniaturized Master-Slave Hyper Finger in real size (Mark-2 with 7 D.O.F.)

In addition, the friction loss is very small due to no wire folding at each joint. Therefore, there are no differences in drive characteristics between vertical and horizontal directions, and so this new joint system provides smoother drive compared with the active universal joint described in our previous reports.

Owing to its simple structure, the diameter is successfully reduced to 10 mm, which is sufficiently small for laparoscopic surgery.

4.2   Compensation Mechanism for Wire Elongation

In a wire drive system, repeated stress generally causes wire elongation, which reduces the accuracy of positioning. The new mechanism devised by Hirose et al., which compensates for the wire elongation, was adopted to solve the problem [3].

Figure 6 shows the scheme of the compensation mechanism for wire elongation. When the wire is under high tension during driving, the static friction between the friction bar and the wire moves the pedestal so that the route length of the wire is kept constant. At the same time, the tension pulley and the coil springs stay still on the pedestal and do not affect driving. On the contrary, when the wire elongates to reduce the tension, the friction with the friction bar decreases, the spring rolls up the elongated wire and thus the mechanism keeps the route length constant. This mechanism improves the positioning accuracy and ensures long-time stable driving.

4.3   Unit-Type Regular Hexagonal Pyramid Structure

A drive mechanism having one degree of freedom consists of a motor, a potentiometer and a elongated wire compensation mechanism. Six units were configured to create a regular hexagonal pyramid. The completed module is shown in Fig. 3.

Since the six units are attached to the hexagonal pyramid frame, the whole module is very light and can be mounted on a basic camera tripod. Robots must be small to fit in operating rooms which are packed with various precision machines; there is no small, light surgery robot system that can rival our system.

Moreover, the friction loss is very small due to the direct wire insertion from each unit to the arm, which requires no wire folding, and also the number of degrees of freedom can be easily increased thanks to the unit-type structure.

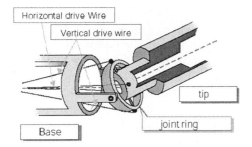

Fig. 4. Schematic design of active ring joint driven by decoupled wire drive mechanism

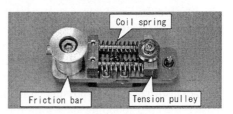

Fig. 5. Compensating elongated wire mechanism

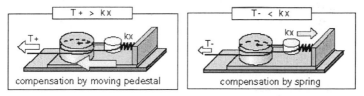

Fig. 6. Schematic design of compensating elongated wire mechanism

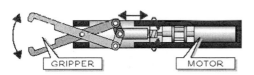

Fig. 7. (a) Schematic design of gripper mechanism installable on Hyper Finger

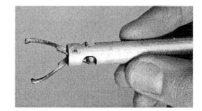

Fig. 7. (b) Gripper installable on Hyper Finger

4.4 Detachable Gripper Mechanism

A prototype gripper mechanism was developed as an end-effector because gripper mechanisms are used very often in laparoscopic surgery. A schematic design of the gripper mechanism is shown in Fig. 7.

The small motor in the mechanism enables the gripper to be driven independently and to be easily attached to a Hyper Finger. To ensure hygiene and prevent infection, sterilization of the gripper unit and making it disposable will need to be considered.

Using a link mechanism, the gripper can widely open up to about 40 degrees. Furthermore, the screw mechanism of the gripper gives the gripper sufficient holding power to maintain posture and force, to reduce errors such as slipping off an organ.

5 Control System

The block diagram of the control system is shown in Fig. 8. The system consists of a master Hyper Finger controlled by the doctor, a slave Hyper Finger inserted in the abdominal cavity for operation, and a control PC. The master has as many potentiometers to read the arm angles as degrees of freedom. The slave has as many potentiometers, drive motors and their motor drivers as degrees of freedom.

Backlash-free drive is possible at the master, and by manipulating each joint of the master, the corresponding slave joint follows the master.

Unilateral control, the most simple master-slave control system, is adopted for the present control system. By mounting force sensors, the system can easily be evolved to a bilateral control system in the future. Both the master and the slave adopt decoupled wire drive mechanisms, so there is no need for complicated calculations.

6 Driving Experiments

A position tracking experiment was conducted with this master-slave system. Fig.9 shows the position tracking result of the slave, which follows the master. The master was manually made to follow a sine wave with ±40 deg. joint amplitude per cycle of about 10seconds. From viewpoint of response and deviation, all joints showed excellent tracking characteristics, even though the worst delay was 0.4 sec in base joint.

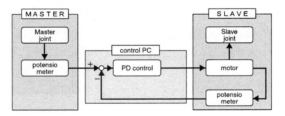

Fig. 8. Total control system for master-slave Hyper Finger

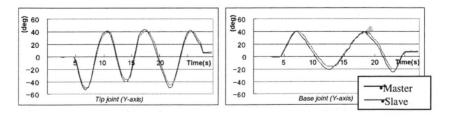

Fig. 9. Master-slave control of each active joint

7   In-vivo Experiment by Surgeons

The effectiveness of the surgical Hyper Finger with the new mechanism was tested on an animal. The experiment was conducted using an anesthetized pig by the lifting method under nearly the same conditions as practical laparoscopic surgery. In the experiment, the doctor manipulated the master while watching the endoscopic image on the monitor and conducted slave operations in the abdominal cavity such as lifting an organ. Figure 10 shows the experiment in progress.

The results and discussion are summarized below.

The Hyper Finger had no problems in term of movement area and drive speed. The Hyper Finger was also able to lift the liver to secure space for surgery with the gripper mechanism on the end-effector, thus verifying that the holding force of the Hyper Finger is sufficient for surgery. Moreover, the Hyper Finger could be attached to a camera tripod, enabling it to be placed anywhere and thus avoid interference with other surgical instruments and any spatial problems.

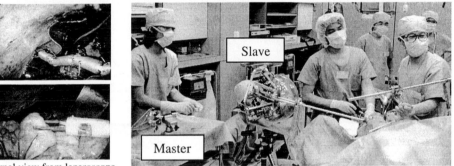

internal view from laparoscope

Fig. 10. In vivo surgical experiments with anesthetized pig

8   New Hyper-finger (Mark-3) for Clinical Use

A further miniaturized version with higher degree of freedom of hyper finger for clinical testing was developed. This model has the following new functions suitable for minimally invasive operation in deep sites.

1) Nine degrees of freedom
2) Rotating gripper with wire drive
3) Detachable finger mechanism
4) Small and light weight suitable for remote surgery by plural doctors

These additional new functions were verified through in-vivo experiment by doctors. All of the unique mechanisms verified by Hyper Finger (Mark 2) were introduced in the new version.

Figure 11 shows the clinical size Master-slave New Hyper Finger (Mark 3). Both the master and slave have been made far smaller. The diameter of the slave finger is

10mm and it is sufficiently light to be set on a camera tripod. Several types of end-effector have been developed and can easily be replaced during surgery because each finger is detachable as shown in Fig. 12.

Figure 13 shows the new driving mechanism of the wire drive gripper satisfying rotational operation with enough torque. , Since rotation of only a tip part is possible, this gripper makes it much easier to perform a suture in a deep site.

Figure 14 shows the surgical experiment using the miniaturized Hyper Finger (Mark-3). The doctor could maneuver the master finger with the same nine degrees of freedom. Suturing of a deep organ was done without much difficulty. According to the doctor's opinion after remote operation of the pig, the force and torque were sufficiently high and the feeling of maneuvering was very smooth.

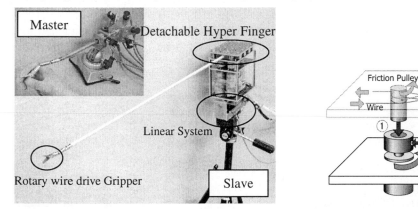

Fig. 11. Clinical size prototype Hyper Finger (Mark-3 with 9 D.O.F) set on camera tripod

Fig. 12. Drive mechanism of Detachable Hyper Finger

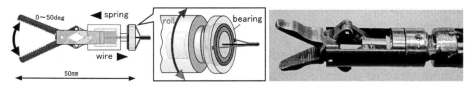

Fig. 13. Rotary wire drive Gripper

9   Conclusions

A new robotic system named Hyper Finger for minimally invasive surgery in deep organs has been developed. The finger size of the latest version is 10 mm and the entire system is much smaller and lighter, and can be set up on a camera tripod. This is one of the smallest master-slave robots in medicine. Each finger has nine degrees of freedom and several unique mechanisms are employed to solve the fundamental issues of conventional wire drive manipulators. The new concept and system were verified successfully by in-vivo remote minimally invasive surgery. Further improvements of the system toward a clinical version are now underway.

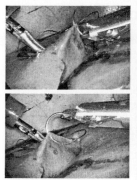

internal view from laparoscope

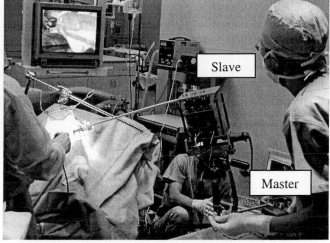

Fig. 14. In-vivo surgical experiments using clinical sized Hyper Finger Mark-3

Acknowledgments

The authors thank Dr. Daijou Hashimoto and Dr. Kazuhiro Shinohara at Saitama Medical School for their assistance in the animal experiment. We also acknowledge the assistance of Shinko Senda at Nagoya University and all contributors.

References

1. K.Ikuta, M.Nokata, S.Aritomi, "BIOMEDICAL MICRO ROBOTS DRIVEN BY MINIA-TURE CYBERNETIC ACTUATOR", Proc. of International Workshop on Micro Electro-mechanical Systems (MEMS'94) , pp263-268, 1994
2. K.Ikuta, F.Higashikawa, K.Ogata "Study on Hyper Finger for Remote Minimal Invasive Surgery" Plenary Proc. of 1999 JSME Conference on Robotics and Mechatronics (RO-BOMEC 99),1P2-10-005,1999
3. Shigeo Hirose, Richard Chu; Development of a light weight Torque Limiting M-Drive Actuator for Hyper Redundant Manipulator Float Arm, To be appeared in Proc.IEEE Int.on Robotics and Automation, 2831-2836,1999

Safety-Active Catheter with Multiple-Segments Driven by Micro-hydraulic Actuators

Koji Ikuta, Hironobu Ichikawa, and Katsuya Suzuki

Nagoya University, Graduate School of Engineering,
Department of Micro System Engineering,
Furo-cho, Chikusa-ku, Nagoya, Aichi, 464-8603, Japan
Tel: +81 52-789-5024, Fax: +81 52-789-5027
ikuta@mech.nagoya-u.ac.jp

Abstract. We proposed and developed an innovative active catheter with multi-segments that can bend in the narrow blood vessel. Micro hydraulic actuator system based on new principle has been developed by the authors. Moreover, new micro fabrication method named hybrid stereolithograpy (IH process) requiring any assemble process is introduced for leakage-free packaging catheter. Total system with pressure control system was made. Good safety and drive performance were verified experimentally. We also devised theoretical models of these valves to facilitate quantitative design and to extend applications for safe medical tools.

1 Introduction

Non-invasive or minimally invasive examinations and medical treatments are increasing in number as society ages. Catheterization is a typical minimally invasive medical technique. A catheter is a thin tube which is inserted into a peripheral vessel in an upper or lower limb for diagnosis or treatment of vascular system diseases; it is mainly used to measure internal pressure of the cardiovascular system, collect blood samples and inject contract medium for angiography. Catheterization is popular in clinical surgery because it allows minimally invasive diagnosis.

However, it is very difficult to insert a catheter with a guide wire which is now widely used, due to not only small inner diameter but also bending, twisting and frequent branching of vessels. Therefore, there is a need to develop an active catheter which can bend and twist its shaft in any direction and choose a direction at a branch point of a vessel [1][2][3]. These studies attached electric actuators on the parts to be inserted into the body, such as SMA or a special polymer that requires a high electric current of several amperes; this could be dangerous, with a risk of electric leakage in case of an accident such as breakage. There are also other problems that prevent practical application such as poor durability due to the complex internal mechanism of a catheter, and increasing lines associated with increasing joints [4].

To solve these problems, this study employed normal physiological salt solution for both drive and drive signal transmitter, and proposed a concept of a novel, safety-active catheter with simple mechanism using a hydraulic actuator. A prototype of a new type of microvalve, which is the key to this catheter, was developed and examined. The valve was then miniaturized to fit into an actual catheter. The control system was developed and safe actuation in the model blood vessel was verified.

T. Dohi and R. Kikinis (Eds.): MICCAI 2002, LNCS 2488, pp. 182–191, 2002.
© Springer-Verlag Berlin Heidelberg 2002

2 Proposal of Hydraulic Active Catheter

Figure 1 shows the concept of the hydraulic active catheter proposed in this study. The features of this system are as follows:

1) Electricity is not used on any part to be inserted into the body.

2) The drive fluid also works as a signal transmitter.

3) The number of diving lines will not increase with the number of active joints due to the single drive system.

In summary, this system consists of bellows as an actuator at each joint and a drive tube to control the bellows as shown in the figure.

Each joint is designed to bend while a bellows, as an actuator, is extended by fluid supply. Since normal saline is used as the drive fluid, safety is ensured because only harmless normal saline, instead of an electric leak, would leak if the catheter were to break inside the body.

The problem is how to achieve compact wiring in designing micromachinery. If a signal line is required for each new joint, reliability is impaired due to complicated signal lines at the proximal end, especially in the case of a long, thin system like a catheter. Our proposed single drive system allows a multi-joint design, free from complicated signal lines.

3 Band Pass Valve (BPV)

In this study, we developed a so-called "Single-input, multi-output" control mechanism which uses drive fluid that can also act as a signal transmitter and which controls each bellows (valve) independently through the drive fluid. We invented a static pressure Band Pass Valve (BPV) for independent active drive to ensure a simple mechanism and ease of control.

The concept of the BPV drive is shown in Fig. 2. This valve consists of a pair of valves: a High Pass Valve (HPV) and a Low Pass Valve (LPV). When the inner pressure of the tube (a drive system) reaches specific pressure P1, the lower valve (HPV) opens to make BPV open, and therefore drive fluid is supplied to the bellows (a drive actuator). When the inner pressure increases to P2, the upper valve (LPV) shuts to make BPV shut, and therefore the mechanism stops supplying fluid to the bellows.

Through these actions, BPV remains open within the preset specified pressure range only (from P1 to P2 of inner tube pressure in the figure) and BPV supplies drive fluid into the bellows.

Figure 3 shows the general scheme of the single-input, multi-output control mechanism of multi-joint active catheter using this BPV. The application of three joints is shown in this figure. A set of bellows (an actuator) and BPV corresponds to a joint, and they are arranged parallel to the drive tube. The drive pressure range of BPV on each joint is set to be different from each other.

By increasing the inner pressure of the drive tube stepwise to the activation pressure band of each valve, only the target valve opens and fluid is discharged each time. Therefore, only the target bellows connected to the valve is supplied with fluid and extended, and only the target joint will bend.

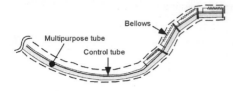

Fig. 1. Basic concept of Micro Hydraulic Active Catheter with Multi-degrees of Freedom

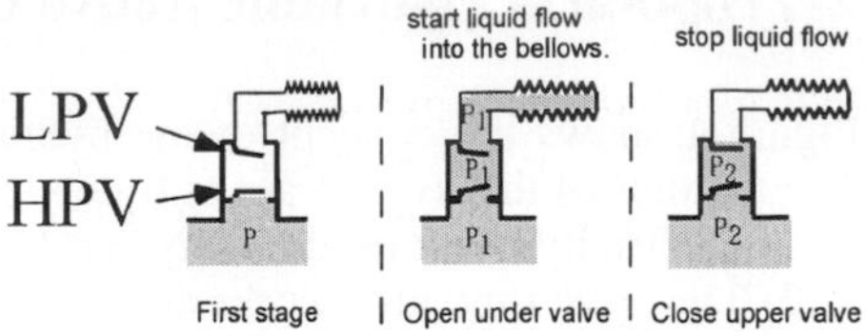

Fig. 2. Basic Principle of Band Pass Valve

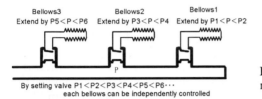

Fig. 3. The one input multi-output control mechanism

In this way, any valve state can be controlled by regulating the inner pressure of one drive tube using the Band Pass Valve (BPV), and so each associated joint can be controlled.

4 Design and Development of a Prototype Band Pass Valve (BPV)

To configure the proposed BPV, it is necessary to develop a pair of valves as mentioned above, HPV and LPV.

4.1 Design of HPV

Figure 4 shows the basic structure of the High Pass Valve (HPV). This valve is structured to block the flow path with a core material which is pressed by an elastic membrane.

No leakage occurs from HPV in its closed state due to the complete blocking of the flow path with the core material. When the inner pressure exceeds the elastic membrane pressure against the core material, the valve opens as the core material is lifted, and fluid is discharged.

4.2 Design of LPV

Figure 5 shows the basic structure of the Low Pass Valve (LPV). This valve is structured such that its elastic membrane covers a keyhole shaped channel.

When the inner pressure is low, fluid discharges from the gap between the flow path and the elastic membrane. When the inner pressure increases, the elastic membrane is pressed to block the flow path and thus fluid discharge is stopped.

4.3 Development of a Prototype Band Pass Valve (BPV)

Prototypes of HPV and LPV were developed as to verify the mechanism based on the valve designs described in sections 4.1 and 4.2. Then, by connecting these two proto-type valves, a prototype BPV was made as shown in Fig. 6.

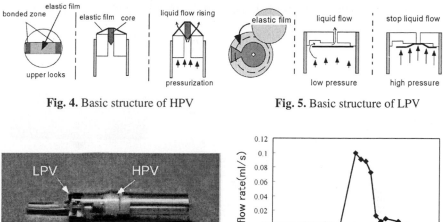

Fig. 4. Basic structure of HPV   **Fig. 5.** Basic structure of LPV

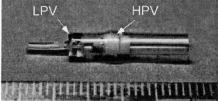

Fig. 6. Prototype of BPV

Fig. 7. Experimental evaluation on Pressure dependent flow rate of BPV

4.4 Characteristic Evaluation of BPV

The characteristics of the prototype BPV were evaluated. Figure 7 shows the test results of the relationship between the inner pressure and the outflow discharge of the prototype BPV. These data verified showed that in the band pass drive, fluid passed through the valve only when a specific pressure was applied.

5 Construction of Theoretical Model for Quantitative Design

Theoretical models of two component valves of BPV, the LPV and HPV, were con-structed in order to design the BPV quantitatively. In addition, an experiment to verify the constructed model was conducted.

5.1 Theoretical Model of LPV

First, the theoretical model of LPV was developed as shown in Fig. 8. Bernoulli's theorem was applied to this model to derive Eq. (1). Let k represent the modulus of elasticity of a circular elastic membrane of 1 mm diameter. This equation states that the pressure difference to close the valve (P_{close}) is inversely proportional to the cube of the diameter d of the elastic membrane.

5.2 Theoretical Model of HPV

Next, the theoretical model of HPV was developed as shown in Fig. 9. Equation (2) was derived by considering the force balance on the valve. (F is a bias force applied to core from elastic film.)

This equation states that the pressure difference to open the valve (P_{open}) is directly proportional to the modulus of elasticity of the membrane.

$$\Delta P_{close} = \frac{64\,h^3 k}{d_0^2 \pi} \cdot \frac{1}{d^3} \quad (1) \qquad \Delta P_{open} = \frac{k \cdot (l + l_0) + F}{A} \quad (2)$$

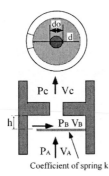

Fig. 8. Theoretical model of LPV

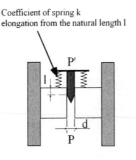

Fig. 9. Theoretical model of LPV

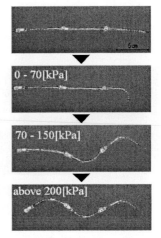

Fig. 11. First prototype of an active catheter with four active segments for verification of basic principle

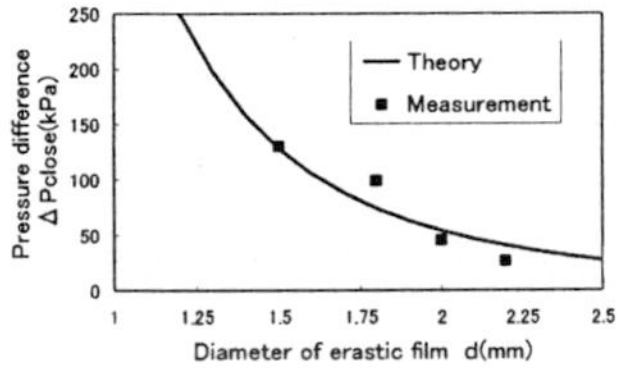

Fig. 10. The comparison of experimental result and theoretical model

5.3 Verification Experiment of Basic Principle

An experiment was conducted using a prototype LPV to verify our theoretical model. Measurement data were collected on the relationship between the diameter of the elastic membrane which blocks the flow path and the pressure difference when the valve is closed in this experiment. The results are shown in Fig. 10. The chart indicates that the data are very close to the ideal curve, and hence this theoretical formula enables the LPV to be quantitatively designed to close at a given pressure.

However, the theoretical model of the HPV could not be verified because of difficulty of quantitatively measuring the modulus of elasticity of the membrane. Nevertheless, the quantitative design with the developed model is sufficiently practical owing to the very simple operation mechanism of the HPV.

6 Driving Experiment of the First Prototype

A prototype of a hydraulic active catheter was developed which has three joints with BPV of the prototype verification model. A driving experiment was conducted with this catheter on a single-input, multi-output control mechanism (Fig. 11).

The results confirmed that each joint was driven independently by the pressure control on one drive tube, verifying that a single-input, multi-output control mechanism using drive fluid as a signal transmitter has been achieved.

7 Miniaturization of Band Pass Valve

The driving experiments proved the usefulness of the Band Pass Valve (BPV). However, the maximum diameter of the prototype active catheter used in the driving experiments was 6 mm, which is sufficient for experiments but too large for catheter use, and therefore it should be made smaller. To do this, the size of the valve must be reduced.

7.1 Problems for Miniaturization

Generally, miniaturization involves the following problems:
  1) Assembly operation
  2) Bonding part
In this system, each part should be made smaller to reduce the size of the valve. However, it is difficult to assemble such micro parts, and furthermore, the bonding part for valves hinders miniaturization. Airtightness is another important issue as the fluid must not leak from the valve.

To solve these problems, we devised the Hybrid IH process [5] .

7.2 New Fabrication Method Using Hybrid Micro-stereolithography (IH Process)

The Hybrid IH process is a shaping method developed in our laboratory, by the process shown in Fig.12. In this shaping method, first, UV curable epoxy resin is cured by laser and laminated as in the usual shaping method. Next, a part made from a different material is loaded in the middle of the shaping process, and a single piece is formed.

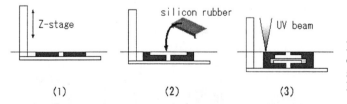

Fig. 12. Fabrication process of Hybrid micro stereolithography (IH Process)

The features of the Hybrid IH process are as follows:
  1) No need for assembly operation and bonding
  2) High airtightness
  3) 3D structures can be produced.

A leak-free miniature 3D structure can thus be easily produced by the Hybrid IH process.

7.3 Design of Micro-HPV and Micro-LPV

The following factors were taken into consideration to produce microvalves by the Hybrid IH process.

1) Selection of desirable materials for Hybrid IH process

2) Appropriate design for a single-piece style

Considering these points, the LPV and HPV are designed to make the most of the characteristics of the Hybrid IH process.

The LPV in the verification model had a keyhole shaped flow path covered with the circular elastic membrane. The shapes of the flow path and the elastic membrane were modified for miniaturization as shown in Fig. 13. The material of the elastic membrane was replaced with silicone rubber and formed into a platy, legged shape. There is no need for a bonding surface because the part is held in an insertion structure. The drive mechanism is the same as that in the verification model: when the inner pressure increases, the silicone rubber part changes shape, plugs the fluid path and stops the fluid discharge.

As for the HPV, the core material and the elastic membrane blocked the flow path in the verification model. Therefore it consisted of many parts and also the assembly was complex. These parts were therefore integrated into one silicone rubber part in the miniaturized model (Fig. 14); again, no bonding part is needed because the silicone rubber part is held in an insertion structure. The drive mechanism is also the same as that in the verification model. No leakage occurs in the closed state due to the complete blocking of the flow path. When the inner pressure increases, fluid is discharged from a gap which is formed by distortion of the silicone rubber part.

Since the mounting location on the drive tube is taken into consideration in designing both valves, the whole system is sleek even after mounting the valves to the tube.

7.4 Fabrication of a Prototype Micro-BPV

Miniaturized prototypes of the LPV and HPV having the designs described above were combined to make the BPV. Figure 15 shows a comparison of a micro-BPV made by the Hybrid IH process and a BPV unit used as a verification model in the driving experiment.

The valve diameter is reduced from 6 mm in the verification model to 3 mm using the Hybrid IH process as the figure shows.

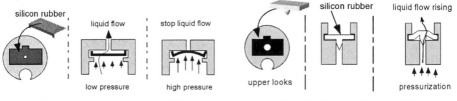

Fig. 13. Design of micro LPV   **Fig. 14.** Design of micro HPV

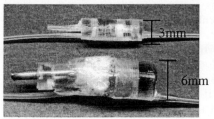

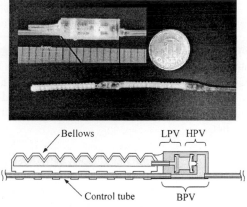

Fig. 15. Prototype of BPV and minia-turized BPV in 3mm diameter

Fig. 16. Cross section of an one segment of active catheter

8 Prototyping Two-Segments Active Catheter

A two-segments active catheter was constructed using the developed micro-BPV. The bellows and BPV are arranged along the drive tube. The size of a joint is 40 mm in length and 3 mm in diameter. The bellows as an actuator is made from silicone rubber; it extends easily on one side but not on the other, so supplied fluid readily bends it.

Figure 17 shows an prototyped active catheter on the finger tip. Each segment can be bent independently as shown in this figure. Master-slave pressure control system shown in Figure 18 was made for simple control by the doctors. Pressure range is enough low so as to decrease risk of break.

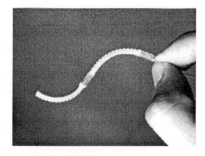

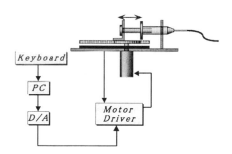

Fig. 17. Miniaturized hydraulic active catheter with two segments

Fig. 18. Pressure control system for master-slave bending of each segment

9 Insertion Experiment

An insertion experiment was performed using the constructed active catheter with two segments

The pathway for this insertion experiment is 5 mm in width and 5 mm in depth. Figure 19 shows a running insertion experiment, confirming that the two-segments active catheter is inserted smoothly. Moreover, it can easily be inserted into places where one-joint catheters are difficult to insert. In another experiment in the branched blood vessel, the active bending ability of this tool was verified as shown in Fig.20. It was much easy to select direction at the branching point.

Even a 3-mm diameter catheter can be used if the sites are confined. For future application to thin blood vessels such as capillaries, the system needs to be made even smaller.

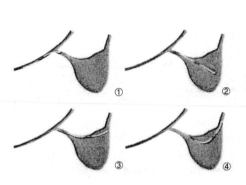 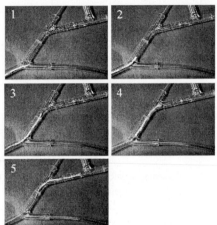

Fig. 19. Insertion experiment into blood vessel model

Fig. 20. Selecting direction at in the branched blood vessel model

10 Conclusion

An innovative hydraulic micro actuator system that controls multiple segments independently with single-input signal through fluid as a signal transmitter for safe medical tools was developed. And the prototype hydraulic active catheter using this mechanism was developed successfully. A driving experiment was conducted with the prototype active catheter and the results were favorable. Verification experiments of the theoretical models of valves confirmed that quantitative design was made. Moreover, a valve unit having the same function was made smaller using the Hybrid micro streolithography (IH process), involving micromachining technology developed by the authors, and an actual-size two-segment active catheter was constructed with these valves. The usefulness and safety feature of the developed active catheter was demonstrated by an insertion experiment.

References

1. Shuxiang Guo, Toshio Fukuda, Fumihito Arai, Makoto Negoro, Keisuke Oguro, A Study on Active Catheter System Structure Experimental Results and Characteristic Evaluation of Active Catheter with Multi DOF, Journal of the Robotics Society of Japan, Vol.14 No.6, pp.820-835, 1996.

2. M.Tanimoto et al, Improvement of Safety in Telemedicime System, Proc. of 3rd Robotics Symposia, pp.139-144,1998.
3. M.Esashi,Moption Control System by Micromachining, Plenary Proc. of 1998 JSME Conference on Robotics and Mechatronics (ROBOMEC 98), pp.5-13, 1998.
4. K Ikuta, M.Nokata, Minimum Wire Drive of Multi Micro Actuators Journal of the Robotics Society of Japan, Vol.16, No.6, pp.791-797, 1998.
5. K. Ikuta, S. Maruo, T. Fujisawa and A. Yamada, "Micro Concentrator with Opto-sense Micro Reactor for Biochemical IC Chip Family - 3D Composite Structure and Experimental Verification -," Proceedings of the IEEE International Workshop on Micro Electro Mechanical Systems(MEMS99), 376-381, 1999.

A Stem Cell Harvesting Manipulator with Flexible Drilling Unit for Bone Marrow Transplantation

Kota Ohashi[1], Nobuhiko Hata[1], Tomoko Matsumura[2],
Naoki Yahagi[2], Ichiro Sakuma[3], and Takeyoshi Dohi[1]

[1] Graduate School of Information Science and Technology, the University of Tokyo,
7-3-1 Hongo Bunkyo-ku Tokyo 113-8656, Japan
{kotaoha,noby,dohi}@atre.t.u-tokyo.ac.jp
http://www.atre.t.u-tokyo.ac.jp
[2] Graduate School of Medicine, the University of Tokyo,
7-3-1 Hongo Bunkyo-ku, Tokyo 113-8656, Japan
Naokiyah@aol.com, tmatsumu-tky@umin.ac.jp
[3] Graduate School of Frontier Sciences, the University of Tokyo,
7-3-1 Hongo Bunkyo-ku, Tokyo 113-8656, Japan
isakuma@k.u-tokyo.ac.jp
http://miki.pe.u-tokyo.ac.jp/lab.html

Abstract. We present the development of an innovative device (*Stem Cell Harvesting Manipulator*) to get hematopoietic stem cells for bone marrow transplantation. By using this manipulator, stem cells are harvested from the iliac bone of the donor with minimal puncture. Additionally, the time for carrying out harvesting and the contamination of T cells can be minimized. In this paper, we report the development of a prototype of the *Stem Cell Harvesting Manipulator with Flexible Drilling Unit*. The manipulator is inserted into the medullary space from the iliac crest and aspirates the bone marrow while an end-mill on the tip of the *Flexible Drilling Unit* drills through cancellous bone to create a curved path. We found that the manipulator can be inserted into the medullary space of the pig iliac bone 131 mm by 32.1 mm/min and harvests a phantom of bone marrow about 6 times as much in mass as the conventional Aspiration Method. Further consideration regarding whether or not this device can harvest viable hematopoietic stem cells should be considered through experiments using laboratory animals.

1 Introduction

Over the past three decades, Bone Marrow Transplantation (BMT) has been established as a curative form of therapy for various acquired hematological malignancies and congenital immune deficiencies such as leukemia or lymphoma [1,2]. On the other hand, the number of cases of BMT has been increasing so rapidly that it has become a problem to harvest hematopoietic stem cells from donors' bone marrow in the iliac bone invasively by means of the conventional "Aspiration Method" using bone marrow needles [3]. Though animal studies have been made on harvesting

T. Dohi and R. Kikinis (Eds.): MICCAI 2002, LNCS 2488, pp. 192–199, 2002.

methods from the long bone [4,5], alternatives to the Aspiration Method, how to collect stem cells from a donor's iliac bone, have not been examined to this time.

Briefly stated, there are problems with the"Aspiration Method": the invasiveness of punctures by bone marrow needles and the low density of harvested graft [6]. Doctors generally aspirate about 10cc of bone marrow to be used as graft with each puncture and totally 500-1200cc from donors' iliac bone. That is to say, donors have to be punctured about 50-120 times by a series of harvest. Moreover, the density of harvested graft is so low that doctors aspirate much more graft than required. In other words, the harvested graft includes much contamination from peripheral blood, which contains greater than 20% of T cells that can cause acute graft-versus-host disease (GVHD, a sort of acute rejection) [3].

To tackle the issues, we propose a device (*Stem Cell Harvesting Manipulator*) to approach medullary space with flexible drill to create a curved path (*Flexible Drilling Unit*) and harvest graft using negative pressure generated by an actuator. *Flexible Drilling Unit* like catheter is inserted into medullary space of the iliac bone through a bone marrow needle as a trochanter while an end-mill on the tip of the unit drilled cancellous bone to create a curved path. Then *Stem Cell Harvesting Manipulator* generates negative pressure to harvest viscous bone marrow efficiently that contains stem cells (Fig.1). By using this method, dense hematopoietic stem cells are harvested within minimal puncture.

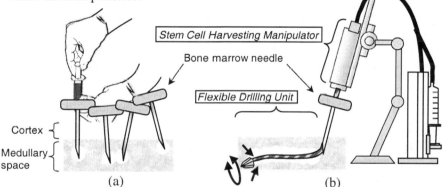

(a)   (b)

Fig. 1. Concept of the *"Stem Cell Harvesting Manipulator"* vs. the conventional "Aspiration method" (a) Aspiration Method [7]: To aspirate viscous bone marrow, doctors pull the syringe connected to the bone marrow needle as fast as possible to generate negative pressure. Stem cells only around the tip of the needle, however, can be harvested by a puncture. So, doctors have to puncture for many (50-120) points. (b) A new method for stem cell harvesting using *"Stem Cell Harvesting Manipulator"*: First, the end-mill on the tip of the *Flexible Drilling Unit* is inserted into medullary space and drills cancellous bone to create curved path. Then, the unit is inserted through the path and harvests graft

The clinical contribution of this study is to minimize invasiveness of donors by means of harvesting denser graft from wider area of the iliac bone with minimal punctures. Additionally, patients and doctors take benefits because risks of the GVHD and time needed for harvesting can be minimized.

The engineering contribution of this study is to develop a small device to drill into cancellous bone while creating a curved path with the *Flexible Drilling Unit*, and to generate negative pressure enough to harvest viscous bone marrow efficiently.

First of all, we have produced a prototype of *Stem Cell Harvesting Manipulator with Flexible Drilling Unit* and carried out in vitro experiments for evaluation using the iliac bone of the pig.

2   Methods

2.1   System Requirements

To design the prototype of the *Stem Cell Harvesting Manipulator*, we referred to a model of adult female human iliac bone. It is 5 to 24 mm in thickness and 153 mm in width. In order to insert the *Flexible Drilling Unit*, the unit is limited to less than 5 mm in diameter and more than 100-150 mm in length. The radius of curvature of the iliac bone is more than 60 mm.

The iliac bone is so curved that the *Flexible Drilling Unit* has to create a curved path; therefore the unit has to be flexible. Though a variety of new surgical tools with active bending mechanism are currently under development as part of computer assisted surgery (CAS) and stand-alone devices [8-13], it is not necessary for this unit to bend actively controlled by doctors because of the structure of the iliac bone. Once the unit reaches through the bone marrow needle to medullary space where stem cells are stored, the unit can move within only medullary space enclosed by cortical bone that is hard to drill through. In other words, cortical bone works as a guide.

2.2   System Overview

The prototype of Stem Cell Harvesting Manipulator consists of three units, the *Stem Cell Harvesting Manipulator* itself, the *Flexible Drilling Unit* and the power unit (Fig.2). The power unit generates negative pressure to harvest stem cells and rotation to drill cancellous bone. The *Stem Cell Harvesting Manipulator* is attached to an retainer that is generally used for clinical application. Harvested graft from the tip of the *Flexible Drilling Unit* is collected into a bag with an anticoagulant. Actuators on the power unit and an optical fiber photoelectric switch on the manipulator are controlled by a stored programmable motion controller (EMP2002-V1, Oriental Motor, Japan).

2.3   Flexible Drilling Unit

A flexible rod made of high carbon steel 0.8 mm in diameter transmits rotation to the end-mill on the tip of the *Flexible Drilling Unit* (Fig.3a). A liner tube made of helical stainless sheet and coated with PVC operates as a path of harvested graft. To drill through fragile cancellous bone, we selected a tip of the self-drilling screw as the end-mill 3.5 mm in diameter (Fig.3b). In order to generate strong flow on the tip of it, inner diameter of the tube is 2.2 mm, much larger than normal bone marrow needles, 1.6 mm. The length is 250 mm, total length of a bone marrow needle and insertion.

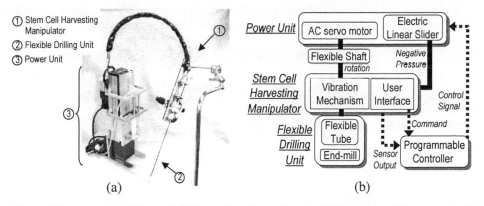

① Stem Cell Harvesting Manipulator
② Flexible Drilling Unit
③ Power Unit

(a)   (b)

Fig. 2. The prototype of *Stem Cell Harvesting Manipulator*: (a) Overview of the system: (b) System configuration: it consists of three units, the *Stem Cell Harvesting Manipulator*, the *Flexible Drilling Unit* and a power unit controlled by stored programmable controller

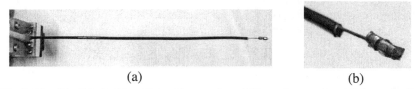

(a)   (b)

Fig. 3. The *Flexible Drilling Unit*: (a) overview: 250 mm in length and 3.5 mm in diameter (b) the end-mill on the tip of the unit: It rotates and vibrates axially. Graft is harvested from an aperture between flexible tube and the rod of the end-mill

2.4 Stem Cell Harvesting Manipulator

There are mainly two functions in the *Stem Cell Harvesting Manipulator* (Fig.4a). One is transmission of rotation and negative pressure from the power unit to the *Flexible Drilling Unit*. The other is user-interface to control linear movement of the manipulator and collection of graft manually by doctors. The rotation from the power unit transmits to the end-mill through the intermediary of the vibration mechanism (Fig.4b).

By means of collisions between hammering parts of the mechanism, the end-mill vibrates axially 16.7 Hz by 250 rpm to crush and drill cancellous bone. Additionally, not to drill through cortical bone accidentally and injure internal organs, the mechanism doesn't transmit power until the end-mill receive valid axial counter force from cancellous bone detected by an optical fiber photoelectric sensor.

2.5 The Power Unit for Negative Pressure and Drilling

To generate negative pressure, the power unit contains an electric linear slider. The slider is equipped with a 60cc syringe normally used in clinical field and pulls it like a syringe pump. The stroke of the slider is 100 mm. A tube to transmit negative pressure is connected from the syringe to the *Stem Cell Harvesting Manipulator* through check valves not to generate backward flow accidentally.

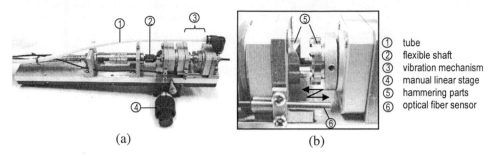

①	tube
②	flexible shaft
③	vibration mechanism
④	manual linear stage
⑤	hammering parts
⑥	optical fiber sensor

(a)   (b)

Fig. 4. the *Stem Cell Harvesting Manipulator*: (a) overview: the manipulator is fixed on a linear stage the stroke of which is 300 mm. (b) the vibration mechanism: By means of collisions between hammering parts, the end-mill vibrates axially to crush and drill cancellous bone

The power unit also generates rotation for end-mill by an AC servo-motor. The shaft of the motor is connected with the vibration mechanism of the Manipulator through the intermediary of a flexible shaft that is 800 mm in length and 8.0 mm in diameter.

3   Results

3.1   In vitro Experiment of Drilling

We had experiments for evaluation about mechanical performance of drilling using iliac bone of the pig, which is similar to that of human in respect of cutting [14]. The prototype was inserted into medullary space from a spot in the iliac crest.

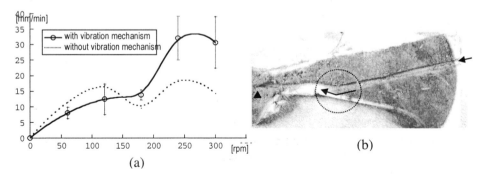

(a)   (b)

Fig. 5. Results of experiments for evaluation about mechanical performance of drilling using iliac bone of the pig: (a) the relation between rotation speed and the velocity of insertion: It is found that drilling with the vibration mechanism (*solid line*) had an advantage of that without the mechanism (*dotted line*) in velocity of insertion especially over 200 rpm. (b) a cross section of the curved path created by the *Flexible Drilling Unit*: It is 131 mm in length and 3.9 mm in diameter. The turning point (*dotted circle*) can be seen

Firstly, we measured the relation between the velocity of insertion and rotation speed both with and without the vibration mechanism (Fig.5a). The velocity rose continuously and slightly till 200 rpm and rose rapidly between 200-250 rpm. Additionally, it is found that drilling with vibration mechanism had an advantage of that without the mechanism in velocity of insertion especially over 200 rpm.

Secondly, we tried inserting the unit into medullary space as deep as possible and measure the depth to estimate whether the unit can drill cancellous bone and approach wide area of iliac bone (Fig.5b). It was found that the unit could create a path over 75.0 mm to 131 mm in length while cortical bone worked as a guide and changed the direction of the end-mill. The path connected from the point of the iliac crest to the acetabulum.

3.2   Phantom Experiment of Harvesting

We had experiments for evaluation about mechanical performance of harvesting using agar as a phantom of the bone marrow. The phantom was harvested by two methods, the Aspiration Method using bone marrow needle and our method using the *Stem Cell Harvesting Manipulator* (Fig.6). Then, We measured both of the weight of the harvested phantom. As a result, the graft harvested by a puncture is 3.10 g by Aspiration Method on average and 18.8 g by our method.

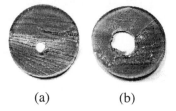

(a)   (b)

Fig. 6. Comparison of the harvested phantoms (made of agar) between conventional Aspiration Method and *Stem Cell Harvesting Manipulator*: (a) the phantom harvested by the Aspiration Method: It is 8.54 mm in diameter and 3.10 g in weight. (b) the phantom harvested by the *Stem Cell Harvesting Manipulator*: It is 20.4 mm in diameter and 18.8 g in weight on average. That is, the manipulator can harvest graft from wider area

4   Discussion

4.1   Mechanical Performance

On the basis of the results of the experiments, it is found that the prototype has possibility to drill into iliac bone. As I mentioned before, the width of human iliac bone is less than about 150 mm, enough for the prototype to create curved path. Additionally, the vibration mechanism on the Flexible Drilling Unit showed adequate performance as a drilling mechanism for iliac cancellous bone though there was much dispersion. To optimize the mechanism for drilling, further study about modeling of interaction between end-mill and bone [15].

According to the experiment of harvesting, it can be said that the new method has capacity to harvest graft from wider area; however, we must take much consideration about the difference of mechanical behavior between the phantom made of agar and real bone marrow. In addition, stem cell is stored in vacancies of cancellous bone, much different from the phantom. We will reconsider these points and optimize the mechanical performance through animal experiments.

4.2   Perspective

Further consideration should be given whether our new method using the *Stem Cell Harvesting Manipulator* can collect viable hematopoietic stem cells enough to be used as graft for bone marrow transplantation. To confirm it, we should test the harvested graft for some biological tests by means of colony assay and flow cytometry.

It is true that peripheral blood stem cell transplantation (PBSCT, harvesting stem cells from peripheral blood) has been increasing, but some troubles about donors have been reported recently [3]. On the other hand, methods for stem cell ex vivo expansion are developing [16,17], but they were still used for few cases so far. Indeed, the Stem Cell Harvesting Manipulator would work in cooperation with these methods.

Today, the significance of bone marrow cells has been increasing rapidly from the viewpoint of not only cure for immune deficiencies and hematological malignancies [18] but also tissue engineering [19,20]. It can be said that the method for stem cell harvesting will play a more important part in the near future.

5   Conclusion

First, we have developed a new method for stem cell harvesting for bone marrow transplantation using an innovative device, *Stem Cell Harvesting Manipulator* with *Flexible Drilling Unit*. By using this manipulator, dense stem cells are harvested from iliac bone of the donor within minimal puncture.

Then, we produced a prototype of the manipulator and did experiments for estimation whether it can create curved path and harvest phantom of bone marrow. Through the experiments using pig iliac bone, the manipulator is inserted into the medullary space from the iliac crest 75.0-131 mm by 32.1 mm/min, enough to sweep the iliac bone. Moreover, the prototype aspirated the phantom of bone marrow 18.8 g by one puncture, about six times as much as the conventional Aspiration Method.

It has been clear that the *Stem Cell Harvesting Manipulator*, inserted into medullary space curvedly using the *Flexible Drilling Unit* and harvesting stem cells mechanically, have possibility to become an alternative of the Aspiration Method and minimize the invasiveness to donors and patients.

References

1. E. D. Thomas: Does bone marrow transplantation confer a normal life span. , N. Engl. J. of Med. (1999) 341, pp. 50-51

2. J. M. Rowe, H. M. Lazarus and A. M. Carella: Handbook of Bone Marrow Transplantation, Martin Dunitz, London (1997) vii

3. S. J. Forman, K. G. Blume and E. D. Thomas: Bone Marrow Transplantation, Blackwell Scientific Publications, Boston (1999) ch.21, pp. 259-269

4. T. Kushida, M. Inaba, K. Ikebukuro, T. Nagahama, H. Oyaizu, H. Lee, T. Ito, N. Ichioka, H. Hisha, K. Sugiura, S. Miyashima, N. Ageyama, F. Ono, H. Iida, R. Ogawa and S. Ikehara: "A New Method for Bone Marrow Cell Harvesting", Stem Cells, Vol. 18, No.6 (2000) pp. 453-456

5. K. Ohashi, T. Shibata, N. Hata, N. Yahagi, T. Matsumura, E. Kobayashi, I. Sakuma and T. Dohi: "Development of Minimally Invasive Bone Marrow Cell Harvester", Proc. of The 10th Meeting of JSCAS (2001) pp. 101

6. H. J. Deeg, H. –G. Klingemann, G. L. Phillips and G. Van Zant: A Guide to Blood and Marrow Transplantation 3rd edn, Springer-Verlag, Berlin Heidelberg (1999) ch. 2, pp. 75-80

7. Islam: Manial of Bone Marrow Examination, harwood academic publishers, Amsterdam (1990) ch. 2, pp. 5-29

8. P. Dario: A Novel Mechatronic Tool for Computer-Assisted Arthroscopy, IEEE Trans. on Information Technology in Biomedicine Vol.4, No.1 (2000) pp. 15-28

9. R. Nakamura, T. Oura, E. Kobayashi, I. Sakuma, T. Dohi, N. Yahagi, T. Tsuji, D. Hashimoto, M. Shimada and M. Hashizume: Multi-DOF Forceps Manipulator System for Laparoscopic Surgery, Proc. of 4th MICCAI (2001) pp. 606-613

10. P. Dario, C. Paggetti, N. Troisfontaine, E. Papa, T. Ciucci, M. C. Carrozza and M. Marcacci: A miniature steerable end-effector for application in an integrated system for computer-assisted arthroscopy, Proc. of ICRA Vol.2 (1997) pp. 1573-1579

11. T. Fukuda, S. Guo, K. Kosuge, F. Arai, M. Negoro and K. Nakabayashi: Micro active catheter system with multi degrees of freedom, Proc. of ICRA (1994) pp. 2290-2295

12. H. Rininsland: ARTEMIS. A telemanipulator for cardiac surgery, Europian J. of Cardiothoracic Surgery 16 Suppl.2, (1999) pp. s106-s111

13. K. Ikuta, T. Kato, S. Nagata: Micro active forceps with optical fiber scope for intra-ocular microsurgery, Proc. of the IEEE MEMS (1996) pp. 456-461

14. S. Itoh: Bull. of Japan Society of Mechanical Engineers 26-222 (1983) pp. 2295

15. V. G. Kaburlasos, V. Petridis, P. Brett and D. Baker: Learning a linear association of drilling profiles in stapedotomy surgery, Proc. of ICRA Vol.1 (1998) pp. 705-709

16. J. Jaroscak: A phase 1 trial of augment of unrelated umbilical cord blood transplantation with ex-vivo expanded cells, Blood Suppl.1, (1998) pp. 646a

17. X. Sui: gp130 and c-Kit signalings synergize for ex vivo expansion of human primary hematopoietic progenitor cells, Proc. of Natl. Acad. Sci. USA 92 (1995) pp. 2859-2863

18. M. Marmont: Immune ablation followed by allogeneic or autologous bone marrow transplantation: a new treatment for severe autoimmune diseases? , Stem Cells Vol.12 (1994) pp. 125-135

19. J. Kohyama, H. Abe, T. Shimazaki, A. Koizumi, K. Nakashima, S. Gojo, T. Taga, H. Okano, J. Hata and A. Umezawa: Brain from bone: efficient "meta-differentiation" of marrow stroma-derived mature osteoblasts to neurons with Noggin or a demethylating agent. , Differentiation Oct;68 (4-5) (1996) pp. 235-44

20. P. Bianco, M. Riminucci, S. Gronthos, PG. Robey: Bone marrow stromal stem cells: nature, biology, and potential applications, Stem Cells, 19(3) (2001) pp. 180-92

Liver Tumor Biopsy
in a Respiring Phantom with the Assistance
of a Novel Electromagnetic Navigation Device

Filip Banovac[1,2], Neil Glossop[3], David Lindisch[1],
Daigo Tanaka[1], Elliot Levy[1,2], and Kevin Cleary[1]

[1] Imaging Sciences and Information Systems Center (ISIS), Department of Radiology,
Georgetown University, 2115 Wisconsin Avenue, Suite 603, Washington, DC, U.S.A.
{Banovac,Lindisch,Tanaka,Levy,Cleary}@isis.imac.georgetown.edu
[2] Georgetown University Hospital, 3800 Reservoir Road, N.W., Washington, DC, U.S.A.
[3] Traxtal Technologies LLC, 5116 Bissonnet, Bellaire, TX 77401

Abstract. The purpose of this study was to evaluate our ability to insert magnetically tracked needles into liver phantom tumors which move simulating physiologic respiration. First, a novel image-guided platform based on a new magnetic tracking device (AURORA™) was constructed. Second, an accuracy evaluation of a compatible magnetically tracked needle (MagTrax) was performed. Finally, 16 liver tumor punctures were attempted using only the image-guided platform for guidance. The inherent MagTrax needle positional error was 0.71±0.43 mm in the non-surgical laboratory setting. Successful puncture of liver tumors was achieved in 14 of 16 attempts (87.5%) by two users. The average time of each procedure was short (163±57 seconds.) The system adequately displayed the moving liver allowing for tumor target visualization and targeting. The AURORA based navigation platform and the compatible MagTrax needle appear promising for more rigorous phantom accuracy studies and *in vivo* tumor puncture testing in a respiring animal.

1   Introduction

Image-guided systems for intervention in the thorax and abdomen have not been developed, in part because of problems related to organ motion induced by respiration. The internal organs are not rigid nor directly accessible and therefore difficult to track and register for purposes of image guidance. This is in contrast to intracranial and musculoskeletal interventions where image-guided systems based on bony landmarks have been developed by many researchers and commercial systems are available.

In particular, the need for organ tracking and precision instrument placement in liver procedures has multiple clinical justifications. Tumor biopsy, radiofrequency ablation of tumors, portal and hepatic venous access for intrahepatic shunts, and billiary access for drainage all require precision for procedural success. The liver predominately moves in a cranio-caudal direction during quiescent physiologic breathing exhibiting displacements from 10 to 25 mm [1, 2]. For open surgery, Herline et al. explored the feasibility of surface based registration methods for intraoperative liver tracking [3]. They also showed the feasibility of liver tracking in open and laparoscopic procedures [4]. However, for percutaneous minimally invasive procedures, the only clinically accepted methods are direct visualization with fluoroscopy or ultrasound, each of which has its own shortcomings.

T. Dohi and R. Kikinis (Eds.): MICCAI 2002, LNCS 2488, pp. 200–207, 2002.

Several image-guided surgical systems based on magnetic position tracking are currently commercially available. BioSense Webster, a Johnson and Johnson company, offers two navigational systems for cardiac catheterization and mapping, the NOGA™ and CARTO™ systems. This product has been used in early clinical studies showing feasibility for intracranial neuro-navigation [5] and cardiac mapping in treatment of arrhythmias [6]. Solomon et al. used the Biosense system to assist in placement of a transjugular intrahepatic portosystemic shunt (TIPS) in swine [7]. For endoscopic sinus surgery, Visualization Technologies Inc. a subsidiary of General Electric (Lawrence, MA) sells the InstaTrack 3000® image-guided surgery system.

A magnetic positioning guidance system that is targeted at intra-abdominal interventions is the UltraGuide1000 (UltraGuide, Tirat Hacarmel, Israel). The UltraGuide device was introduced to complement currently used sonographic guidance techniques, especially to enhance the freehand techniques. The device uses small magnetic sensors attached to the hub or the shaft of the needle to help the user navigate the needle to the target. Howard et al. and Krombach et al. independently reported the successful use of UltraGuide to perform liver and kidney percutaneous procedures respectively [8, 9]. Wood et al. reported the use of the same device in RF ablation of renal cell carcinoma [10].

The purpose of this study was to evaluate the usefulness of magnetic tracking and image guidance for precision biopsy of simulated lesions in a moving liver phantom. This study was based on a liver respiratory motion simulator developed by our group and the AURORA magnetic tracking system under development by Northern Digital Inc., Ontario, Canada. An accuracy evaluation of a newly developed, commercially available and AURORA compatible needle was also performed.

2   Materials and Methods

2.1   Liver Respiratory Motion Simulator

To evaluate magnetic tracking for minimally invasive abdominal interventions, the Georgetown group has developed a liver respiratory motion simulator. The simulator includes a synthetic liver mounted on a motion platform. The simulator consists of a dummy torso, a synthetic liver model, a motion platform, a graphical user interface, the AURORA magnetic tracking system, and a magnetically tracked needle and catheter as previously described [11, 12].

2.2   Liver Phantom

A human torso model containing a liver phantom was modified from our previously described prototype [12]. The liver phantom was made from a two part flexible foam (FlexFoam III, Smooth-On, Easton, PA) which was cast from a custom made mold. The foam material was cured to approximately simulate liver tissue resistance to needle puncture. Two spiculated, silicone, elliptical tumors (maximum diameters of 3.1 and 2.2 cm) containing radio-opaque CT contrast were incorporated into the liver model prior to curing to serve as tumor targets. The liver was attached to a linear motion platform at the base of the torso's right abdomen (Figure 1).

The platform can be programmed to simulate physiologic cranio-caudal motion of the liver with options for respiratory rate control, breath depth, and breath pause (breath hold). A ribcage and single layer latex skin material (Limbs and Things, Bristol, UK) were added for aesthetic and physical reality.

2.3   Magnetic Tracking Device and Sensors

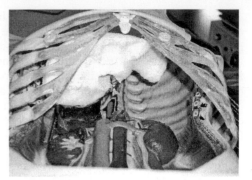

Fig. 1. A foam liver model (white) mounted on a linear platform inside the torso model

A prototype of a new magnetic field based tracking system, the AURORA, was used in the experiments. The system consists of a control unit, sensor interface device, and field generator as shown in Figure 2.

The AURORA uses cylindrically shaped sensors that are extremely small (0.9 mm in diameter and 8 mm in length). This enables the sensors to be embedded into surgical instruments. We used two magnetically tracked instruments in these experiments: 1) A prototype 5-French catheter with an embedded sensor coil was provided by the manufacturer; and 2) A needle/probe combination (MagTrax) as shown in Figure 3.

The MagTrax (Traxtal Technologies, Houston, Texas) needle/probe consists of a 15 cm stylette with a magnetic sensor at its tip and an 18-gauge trocar. This instrument was used in the study to puncture the tumors.

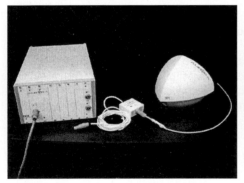

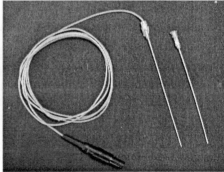

Fig. 2. AURORA control unit and field generator (courtesy of Northern Digital Inc.)

Fig. 3. MagTrax needle/probe with a stylette containing a magnetic sensor in its tip and leads exiting the hub. An 18-gauge trocar is seen on the right.

2.4   Guidance System and Software

A PC-based software application called ROGS (Respiring Organ Guidance System) was developed to assist the physician in performing the puncture of the liver parenchyma and needle guidance into the liver tumors. The system incorporates a graphical user interface [13] shown in Figure 4. The ROGS software allows for the loading of serial axial CT images, pre-procedural planning to the target of interest, tracking of respiratory motion, and real-time display of the biopsy needle as it approaches the target tumor. The sequence of steps in path planning and needle placement is shown in Figure 5.

2.5   MagTrax Needle/Probe Accuracy Evaluation

A MagTrax needle/probe containing a single five degree of freedom magnetically tracked sensor was solidly fixed to two passive optically tracked rigid bodies (small 50 x 50 mm and large 95 x 95 mm). The sensor assembly was moved randomly through 101 positions in a volume of 36 mm x 36 mm x 47 mm. At each location the sensor assembly was clamped and 10 samples from each of the targets were collected by the POLARIS optical system (Northern Digital Inc, Ontario, Canada) and AURORA magnetic system. The data sets were aligned by mathematical transformations and the difference in position and orientation of the two POLARIS sensors (control) versus the larger POLARIS sensor and MagTrax probe were calculated over the 101 positions. The experiment was performed in the absence of ferromagnetic interference.

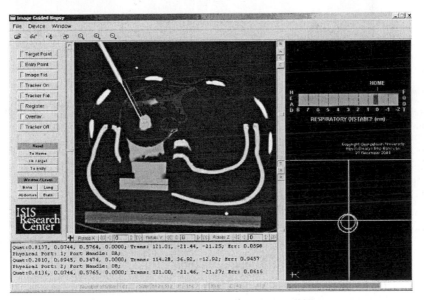

Fig. 4. Graphical user interface (center window shows probe overlaid on image, respiratory tracking in upper right, targeting window in lower right, *patent pending 2001-2002*)

2.6   Real-Time Tumor Biopsy Evaluation

A series of tumor targeting experiments were performed to test the usefulness of the system in accurately guiding a user to a target while the phantom resumes physiologic respiration. Two users (F.B. and D.L) independently performed 8 punctures each. The experimental design was divided into three stages as follows:

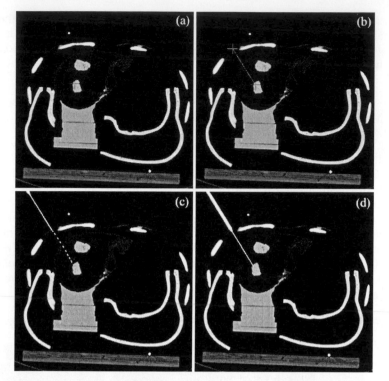

Fig. 5. Target tumor on an axial image of the phantom torso is selected by the radiologist (a); subsequently, the radiologist selects the skin entry point (b) and a planned path appears on the reconstructed image; the needle/probe is placed at the skin entry point (c) using cross hairs targeting window (Fig 4. lower right); finally, the needle is driven into the tumor (d) along the planned path indicated by the dotted line

Stage 1: CT Scanning and Registration

1. A magnetically tracked catheter was wedged in the hepatic vein of the liver. Several skin fiducials (multimodality markers, IZI Medical, Baltimore, Maryland) were placed on the rib cage.
2. A series of 3 mm axial slices with 1 mm axial reconstructions were obtained on CT VolumeZoom (Siemens, Erlangen, Germany) from the base of the lungs through the liver while the liver was kept in end-inspiration (simulating the breath-hold technique used in clinical practice).
3. The images were transferred to the ROGS using the DICOM standard.
4. The tracking catheter was left in the hepatic vein and the simulator was moved to the interventional radiology suite. The magnetic field generator was positioned near the phantom above the chest.
5. The position of the wedged catheter was read in the magnetic coordinate system. The position of the skin fiducials were read in the magnetic coordinate system by touching each fiducial with the MagTrax needle.
6. The position of the catheter and fiducials was determined in CT coordinate space by prompting the user to select these same points on the CT images.

7. A least-squares fit registration algorithm was invoked to determine the transformation matrix from magnetic space to CT space.

Stage 2: Biopsy Path Planning Phase
8. Each user was allowed one practice "planning phase" and "puncture (biopsy) phase" to get familiarized with the ROGS.
9. The user selected the target and a suitable skin entry point by scrolling through the axial images (figure 5a and 5b) thus selecting a biopsy path.
10. Simulated respirations were initiated at 12 breaths per minute with 2 cm cranio-caudal liver excursion.

Stage 3: Biopsy Phase
11. The MagTrax needle/probe was positioned on the skin entry point as determined in the "planning phase" and displayed by the ROGS overlay.
12. A real-time display of the current liver position was displayed by the ROGS system based on the position of the magnetically tracked catheter.
13. The MagTrax needle was tracked in real-time and the transformation matrix computed in step 7 was used to compute the overlay of the probe on the CT images which were reconstructed so to show the planned path of the needle.
14. When satisfied with the target position relative to the planned path, the user would initiate temporary cessation of respiration (simulating a 20 second breath hold in clinical practice). If the allotted time was exceeded, the phantom would continue spontaneous respirations for a minimum of 20 seconds (hyperventilation in clinical practice). Any partially inserted needle would be left in place as is frequently done during biopsy procedures.
15. Repeating step 14 the user would keep making minor adjustments to the needle until satisfied with the needle position as displayed on ROGS.
16. The time for each "planning phase" and "biopsy phase" were recorded. Multi-projection fluoroscopic images were taken at the end of each needle placement to ascertain whether the target tumor was successfully punctured.

3 Results

3.1 Accuracy Evaluation of the MagTrax Needle

Using the optical passive tracking system as the gold standard as described in the methods in Section 2.5, the mean measurement error and standard deviation of the MagTrax needle/probe using the AURORA system was 0.71 ± 0.43 mm (n=101) in a non-surgical environment. The maximum error noted was 2.96 mm.

3.2 Tumor Biopsy Evaluation

The targeted tumor was successfully punctured in 14 out of 16 biopsy attempts (87.5%). This was done without any additional real-time imaging guidance such as fluoroscopy. Instead, fluoroscopy was used to confirm the final location of the needle and evaluate accuracy.

Each user missed the target tumor once. In those instances, the maximal tangential distance from the lesion to the needle was 3.98 mm. On most occasions, the user was able to reach the tumor in a single continuous puncture after the needle was positioned on the skin entry point.   This was done within a single 20 second breath hold (pause in liver motion) in end-inspiratory liver position.   More than two breath hold cycles with intervening period of hyperventilation were needed on only 1 out of 16 experimental trials. The time needed for registration ranged from 173-254 seconds. The planning time, needle manipulation time, and total procedure times for the 16 trials are presented in Table 1.

Table 1. Planning, needle manipulation and total procedure times for ROGS assisted biopsy of tumors in a respiring liver phantom

	Mean Planning Time (s) ± SD	Needle Manipulation Biopsy Time (s) ± SD	Total Procedure Time (s) ± SD
User 1	72 ± 35	79 ± 40	151 ± 59
User 2	61 ± 31	111 ± 41	172 ± 43
Overall	71 ± 36	93 ± 43	163 ± 57

4   Discussion

Image-guided surgery is now an established practice for brain, ENT, and spinal procedures. These systems are based on optical tracking and bony landmarks. The introduction of a new magnetic tracking system with sensor coils small enough to be embedded into instruments may enable the development of image-guidance for abdominal and thoracic internal organs.

The overall goal of the research described here is to develop magnetic tracking for internal organs, including methods of compensating for respiratory motion. The initial results presented here show the feasibility of magnetic tracking, but much work remains to be done before this technology can implemented in clinical practice.

The accuracy of the MagTrax needle/probe used with the AURORA was measured as 0.71 mm. This should be sufficient for clinical practice. Additionally, the location of the magnetic sensor in the tip of the needle/probe means the instrument is not subject to errors introduced by needle bending unlike those used in the UltraGuide system where the proximal end of the needle is tracked [8].

The ROGS interface allowed a high success rate (87.5%) for needle puncture of the two small to medium sized simulated tumors. Most notably, the procedure was done while actively tracking the physiologic motion of the liver.   To our knowledge, ROGS is the first system that allows real-time compensation for the moving intra-abdominal target and subsequent compensated guidance for the needle puncture. The system was easy to use requiring only a single practice attempt to attain a satisfactory comfort level. The entire average procedure time lasted less than three minutes which is shorter than the time needed to perform this task during a conventional CT guided biopsy. These initial results are promising towards the development of a clinically useful system. Further experiments and animal studies are planned.

Acknowledgements

This work was funded by U.S. Army grant DAMD17-99-1-9022, an NIH National Research Service Award Fellowship (F32HL68394-01), and a CIRREF Academic Transition Award.. The content of this manuscript does not necessarily reflect the position or policy of the U.S. Government. The authors would like to thank Northern Digital, Inc., for the loan of the magnetic tracking system. The software was developed by Daigo Tanaka of Georgetown University and Sheng Xu, a graduate student in the NSF-funded Center for Computer Integrated Surgical Systems and Technologies at Johns Hopkins University.

References

1. Davies, S.C., et al., Ultrasound quantitation of respiratory organ motion in the upper abdomen. Br J Radiol, 1994. **67**(803): p. 1096-102.
2. Suramo, I., M. Paivansalo, and V. Myllyla, Cranio-caudal movements of the liver, pancreas and kidneys in respiration. Acta Radiol Diagn (Stockh), 1984. **25**(2): p. 129-31.
3. Herline, A.J., et al., Surface registration for use in interactive, image-guided liver surgery. Comput Aided Surg, 2000. **5**(1): p. 11-7.
4. Herline, A.J., et al., Image-guided surgery: preliminary feasibility studies of frameless stereotactic liver surgery. Arch Surg, 1999. **134**(6): p. 644-9; discussion 649-50.
5. Zaaroor, M., et al., Novel magnetic technology for intraoperative intracranial frameless navigation: in vivo and in vitro results. Neurosurgery, 2001. **48**(5): p. 1100-7
6. Gepstein, L., G. Hayam, and S.A. Ben-Haim, A novel method for nonfluoroscopic catheter-based electroanatomical mapping of the heart. In vitro and in vivo accuracy results. Circulation, 1997. **95**(6): p. 1611-22.
7. Solomon, S.B., et al., TIPS placement in swine, guided by electromagnetic real-time needle tip localization displayed on previously acquired 3-D CT. Cardiovasc Intervent Radiol, 1999. **22**(5): p. 411-4.
8. Howard, M.H., et al., An electronic device for needle placement during sonographically guided percutaneous intervention. Radiology, 2001. **218**(3): p. 905-11.
9. Krombach, G.A., et al., US-guided nephrostomy with the aid of a magnetic field-based navigation device in the porcine pelvicaliceal system. J Vasc Interv Radiol, 2001. **12**(5): p. 623-8.
10. Wood, B.J., et al., Percutaneous radiofrequency ablation with three-dimensional position sensor guidance. Cardiovasc Intervent Radiol, 2001(in print).
11. Cleary, K., et al. Development of a Liver Respiratory Motion Simulator to Investigate Magnetic Tracking for Abdominal Interventions. in SPIE Medical Imaging. 2002. San Diego, CA.
12. Banovac, F., et al. Design and Construction of a Liver Phantom for CT Imaging and Interventions that Simulates Liver Motion Seen During Respiration. in Radiologic Society of North America. 2001. Chicago, IL.
13. Cleary, K., et al. Feasibility of Magnetic Tracking for Image-Guided Abdominal Interventions Based on a Liver Respiratory Motion Simulator. submitted to IEEE International Symposium on Biomedical Imaging. 2002. Washington, DC.

Non-invasive Measurement of Biomechanical Properties of *in vivo* Soft Tissues

Lianghao Han, Michael Burcher, and J. Alison Noble*

Medical Vision Lab, Department of Engineering Science, Oxford University
{lhhan,burcher,noble}@robots.ox.ac.uk

Abstract. Quantitative descriptions of *in vivo* biomechanical properties of soft tissues are necessary for tissue evaluation and a meaningful surgical simulation. A hand-held ultrasound indentation system that can acquire force-displacement response in vivo has been developed. Using this system, non-invasive measurements of in vivo biomechanical properties of tissues are described in this paper. First, a linear elastic model was used to describe a porcine phantom material. Its Young's modulus was estimated via a mathematical solution from force-displacement curves. The estimated value of Young's modulus was in good comparison with those from a material test machine and 2D and 3D finite element simulations. Secondly, a finite element-based inverse scheme was used to reconstruct Young's modulus distribution of a three-layer phantom based on the displacement field measured from 2D continuous ultrasound images. Finally, in our primary study a pseudo-elasticity model was used to fit the experimental data of in vivo breast tissue.

1 Introduction

Soft tissue abnormalities are often correlated to a local change in mechanical properties. For instance, physicians use palpation widely as a qualitative diagnostic tool for breast cancer. However, this technique is subjective. More quantitative descriptions of *in vivo* biomechanical properties of soft tissues are needed for successful clinical applications in surgical simulation and planning, minimally invasive and tele-surgery, and image guided surgery and diagnosis. The biomechanical properties of soft tissues vary significantly from one individual to another, and can take on different values depending on whether they are measured *in-vivo* or *in vitro*. Unfortunately, most research has been focused on *in vitro* measurements of soft tissue under different loading conditions [1,2]. Very little quantitative information is available on the biomechanical properties of soft tissue *in vivo* in the literature [3,4].

A common method of assessing biomechanical properties involves using an indentation test, a procedure where an indenter depresses the tissue and the resulting deformation of the external surface is recorded. Indentation tests have been widely used for measuring material properties of soft tissues [4,6,7]. Because tissue's thickness will affect the indentation response [8,9], it is necessary to measure it. Using a combination of ultrasound techniques and some theoretical models [8,9], hand-held

---

* Correspondence to: Dr J.A. Noble

T. Dohi and R. Kikinis (Eds.): MICCAI 2002, LNCS 2488, pp. 208–215, 2002.
© Springer-Verlag Berlin Heidelberg 2002

ultrasound indentation devices [5,10] have been proposed to measure in vivo biomechanical properties of soft tissue, in which ultrasound techniques were used to measure tissue's thickness. The above indentation devices with a single element transducer were restricted to one-dimensional testing, and limited in investigating internal components of tissues. Recently, some reconstruction approaches [11,12,13,14] under the framework of inverse-problem solutions have been proposed to quantitatively reconstruct the material properties of tissues based on 2D internal deformation (displacement or strain) fields induced from an externally applied compression. In these methods, the displacement or strain field was obtained from a sequence of medical images (MRI or ultrasound). Combining indentation test devices, imaging devices and reconstruction algorithms, it is possible to investigate biomechanical properties of abnormal and normal components of *in vivo* tissues.

A 3D free-hand ultrasound imaging system with a force transducer was used for deformation correction in ultrasound imaging to produce an improved 3D reconstruction [15]. In the current study, this system was used as a novel hand-held ultrasound indentation system to measure in vivo material properties of tissues. Non-invasive measures of biomechanical properties on simulation material and *in vivo* breast tissue are described in this paper.

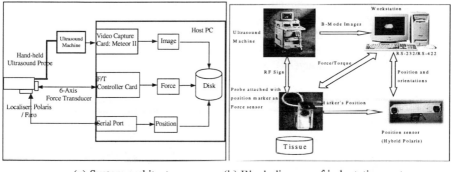

(a) System architecture   (b) Block diagram of indentation system

Fig. 1. Free-hand Ultrasound Indentation System

2 Material and Methods

2.1 System Description

A force transducer (Mini 40, ATI Industrial Automation) was mounted on a 3D free-hand ultrasound system developed in our lab to form an ultrasound indentation test system in which the ultrasound probe attached with a force sensor and 4 infrared LED's (position marker) formed a hand-held indenter. Figure 1(a) shows the system architecture. Figure. 1(b) presents the schematic diagram of the ultrasound indentation system. The ultrasound (B-mode) images were obtained using a conventional ultrasound machine (Sonos 5500(Agilent Technologies)) and a 7.5MHz linear array probe (Hewlett Packard L7540). A meteor II-MC frame grabber (Matrox Imaging, Dorval, Canada) was used to capture frames from the video output of the ultrasound machine. The position and orientation of the probe was recorded using a Polaris hybrid optical tracker (Northern Digital Inc, Ontario, Canada) that uses a stereo camera to measure the position of 4 infrared LED's mounted on the probe.

Software has been written in C++ that interfaces with the hardware components and controls the acquisition. The code is multi-threaded with separate threads acquiring video, position and force data. This allows the recording to occur asynchronously at the maximum rates determined by the acquisition hardware: 25Hz for video, 60Hz for position and force measurements.

2.2   Phantom

Two types of block-shaped phantoms were made to simulate soft tissue. One contained one layer, the other one contains three layers. Each layer was constructed of gelatin powder from porcine skin (G-2500, Sigma Ltd.). The gelatin powder was hydrated with deionized water and heated above its gel point to disperse the collide, clarify the solution and release trapped gases. Then, the liquid gel solution was cooled and poured into a box mould kept in an ice-water bath. While the gel solution was still in liquid form, talcum powder (Johnson's Ltd.) was added to increase the absorption and scattering. The phantoms were then stored at $10°C$. The one-layer phantom was constructed from 5% by weight gelatin. The three-layer phantom was constructed from 6%, 2% and 4% by weight gelatin from top to bottom (Fig.2). The one-layer phantom was of dimensions 120mm wide, 190mm long and 42mm high; the three-layer phantom was of dimensions 120mm wide, 190mm long and total 33.5 mm thick (first layer 8.7mm, second layer 10.8mm, third layer 14mm).

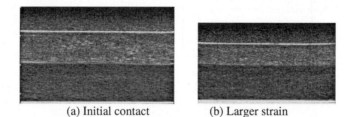

(a) Initial contact   (b) Larger strain

Fig. 2. B-mode images of a three-layer phantom at different compression

2.3   Measurement Procedure

The US-based indentation system was applied to phantoms and the breast of a volunteer. First, the probe was placed on the surface of the specimen with a minimal force. Then, the load was gradually increased manually and then removed. This was repeated a few cycles in each trial. Ultrasonic coupling gel (Parker Laboratories, NJ, USA) was spread on the contact surface of each specimen prior to indentation. The phantom was compressed with indentation rates approximately, 1-2mm/s, 2-3mm/s, and 5-10mm/s to investigate the effect of loading rate on measurement values. The maximum indentation depth was kept to within 20% of the initial thickness. During each experiment, the load, the probe position and 2D B-mode image (Fig.2) measurements were acquired simultaneously and stored to the computer disk. From the position information of the probe obtained with optical tracking system, via a co-ordinate transformation, the indentation depth was obtained. The tissue depth also could be measured from the B-mode images under the assumption that the speed of sound in soft tissue is a constant (1540ms^{-1}). In Fig. 2, B-mode images of one three-layer phantom are shown at different strains. Because there were unknown time delays in the position sensor, force sensor, ultrasound machine and frame grabber recordings, it was necessary to calibrate for the relative time delay between the storage of the ultrasound scan and the position measurement. In this paper, we employed the same method used by Prager et al [16].

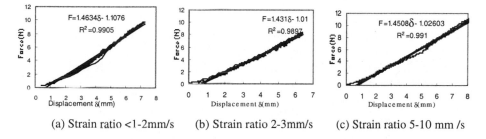

(a) Strain ratio <1-2mm/s   (b) Strain ratio 2-3mm/s   (c) Strain ratio 5-10 mm /s

Fig. 3. The force-displacement curves of a one-layer porcine phantom

3   Results

3.1   Single-Layer Phantom

Figure 3 shows experimental force-displacement curves of the one-layer phantom for three indentation rates. At the beginning of loading, the force-displacement curve shows slightly nonlinear behavior because of the incomplete contact between the probe and the phantom. When the indentation depth increases to about 1.0 mm, the probe and the phantom contact each other completely. The response of phantom to loading is now linear and nearly independent of the indentation rate. This demonstrates that the phantoms behave as elastic materials i.e. the viscous component is negligible.

The Young's modulus E can be calculated using a mathematical solution to the contact problems of a rectangular block on an elastic layer with finite thickness [17,18].

$$E = 2(1 - v^2)(\frac{2ap}{\delta})\kappa(v, {}^{h}\!/_{a}) = 2(1 - v^2)(\frac{F}{\delta})l^{-1}\kappa(v, {}^{h}\!/_{a}) \tag{1}$$

Here, v is Poisson's ratio, F the total applied force, l the probe's length, a the indenter half-width, $p=F/al$, δ the indentation depth, h the tissue thickness, and K a scaling factor. The scaling factor κ provides a theoretical correction for the finite thickness of the elastic layer, and it depends on both the aspect ratio h/a and Poisson's ratio v. Assuming phantoms to be nearly incompressible, the Poisson's ratio is taken to be 0.495 in the study, then $\kappa=ln(2h/a)-0.976+1.02(h/a)^{-2}-1.14(h/a)^{-4}$ [18]. The assumption of near incompressibility was made based on the fact that most tissue fluid would not have enough time to move within the tissue under a quick indentation

[19]. The ratio F/δ is determined by the slope of the load-indentation response shown as Fig.3. The value of Young's modulus of one layer phantom was *28.1KPa* from Eq.(1). The measured Young's modulus *28.6KPa* from a standard material test machine verified the above value.

The experimentally measured Young's modulus was also verified using two finite element(FE) models shown as Fig 4. Because the length(50mm) of contact area between the US probe and the phantom surface is larger than its width(14mm), a 2D FE model under the plane strain assumption was used to find the Young's modulus. A 3D FE model was also used. Four-node elements and eight-node elements (ABAQUS, HKS Inc. Pawtucket, RI) were created for 2D and 3D analysis, respectively. The interface between the US probe and the phantom was assumed to be frictionless because friction has a negligible effect on the indentation process for a thick-layer tissue[18]. Based on an elastic assumption, the Young's modulus of a homogeneous structure has a linear relationship with indentation depth under the same boundary condition. The Young's moduli determined by 2D and 3D FE analysis were *27.2KPa* and *29.8KPa*,respectively.

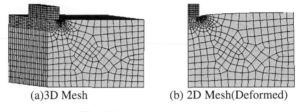

(a)3D Mesh   (b) 2D Mesh(Deformed)

Fig. 4. Finite element meshes

3.2   Multi-layer Phantom

To demonstrate how the same indentation probe can be used to estimate Young's moduli of different components of a tissue, a three-layer phantom as shown in Fig.2 was indented by the ultrasound probe. The internal deformation of three layers was measured by tracking the boundary lines between two different layers from a sequence of B-mode images [20]. The percentage deformation of the three layers is plotted against the total applied force in Fig. 5. Note that the second layer is softer than other two layers, and hence its percentage deformation is the largest. The first layer directly contacts with the probe, it is subject to a much larger local stress. Therefore, although the first layer is harder than the third layer, its percentage deformation is very close to that of the third layer. The Young's modulus of each layer in this phantom cannot be measured directly. To reconstruct the Young's modulus distribution, a finite element based inverse method has been developed [14]. An objective function relating the least-square difference of model-predicted and measured displacement fields from a sequence of 2D B-mode images is minimized with respect to the unknown Young's moduli. The solution can be obtained by iteratively adjusting the Young's moduli in the FE mode until the model-predicated displacements most closely match the measured displacements from ultrasound images. In order to obtain a physically meaningful solution, the Young's moduli are bounded with the lower and upper limits that are not considered in other research groups [11,12,13]. The finite element method acts as a forward problem solver to calculate the displacement field of a simplified 2D plane-strain model. A modified *Levenberg-Marquardt method* and an active set strategy are used to solve this constrained nonlinear optimization problem. For more details on constrained optimization, see [21]. Using this method the ratio of the Young's moduli among three layer materials was reconstructed as 1:0.298:0.562, which was comparable to 1:0.256:0.498 measured from three single-layer phantoms corresponding to three layers of the phantom respectively.

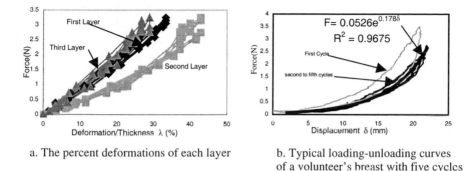

a. The percent deformations of each layer

b. Typical loading-unloading curves of a volunteer's breast with five cycles

Fig. 5. The Force-deformation curves

3.3 In vivo Test on Breast Tissue

Figure 5(b) shows the relationship between the force and external cyclically varying strain under the compression of the probe on the breast of a volunteer. The effect of preconditioning [1] of in vivo breast tissue is evident. With an increased number of cycles of force, the hysteresis decreases while the curve shifts to right. After around 2 cycles a steady state is reached. The breast tissue in vivo exhibited visoelasticity, linear and elastic model was no longer suitable to describe this material. Because the differences between the loading and unloading curves(Fig. 5(b)) after the first cycle are not large, we can describe the properties of the soft tissue by a pseudo-elasticity model[1]. Force and deformation response can be represented as $F(\lambda)=\alpha e^{\beta\lambda}$, in which λ is the stretch ratio δ/δ_0, δ and δ_0 are the compression depth and initial thickness, respectively, and F is the measured force. Taking the derivative $dF/d\lambda=\beta F$ results in parameter β as a measure of the stiffness of the tissue. In Fig. 5(b) the force and indentation response of breast tissue in vivo can be expressed as $F = 0.0526\,e^{0.178\,\delta}$, or $F = 0.0526\,e^{7.12\,\lambda}$ with an initial thickness 40mm at the measured position. The static expression of Eq.(1) can be extended to the dynamic case through the correspondence principle[1], so that Young's modulus is determined as $E=2(1-v^2)\kappa F/\delta l$. If we assume the breast tissue is incompressible, $E(\delta)=0.0526e^{0.178\delta}$. (The unit of Young's modulus is MPa).

4   Discussion and Conclusion

In this study, a hand-held ultrasound indentation system that can acquire force-displacement response in vivo was presented. Non-invasive measures of biomechanical properties of soft tissue derived using this system were described. One novelty of our approach in comparison to others [5,10] is we can quantitatively estimate not only integrated biomechanical properties of soft tissues (i.e. treating soft tissue as a homogeneous material) but also those of their internal components.

We presented phantom and *in-vivo* results. We showed that a linear elastic model could be used to model the phantom material over normal strain levels (up to 20%). The Young's modulus estimated from experimental data via a mathematical solution, showed good agreement with 2D FEA and 3D FEA results, which showed that a plane-strain approximation was valid in this study. Considering the effect of different Poisson's ratios, friction factors, geometry sizes and boundary conditions, more detailed 2D and 3D FE analysis has been doing to define the applicable range of this mathematical solution. *In vivo* testing on breast tissue showed the viscoelasticity of the tissue. A pseudo-elastic model was fit to in vivo indentation data. In the indentation experiment, since the full deformation-time record and force-time record were acquired simultaneously, this meant we could investigate the hysteresis, relaxation and creep of the tissue *in vivo*. Future work will focus on investigating these features of soft tissues such as breast tissue.

In this study, the indentation rates ranged from 1.0mm/s to 10mm/s, which was appropriate for manual control of the hand-held probe. It was shown that the indentation rate was insensitive to gelatin phantom measures. The same results were reported by Krouskop et al [22] for in-vitro tissues and Zheng et al [4] for in vivo plantar foot tissue.

Based on non-invasive ultrasound technique, the internal deformation field of soft tissue can be obtained. Consequently it is possible to evaluate abnormal and normal components of tissues. Both the Young's modulus and the Poisson's ratio can be reconstructed from this algorithm. In a primary study, using a finite element-based inverse reconstruction algorithm, the Young's moduli of a three-layer phantom were calculated. Good comparison was found between the reconstruction algorithms and experiments. This inverse reconstruct algorithm will be applied to clinical data in the future.

In this study, B-mode images were used to measure the displacement field. If raw RF signal data can be accessed from the ultrasound machine, this system can also act as a free-hand elastographic imaging system [23]. Because the force can be measured, quantitative Young's modulus can be determined rather than relative Young's modulus.

References

1. Fung, Y.C., Biomechanics-Mechanical Properties of Living Tissues. Second Edition, Springer-Verlag (1993)
2. Yamada, H., Strength of Biological Materials, Robert E. Krieger Publishing Company Huntington, New York.
3. Wang, B.C., Wang, G. R., Yan, D. H., Liu, Y. P. An Experimental Study on Biomechanical Properties of Hepatic Tissue Using A New Measuring Method. BioMedical Materials and Engineering. 2 (1992) 133-138
4. Zheng, Y.P.; Choi, Y.K.C.; Wong, K.; Chan, S.; Mak, A.F.T. Biomechanical Assessment of Plantar Foot Tissue in Diabetic Patients Using An Ultrasound Indentation System, Ultrasound in Medi.&Biol, 26 (2000) 451-456

5. Zheng, Y.P., Mak, A.F.T. An Ultrasound Indentation System for Biomechanical Properties Assessment of Soft Tissues in-vivo, IEEE Trans. Biomed. Engng. 43 (1996) 912-918

6. Mak, A.F.T., Liu, G.H.W. and Lee, S.Y. Biomechanical Assessment to Below-knee Residual Limb Tissue. J. Rehabil. Res. Dev. 31 (1994) 188-198

7. Miller, K, Chinzei, K., Orssengo G. and Bednarz P. Mechanical Properties of Brain Tissue In-Vivo. Experiment and Computer Simulation, J. Biomechanics, 33 (2000) 1369-1376

8. Hayes,W.C., Keer,L.M., Herrman,G and Mockros,L.F. A Mathematical Analysis for Indentation Tests of Articular Cartilage. J Biomechanics, 5 (1972) 541-551

9. Mak,A.F., Lai,W.M., Mow,V.C. Biphasic Indentation of Articular Cartilage-I. Theoretical Analysis. J. Biomechanics, 20 (1987) 703-714

10. Lyyra T., Jurvelin J., Pitkanem,P., Vaatainen U. and Kiviranta, Indentation Instrument for the Measurement of Cartilage Stiffness under Arthroscopic Control, Med. Eng. Phys. 17 (1995) 395-399

11. Kallel F, Bertrand M. Tissue Elasticity Reconstruction Using Linear Perturbation Method. IEEE Trans Med Imag, 15 (1996) 299–313.

12. Doyley M.M., Meaney P.M. and Bamber J.C., Evaluation of An Iterative Reconstruction Method for Quantitative Elastography, Phys. Med. Biol. 45 (2000) 1521-1540

13. Moulton M.J., Lawrence L.C., Ricardo L.A. An Inverse Approach Determining Myocardial Material Properties, J. Biomechanics 28 (1995) 935-948

14. Han L., J.A. Noble, M. Burcher, The Elastic Reconstruction of Soft Tissues, IEEE International Symposium on Biomedical Imaging: Macro to Nano (2002)

15. 15 Burcher, M., Han, L. and Noble J.A. Deformation Correction in Ultrasound Imaging Using Contact Force Information, Proc. IEEE Workshop on Mathematical Methods in Biomedical Image Analysis (2001)

16. Prager, R.W., Gee A.H., Berman L.. Stradx: Real-Time Acquisition and Visualisation of Freehand 3D Ultrasound, Cambridge University Engineering Dept. Technical Report, 1998.

17. Alblas, J.R, and Kuipers, M. Contact Problems of A Rectangular Block on An Elastic Layer of Finite Thickness, Part I :The Thin Layer, Acta,Mechica, 8 (1969) 133-145

18. Alblas, J.R, and Kuipers,M. Part II :The Thick Layer, Acta, Mechica ,9(1970) 1-12

19. Zhang, M., Zheng, Y.P and Mak, A.F.T. Estimating the Effective Young's modulus of Soft Tissue from Indentation Tests•Nonlinear Finite Element Analysis of Effects of Friction and Large Deformation, Med. Eng. Phys. 19, (1997) 512-517

20. Hayton, P.M., Brady, M., Smith, S. M. and Moore, N. A Non-rigid Registration Algorithm for Dynamic Breast MR Images, Artificial Intelligence, 114 (1999) 125-156.

21. IMSL Math/Library Manual, Visual Numerics, Inc.1997

22. Krouskop, T.A., Wheeler, T.M. Kallel, F. Garra, B.S. and Hall, T. Elastic Moduli of Breast and Prostate Tissues Under Compression. Ultrasonic Imaging 20,260-274 (1998)

23. Moyley, M.M., Bamber, J.C., Fuechsel, F. and Bush, B.L. A Freehand Elastographic Imaging Approach for Clinical Breast Imaging: System Development and Performance Evaluation, Ultrasound in Med.& Biol. 27,1347-1357 (2001).

Measurement of the Tip and Friction Force Acting on a Needle during Penetration

Hiroyuki Kataoka[1], Toshikatsu Washio[1], Kiyoyuki Chinzei[1],
Kazuyuki Mizuhara[2], Christina Simone[3], and Allison M. Okamura[3]

[1] National Institute of Advanced Industrial Science and Technology,
1-2 Namiki, Tsukuba-shi, Ibaraki, 305-8564 Japan
gacha@ni.aist.go.jp, washio.t@aist.go.jp, k.chinzei@aist.go.jp
[2] Dept. of Mechanical Engineering, Tokyo Denki University,
2-2 Nishiki-cho, Kanda, Chiyoda-ku, Tokyo, 101-8457 Japan
mizuhara@cck.dendai.ac.jp
[3] Dept. of Mechanical Engineering, Johns Hopkins University,
322 New Engineering Building, 3400 N. Charles Street, Baltimore, MD 21218, USA
csimone@titan.me.jhu.edu, aokamura@jhu.edu

Abstract. We present the tip and friction forces acting on a needle during penetration into a canine prostate, independently measured by a 7-axis load cell newly developed for this purpose. This experimental apparatus clarifies the mechanics of needle penetration, potentially improving the development of surgical simulations. The behavior of both tip and friction forces can be used to determine the mechanical characteristics of the prostate tissue upon penetration, and the detection of the surface puncture, which appears in the friction force, makes it possible to estimate the true insertion depth of the needle in the tissue. The friction model caused by the clamping force on the needle can also be determined from the measured friction forces.

1 Introduction

Needle insertion is a basic and least invasive method of treatment. However, surgeons must possess considerable skill and experience in order to control the needle path so that the needle may reach a preoperatively determined target inside the tissue. Because thin needles can deflect inside the tissue, and the tissue can also deform, surgeons must predict these deflections and deformations. Since surgeons commonly predict such behavior by feeling the force acting on the needle with their fingers, it is important to train realistic insertion tasks using a force-feedback needle simulator.

In order to simulate the forces acting on a needle, the mechanism of force generation should be clarified and modeled. Considering that the needle shaft rubs against the tissue while the needle tip cuts the tissue, the force on the needle shaft should be distinguished from that on the needle tip. Following this idea, we assumed three different forces acting on the needle as shown in Fig.1: the tip force acting on the needle tip in the axial direction, the friction force acting on the side wall of the needle shaft in the axial direction, and the clamping force acting on the side wall of the needle shaft in the normal direction. The tip force concerns the cutting force when the needle

T. Dohi and R. Kikinis (Eds.): MICCAI 2002, LNCS 2488, pp. 216–223, 2002.
© Springer-Verlag Berlin Heidelberg 2002

is penetrating the tissue, and its magnitude is affected by the shape of the tip of the needle. The Coulomb friction force is defined as the scalar product of the normal force acting on the surface and the coefficient of friction. Viscous friction, the product of a damping coefficient and relative velocity of the two materials, can also affect the total friction force. In the case of the needle, the normal force is determined as the total amount of clamping force. When the needle is inserted into the tissue, the clamping force increases due to the increase of the contact area between the needle and the tissue. The clamping force is the resistance force of the tissue compressed out from the needle path, which is affected by the incision shape in the tissue created by the needle tip, as well as the needle gauge.

The total axial force of the needle is the sum of the tip force and the friction force. Some researchers reported the total axial force of the needle. Hiemenz, et al. [1] and Westbrook, et al. [2] detected the puncture of ligamentum flavum or dura by the peak in the total axial force measured on the penetration. Brett, et al. [3-4] also measured and modeled the total axial force to identify the tissue type on the needle path on spinal anesthesia. All of them measured the total axial force acting on the needle, but did not separate the tip and friction force from the total axial force. Therefore, their data were insufficient to quantify each force even though Brett referred to the friction force in his model. Simone and Okamura [5] separated cutting and friction forces in experiments with liver tissue, but did not measure them simultaneously.

In this study, we independently quantified the tip and friction forces of a needle on penetration with a load cell newly developed for this purpose. Since we are considering the needle simulator of brachytherapy for the prostate, we inserted needles into the prostate of a canine cadaver, and investigated the mechanism of the generation of the tip and friction forces according to the experimental data.

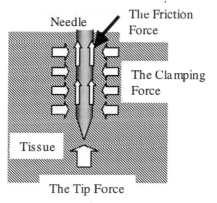

Fig. 1. The forces acting on a needle in tissue

2   Materials and Methods

In order to independently measure the tip and friction forces acting on a needle, a load cell named 7-axis load cell was developed. Figure 2 shows the structure of the 7-axis load cell, and Fig.3 shows the prototype used in the experiments. This load cell consists of an inner needle of 1.15mm diameter with a triangular pyramid tip and a cylindrical outer needle of 1.4mm diameter (similar to biopsy needles). The outer needle is attached to the load cell casing via a 6-axis load cell, and the inner needle is attached to the outer needle via a 1-axis load cell. Since only the tip of the inner needle appears outside the outer needle, the 1-axis load cell outputs the tip force of the inner needle. The 6-axis load cell outputs the total force and torque acting on the both needles. The load capacity of the 7-axis load cell is shown in Table 1. The tip force of this system is measured as the tip force of the inner needle, and the friction force is calculated by subtracting the tip force from the axial force component of the output of the 6-axis load cell.

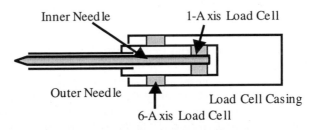

Fig. 2. Structure of the 7-axis load cell

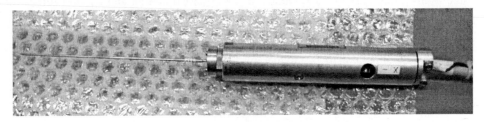

Fig. 3. Picture of the 7-axis load cell

Table 1. Maximum load capacity of the 7-axis load cell

Axis	Maximum Load Capacity
Fx, Fy	20N
Fz	50N
Ftip	10N (for measurement)
Tx, Ty	2Nm
Tz	0.3Nm

A fresh beagle cadaver (31kg weight) was prepared and frozen for 2 weeks until the experiment. After 3 days defrosting, it was laid supine on the operating table and the abdomen was opened to expose the prostate. The 7-axis load cell with a set of needles was attached on a linear stage above the prostate, and driven vertically at a constant speed of 2.95mm/sec. Figure 4 shows the experimental apparatus.

In our penetration procedure, the needle was first positioned 5mm above the surface of the prostate, driven down 25mm, then stopped and remained still in the prostate for 5sec. Finally, the needle was pulled up 20mm. Data from the 7-axis load cell were recorded at a 50Hz sampling rate, together with the trigger signal of the linear stage controller, by a PC computer. The data was analyzed after the experiment. The penetration was performed twice, changing the puncture positions on the prostate surface to prevent the needle from going into the hole created by the previous penetration. The motion of the needle in the cadaver was monitored by a biplane X-ray system during the penetration.

The total amount of the clamping force increases following the increase of the insertion depth of the needle in the prostate. Since the prostate surface is commonly compressed by the needle before its puncture, the true insertion depth of the needle was estimated by subtracting the compressed depth of the prostate surface from the driving distance of the needle by the linear stage.

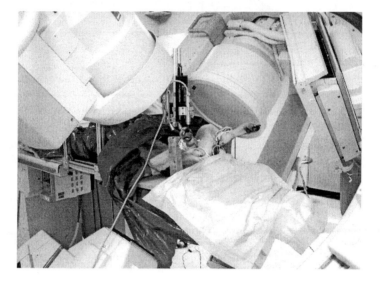

Fig. 4. Overview of the experimental apparatus with a canine cadaver. The tubes above the canine are part of the biplane X-ray system used to monitor the motion of the needle in the canine

3   Results

Figure 5 shows the forces acting on the needle and the position of the needle tip versus time during penetration into the canine prostate. Each force data point was plotted from an average five samples. The step line in the force plot is the trigger signal of the linear stage controller, and the position of the needle tip is plotted according to this signal. The thick lines indicate the total axial forces. The dotted lines indicate the tip forces. The thin lines indicate the friction forces calculated by subtracting the tip forces from the corresponding total axial forces.

The position of the needle tip is presented as 0mm at the prostate surface before the penetration, and positive in the insertion direction. The needle tip positioned at -5mm at the beginning, and touched the prostate surface about at 1.7sec. We defined this period as (A).

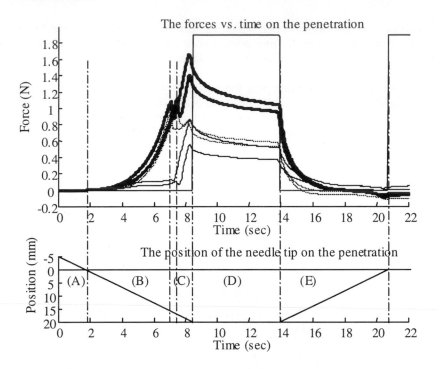

Fig. 5. The total axial, tip and friction forces vs. time together with the trigger signal of the linear stage controller and the position of the needle tip vs. time. The thick line indicates the total axial force, the dotted line the tip force, and the thin line the friction force. The step line indicates the trigger signal, which is high when the needle is stationary. The position of the needle tip is set as 0mm where the surface was before the penetration, and positive in the insertion direction

After the tip touched the prostate surface, the total axial forces increased exponentially and had two peaks. The first peaks were located at 7.2 or 7.5sec. We defined the period following (A) until the first peak as (B). During this period, the tip forces followed the total axial force until the first peak, but the friction forces remained low. The needle tip moved about 16mm during period (B) according to the needle speed. After the first peak the total axial forces decreased about 0.2N, and increased again until the needle stopped. We defined this period as (C). During period (C), the tip forces followed this decrease at the beginning, and remained constant with some noise. In contrast, the friction force increased proportionally to time. We defined the period following (C) until when the needle started to be pulled up as (D). During this period, all of the forces decreased exponentially, and the tip forces remained positive without being zero. The following period until the needle stopped again was defined as (E), where the forces decreased more drastically. The tip forces became negative at the end of (E).

After the whole procedure completed, it was observed that the needle tip was still inside the tissue even when the tip position was at the location of the prostate surface before penetration. At this time, the prostate surface was raised.

In these procedures, needle deflection was not observed on the X-ray monitors, and the transverse force of the needle, which was also measured together with the axial forces, was almost zero. Therefore, we ignore the transverse force in this report.

4   Discussion

Since the tip forces traced the total axial forces during period (B), and the friction forces remained low while they increased during period (C), it is considered that only the needle tip touched to the surface without insertion into the prostate during (B). This means that the first peak revealed the puncture of the prostate surface, and the needle just compressed the surface until the tip force reached the magnitude required for puncturing the surface membrane. Since this magnitude would change due to the shape and sharpness of the needle tip, needle simulators should differentiate the peak value according to the needle tip. The tip forces in (B) increased exponentially. This means that the behavior of the prostate tissue under compression by a point is not linear elastic. It is possible that this characteristic was caused by the non-elasticity of the tissue or the effect of shear stress on the surface membrane. Since the needle penetration into a swine hip muscle without skin revealed the same characteristic in our previous experiment [6], we suppose that the latter hypothesis has higher possibility. Further investigation is required.

The tip forces during period (C) decreased at first. This occurs because the force required to cut the tissue inside the prostate was less than that required to puncture the surface membrane of the prostate. The tip force slightly increased after the decrease. Assuming that the tissue inside the prostate is uniform, it is expected that the tip force remained constant after the decrease. We consider that this increase was caused by the resistance force of the tissue below the prostate against its compression, therefore the increase can be ignored for simulating the reaction of the prostate itself. The linearity of the increase of the friction force in (C) means that the friction force was proportional to the true insertion depth of the needle, since the true insertion depth also increased linearly with time due to the constant speed of the needle. The true insertion depth can be obtained by subtracting the 16mm surface motion of the prostate in (B) from the driving distance of the needle by the linear stage. Assuming that the uniform diameter of the needle generates the uniform clamping force along the axis, it is expected that the distribution of the friction force is also uniform along the axis. The linearity between the friction force and the true insertion depth encourages this assumption. Penetration with needles of different diameters is planned in order to investigate the relation between clamping force and needle diameter. It is expected that the slope of the friction force will increase following the increase of the needle diameter. In a needle simulation, the total axial force in this period will be represented as the sum of the tip force, which decreases at the beginning from the value for the surface puncture to the value for the cutting force of tissue and remain constant, and the friction force, which increases proportionally to the true insertion depth according to the needle diameter.

The decrease of all the forces in (D) is supposed to be caused by the viscosity of the tissue. Since the tip forces were not zero, the needle tip still compressed the tissue even when it did not cut the tissue. The decrease of the friction force was caused by the decrease of the dragging-up force of the tissue edge facing to the needle, not by the decrease of the contact area on the needle surface to the tissue, because it was observed that the prostate surface did not move during (D) in the X-ray images. Since it is considered that the decrease of both the tip and friction forces were governed by the same viscosity model, the total axial force in the simulation will be also represented by that viscosity model.

During period (E), the needle was drawn out from the tissue, and the tissue was also stretched simultaneously by releasing the compression. Considering that the tip force remained positive in the former part, it is possible that the stretch of the tissue started first, then the drawing of the needle followed, because the drawing of the needle would drastically reduce the force to zero or negative. The decrease of static friction force by the dragging-up force at the tissue edge facing to the needle (an exponential function of time) and the decrease of the dynamic friction force by the drawing of the needle (a linear function of time) occurred simultaneously. Thus, it is difficult to distinguish them. The reason that the tip force remained negative at the end of (E) is that the tissue was still held on the needle and the raised tissue pulled down the needle tip even when the needle at the location of the surface before penetration. For a simulation model in this period, the tip force will decrease exponentially in the same order as in period (B) until it reaches a negative value, which will be determined by the maximum true insertion depth. This depth is determined by the amount of the held tissue on the needle, and the friction force will also decrease, where the same exponential function as the tip force and the linear function for drawing out are added.

5   Conclusions

The tip force and the friction force on a needle during penetration into a canine prostate were independently measured by a newly-developed 7-axis load cell, and each force was related to the mechanical behavior of the prostate tissue. The change of the behavior of friction force during penetration revealed the puncture of the surface, and the true insertion depth of the needle in the tissue was also estimated from the puncture of the surface. The linearity of the friction force during the insertion imply that the friction force was generated uniformly along the axis by the constant clamping force depending on the needle diameter. The tip and friction force when the needle stopped revealed the viscosity of the tissue, and it was suggested that the tissue stretch is prior to the needle drawing when the needle was released. The overview of the needle simulation model was also revealed as the combination of an exponential function and a linear function. Additional experiments with the needles of different diameter and with different true insertion depths will be performed in near future.

Acknowledgement

This work is supported by AIST grant for international collaborative research and National Science Foundation grant ERC 9731748. The authors thank Dr. Rand Brown, DVM and Dr. Gabor Fichtinger for their assistance with experiments.

References

1. Hiemenz, L., Stredney, D., and Schmalbrock, P., "Development of the force-feedback model for an epidural needle insertion simulator," Medicine Meets Virtual Reality 6, pp. 272-277, 1998.
2. Westbrook, J. L., Uncles, D. R., Sitzman, B. T., and Carrie, L. E. S., "Comparison of the Force Requied for Dural Puncture with Different Spinal Needles and Subsequent Leakage of Cerebrospinal Fluid," Anesth Analg, Vol.79, pp.769-72, 1994.
3. Brett, P. N., Harrison, A. J., and Thomas, T. A., "Schemes for the Identification of Tissue Types and Boundaries at the Tool Point for Surgical Needles," IEEE Trans on Info Technol Biomed, Vol.4, No.1, pp.30-36, 2000.
4. Brett, P. N., Parker T. J., Harrison, A. J., Thomas, T. A., and Carr, A., "Simulation of resistance forces acting on surgical needles," Proc. Instn Mech Engrs, Vol. 211, Part H, pp.335-347, 1997.
5. Simone, C. and Okamura, A.M., "Haptic Modeling of Needle Insertion for Robot-Assisted Percutaneous Therapy," Proc. IEEE International Conference on Robotics and Automation, pp. 2085-2091, 2002.
6. Kataoka, H., Washio, T., Chinzei, K., Funamoto, Y., and Mizuhara, K., "Experimental Analysis of Resistance Acting on a Surgical Needle," Proc. NordTrib2002, Stockholm, June, 2002.

Contact Force Evaluation of Orthoses for the Treatment of Malformed Ears

Akihiko Hanafusa[1], Tsuneshi Isomura[1], Yukio Sekiguchi[1],
Hajime Takahashi[2], and Takeyoshi Dohi[3]

[1] Department of Rehabilitation Engineering, Polytechnic University
4-1-1 Hashimotodai, Sagamihara, Kanagawa 229-1196, Japan
hanafusa@uitec.ac.jp
[2] Department of Plastic Surgery, Tokyo Metropolitan Toshima Hospital
33-1 Sakaemachi, Itabashi-ku, Tokyo 173-0015, Japan
hajime-t@toshima-hp.metro.tokyo.jp
[3] Graduate School of Information Science and Technology, The University of Tokyo
7-3-1 Hongou, Bunkyou-ku, Tokyo 113-8654, Japan
dohi@miki.pe.u-tokyo.ac.jp

Abstract. In most cases, malformed ears of neonates can be effectively treated by fitting a suitably shaped orthosis. In this study, a finite element analysis system was developed to evaluate the contact force between the orthosis and auricle. In order to reduce the contact force, two methods for modifying orthosis shape were developed. One entailed the addition of a detour curve, while the other canceled out the insertion of the nodal point where maximum force exceeded the limit during the incremental step of finite element analysis. Moreover, two small sensors were developed, one using a silicon tube and the other a strain gauge, for mounting on the orthosis and measuring contact force. Straight, curved and maximum force-restricted orthoses were manufactured for an adult auricle. Simulation and insertion experiments using silicon tube and strain gauge sensors were performed. Results demonstrated that the strength of contact force between the orthosis and auricle decreased from straight type, through curved type to the maximum force-restricted type.

1 Introduction

Most cases of malformed ears of neonates can be treated by mounting an appropriately shaped orthosis in the auricle [1]. Currently, the authors use orthoses made of nitinol shape memory alloy wire covered with an expanded polytetrafluoroethylene tube. Examples of both a straight orthosis mounted on cryptotia and a curved orthosis mounted on a folded helix are shown in Fig.1. We have recently developed a computer-assisted design system [2] for use in constructing the orthosis.

It is essential to control the contact force between the orthosis and auricle, to ensure that it is sufficient to correct the auricle shape, while not excessive to the degree that it may cause a decubitus-like inflammation on the auricle. This paper describes the simulation results of finite element analysis, developed using MATLAB (The Math Works Inc.), to evaluate the contact force. Moreover, methods that could potentially reduce the contact force were tested using sensors mounted on the orthosis to measure this force.

T. Dohi and R. Kikinis (Eds.): MICCAI 2002, LNCS 2488, pp. 224–231, 2002.
© Springer-Verlag Berlin Heidelberg 2002

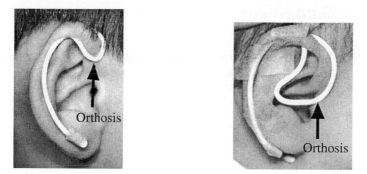

(a) Straight orthosis mounted on a cryptotia   (b) Curved orthosis mounted on a folded helix

Fig. 1. Examples of orthoses made of nitinol shape memory wire

2   Finite Element Analysis of Contact Force [3]

2.1   Methods

Finite element analysis is widely used to simulate deformation or determine strength of the structure. There are numerous examples of use of this analysis in the biomedical field, including simulation of maxillofacial functions [4], and pressure at the below-knee socket. To evaluate contact force between the orthosis and auricle, one should consider the following:
– The material property of an auricle is nonlinear.
– Both auricle and orthosis deform on contact with each other.
To contend with the former concern, an incremental method was employed, whereby force or displacement was increased step by step, and moving to the next step was dependent upon a relationship between stress and strain in the current step. Displacement was increased by inserting the orthosis gradually. Moreover, a tensile test using pig's auricular cartilage was performed, and the resultant strain-stress diagram applied to the material properties.

Multiple points' constraints were also used to represent the contact deformation of auricle and orthosis. The constraint was that the orthosis nodal point never penetrated the auricle and at most on the surface of the auricular element. Using the incremental method, the constraint condition should be updated at each insertion step. In some cases, surplus constraint may occur. At the surplus constrained nodal points, the constrained force pulls the auricle inward. These constraints should be canceled and the stiffness equation should be recalculated.

A function was added that can automatically modify the orthosis shape so as to avoid excessive contact force. Briefly, we adopted a simple method that canceled the insertion of the nodal point in an incremental step where the force exceeded the limit. As the cancellation of some nodal points may change the condition of multiple points' constraint and cause excessive force at other nodal points, the condition and force should be recalculated in the insertion step.

2.2   Simulation Examples

An adult male auricular model was constructed using multiple three dimensional data measured by the non-contact laser measurement system. Contours of the helix and auriculotemporal sulcus were extracted and approximated by spline using eight control points. Orthosis shape was produced by moving the third control point outward so that the top of the orthosis projected over the helix by 4 mm. Models for finite element analysis were made under the following conditions:

- The auricle was modeled by 1093 triangular shell elements. Results of a tensile test using pig's auricular cartilage were applied to the material properties.
- The orthosis on the helix side was modeled by 33 beam elements. Results of a tensile test using nitinol shape memory wire were applied to the material properties.
- Each nodal point had six degrees of freedom.

The orthosis was inserted in the helix in 8 steps increasing by 0.5 mm each. The start edge of the orthosis and auriculotemporal sulcus of the auricle were clipped. Fig.2(a) shows the orthosis deformation and the force produced by the contact, and Fig.2(b) shows distribution of the contact force on the auricle. The bright area at the top of auricle and along the clipped auriculotemporal sulcus highlights where a larger force is generated. As the orthosis is inserted, it is bent backwards. The contact force between the orthosis and the auricle is concentrated in two elements. Forces at the 12th, 13th and 14th nodal points were 0.33, 0.18 and 0.21 N respectively with a total force of 0.72 N. The force at the clipped first nodal point was 0.79 N.

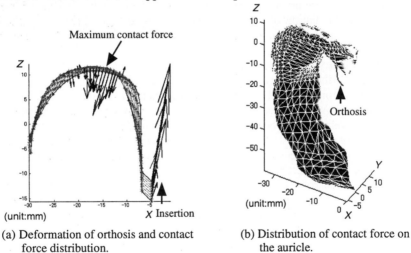

(a) Deformation of orthosis and contact force distribution.

(b) Distribution of contact force on the auricle.

Fig. 2. Results of finite element analysis when the original straight type orthosis is inserted

To relax the force, two types of orthosis were constructed, a curved type and a maximum force-restricted type (Fig.3). In the former case, a detour curve was added to the start of the helix side to permit bending and thus reduce the force. With regards the maximum force-restricted type, the previously described method for automatic modification to cancel insertion of nodal points where the force exceeded the limit of 0.15 N was applied.

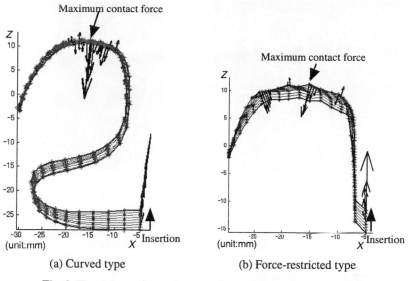

(a) Curved type   (b) Force-restricted type

Fig. 3. The deformation and contact force of finite element analysis

Fig.3 shows the deformation and contact force of finite element analysis performed under the same condition with the original straight type. With respect to the curved type, a maximum force of 0.40 N was generated at the two points backward in relation to the position of original shape. The maximum total force of the two elements was 0.52 N. The force of the clipped first nodal point was also 0.52 N. Deformation occurred mainly at the curved part, and that at the top was relatively small. With respect to the maximum force-restricted type, a maximum force of 0.18 N was produced at the same point as with the curved type. The backward deformation was smaller than that of the original straight type orthosis.

3   Sensors to Measure Contact Force

In order for a sensor to be mounted on an orthosis, it is required to be both small and thin. A sensor system was constructed using either a silicon tube or strain gauge. Straight, curved type and maximum force-restricted type orthoses were manufactured and either a silicon tube or strain gauge sensor was mounted, as illustrated in Fig.4. The sensor was positioned at the point of maximum contact force, as determined by the finite element analysis.

3.1   Silicon Tube Sensor

The silicon tube sensor functions based on the phenomenon that the air flow in a tube decreases when it is compressed. The inside diameter of the silicon tube was 1.0 mm, and outside diameter 1.5 mm. The sensor was bent over with slight tension and bonded to the orthosis. As the tube was compressed, the thickness and width of the sensor was in the order of 0.5 mm and 2.0 mm respectively.

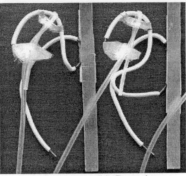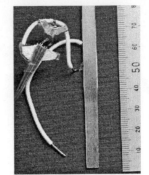

(a) Straight type   (b) Curved type   (c) Maximum force restricted type
(Silicon tube sensor)   (Strain gauge sensor)

Fig. 4. Orthoses with sensors mounted

The sensor calibration system was constructed as shown in Fig.5. Firstly, air was pumped into the air tank and the valve was opened. The air flowed through the sensor and the change in pressure in the air tank was measured using the pressure sensor. The sensor part on the orthosis was compressed by the load sensor on the table. On the tip of the load sensor push rod, a 2.5 x 2.5 mm silicon plate was mounted. The higher the load, the slower the air moved through the sensor and the slower the change in pressure.

The relationship between load and time constant of decreasing air pressure is illustrated in Fig.6. As load is increased, time constant also increases exponentially. The curve approximated by the quadratic equation of the natural logarithm of time constant can be used to derive the load.

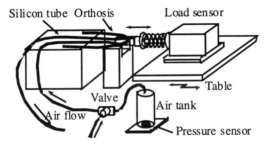

Fig. 5. Configuration of sensor calibration system

3.2   Strain Gauge Sensor

The strain gauge sensor functions based on the phenomenon that the gage is deformed and electric resistance is changed when compressed. The base size and grid size of the gauge were 4.2 x 1.2 mm and 1.0 x 0.68 mm respectively, and the thickness was 0.1 mm. Two gauges were bonded back-to-back to limit the influence of temperature. These gauges were then bonded onto the orthosis and covered with Teflon tape of thickness 0.1 mm. Thus, the total thickness of the sensor was 0.3 mm. Although double gauges were used, coefficients of the temperature were still -0.0073 to 0.0046 (V/°C) when there was no load. A thermistor was used to measure the temperature, and correct the sensor output voltage by subtracting the value at the same temperature as when there was no load.

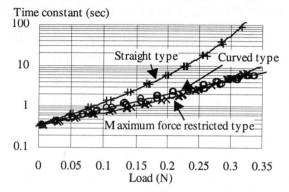

Fig. 6. Relationship between load and time constant of decreasing air pressure

Using the same calibration system illustrated in Fig.5, the relationship between load and sensor output voltage was measured. Fig.7 shows the results after temperature compensation. As the load was increased, the sensor output voltage decreased. The curve approximated by the quadratic equation of the sensor output voltage was used to derive the load.

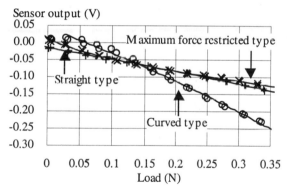
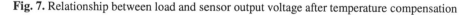

Fig. 7. Relationship between load and sensor output voltage after temperature compensation

4   Insertion Experiment for an Adult Auricle

An insertion test for an adult auricle, used to generate orthosis shape, was performed using six orthoses of the three previously described shapes and with two types of sensors. An aluminum plate attached to the orthosis was used to define the position on the cheek by marking the boundary of the plate. Fig.8(a) shows the results obtained using an original straight orthosis overlaid with a simulation result. Fig.8(b) shows the results obtained using a curved orthosis and (c) shows the results obtaining using a maximum force-restricted type orthosis. The overlay shows orthoses shape before and after insertion. The straight and almost vertical line is the boundary of the aluminum plate and the 10mm square is a reference indicator. In the case of the curved orthosis, the experimental result was in close agreement with the simulation result. Using the straight or maximum force-restricted types, orthoses were bent two or three degrees extra compared to those shown in the simulation results. The reason for the difference is that the orthosis edge of the helix side was clipped in the simulation, and the edge is only pushed onto the cheek in the insertion experiment.

The insertion and removal experiment was performed 15 times and the contact force measured using the silicon tube and strain gauge sensors. Fig.9 shows the average force and range measured during the insertion experiment. The average contact forces measured by the silicon tube sensors on straight, curved and maximum force-restricted orthoses were 0.238, 0.140 and 0.080 N respectively, while those measured by strain gauge sensors were 0.295, 0.183 and 0.045 N respectively. The difference ranged from -0.035 to 0.057 N. As the range of values measured by the two sensors overlapped, it is estimated that the actual value is around the overlapped value. In the simulation studies, the total forces on the two elements that included the nodal point where maximum contact force was produced and the sensors were mounted were 0.72, 0.52 and 0.19 N respectively. The measured force corresponded to about 0.35 times that of the simulated value. To get a more accurate simulation result, a finer and more precise model that incorporates not only the auricular cartilage but also skin and muscle is necessary. Moreover, it is essential to know the material properties of the tissue. The results of the current study demonstrate that both a modified curved type and maximum force-restricted type orthoses can reduce the contact force to a greater degree than the original straight orthosis.

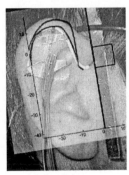 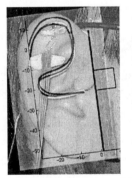 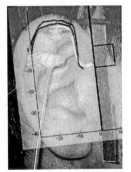

(a) Straight type   (b) Curved type   (c) Maximum force-restricted type

Fig. 8. Insertion results overlaid with simulation results

5   Conclusion

A finite element analysis system was developed to evaluate the contact force between the orthosis and auricle. Two methods were developed to reduce the contact force; modifying the orthosis shape by adding detour curve; and canceling the insertion of nodal point where maximum force exceeds the limit during the incremental step of finite element analysis. Also, sensors using either silicon tube or strain gauges were developed to be mounted onto an orthosis and measure the contact force.

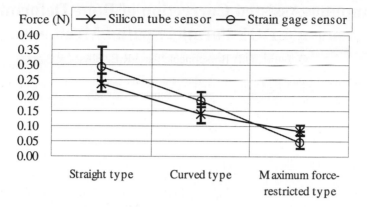

Fig. 9. Force measured during the insertion experiment for the adult auricle

Straight, curved and maximum force-restricted orthoses were made for an adult auricle. Simulation and insertion experiments using silicon tube and strain gauge sensors were performed and the results demonstrated that the strength of contact force decreased from straight type, through curved type to the maximum force-restricted type. The difference in measured contact force between the silicon tube and the strain gauge sensor ranged from -0.035 to 0.057 N. The measured contact force corresponds to about 0.35 times that of the total simulated value along the two elements that included the nodal point where maximum contact force was produced.

References

1. Matsuo K, Hirose T, Tomono T, Iwasawa M, Katohda S, Takahashi N, Koh B : Nonsurgical Correction of Congenital Auricular Deformities in the Early Neonate, Plast. Reconstr. Surg. 73 (1984) 38-50.
2. Hanafusa A, Takahashi H, Akagi K, Isomura T : Development of Computer Assisted Orthosis Design and Manufacturing System for Malformed Ears, Computer Aided Surgery 2 (1997) 276-285.
3. Hanafusa A, Isomura T, Sekuguchi Y, Takahashi H, Dohi T: Computer Assisted Orthosis Design System for Malformed Ears -Automatic Shape Modification Method for Preventing Excessive Corrective Force-, Proc. of the World Congress on Medical Physics and Biomedical Engineering Chicago 2000 (2000) 1-3.
4. Maki K, Inou N, Mikasa M, Tanaka T, Usui T, Toki Y, Shibasaki Y: Computer-Aided Biomechanical Simulations for the Diagnosis of Maxillofacial Functions, Proc 12th International Symposium CAR and CAS (1998) 819-823.

Computer-Assisted Correction of Bone Deformities Using a 6-DOF Parallel Spatial Mechanism

O. Iyun[1], D.P. Borschneck[3], and R.E. Ellis[1,2,3]

[1] School of Computing   [2] Mechanical Engineering   [3] Surgery
Queen's University at Kingston, Canada
ellis@cs.queensu.ca

Abstract. The Ilizarov method is used to correct bone deformities by using an adjustable frame to simultaneously perform alignment and distraction of an open-wedge osteotomy. We have adapted the idea of fixation-based surgery, which requires computer-assisted planning and guidance, to the Ilizarov method with the Taylor frame.

This work incorporates the kinematics of the Taylor frame (a Stewart platform) into the planning and application phases of surgery. The method has been validated in laboratory studies. The study shows that the method requires almost no intraoperative X-ray exposure and that complex corrections can easily be achieved.

1   Introduction

In previous work [2] we introduced the idea of fixation-based surgery, using a fixed plate to distract, align, and fixate bone fragments during corrective wrist surgery. The Ilizarov method also requires distraction, alignment, and fixation but with an adjustable external-fixation frame (rather than with a simple plate). The fundamental concept here is similar to assembly of manufactured components: fixation holes are drilled in the bone fragments, the frame is attached to the bone, the bone is cut, and the frame is adjusted to move the fragments into a new alignment.

Here, we show that fixation-based surgery can be used to improve the Ilizarov method when using a six-degree-of-freedom parallel mechanism, the Taylor spatial frame. We planned a corrective procedure, used the inverse of the plan to compute the kinematics of the Taylor frame, and used computer guidance to help a surgeon apply the frame to a deformed bone. This is a new way of performing complex corrections of deformities of the extremities.

1.1   The Ilizarov Method

The Ilizarov method of osteogenesis by distraction and fixation, developed in 1951 by Russian orthopædic surgeon Gavril Abramovich Ilizarov, is used to correct rotational and translation deformities in the three axes of motion. The Ilizarov method is done by performing osteotomies on the healthy portions of the deformed bone and distracting at a regulated rate to promote bone growth [6]. The method eliminates the need to destroy tissue, insert permanent artificial screws or metals, inject compounds or immobilize bones for months in a cast, and has been found to be highly successful in the treatment of angular deformities, malunions, non-unions, pseudoarthroses, bone infections, open fractures, post-traumatic osteomyelitis, limb lengthening, bone gaps, poliomyelitis, club

T. Dohi and R. Kikinis (Eds.): MICCAI 2002, LNCS 2488, pp. 232–240, 2002.

foot, congenital and acquired disorders of the limbs, dwarfism, skeletal defects, stump elongation and joint contractions [6, 1, 4, 12, 9, 8].

Preoperative planning is done by using X-ray images to measure angular and translational discrepancies in the anterior-posterior and medio-lateral views, and clinical examination to measure rotational and translational deformity in the axial direction. These measurements are used to determine the initial and final shapes of a distraction frame (the Taylor frame is one of many frames used in the method).

Intraoperatively, the surgeon applies the frame to the patient with the aid of fluoroscopic images and performs a low-energy cortical osteotomy. The patients are usually discharged after a few days and scheduled for outpatient visits for both physical therapy and a monitoring of the healing process. The frame is used to rotate and translate the bones at up to 1mm per day. The distraction of the bones induces the growth of new cortical bone. With the use of additional X-ray images, the surgeon can change the configuration of the Ilizarov frame to ensure adequate correction of the problem.

1.2 The Taylor Spatial Frame

The Taylor Spatial Frame, invented by Dr. John Charles Taylor, is an external orthopedic fixator device used to implement the Ilizarov method. The device is kinematically equivalent to a Stewart platform [10, 3], consisting of two circular bases or rings, six telescopic linkage rods (also called struts), and twelve universal joints that connect the struts to the rings [11]. The six measurements used to characterize deformities are related to the displacements on the struts by inverse kinematics.

Preoperatively, a surgeon determines the desired correction and specifies the *neutral* shape of the frame, which is the intended shape when the distraction schedule is complete. A computer program then calculates the strut lengths in the initial and final desired shapes. Intraoperatively, as with other Ilizarov frames, the Taylor frame is attached to the deformed bone with wires, full pins, or half pins. Postoperatively, after the correction schedule has been completed, any residual deformity can be corrected. This is done by developing a new plan that will change the Taylor frame from a *neutral* shape to a final shape which is similar to the initial shape of the first correction. This final shape is dependent on the residual deformity present. A new correction schedule can also be calculated. The Taylor frame, in its initial and neutral shapes, can be seen after application to a plastic bone model in Figure 2.

1.3 The Problem and the Approach

Error in preoperative planning is the most important factor in poor results from use of the Ilizarov method [9]. A secondary source of error is "mis-application" of the frame, which is the failure to place the frame in the intended position and orientation.

We seek to improve the accuracy of Ilizarov's method by (a) planning the correction from a patient-specific CT scan, and (b) using image-guidance technology to apply the frame to a patient. We use many of the same ideas from our fixation-based method of distal radius osteotomy: both that work and the Ilizarov method employ fixation as an essential part of distraction and alignment of bone fragments [2].

2   Materials and Methods

Our laboratory study compared results of conventional application of the Taylor frame with computer-assisted planning and application. This section describes the surgical techniques and the analytical methods used in the study.

2.1   Conventional Technique for the Taylor Frame

The surgeon first planned the procedure by determining the nature of the deformity and the specific mechanical parameters of the Taylor frame. The rotational parameters were angles θ, ϕ and δ[1]. The parameter θ was the lateral angulation, taken from an AP view; ϕ was the angulation, taken from a lateral view; and δ was the axial rotation, usually determined by clinical examination.

The three translational parameters were determined similarly. The surgeon then determined the mechanical parameters, which were the size of the moving ring and the base ring, the *neutral* shape of the frame, and the XYZ position of the frame with respect to the osteotomy. The neutral shape was a symmetric configuration in which all struts have the same length, e.g., 145mm.

These parameters combined to determine the initial and neutral lengths of each strut, from which a daily schedule of strut lengths could be calculated. The calculations were performed by a program that is supplied by the manufacturer of the Taylor frame. These calculations determined the coordinates of each ring in the coordinate frame of the deformity (at the osteotomy site). One ring was the base ring, and had a constant pose that was determined from the XYZ position of the frame with respect to the osteotomy. The neutral pose of the mobile ring was initially a simple translation from the pose of the base ring, e.g., if a neutral strut length of 145mm is chosen then the height of the frame was found by simple trigonometry.

To find the initial strut lengths, a rotation matrix R and a translation vector t were calculated from the rotational and translational parameters. The mobile ring was rotated about the origin of the anatomical coordinate system and translated to its initial position. If the point where the ith strut inserts into the base ring is S^b and the point where the ith strut inserts into the mobile ring in the neutral shape is S_n^m then the point where the ith strut inserts into the mobile ring in the initial shape is

$$S_i^m = RS_n^m + t$$

and the initial length of the ith strut is

$$L_i = \|S_i^m - S^b\|$$

Finally, a daily schedule of strut lengths was calculated. The maximum absolute strut change, in millimeters, is the number of days for the frame to be changed from its initial shape to its neutral shape, because the bone callus can be distracted at a maximum rate of 1mm per day. The lengths of each strut could thus be determined by linear interpolation.

---

[1] These are similar to, but not identical with, Cartesian or Grood-Suntay angular parameters [5]. The difference is that, for the Taylor frame, the angles are coupled because they are specified independently from the X-ray images rather than consecutively about axes.

We have shown[2] that rotation matrix can be reduced to

$$R = \begin{bmatrix} ec - bf & d & a \\ dc - af & e & b \\ db - ae & f & c \end{bmatrix}$$ (1)

where

$$a = c \cdot \tan(\theta)$$

$$c = \sqrt{1/\left(1 + \frac{1}{\tan^2 \theta} + \frac{1}{\tan^2 \phi}\right)}$$

$$b = c \cdot \tan(\phi)$$

$$e = \sqrt{\frac{c^2 \eta^2}{c^2(1 + \eta^2) + a^2 + 2ab\eta + b^2 |eta^2}}$$

$$\eta = \tan(\pi/2 + \delta)$$

$$f = \frac{-1}{c} e(\frac{a}{\eta} + b)$$

$$d = e/\eta$$

2.2   Computer-Assisted Technique for the Taylor Frame

Our surgical technique changed the conventional technique in two ways. First, we planned both the correction and the fixation preoperatively, with a computerized planning system. To mimic the intraoperative phase, we used computer guidance to implant the fixation pins in the desired locations and to guide the osteotomy.

The preoperative planning stage can be conducted in seven steps:

1. Develop a surface model of the deformed bone from a CT scan;
2. Determine the anatomical frame of reference (usually distal to the deformity);
3. Perform "virtual surgery" by cutting the deformed model and moving one fragment into a corrected position and orientation;
4. Position a model of the fixation pins, for a *neutral* Taylor frame shape, through the fragments;
5. Calculate the rotational and translational components of the correction;
6. Calculate the *initial* Taylor frame shape;
7. Calculate the *initial* positions of the fixation pins.

Figure 1 shows a CT-derived model of the deformed femur and a plan.

We used homogeneous coordinates to describe all spatial motion. A transformation from frame j to frame k was represented as

$$^kT^j = \begin{bmatrix} ^kR^j & t^j \\ 0^T & 1 \end{bmatrix}$$ (2)

Using this notation, the planned correction in CT coordinates was $M^p = {}^cT^p$ and the location of the anatomical coordinate frame in CT coordinates was T^a. Thus, the plan in anatomical coordinates was

$$P^a = {}^aT^c \cdot (M^p)^{-1} \cdot {}^cT^a$$ (3)

---

[2] Contact the Corresponding Author for the mathematical proofs.

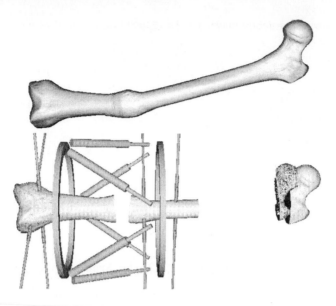

Fig. 1. A model of the deformed femur and a plan. The deformed femur has been cut, with the proximal fragment aligned to the model of the normal femur (shown as a green mesh) and lengthened by 25mm. The long cylinders indicate the planned placement of the fixation half-pins for the frame in its neutral shape (all struts at 145mm length).

The rotation matrix of this transformation was used directly to determine the positions of the initial struts on the mobile ring[3]. The matrix could also be decomposed to find the parameter angles θ, ϕ and δ as

$$
\begin{aligned}
\theta &= \tan^{-1}(a/c) = \tan^{-1}(R_{13}/R_{33}) \\
\phi &= \tan^{-1}(b/c) = \tan^{-1}(R_{23}/R_{33}) \\
\delta &= \tan^{-1}(e/d) - \pi/2 = \tan^{-1}(R_{22}/R_{12}) - \pi/2
\end{aligned}
\tag{4}
$$

so that the manufacturer's programs could be used to determine the daily schedule of strut lengths.

2.3   A Laboratory Study

Fourteen identical polyurethane-foam models of a single deformed femur (model #1164, Pacific Research Laboratories, Bellingham, WA) and one normal femur (model #1120) were used for the study. The normal femur was scanned by CT to represent the template for correction. Seven corrections were performed using the traditional procedure using fluoroscopy and seven using the computer planning and navigation system.

In each of the procedures, a fresh deformed femur was instrumented with two "target" plates containing infrared emitting diode (IRED) markers, one attached distal bone fragment and the other to the femoral shaft. The bone surface was registered to the base

---

[3] This was the planned correction, so the transformation of the mobile ring is actually the inverse of the planned correction.

target by a robust surface-point registration algorithm [7] so that the location of the anatomical coordinate system could be determined.

The locations of the two markers were captured before and after the procedure and used to analyze the overall correction established. Representing the initial poses of the base and mobile targets in the tracker frame as $^{b}T_{0}^{t}$ and $^{m}T_{0}^{t}$, the final poses as $^{b}T_{1}^{t}$ and $^{m}T_{1}^{t}$, and the registration as $^{c}T^{b}$, the relative motion of the mobile target in anatomical coordinates was calculated as

$$M^{a} = {}^{a}T^{b} \cdot {}^{b}T_{0}^{t} \cdot {}^{t}T_{0}^{m} \cdot {}^{m}T_{1}^{t} \cdot {}^{t}T_{1}^{b} \cdot {}^{b}T^{c} \cdot {}^{c}T^{a} \tag{5}$$

and so the residual error, which was the difference between the planned motion of Equation 3 and the actual motion of Equation 5, was

$$E^{a} = (P^{a})^{-1} \cdot M^{a} \tag{6}$$

The errors were extracted from the matrix as the rotational and translational values used in determining the shape of the Taylor frame. The mean, standard deviation, and range were computed in Matlab (The Mathworks, Natick, MA). For accuracy, the mean translations and rotations were analyzed using Student's t-test. For repeatability, standard deviations were analyzed using the two-sample F-test.

3   Laboratory Results

One of us (DPB), a practising orthopædic surgeon trained in the Ilizarov method, measured the deformed femur and planned a correction. As Table 1 shows, this differs substantially from the CT-based plan.

Table 1. Plans from traditional examination and CT-based computer-assisted technique.

Source	Angles (deg)			Translations (mm)		
	x	y	z	θ	ϕ	δ
Traditional	20	10	0	0	0	25
Computer-Assisted	13.2	7.5	1.1	7.0	9.3	26.5

Figure 2 shows a deformed femur during one test run of the laboratory study, in which four pins and the osteotomy were performed with computer assistance. The visual agreement of the plan and the achieved result is excellent.

The residual error matrix of Equation 6 was decomposed into its six independent components for analysis. Table 2 gives the angular and translational residuals for fluoroscopic guidance. Table 3 gives the angular and translational residuals for computer-assisted guidance. For both techniques, the mean and standard deviations of the residuals is shown.

Statistical analysis shows that there is a significant difference in the individual angular residuals for θ ($p<0.012$), ϕ ($p<0.001$) and δ ($p<0.0001$). There is no significant

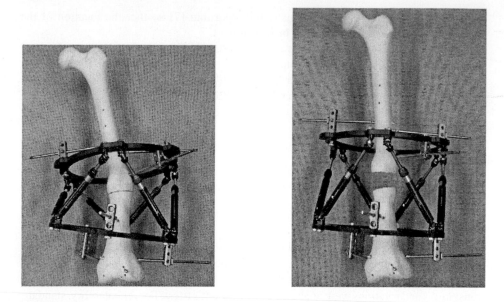

Fig. 2. The plastic model of a deformed femur from a trial using computer-assisted guidance. The Taylor frame is in the initial shape on the left and in the neutral shapes on the right.

difference between the individual or total translational residuals ($p<0.765$). Using the f-test for repeatability shows that the repeatability is nearly significant for translational corrections ($p=0.0975$) and not significant for angular corrections ($p=0.661$).

It is apparent that much of the difference between the residuals is in the first run using fluoroscopic guidance. If this run is discarded, the results are not statistically distinguishable.

4   Discussion

We have developed a technique for planning and performing the Ilizarov method with computer assistance. Our technique allows a surgeon to plan the 3D correction from a patient-specific CT scan, automatically calculate the kinematics of the Taylor frame to find both a distraction schedule and the planned location of fixation pins, and to use computer guidance to apply the frame intraoperatively to a patient. In a laboratory study, the difference between a traditionally derived plan and the 3D plan was substantial: in use, the patient would have needed an extra week of distraction therapy to correct for this difference.

In a test that compared fluoroscopic guidance with computer-assisted guidance, the computer-assisted technique was significantly better than the traditional technique. Both techniques had low residuals, but fluoroscopic guidance produced somewhat greater variances (less repeatable outcomes). Much of the difference is due to a single poor surgery, in which an overall angular error of about 6° produced large (25mm) translational errors because the kinematics of the Taylor frame couples rotations and translations intimately.

Table 2. Residual errors for corrections performed with traditional technique.

Run	Angular Differences (deg)				Translational Differences (mm)			
	θ	ϕ	δ	ψ_{total}	x	y	z	d_{total}
1	-3.6	-4.3	-1.7	5.9	-1.7	4.8	23.9	24.4
2	-1.2	1.1	-0.9	1.9	-2.7	-2.1	-4.0	5.3
3	-0.8	-1.2	0.4	1.5	-0.2	1.5	-0.4	1.6
4	-1.1	-2.1	-0.9	2.6	-4.8	2.7	0.1	5.5
5	-0.7	-2.9	-1.3	3.3	-0.3	2.1	1.2	2.4
6	0.3	-0.3	0.2	0.5	-1.6	1.7	-0.2	2.3
7	-1.3	-2.1	-1.1	2.7	-1.8	0.8	-1.5	2.5
Mean	-1.2	-1.7	-0.8	2.6	-1.9	1.6	2.7	6.3
σ	1.2	1.8	0.8	1.7	1.6	2.1	9.5	8.1

Table 3. Residual errors for corrections performed with computer-assisted technique.

Run	Angular Residuals (deg)				Translational Residuals (mm)			
	θ	ϕ	δ	ψ_{total}	x	y	z	d_{total}
1	1.4	2.2	1.4	3.0	-1.5	1.2	-6.1	6.4
2	1.7	3.1	1.1	3.7	-3.5	0.8	-7.8	8.6
3	0.9	1.6	1.4	2.3	-1.7	2.2	-3.6	4.6
4	-1.2	0.6	1.5	2.1	-3.3	2.3	-0.0	4.0
5	2.7	3.2	0.5	4.2	-3.0	-0.2	-4.2	5.2
6	0.9	3.5	1.4	3.9	-0.0	-2.5	-1.5	2.9
7	1.9	2.7	0.7	3.4	-2.3	-2.8	-4.6	5.9
Mean	1.2	2.4	1.1	3.2	-2.2	0.2	-4.0	5.4
σ	1.2	1.0	0.4	0.8	1.2	2.1	2.6	1.8

This study is limited by the relatively small number of runs (seven): many more samples are needed to eliminate the likelihood of Type II errors. The planning process was carried out under ideal conditions, with no soft-tissue obstacles such as nerves or blood vessels to complicate the process. The fluoroscopic guidance was extremely easy, also because of the very clean X-ray images available from phantoms.

Computer technology appears promising for reducing planning errors, which are a prominent concern in traditional technique [9]. Computer-assisted guidance appears to be significantly superior to fluoroscopic guidance, and is certainly no worse than traditional technique even if the one poor run is discarded. We are planning to conduct an approved clinical trial of our new technique for the Ilizarov method to study the outcomes for patients with complex bone deformities.

Acknowledgments

This research was supported in part by Communications and Information Technology Ontario, the Institute for Robotics and Intelligent Systems, the Ontario Research and Development Challenge Fund, and the Natural Sciences and Engineering Research Council of Canada. We gratefully acknowledge the assistance of Shawn Leclaire in conducting the laboratory studies.

References

1. R. Cattaneo, M. Catagni, and E. Johnson. "The treatment of infected nonunions and segmental defects of the tibia by the methods of ilizarov". *Clinical Orthopaedics and Related Research*, 280:143–152, 1992.

2. H. Croitoru, R. E. Ellis, C. F. Small, R. Prihar, and D. R. Pichora. "Fixation-based surgery: A new technique for distal radius osteotomy". *Journal of Computer Aided Surgery*, 6:160–169, 2001.

3. E. Fichter. *A Stweart platform-based manipulator: General theory and practical construction*, pages 165–190. MIT Press, Cambridge, MA, 1987.

4. S. Green. "Editorial comment". *Clinical Orthopaedics and Related Research*, 280:2–6, 1992.

5. E. S. Grood and W. J. Suntay. "A joint coordinate system for the clinical description of three-dimensional motions: application to the knee". *ASME Journal of Biomechanical Engineering*, 105:136–144, May 1983.

6. G. Ilizarov and V. Ledyaev. "The replacement of long tubular bone defects by lengthening distraction osteotomy of one of the fragments". *Clinical Orthopaedics and Related Research*, 280:7–10, 1992.

7. B. Ma, R. E. Ellis, and D. J. Fleet. "Spotlights: A robust method for surface-based registration in orthopedic surgery". In *Medical Image Computing and Computer-Assisted Intervention – MICCAI'99*, pages 936–944. Springer Lecture Notes in Computer Science #1496, 1999.

8. D. Paley, M. Catagni, F. Argnani, J. Prevot, D. Bell, and P. Armstrong. "Treatment of congenital pseudoarthrosis of the tibia using the ilizarov technique". *Clinical Orthopaedics and Related Research*, 280:81–93, 1992.

9. N. Rajacich, D. Bell, and P. Armstrong. "Pediatric applications of the ilizarov method". *Clinical Orthopaedics and Related Research*, 280:72–80, 1992.

10. D. Stewart. "A platform with six degrees of freedom". *Proceedings of the Institute of Mechanical Engineers*, 180(1):371–386, 1965.

11. J. Taylor. "A new look at deformity correction". *Distraction, The Newsletter of ASAMI-North America*, 5(1), 1997.

12. H. Tucker, J. Kendra, and T. Kinnebrew. "Management of unstable open and closed tibial fractures using the ilizarov method". *Clinical Orthopaedics and Related Research*, 280:125–135, 1992.

Development of 4-Dimensional Human Model System for the Patient after Total Hip Arthroplasty

Yoshito Otake[1], Keisuke Hagio[2], Naoki Suzuki[1], Asaki Hattori[1],
Nobuhiko Sugano[3], Kazuo Yonenobu[4], and Takahiro Ochi[2]

[1] Institute for High Dimensional Medical Imaging, Jikei University School of Medicine,
4-11-1, Izumi Honcho, Komae-shi, Tokyo, Japan
{otake,nsuzuki,hat}@jikei.ac.jp
[2] Department of Computer Integrated Orthopaedics,
Osaka University Graduate School of Medicine,
2-2 Yamadaoka, Suita 565-0871, Osaka, Japan
k-hagio@caos.med.osaka-u.ac.jp, ochi@ort.med.osaka-u.ac.jp
[3] Department of Orthopaedic Surgery, Osaka University Graduate School of Medicine,
2-2 Yamadaoka, Suita 565-0871, Osaka, Japan
sugano@ort.med.osaka-u.ac.jp
[4] Department of Orthopaedic Surgery, Osaka Minami National Hospital,
2-1 Kidohigasi-machi, Kawachinagano 586-0008, Osaka, Japan
yonenobu-k@umin.ac.jp

Abstract. In total hip arthroplasty(THA), complications such as dislocation, loosening, or wearing of the sliding surface are serious clinical problem, and the daily motion of patients has been limited to some extent. However, it is hard to recognize the situation of the components during movement and to predict complications. We have developed the 4-dimensional human model that can visualize the motion of the patient's skeleton and estimate the risk of complications using computer simulation. At first we constructed a 3-dimensional skeletal model of the patient's lower limb from CT data. Then we acquired motion capture data from an infrared position sensor (VICON512, VICON Motion Systems, UK), and drove the patient's skeletal model corresponding to the captured data. Thus we were able to predict the prognosis after the installation of the artificial hip joint, and we have examined the accuracy of the measurements in this system following an experiment using an open MRI.

1 Background

Generally, the daily motion of patients who underwent total hip arthroplasty (THA) has been limited to some extent in order to prevent complications such as dislocation, loosening, or wearing[1][2][3][4]. However the causes of these complications are related to the individual patient's information regarding the position and alignment of the components, skeletal structure, and characteristics of the daily motion. Therefore to give a precise guidance of postoperative daily motion for each patient is difficult for a clinician. The effects of the component alignment on the range of hip motion were reported previously[5][6], but the relative position of the components and skeletal structures during movement has not been reported.

T. Dohi and R. Kikinis (Eds.): MICCAI 2002, LNCS 2488, pp. 241–247, 2002.
© Springer-Verlag Berlin Heidelberg 2002

2   Purpose

The purpose of this study is (1)to develop a 4-dimensional motion analysis system
that can visualize the patient's skeletal structure and analyze the motion of the components and bones during movement, and (2)to examine the accuracy of the measurement error at the methods of motion capture in this system.

3   Methods

3.1   4-Dimensional Human Model for the Patient after THA

We used skeletal structure data from CT (HiSpeed CT, GE Medical Systems, Milwaukee, WI). 15 reflective markers for infrared-light were attached to characteristic
points on the body surface of the patient and CT images were obtained of the whole
lower limb. Then 3-D model of each bone was reconstructed from that CT dataset. To
achieve accurate model with minimum exposure, we scanned joint periphery part with
3mm intervals and the other part with 5mm-30mm intervals. Accuracy of the model
around the artificial joint falls off from the influence of the metal artifact, therefore
we registered the CAD data of the patient's implant to the reconstructed 3-D model
using the algorithm of 3-D surface registration (ICP algorithm[7]).

Next we acquired motion capture data of the patient. We conducted motion capture
by tracking reflective markers attached to the skin using the VICON system, and regarding the motions that we could not capture due to occlusion, we used magnetic
3-D position sensors (FASTRAK, Polhemus, USA). By acquiring the relative positions between bones and markers from CT data, the movement of the skeletal structures could be calculated from the movement of the markers. As a result, we visualized the skeletal movement on the basis of this data, and analyzed various motion
parameters such as hip joint angle, range of motion, impingement point between
bones and/or implants and so on. We also calculated the distance that each point on
the femoral head component moves over the sliding surface of the acetabular component during one motion cycle, because this distance may exert some influence on the
extent of the wearing of the sliding surface.

In order to easily recognize the correlation between the skeletal movement and the
patient's behavior, we superimposed the skeletal model onto the video footage that
was captured by digital video camera in sync with the motion capture system. For the
purpose of displaying the video footage and the skeletal model on the same coordinate
system, estimating the camera parameter, including the position and orientation of the
camera and the focus length or the principal point of the camera coordinate, is necessary. We obtained these information by using a camera calibration algorithm[8] from
the correspondence of the skin marker position on the 3D coordinates with the 2D
image coordinate. By superimposing the skeletal model onto the video footage, we
were able to observe the movement of the skeletal structures and patient's outward
appearance simultaneously.

3.2   Examination of the Accuracy

We carried out an experiment to examine the accuracy of this system. The accuracy of the joint angle measurements in this system mainly depends on the rigidity between the reflective markers and the underlying bones, and therefore movements of the skin markers against the bones during motions are the source of measurement errors. To validate these measurement errors, relative positions of the skin markers against the bones in various postures was evaluated using an open MRI (SIGNA SP 0.5 T, GE Medical Systems, Milwaukee, WI).

   5 reflective markers were attached to the volunteer's skin and MR images (SIGNA Horizon LX HiSpeed 1.5T, GE Medical Systems, Milwaukee, WI) were obtained from the pelvis to the femur to acquire the bone structure and the relative position of the reflective markers. As well, 3-D models of the bones and markers were reconstructed from MRI data. Next the volunteer with the reflective markers was ordered to rest for 12 static postures for a few minutes in the valid area of the open MRI, and the structure data of the bones around the hip was obtained. Simultaneously, the positions of the markers were also tracked and captured by the VICON sensor. By matching the 3-D models from the open MRI images to the models from the MRI images for each posture, the relative position between the pelvis and the femur was obtained and was used for the gold standard of measurements. The relative position between the pelvis and the femur was also calculated by combining the 3-D models with the data of marker position captured by the VICON sensor for each posture. After comparing these data to the gold standard data, we estimated the errors in the measurement by skin marker.

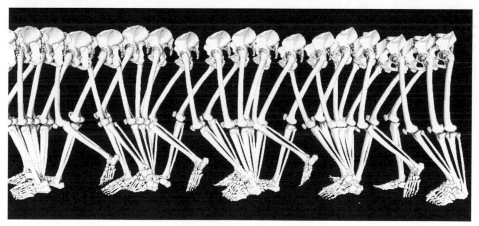

Fig. 1. Time sequential images of the patient's skeletal structures during walking

4   Result

Fig.1 shows the time sequential images of the patient's (female, age 51yr, height 150cm, weight 44kg) skeletal structures of whole lower limb during walking. Fig.2, Fig.3 and Fig.4 show the motion analysis using this system while getting up and down from a chair. The height of the chair was adjusted to be equal to the distance from the head of fibula on the operated side to the floor. Fig.2 represents the display of this system. By displaying bones transparently, a clinician can grasp the movement of the components during motions intuitively. Fig.3 represents the blended images of the patient's skeletal model and the captured video footage. Fig.4 shows the estimated distribution of the extent of the wearing and the safe range of hip motion. Fig.5 indicates the measurement errors of the hip joint flexion angle. For each static posture, the measurement errors of the hip angle using current system were within about ±10 degrees for flexion, adduction, and internal rotation.

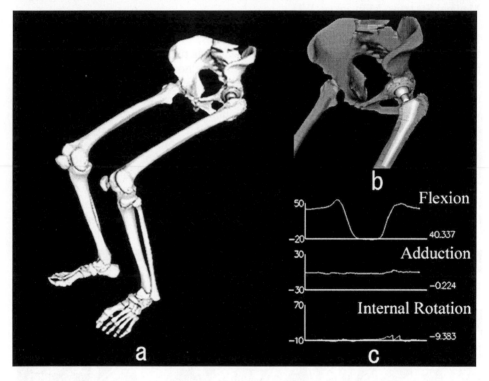

Fig. 2. The display of this system. (a) indicates the skeletal structures of the whole lower limb during sitting. (b) depicts geometry and orientation of the components. (c) shows the time sequential graph of the hip joint angle during sitting

5   Conclusion

Daily motion of the patients who underwent THA has been limited mainly based on intraoperative findings about hip stability in order to prevent complications of the hip joint in postoperative daily motion. However, it is difficult to give precise guidance for each patient in postoperative daily motion in terms of individual differences of alignment of components, skeletal structure and characteristics of daily motion.

This system revealed the movement of the patient's skeletal structures and components during various motions by integrating the patient specific 3-D model from CT

data and the patient's motion capture data. From this model we could recognize the movement of the components intuitively and also quantitatively. Consequently, this system enables dynamic analysis in terms of not only alignment of components and bones of each patient but also individual differences of the characteristics of daily motion.

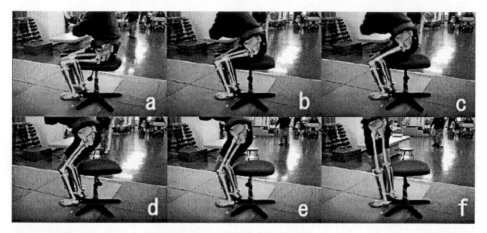

Fig. 3. Blended images of the patient's skeletal model and the captured video footage while getting up and down from a chair. The images laid out time sequentially (a) to (f). These images are visualizing the inner skeletal structures of the patient and his outward appearance simultaneously

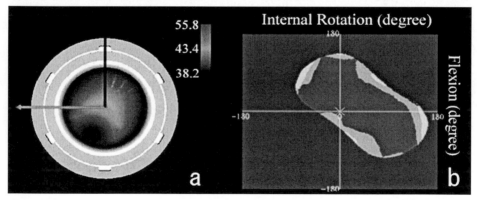

Fig. 4. (a) shows estimated distribution of the extent of the wearing at the sliding surface of the acetabular component while the patient get up and down from a chair. (b) indicates the safe range of hip motion at the movement on the sagittal plane

By using several applications, by which we can calculate various motion parameters of the hip joint, we were able to assess the safe range of component alignment for the hip dislocation and predict the wearing of the sliding surface on the acetabular implant.

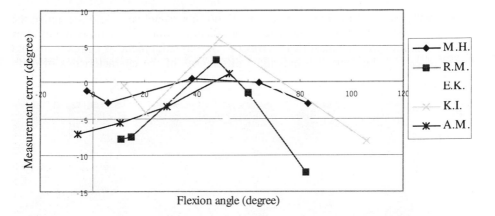

Fig. 5. Measurement errors of the flexion angle. The flexion angles from –5 degrees to 105 degrees are examined, and the errors are within about ±10 degrees. Almost the same tendency was acquired for adduction and internal rotation angle

The maximum degree of the hip angle measurement error for the current system was within ±10° for flexion, adduction, and internal rotation. From the viewpoint of the degree of angle, reducing the error wherever possible is preferable. However, as long as the skin marker is used, the error induced by the changes of the marker position with respect to the underlying bones is inevitable. On the other hand, currently the method by using skin markers is the only way to capture human motion non-invasively. And according to a clinician, this degree of error is quite acceptable to enable the use of this system in a clinical setting to provide useful information regarding each patient and the corresponding safe daily motion to prevent complications of the hip.

This system helps the patient to understand the state of the components in his body, and also helps clinicians to give advice regarding the limitations of daily motion to the patient. More investigation with this system will enable to estimate the safe motion preventing hip dislocation precisely, and lead to more precise guidance of each patient in postoperative daily motion.

References

1. Richard C. Johnston, Gary L. Smidt: Hip Motion Measurements for Selected Activities of Daily Living, Clinical Orthopaedics and Related Research Number 72 (1970) 205-215
2. Ronald Y. G. Woo, Bernard F. Morrey, Rochester, Minnesota: Dislocations after Total Hip Arthroplasty, The Journal of Bone and Joint Surgery vol. 64-A No.9 (1982) 1295-1306
3. F. Pierchon, G.Pasquer, A. Cotton, C. Fontaine, J. Clarisse, A. Duquennoy: Causes of Dislocation of Total Hip Arthroplasty, The Journal of Bone and Joint Surgery vol. 76-B No.1 (1994) 45-48
4. A.Wang :A unified theory of wear for ultra-high molecular weight polyethylene in multi-directional sliding, Wear 248 (2001) 38-47

5. D'Lima DD.,et al.: The effect of the orientation of the acetabular and femoral components on the range of motion of the hip at different head-neck ratios, The Journal of Bone and Joint Surgery 82- A (2000) 315-321
6. Anthony M. DiGioia, et al: Image Guided Navigation System to Measure Intraoperatively Acetabular Implant Alignment. Clinical Orthopaedics and Related Research 355 (1998) 8-22
7. P.J. Besl, and N.D. McKey: A method for registration of 3-D shapes, IEEE Trans. Patt. Anal. Machine Intell. vol. 14 no.2 (1992) 239-256
8. Roger Y. Tsai: A Versatile Camera Calibration Technique for High-Accuracy 3D Machine Vision Metrology Using Off-the-Shelf TV Cameras and Lenses, IEEE Journal of Robotics and Automation vol. RA-3 No.4 (1987) 323-344
9. Y. Otake, Eun S. S., N. Suzuki, A. Hattori, Y. Yamamoto, M. Abo, S. Miyano: Development of 4-Dimensional Whole Body Musculoskeletal Model "Digital Dummy", The 1st World Congress of the International Society of Physical and Rehabilitation Medicine (2001) 47-52

Development of a Training System
for Cardiac Muscle Palpation

Tatsushi Tokuyasu[1], Shin'ichiro Oota[1], Ken'ichi Asami[1], Tadashi Kitamura[1],
Gen'ichi Sakaguchi[2], Tadaaki Koyama[2], and Masashi Komeda[2]

[1] Kyushu Inst. of Tech., Dept. of Mechanical Systems Eng.,
680-4 Kawazu, Iizuka, Fukuoka 820-8502, Japan
{toku,oota,asami,kita}@imcs.mse.kyutech.ac.jp
http://www.imcs.mse.kyutech.ac.jp/
[2] Kyoto Univ., Dept. of Cardiovascular Surgery, Konoe-cho, Yoshida,
Sakyo-ku, Kyoto 606-8501, Japan
{tadaakik,sakaguti,masakom}@kuhp.kyoto-u.ac.jp
http://www.kuhp.kyoto-u.ac.jp/~Cardiovasc-Surg/index.html

Abstract. Touching the cardiac muscle is necessary to get mechanical conditions of muscle before cardiac surgery. The cardiac palpation is the only way to make surgical plans for left ventricular plastic surgery. The training system for cardiac palpation we have developed consists of a MRI-based virtual left ventricular image and a one-dimensional manipulator as a haptic device. Mechanical properties of the cardiac muscles of a dog and a pig are embedded in the virtual heart. Our experiments show that the developed training system enables users to feel the reactional force to the virtual heart surface from the manipulator in real time.

1   Introduction

In order to put into a surgical operation for ventricular plastic surgery, the cardiac surgeon needs to touch the cardiac muscle to recognize where thin and soft regions of the muscular wall due to myocardial infraction and dilate cardiomyopathy are located. Qualitative estimation of partial geometric properties for the heart can be made from cardiac medical image data such as MRI, UT and XCT, which are available in the diagnostic process before the operation. But any medical imaging techniques and instruments provide neither mechanical information nor satisfactorily wall thickness information of the diseased ventricle. Namely, the opportunity to inspect the beating heart based on feels is limited to the scene of the operating room. Therefore training systems for cardiac muscle palpation are desired to the cardiac surgeon.

In this study, a virtual heart model is proposed to design and build a training system for the cardiac muscle palpation. We focus on the importance of dynamic mechanical properties of the cardiac muscle that is reflected on a 3D image of the left ventricle interactively responding to the user's finger force. Thus the proposed training system enables to (1) visualize the virtual heart model including the mechanical characteristics for cardiac muscle, and (2) feel the elasticity of the virtual heart through the haptic-device to transmit the reactional force to the finger. The goal of our system initially offer an opportunity for inexperienced surgeons to palpate the cardiac muscle is provided. The proposed training system would make a benefit of the clinical

T. Dohi and R. Kikinis (Eds.): MICCAI 2002, LNCS 2488, pp. 248–255, 2002.

use if either real measurements or estimates of mechanical properties of each individual diseased heart are available. This paper reports the modeling of the virtual heart and determining the mechanical parameters of the heart and discusses these techniques.

In the following section, the system structure of the palpation training system is described. In the third section, the method of modeling the virtual left ventricle is presented. In the fourth section, the manipulator structure for transmitting the elasticity of the virtual heart is presented. In the fifth, sixth and final sections, experimental results, discussions and conclusions will be given respectively.

2   System Descriptions

Fig.1 shows the schematic diagram of the proposed training system for cardiac palpation, which consists of two PCs and the haptic device. The one computer processes the virtual heart motion based on the dynamic model graphically with use of OpenGL graphics library. The other computer controls and measures the values of electric current of the manipulator through AD/DA conversion board, where the input-output data are processed in real time. These two PCs are connected via a data communication board and a one-dimensional manipulator as a haptic-device. The sampling rate of the control drive is 1000 [Hz].

The virtual heart model is connected to a simple systemic circulatory system model as Windkessel model. The left atrial pressure of 9 [mmHg], the right atrial pressure of 7 [mmHg], and the means of aortic pressure of 100 [mmHg] are assumed as the normal condition of the virtual heart. The vascular resistance depends on the body weight. Here the body weight is assumed to be 25 [kg] of the dog. The trainee can adjust these parameters depending on the situations.

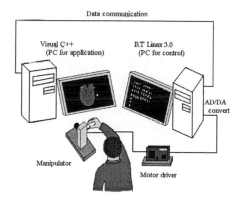

Fig. 1. Schematic diagram of the training system for cardiac palpation

3   Virtual Heart Modeling

3.1   Graphical Modeling

The virtual heart is built using the human MRI image in the textbook [1]. The MRI image includes the wire graphics for the left ventricle over 5 time frames from end-diastole to end-systole. We expanded the 5 time frames in the 21 time frames, and made the movie image of the virtual beating heart. The 21 time frames include the 8 frames of contractile period and the 13 frames of relaxational period, and both ratios are 1:1.7 because of the correspondence to the pulsational duration. In order to draw the smooth curve for the surface of heart, the method of a spline interpolation is applied to the virtual heart graphics.

3.2   Mechanical Modeling

The mechanical model for the virtual heart is developed for the real time linkage between the virtual and actual motions. Since the mechanical modeling of 2th order allows computing the possible behavior of cardiac muscular surface in the case of giving an external force, a method of simulating some complex shape such as F.E.M. is avoided. Here the patch is defined as the part where the finger pushes the virtual heart. The dynamic model is assigned to the patch. Fig.2 shows the schematic diagrams of dynamic and formal models for cardiac muscle, where the dynamic model is composed of mass, spring, and damper as the muscle element. The previous muscular models [2] which compose of parallel damper and spring are unsuitable to analyze the ventricular pressure data of a dog for identifying the mechanical parameters, so that more complex cardiac model is adopted in the horizontal muscle model. In addition, the contractile elements depending on a canine cardiac elastance are used in the horizontal direction.

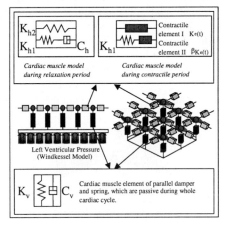

Fig. 2. Schematic diagrams of dynamic models for cardiac muscle

3.3   Mechanical Parameters of Vertical Element

The mechanical coefficients in the vertical direction to the heart surface are measured from the cardiac muscle extracted from a pig by using the lab-made instrumental for position and force instrument. The whole weight of a pig's heart is 310[g]. A lab-made instrument is composed of two arms of aluminum, an angular sensor, and a force sensor. The method how to measure the cardiac characteristics is to fasten the left ventricle to the force sensor attached on the arm. The measured values represent the elasticity $K_v[N/m]$ for the certain ventricular region. When the finger pushes the virtual heart, the reactional force is obtained at the contact area.

The viscosity $C_v[Ns/m]$ is identified by a simple rapid-released technique, where the restoration time from the depression is measured and simulated by using the vertical muscle model. The value of C_v is obtained from restoration time of the depression by a stick.

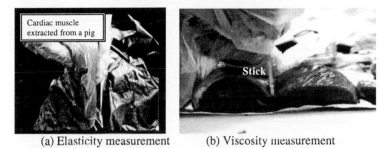

(a) Elasticity measurement   (b) Viscosity measurement

Fig. 3. Measurements of elasticity and viscosity for vertical elements of cardiac muscle of a pig

3.4   Mechanical Parameters of Horizontal Element

The mechanical characteristics in the horizontal direction to the heart surface are measured from the beating heart of an anesthetized dog in the experimental animal room at Kyoto University. The body weight of the dog is about 25[kg]. The mechanical coefficients in the horizontal direction are important for the virtual heart because they govern the whole feature of the virtual heart. As the cardiac characteristics, the left ventricular pressure, left atrial pressure, and the cardiac output are measured from the left ventricle restrained by the same lab-made force and position measurement instrument. The beating motion is captured by the digital video tape recorder (Fig.4 (a)). By using the cardiac muscular contraction and the cardiac output data, the volume of one pulsation for the left ventricle is estimated. Fig.4 (b) shows the pressure-volume diagram plotted by using the measured data.

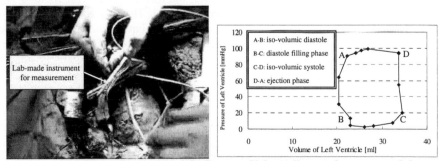

(a) Measurement state   (b) Pressure-Volume diagram from an actual data

Fig. 4. Results of measurement for the cardiac characteristics from an anesthetized dog

The cylindrical model for the horizontal element is developed for the left ventricle because the measured data depend on the whole characteristics of the left ventricle.

Fig.5 (a) shows the schematic diagrams of the cylinder model of the left ventricle during relaxation phase, and (b) for contraction one.

By using the data of the left ventricular pressure during relaxation phase, so that the mechanical coefficients in the horizontal element are determined in the model (a). In the models of (a) and (b), a change of the left ventricular volume is given by the following equation (1).

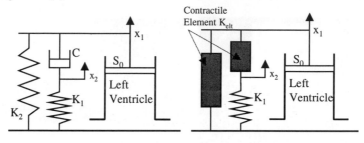

(a) During relaxation phase   (b) During contraction phase

Fig. 5. Schematic diagrams of the cylindrical model of the left ventricle

$$\dot{V}_{LV}(t) = S_0 \dot{x}_1 . \tag{1}$$

The x_2 is dynamic during iso-volumic relaxational phase. For the series element composed of damper C and spring K_1 in the model of (a), the balance of force derives the equation (2).

$$P_{LV}(t) = P(0)e^{-\frac{K_1}{C}t} . \tag{2}$$

Since both x_1 and x_2 are dynamic during diastolic filling phase, the calculated elasticity is given by the following equation (3).

$$f(t) = -K_2 x_1 - C(\dot{x}_1 - \dot{x}_2) . \tag{3}$$

$$J(t, K_1, K_2) = \int_0^\tau (f(t) - \hat{f}(t, K_1, K_2))^2 dt . \tag{4}$$

In order to determine horizontal parameters, the mean square error method is applied under the criterion to be minimized equation (4). The above techniques for the identification are applied to the measured data of the base, middle, and apex parts respectively. The calculated parameters are shown in the table 1. Here the letter v indicates vertical and h for horizontal.

Table 1. Mechanical properties of dynamic model

	Base	Middle	Apex
K_{h1}:[N/m]	30.1	164.8	98.9
K_{h2}:[N/m]	766.5	709.6	655.4
C_h:[Ns/m]	4.6	2.1	8.2
K_v:[N/m]	90	75	45
C_v:[Ns/m]	72	60	51

During contractile phase, spring and damper are replaced to the contractile element, which depends on the elastance for the left ventricle. The effective area determined from the equation (5) shows the spatial reduction of the patch in the left ventricle during contractile phase. Finally the spring of the contractile element is determined by the equation (6). Here parameter α is a compensational coefficient and is given in accord with the part of the diseased heart.

$$S_n(t) = \frac{1}{T_S} \int \left(\frac{V_e(t)}{L_0(t)} \right) dt \ .$$
(5)

$$K_e(t) = \alpha S_n S(t) E_{lt}(t) \ .$$
(6)

The meanings of the variables are shown as follows,

T_s : Contractile period [s],
V_e : Effective volume of the left ventricle [ml],
L_0 : Effective length of the left ventricle [m],
S : The contact area of virtual finger [m^2],
E_{lt} : Elastance of the left ventricular muscle [mmHg/ml].

4   Manipulator for Force Feedback

In this training system, the force between the virtual heart and the user's finger is transmitted through the manipulator. The trainee can touch the virtual heart with operating the manipulator and get the pulsatile elasticity of the cardiac muscle. The previous work shows the technique for transmitting the minute torque [3]. The method of hybrid control achieves to transmit the minimum force of 5 [gf]. Fig.6 shows the overview of the manipulator, which is composed of a DC servomotor, a single lever, and an angular sensor. This training system converts the circular movement of the lever into the straight movement in the computational graphics.

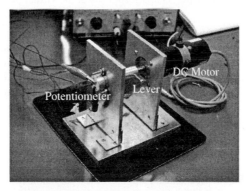

Fig. 6. Manipulator for force transmission

5   Results

Fig.7 (a) shows the graphics image of the virtual left ventricle on the computer display. The trainee is able to rotate and expand the virtual heart by changing the viewpoint. For the patch, he/she can push the affected part by the virtual finger through the manipulator. The patch becomes depressed when the virtual heart is pushed 8 [mm]. Fig.7 (b) shows the diagram for pressure and volume of the virtual heart, where the one graph shows the natural condition of the virtual heart for one pulsation and the other graph for when the virtual finger pushes the virtual heart. For the relaxational phase, the left ventricular pressure does not increase because the left atrium pressure is fixed. As the result, the cardiac output decrease in about 74 [%] when the virtual heart is pushed 8 [mm].

Fig.8 shows the performance for the response of the palpation system. In accord with the displacement of the manipulator operation, the reactional force from the virtual heart is obtained with calculating the beating elasticity of the cardiac muscle. In this experiment, it is assumed that the cardiac palpation is carried out under the low ventricular pressure by adjusting the input value for the left atrial pressure, because the high ventricular pressure prevents feeling the elasticity of the cardiac muscle. The first author Tokuyasu recognizes that the feel of pressing the virtual heart is close to his feel for the dog heart we used for the experiment.

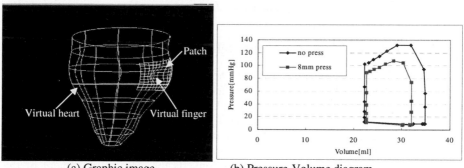

(a) Graphic image   (b) Pressure-Volume diagram

Fig. 7. Experimental responses of the virtual heart

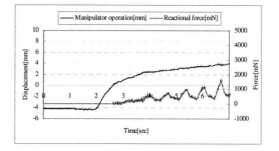

Fig. 8. Mechanical response of the palpation system

6   Discussions

The cardiac palpation is important for the surgeon to make a surgical plan on the basis of feels of the diseased heart. Any diagnostic methods and instruments do not provide mechanical information about the heart so enough to make a surgical plan as palpation on the operative scene. Therefore the mechanical modeling and the training system for cardiac palpation are strongly desired from cardiac surgeons. Thus the proposed training system with the virtual left ventricle has an advantage of cardiac plastic surgery.

Modeling the whole heart consisting of left and right ventricles and atriums are desired to get better virtual reality for the more practical palpation training system. But there was a problem of determining the mechanical parameters because of the limitation of measurements of real hearts by the measuring instrument. To solve this problem, the mechanical parameters should be measured for more and smaller spots on the cardiac muscle with a smaller force-measuring probe. The proposed modeling technique of the left ventricle facilitates to create infarcted regions with high compliance by changing the spring constants.

For clinical applications, a knowledge database for estimating mechanical parameters of each individual diseased heart will be needed reflecting the surgeon's experience about the correspondence between the mechanical characteristics of past patients' hearts and their feels. MR-elastography [4], which can non-invasive measure elastic properties of a living tissue, if completed, would immediately enable our system to be used for planning the surgery of each individual patient before the operation.

The one-dimensional manipulator allows the finger only to push the patch. However the actions to rub and hold the heart are necessary to simulate real cardiac palpation. Therefore the development of a manipulator will be needed to detect the motion of plural fingers and feedback their forces to the fingers.

7   Conclusions

We undertook the development of the palpation system in accord with the cardiac surgeon's request. The virtual heart model provides the real time response modeling a local area of the left ventricle in terms of the dynamic model for the cardiac muscle. The obtained force from the manipulator is corresponding to the feels of the canine cardiac elastance we used for the measurement. These results satisfy basic required conditions for the development of the palpation system. The functions to be added to the palpation system include modeling of the blood flow due to the large cardiac deformation by touching. Moreover the multiple touching points on the virtual heart and the haptic device corresponding plural fingers should be added.

References

1. Dimitris N. Metaxa, Physical-based Deformable Models Applications to Computer Vision, Graphics and Medical Imaging, page 211, 1997.
2. T.Tokuyasu,. et al., Development of A Training System for Cardiac Muscle Palpation with Real-Time Image Processing and Force Feedback, Proc. JCAS The 10th Japan Society of Computer Aided Surgery, pp.129-130, 2001.
3. T.Tokuyasu, T.Kitamura, A study on Minute Torque Transmission for Tele Microsurgery. Proc. of JSME Robomec2001, CD-ROM, 2001.
4. Muthupillai R, and Ehman RL., Magnetic resonance elastography, Nat Med 2:601-603b, 1996.

Preliminary Results of an Early Clinical Experience with the Acrobot™ System for Total Knee Replacement Surgery

Matjaž Jakopec[1], Simon J. Harris[1], Ferdinando Rodriguez y Baena[1], Paula Gomes[1], Justin Cobb[2], and Brian L. Davies[1]

[1]Imperial College of Science, Technology and Medicine, Exhibition Road, London, SW7 2AX, UK; [2]The Middlesex Hospital, Mortimer Street, London, W1N 8AA, UK

Abstract Early clinical experience with a "hands-on" robotic system for total knee replacement surgery is presented. The system consists of a pre-operative CT based planning software, a small special purpose robot called Acrobot (active constraint robot) mounted on a gross positioning device and special leg fixtures. The surgeon guides the Acrobot under active constraint control, which constrains the motion into a predefined region, and thus allows surfaces of the bones to be machined safely and with high accuracy. A non-invasive anatomical registration method is used. The system was clinically tested on 7 patients with encouraging results.

1 Introduction

Total knee replacement (TKR) surgery is a common orthopaedic procedure with the purpose of restoring functionality and reducing the pain caused by injury or by degenerative bone disease in the elderly. Damaged surfaces of the knee bones are replaced with a knee prosthesis, which typically consists of three components: tibial, femoral and patellar. To implant the prosthesis successfully, the bone surfaces must be precisely machined to a specific shape to match the prosthesis components. Typically, a single flat plane is cut across the tibia and the patella, while five planes are required on the femur.

Conventionally, the surgeon uses a complex set of jigs and fixtures in an attempt to accurately position the cutting guides, which are then used to guide the blade of an oscillating saw to cut the flat planes. It is very difficult to achieve a good fit and proper placement of the prosthesis, even by a skilled surgeon using state-of-the-art tools. Poor quality of fit and improper alignment of the prosthesis can lead to pain and reduced functionality of the joint, as well as accelerated wear and loosening of the components, and subsequent need for a revision surgery. A clinical study into conventional TKR surgery [1] reported that the deviation from the ideal prosthesis alignment is over 9° in 7% of cases, and over 5° in 34% of cases.

To overcome the problems and improve the results of the procedure, a robotic surgery system has been developed at Imperial College , and is currently undergoing clinical trials [2]. In contrast to other orthopaedic robotic systems, such

T. Dohi and R. Kikinis (Eds.): MICCAI 2002, LNCS 2481, pp. 256–263, 2002.

as Robodoc [3] or Caspar [4], which use modified industrial robots, a small, low-powered, special-purpose robot called Acrobot (active constraint robot) has been built to ensure safe use in a crowded sterile operating theatre environment. In addition, a novel type of control — active constraint control — has been developed [5,6], where there is a synergy between the surgeon and the robot. The surgeon guides the robot by pushing on the force controlled handle at the tip of the Acrobot, and is thus kept in the control loop, while the robot constrains the motion into a predefined region. This "hands-on" approach allows the surgeon to use his/her sensory capability and understanding of the overall situation to dictate the pace and direction of the procedure, while the robot ensures that the pre-operative plan is executed safely, and with high accuracy.

2   Acrobot TKR System

The Acrobot surgical procedure is divided into two phases: pre-operative planning and intra-operative robotic procedure. An early Acrobot prototype has been successfully tested on plastic phantom bones and cadaveric legs, using fiducial markers for registration [7]. A very good fit of the prosthesis onto the bones was observed, with correct alignment of the leg achieved. The system was subsequently adapted to make it more suitable for the demanding operating theatre environment, and an anatomical registration procedure was introduced to avoid the invasive fiducial marker placement.

2.1   Pre-operative Planning

The pre-operative planning software runs on a standard PC computer, and allows the surgeon to interactive plan the procedure. First, the CT images are processed and the knee bones are segmented in a semi-automatic process. The 3-D models of the bones are built and the bone axes are determined. The surgeon then interactively decides the prosthesis size and placement of the tibial and femoral components onto the bones. The surface of the patella is prepared as in conventional surgery, as the manual preparation is thought to be accurate enough. A number of different 3-D views of the leg and the implant are provided to aid the surgeon to place the components to ensure the correct alignment of the leg (see Figure 2). Once the surgeon is satisfied with the plan, the software generates a constraint boundary for each of the cutting planes (five on the femur and one on the tibia), and a number of locating hole boundaries (for stems and locating features of the prosthesis components). The software also generates bone surface models, which are used intra-operatively for anatomical registration. The planning data is then transferred to the intra-operative system.

2.2   Intra-operative Robotic System

The intra-operative robotic system consists of the Acrobot, a gross positioning manipulator and leg fixtures. The Acrobot is a special-purpose robot with 3 orthogonal axes (Yaw, Pitch and Extension), with a relatively small range of motion. This ensures accurate and safe operation with low-powered motors over a small region. A force sensor handle is mounted near the tip of the Acrobot. The surgeon holds onto this handle and is able to move the robot with low guiding force, due to Acrobot's low mechanical impedance. The guiding force signal is used as part of the active constraint control algorithm to apply a compensating force to stop the motion at the boundary of the pre-defined region. A high-speed orthopaedic cutter system (Stryker Instruments) is used to mill the bone tissue away.

Due to the small workspace of the Acrobot, it is placed on a gross positioning device (see Figure 1), which allows the knee to be accessed from different directions (depending on the plane being cut). The device (manufactured by Armstrong Healthcare Ltd.) is built around a 6-axes robot, with secondary encoders and limited velocity to ensure safe operation. Furthermore, the device is locked-off when the bone is machined, and is only powered-on for a short period between cutting two consecutive planes to move the Acrobot to the next optimal cutting location. The gross positioning manipulator is mounted on a trolley, which allows quick placement and removal of the system. During the procedure, the trolley is clamped to the operating table and its wheels are locked. To ensure sterility, the Acrobot and the gross positioning device are covered with sterile drapes. Only the cutter is autoclaved and mounted through sterile drapes at the start of the procedure.

During the surgery, the tibia and the femur are immobilised with respect to the operating table. This is achieved with two special bone clamps (manufactured by Finsbury Instruments Ltd.), which are rigidly clamped to the exposed parts of the tibia and the femur. Each of the two clamps is fixed to the operating table by means of three telescopic links, connected to the base frame mounted onto the side rails of the operating table. The ankle is placed into a special foot support mounted on the operating table. The weight of the patient has proven enough to immobilise the femur at the hip joint. The bone fixtures are sterilised before the surgery.

3   Clinical Application

The Acrobot TKR system was first tested on plastic phantom bones, to analyse the performance of the overall system, the suitability of the devised surgical protocol, and the accuracy of the anatomical registration. Having obtained very good results with plastic phantoms, the system was brought into the operating theatre and is currently undergoing clinical trials. 7 clinical trials have been performed to date. The first two cases were performed to test the surgical protocol and anatomical registration, but without cutting the bone. The third case involved using the robot to cut the femur only. Full robotic assisted surgery was performed in the rest of the cases.

The procedure was similar in all cases: A CT scan of the patient's leg was taken a few days before the surgery. The CT slices were taken at 1mm intervals

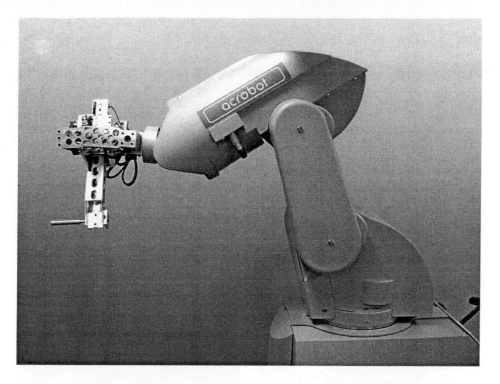

Figure 1. The Acrobot mounted on a gross positioning device

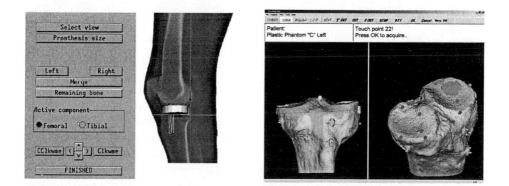

Figure 2. User interface of the planning software (left) and intra-operative user interface during anatomical registration (right)

in the region of the knee and 5 mm intervals for the rest of the leg. The procedure was planned using the planning software, and the intra-operative data was generated.

Intra-operatively, the knee was exposed and the bones were immobilised using the leg fixtures (see Figure 3). During the first trial it was noted that the tibial knee clamp could be improved upon, and it was subsequently modified, which substantially reduced the time required to fit the clamp onto the bone. The robot was covered with sterile drapes and wheeled next to the operating table and clamped to it.

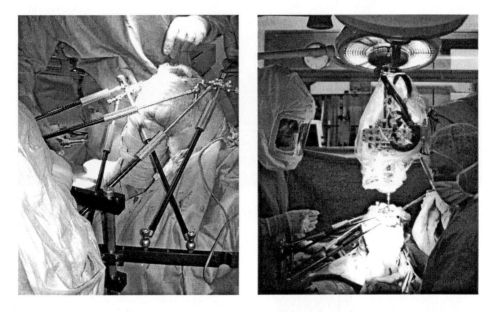

Figure 3. Clinical trial: leg fixtures in place (left) and preparation for registration (right)

Each of the bones was then registered and cut. Registration was performed by first acquiring 4 pre-operatively defined landmarks to obtain an initial registration estimate. The points were acquired by the surgeon moving the Acrobot with a special registration probe (1 mm diameter ball) mounted in the cutter motor. The surgeon then acquired a set of points (typically 20-30) spread over the surface of the exposed bone. An iterative closest point (ICP) algorithm [8,9] was then used to compute the registration transformation. The accuracy of the registration was then verified by using the on-screen colour coded display of the point-set matched onto the surface model, and by touching various landmarks and checking their position on the real-time display (see Figure 2). In case of unsatisfactory registration, the ICP procedure was repeated with a new set of points. The registration results are shown in Tables 1 and 2.

Patient	Sequence	Num. of points	RMS err (mm)	Std Dev (mm)	Max err (mm)	Min err (mm)
A	Initial	4	9.99	—	—	—
	ICP 1	29	0.61	0.361	1.71	0.04
	ICP 2	40	0.59	0.366	1.59	0.01
	ICP 3	36	0.38	0.240	0.85	0.01
B	Initial	4	1.13	—	—	—
	ICP 1	26	0.57	0.352	1.31	0.02
	ICP 2	13	0.27	0.178	0.72	0.01
D	Initial	4	18.58	—	—	—
	ICP 1	17	0.40	0.269	1.01	0.00
E	Initial	4	10.04	—	—	—
	ICP 1	18	1.69	1.255	5.37	0.07
	ICP 2	18	0.71	0.356	1.33	0.01
F	Initial	4	6.20	—	—	—
	ICP 1	17	0.67	0.369	1.20	0.00
	ICP 2	20	0.41	0.226	0.77	0.01
G	Initial	4	15.87	—	—	—
	ICP 1	14	0.36	0.218	0.96	0.02

Table 1. Registration sequences for the tibia

Patient	Sequence	Num. of points	RMS err (mm)	Std Dev (mm)	Max err (mm)	Min err (mm)
A	Initial	4	0.60	—	—	—
	ICP 1	34	0.80	0.537	2.33	0.01
	ICP 2	29	0.21	0130	0.50	0.01
B	Initial	4	2.56	—	—	—
	ICP 1	22	0.96	0.615	2.95	0.09
	ICP 2	19	0.52	0.264	1.13	0.12
	ICP 3	12	0.17	0.116	0.35	0.00
C	Initial	4	5.71	—	—	—
	ICP 1	26	0.85	0.620	3.19	0.11
	ICP 2	24	0.44	0.280	1.16	0.04
D	Initial	4	5.46	—	—	—
	ICP 1	16	0.67	0.498	2.20	0.05
E	Initial	4	23.70	—	—	—
	ICP 1	20	0.86	0.534	2.09	0.06
	ICP 2	17	0.61	0.461	1.43	0.00
F	Initial	4	145.27	—	—	—
	ICP 1	18	0.74	0.462	1.76	0.01
	ICP 2	23	0.39	0.210	0.74	0.00
G	Initial	4	4.56	—	—	—
	ICP 1	18	0.99	0.640	1.97	0.03
	ICP 2	18	0.38	0.228	0.75	0.01

Table 2. Registration sequences for the femur

Once successfully registered, the registration probe was replaced with a drum cutter (7.8 mm diameter) and the surfaces of the bone were machined (see Figure 4). After the surfaces on both the tibia and the femur were prepared, the robot and the leg fixtures were removed from the operating table (see Figure 4). The surgery then proceeded in a conventional way: The knee function was checked with prosthesis trial components in place, the surface of the patella was manually prepared, and all three prosthesis components were cemented onto the bone.

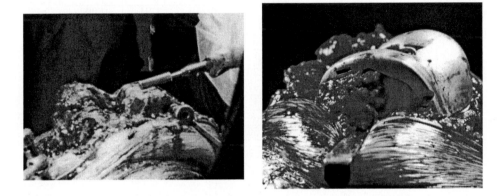

Figure 4. Cutting a plane on the femur (left) and femoral trial in place (right)

In all cases involving cutting the bone with the aid of the robot, the fit of the femoral and tibial components onto the bone was very good, with no femoral notching. The two components were found to mate correctly, giving proper bone alignment and a good range of motion.

4   Conclusions

A "hands-on" robotic system for TKR surgery was successfully applied clinically. The pre-operative planning system was found easy to use, providing an accurate plan for the surgery. The planning alone improved the surgery by giving the surgeon accurate quantitative information about the knee that is unavailable in conventional surgery.

Two preliminary clinical trials were successfully performed to test the suitability of the surgical protocol and the performance of the anatomical registration. All parts of the robotic system performed very well, and the registration results were encouraging. However, the bones were not cut and the procedure was completed in a conventional way.

A further five clinical trials were then performed, which included cutting the bones with the robot. A very good prosthesis fit and proper functioning of the knee was achieved in all cases. However, the time required for the robotic procedure was longer than in conventional surgery, due to added time for leg fixtures setup and registration, and the time spent verifying the progress at each step of the procedure. The robotic system was found easy to use, and its high accuracy and active constraint control, which prevented damage and inaccurate cuts, were welcome improvements over the conventional procedure. No deviation of the prostheses placement from their planned location could be measured on the post-operative CT scans.

More extensive trials are planned, to assess the accuracy of the overall procedure with post-operative CT scans. As a result of these clinical trials, the surgical protocol will be further refined, which will substantially reduce the duration of the surgery. It is felt that these early experiences demonstrate the considerable promise of a "hands-on" approach to robotic assisted surgery.

References

1. M. Tew. Tibiofemoral Alignment and the Results of Knee Replacement. *J Bone Joint Surg Br*, (67), 1985.
2. M. Jakopec, S. J. Harris, F. Rodriguez y Baena, P. Gomes, J. Cobb, and B. L. Davies. The First Clinical Application of a "Hands-on" Robotic Knee Surgery System. *Computer Aided Surgery*, (6), 2002.
3. R. H. Taylor, B. D. Mittelstadt, H. A. Paul, W. Hanson, P. Kazandes, J. F. Zuhars, B. Williamson, B. L. Musits, E. Glassman, and W. L. Bargar. An Image-Directed Robotic System for Precise Orthopaedic Surgery. In R. H. Taylor, S. Lavallee, G. C. Burdea, and R. Mösges, editors, *Computer-Integrated Surgery: Technology and Clinical Applications*. The MIT Press, 1996.
4. C. O. R. Grueneis, R. H. Ritcher, and F. F. Hening. Clinical Introduction of the CASPAR system. In *Proc. of 4th International Symposium on Computer Assisted Orthopaedic Surgery*, Davos, Switzerland, March 1999.
5. S. C. Ho, R. D. Hibberd, and B. L. Davies. Robot Assisted Knee Surgery. *IEEE Engineering in Medicine and Biology*, 14(3), May/June 1995.
6. S. J. Harris, M. Jakopec, J. Cobb, R. D. Hibberd, and B. L. Davies. Interactive Preoperative Selection of Cutting Constraints, and Interactive Force Controlled Knee Surgery by a Surgical Robot. In *Proc. of MICCAI'98*, Cambridge, MA, USA, 1998.
7. S. J. Harris, M. Jakopec, J. Cobb, and B. L. Davies. Intra-operative Application of a Robotic Knee Surgery System. In *Proc. of MICCAI'99*, Cambridge, UK, 1999.
8. Paul J. Besl and Neil D McKay. A Method for Registration of 3-D Shapes. *IEEE Transactions on Pattern Analysis and Machine Intelligence*, 14(2), February 1992.
9. Z. Zhang. Iterative Point Matching for Registration of Free-Form Curves and Surfaces. *International Journal of Computer Vision*, 13(2), 1994.

A Prostate Brachytherapy Training Rehearsal System – Simulation of Deformable Needle Insertion

Asako Kimura (Nishitai)[1,2], Jon Camp[2], Richard Robb[2], and Brian Davis[3]

[1] Graduate School of Engineering Science, Osaka University,
1-3 Machikaneyama-cho, Toyonaka 560-8531, Japan
asa@sys.es.osaka-u.ac.jp
[2] Biomedical Imaging Resource, Mayo Foundation,
Rochester, MN 55902, U.S.A
{nishitai.asako,jjc,rar}@mayo.edu
http://www.mayo.edu/bir/
[3] Radiation Oncology, Mayo Foundation,
Rochester, MN 55902, U.S.A
davis.brian@mayo.edu

Abstract. Prostate cancer is the most common cancer diagnosed in men in the United States. Prostate brachytherapy - an advanced radiotherapy cancer treatment in which radioactive seeds are placed directly in and around the prostate tissues - is complicated by tissue forces that tend to deflect the treatment needles from their intended positions. Medical simulation has proven useful as a technique to enhance surgeons' training and procedure rehearsal. Therefore we are developing a brachytherapy simulation system that includes visual display and haptic feedback, with which a user can see and feel the procedure of the therapy. In this paper, we describe a deformable needle insertion simulation that is a part of our brachytherapy simulation system.

1   Introduction

Since high resolution tomographic image scanners, high performance imaging hardware and comprehensive medical imaging software have become available, interactive 3D visualization of the body, including all organs and their functions is used for accurate anatomy and function mapping, enhanced diagnosis, accurate treatment planning and rehearsal, and education/training [1][2]. Medical simulation is useful to enhance surgeon training and procedure rehearsal. It may also reduce costs and allay ethical concerns. For example, spinal nerve blocks [3], microsurgery [4], endoscopic surgery [5] and catheter insertion [6], can be faithfully simulated using high-resolution graphics, calculated deformation of tissue and organs and haptic feedback.

For a medical simulation system to be useful, realism is one of the most essential factors to consider and provide. However, easy understanding of procedure and intuitive interface, and practice and repeat difficult and critical parts of procedures are also very important. In addition, by measuring and recording the hand movement and associated forces during a simulation, it is possible to make a database of each user's

T. Dohi and R. Kikinis (Eds.): MICCAI 2002, LNCS 2488, pp. 264–271, 2002.
© Springer-Verlag Berlin Heidelberg 2002

technique and habits. This database could help trainees to check whether their hand movement and force is the same as experts. Our objective is to make the simulation system very realistic. From this point of view, we are constructing a brachytherapy simulation system that faithfully incorporates the common tasks used in brachytherapy. The needle insertion procedure in prostate brachytherapy is not very complex, but requires training and skill. Thus this feature is the first step to realize our eventual objective of a complete brachytherapy procedure simulation. In this paper, we describe only this part of the system, namely our deformable needle insertion simulation.

2   Brachytherapy

In the United States, there were 189,000 new cases of prostate cancer estimated during 2002, and 30,200 deaths in 2002 making it the second leading cause of cancer death in men [7]. Since there is an excellent blood test, prostate-specific antigen (PSA), prostate cancer can be diagnosed at a very early stage. Brachytherapy is an advanced cancer treatment using radioactive seeds or sources placed in the tumor itself, giving a high radiation dose to the tumor while reducing the dose to surrounding healthy tissues in the body. Prostate cancer is well suited to it, since the prostate gland is nestled under the bladder and in front of the rectum. This anatomic arrangement makes external beam radiotherapy difficult, and it is imperative that the radiation be focused on the prostate to avoid serious side effects [8].

2.1   Sequence of Brachytherapy - Operation Implant

A prostate brachytherapy includes a three-step process: (1) pretreatment planning, (2) operative implant, and (3) post implant quality evaluation [9]. Since our training rehearsal system supports operative implant procedure, we will explain this procedure in detail.

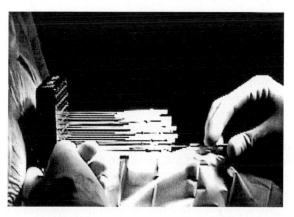

Fig. 1. Brachytherapy Needle Insertion

1) Setting: A fluoroscope, a rectal ultrasound probe in a patient body. The rectal ultrasound is movable so that doctors can check all inserted radiation seed positions, three inches square template is attached to the ultrasound probe. The template has holes every 0.5 cm through which doctors place needles.
2) Calibration: Two non-radioactive seeds are injected as reference markers for calibration between pre-planned prostate position and current prostate position.
3) Needle insertion (Fig.1): Insert hollow needles with a removable metal insert. They are placed through the template, through the skin, and into the prostate gland. The doctors use the ultrasound monitor to check whether the needles are being placed into the correct position or not.
4) Seed injection: Inject seeds throw hollow needles. As during needle insertion, the doctors use the fluoroscopy monitor to check whether the seeds are being injected to the correct position or not.

2.2   Needle Deflection

Since it is imperative in prostate brachytherapy that the radiation is focused not on the other organs but only on the prostate to avoid serious side effects, precise needle positioning is of primary importance.

The problem of needle insertion is needle deflection. It is not easy for surgeons to precisely reach the planned target inside soft tissue with a needle because a thin needle can be deflected in the tissue and the needle also can deform the tissue itself, even if surgeons attempt to lead the needle in a straight direction [10]. Moreover, since the needle path encounters many different tissues of varying resilience, the net deflection is difficult to predict. Therefore a simulation system of a deformable needle insertion is helpful for surgeons and residents for training and rehearsal.

3   Materials and Methods

3.1   System Overview

Our Brachytherapy training rehearsal system consists of a display server and a haptic server (Fig.2). The display server is a SGI workstation (SGI OCTANE) operating under the IRIX6.5. Users can see 3D images of the prostate and other organs, a fluoroscopy image and an ultrasound image on the SGI display (Fig.3). All 3D models of organs are constructed using the medical imaging software Analyze developed in our laboratory, and visualized using OpenGL.

The haptic server is a PC (DELL Precision620) operating under the Windows 2000. We use a PHANToM (PHANTOM Premium 1.5) as a haptic device and GHOST SDK 3.1 as programming software to simulate haptic feedback for needle insertion. In our system, we put a real needle used in a brachytherapy procedure on the end of the PHANToM's stick.

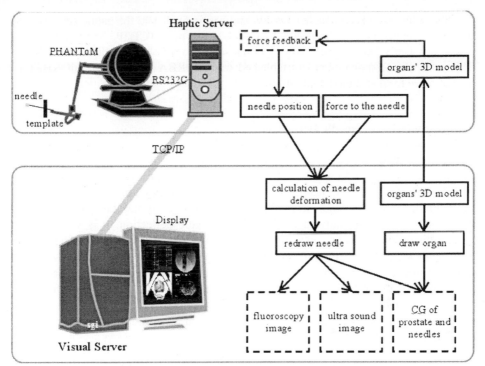

Fig. 2. System architecture

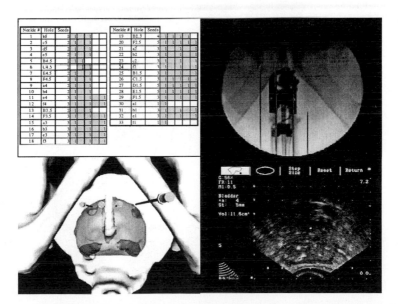

Fig. 3. Visual Display: upper left is planned seed positions, upper right is a fluoroscope image, lower left is a CG of prostate and needles, and lower right is ultrasound image

To synchronize visual needle insertion and haptic feedback, the haptic server sends the latest 3D position of the needle to visual server over TCP/IP. The haptic server also sends user's force to the needle to visual server to simulate needle deformation. This network communication is established with CORBA (AT & T omniORB3.04), the software for distributed computing.

3.2   Simulation of Needle Deflection

Visual Feedback

The prostate lies behind layers of fat, muscle, and soft tissue (Fig.4.). When the needles pass each layer, they encounter varying forces that may gradually deflect them. In addition, the prostate and surrounding tissues are soft, so that the prostate itself is movable. This prostate movement also causes needle deflection. It is very hard to model this needle deflection exactly, since size of prostate, density and thickness of each layer and prostate motility differs widely between patients. Surgeons cannot always estimate how the needle will deform before the insertion, but they check how the needle has deformed, and then remove it halfway and reinsert it. Therefore, our focus is on modeling the appropriate magnitude and direction of deflection forces, rather than predicting the exact deflection forces that a particular insertion path will encounter.

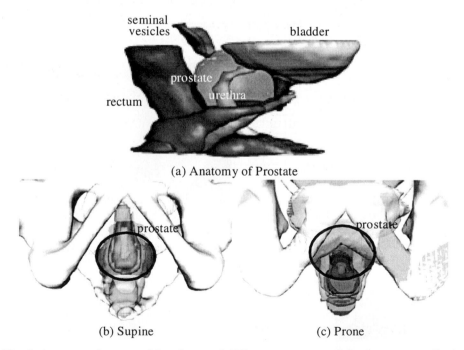

(a) Anatomy of Prostate

(b) Supine   (c) Prone

Fig. 4. Anatomy of prostate: Many layers of different structures and density cause needle deflection

In our initial needle insertion simulation, when the needle passes a new layer, tissues around the needle apply a fixed force. This force is randomly to each layer, and these random series of forces may or may not produce significant needle deflection. On reinsertion, the needle deformation is recalculated based on the previous needle deflection, combined with the force direction and magnitude with which the user pushes the needle to correct the needle position.

In our system, the needle deflection is visible in the ultrasound image and the fluoroscopy image. In a real needle insertion procedure, surgeons don't check needle deflection using the fluoroscopy image to reduce radiation from the fluoroscopy. However, since the fluoroscopy image can show the whole needle deflection image, the user can find needle deflection easier by using both of them. Therefore, in our system, the user can use both images at first, and after they are more experienced, they can turn off the fluoroscopy image.

Fig.5 shows results of needle deflection simulation in the ultrasound image and fluoroscopy image.

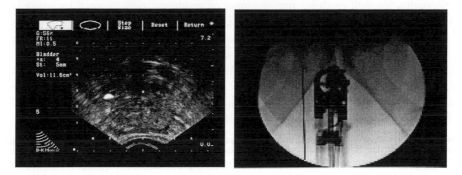

Fig. 5 Visual simulation result of deflected needle in the ultrasound image (left) and a fluoroscopy image (right): A white spot in the ultrasound image is the tip of the needle

Haptic Feedback

Fig.6 shows the haptic feedback in our system. Two kinds of haptic feedback are presented; one is to fingers that push needle into prostate, and another is to fingers of the other hand that corrects needle deflection. When the needle passes each surface between organs, a haptic feedback of puncture is provided to the fingers pushing the needle. During needle reinsertion, half of the needle is already fixed with skin and muscles. Therefore to correct needle deflection, surgeons push on the middle of the needle behind the template with fingers of the other hand. This time, force feedback is presented to the fingers in the opposite direction that the user pushes.

4   Evaluation

We are planning to evaluate our training rehearsal system from two aspects; the reality and the usefulness for training.

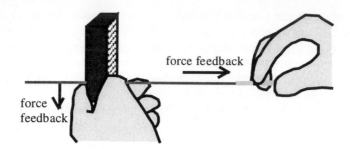

Fig. 6. Two kinds of haptic feedback are presented; one is to fingers that push the needle into prostate, and another is to fingers that correct needle deflection

Firstly, we will have experienced urologists assessed the realism of force magnitudes and needle deformation width and visualization. We will then improve haptic feedback and visual simulation of our initial system.

Secondly, we will evaluate improvement of residents' performance by using our training rehearsal system. Using our system, we will have experienced urologists judge whether needle position is good enough or not. Since our system can measure and save final deflection of the needle, we will gather all data of distance from planned needle positions to inserted needles position, and average them. Based on this result, all new needle deflection can be detected whether their positions are near enough from the planned position. By using this detection, both residents' needle positioning quality and improvement of residents' performance after using our system can be assessed. We will assess improvement of three residents' performance by comparing results between first trial and third trial of our system. We will also discuss usability of our system from the results and the comments from the residents.

5   Conclusions and Future Plans

By using our deformable needle insertion training and rehearsal system, surgeons and residents can train and rehearse needle insertion and correction of deflected needle position by three visual feedbacks, CG of prostate and needles, the ultrasound image and fluoroscopy image, and haptic feedback. We are planning to evaluate realism and usefulness of our training rehearsal system by experienced urologists and residents. Our next step is to complete these two evaluations and to add a seed injection training procedures.

Acknowledgements

We thank Bruce Cameron (Biomedical Imaging Resource, Mayo Foundation, Rochester) for technical advice about network computing and biomedical image visualization.

References

1. R.A. Robb (ed.): THREE-DIMENTIONAL BIOMEDICAL IMAGING. A John Wiley & Sons, Inc. (1998)
2. R.A. Robb (ed.): BIOMEDICSL IMAGING, VISUALIZATION, and ANALYSIS. A John Wiley & Sons, Inc. (2000)
3. D.J. Blezek, R.A. Robb, J.J. Camp, L.A. Nauss, D.P. Martin: Simulation of spinal nerve blocks for training anesthesiology residents. Proceedings of Surgical-Assist Systems, BiOS 98 (1998) 45-51
4. J. Brown, K. Montgomery, J. Latombe, and M. Stephanides: A Microsurgery Simulation System. MICCAI 2001, LNCS2208 (2001) 137-144
5. C. Baur, D. Guzzoni, and O. Georg: A Virtual Reality and Force Feedback Based Endoscopic Surgery Simulator. MMVR1998 (1998) 110-116
6. Zorcolo, E. Gobbetti, G. Zanetti, and M. Tuveri: Catheter insertion simulation with co-registered direct volume rendering and haptic feedback. MMVR2000 (2000) 96-98
7. Cancer Facts and Figures. American Cancer Society (2002) http://www.cancer.org/downloads/STT/CFF2002.pdf
8. http://www.brachytherapy.com/
9. H. RAGDE: Brachytherapy (Seed Implantation) for Clinically Localized Prostate Cancer. Journal of Surgical Oncology, Vol64 (1997) 79-81
10. H. Kataoka, T. Washio, M. Audette, and K. Mizuhara: A Model for Relations between Needle Deflection, Force, and Thickness on Needle Penetration. MICCAI 2001, LNCS2208 (2001) 966-974

A Versatile System for Computer Integrated Mini-invasive Robotic Surgery

Louai Adhami and Ève Coste-Manière

ChIR Medical Robotics group, INRIA Sophia Antipolis (www.inria.fr/chir)

Abstract. This paper presents a versatile system that aims at enhancing minimally invasive robotic surgery through patient dependent optimized planning, realistic simulation and safe supervision. The underlying architecture of the proposed approach is presented, then each component is detailed and illustrated with experimental examples. In particular, an instantiation with the Da Vinci^{TM} [1] robot for performing cardiac surgery is used as a federating case study.

Introduction

Sophisticated robotic simulators and planners are now found in almost any industrial plant. In parallel versatile medical simulators, image manipulation and augmented reality systems exist for research or even in clinical use. However, the combination of medical imaging and robotics in a single system is rarely encountered. In particular, clinically available robotic CIS systems are mainly associated with surgical robots such as ORTHODOC® for ROBODOC® [1] or Carabeamer [2] for Cyberknife®, as well as many neurosurgical systems. The main focus of these systems is on planning and execution through proper registration. Optimized port placement is addressed in [3] where the authors plan a minimally invasive CABG with the Zeus® surgical system; however, they do not integrate the models of the robot in the planner and rely on empirical results from [4] for the port placement. Simulation systems that handle robotics in a clinical background are still under development, or are being built upon existing simulation architecture such as [5]. Results in augmented reality are found in a number of research groups (e.g. [6]). Finally, safety issues have always been a central preoccupation in medical robotics.

The need for an integrated system that can combine medical imaging and robotics in a single versatile system is a recent demand that is rising with the advancements of surgical techniques toward increased mini-invasiveness, and with the introduction of robotic tools in the operating room. As stated by [7]: " ... CIS systems will produce the same impact on surgery that has been realized in computer aided manufacturing", this revolution will go through surgical robotics and will need systems that can efficiently combine the different sources of available information. These needs have formed the major motivation for the work

---

[1] http://www.robodoc.com/eng/robodoc.html

T. Dohi and R. Kikinis (Eds.): MICCAI 2002, LNCS 2488, pp. 272–281, 2002.

presented in this paper : a computer integrated system for robotic mini-invasive surgery (RMIS). The proposed approach addresses these requirements and can be summarized as follows:

1. **Perception**: Gather information about the patient, the robot and the environment.
2. **Port placement**: Determine the best incision sites based on intervention requirements, patient anatomy and endoscopic tools specifications.
3. **Robot positioning**: Determine the best relative position between the robot, the patient and the operating theater.
4. **Verification**: Verify the operating protocol and the corresponding robot logic flow.
5. **Simulation**: Rehearse the intervention using patient and robot data in simulated operating conditions
6. **Transfer**: Transfer the results to the operating room through proper registration and positioning.
7. **Execution**: Execute the planned results with visual and computational assistance.
8. **Monitoring**: Monitor the progress of the intervention and predict possible complications.
9. **Analysis**: Store the settings and history of the intervention for archiving and subsequent analysis.

All the components of this architecture are integrated into a modular single interfaced system. This paper gives a brief overview of each of the aforementioned steps.

1   Perception

A preliminary step to any form of processing is to acquire relevant and usable data. In the case of computer integrated robotic surgery, three sources of information have to be combined. Namely, data about the patient that describes the overall anatomy and gives clear pathologic indications, a model of the robot that can be used to accurately predict its behavior and interaction with its surrounding, and finally a model of the surgical setup or the operating theater that serves to consolidate preoperative planning and simulation with intraoperative execution.

1.1   Patient Model

Patient data is mainly obtained from preoperative radiological imaging. An interactive 3d segmentation system is used to delineate semantically significant entities for further analysis; e.g., ribs must be isolated and numbered for the planning phase described in section 2. Moreover, 3d reconstruction is used to

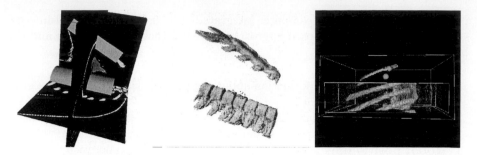

Fig. 1. Interactive 3d segmentation is a successful compromise between versatility and efficiency: (from left to right) 3d manual segmentation of the sternum and backbone, the resulting reconstructed image and an interactive rib growing operation on a volume rendered image.

transform volumetric data into surface data that are easier to visualize and manipulate. Examples of manual and automatic segmentation are shown in figure 1. Under-sampling and triangulation of the segmented data are necessary to enable advanced manipulations such as deformations or active constraints (see section 5).

1.2 Robot Model

The kinematics and shape of the robot are inputted using a simple modeling syntax. Standard DH coordinates are used for kinematic description, whereas the physical envelope of the robot is approximated with basic geometric primitives, namely, regular parallelepipeds, cylinders and spheres. This format accepts any general open-chain multi-armed robotic systems; close chains can also be used but are more difficult to model (see figure 2 for examples). The main originality of the format is its ability to model special surgical robotic features such as an endoscopic arm and a variety of surgical tools. A camera can be added anywhere on the robotic chain, and can take different attributes such as a projection matrix. Likewise, different types of tools can be added to model interactions such as cutting tissue.

1.3 Environment Model

The environment is represented using a geometric model of the operating theater and approximations of the surrounding material. An extra realism can be added through texture mapping views of the operating room, as shown in figure 2.

2 Port Placement

In robotic MIS, a standard endoscopic configuration composed of a left hand, a right hand and an endoscope is used. An optimization algorithm is used to determine the best entry points from a set of previously segmented admissible ports,

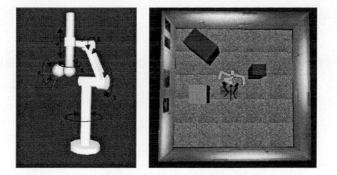

Fig. 2. (left) A prototype of a robot for neurosurgery, (right) Example of an operating room: The surrounding obstacles are important for planning collision free robot movements.

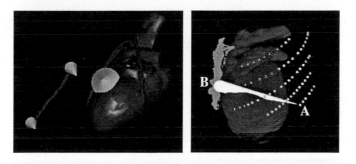

Fig. 3. Optimal port placement: (left) Main syntactic elements (right) Example of a reachability test.

such as the intercostal vectors depicted in figure 3(b). The algorithm is based on a semantic description of the intervention, where the main syntactic elements are target points inserted by the surgeon on the anatomical model of the patient to represent the position, orientation and amplitude of the surgical sites, as shown in figure 3(a). The semantics of the intervention are translated into mathematical criteria that are subsequently used in an exhaustive optimization to yield the most advantageous triplet for the patient, intervention and robotic tools under consideration. The criteria and their mathematical formulation are detailed in [8], they consist of: reachability, dexterity, patient trauma, surgeon effort and factors related to the operative setup. Note that this approach does not depend on the characteristics of the robot, but only on the endoscopic tools. In fact, the same method is currently being used for classical endoscopic interventions (nephrectomy and prostatectomy). Variations to the above configuration can be accommodated either by bypassing the optimization process or adapting it. For instance a fourth port is sometimes used to pull or stabilize an anatomical entity, in which case a segregation in the target vector can be used to assign different role to different tools, while the overall mechanism remains unchanged.

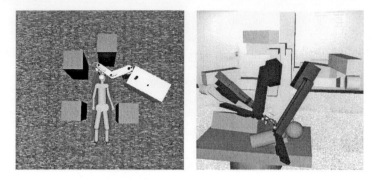

Fig. 4. Pose planning for optimal robot positioning of the SCALPP [11] robot (left) and the Da Vinci™ system (right).

Experimental trials on plastic models have already shown encouraging results [9], and animal trials are currently being conducted to validate and improve the criteria in use.

3   Robot Positioning

Positioning a surgical robot in a typically cluttered operating room for optimal operation is a challenging task. Surgical manipulators are generally designed to have a flexible structure to adapt to the operating environment, and thus have a high number of degrees of freedom (dofs) to position. In mini-invasive interventions, they are also usually subject to additional spatial constraints which are to fixed points that correspond to the entry ports on the patient's skin. Moreover, the planned results should not only guarantee a collision free operation, but should also target a maximum separation form the surrounding obstacles, since this is a critical application, and since the positioning is done in an error prone environment.

A systematic method for the positioning of the passive dofs of a robotic system has been developed and is detailed in [10]. Passive dofs are those not under direct tele-operation or autonomous control, they include the position of the base with respect to the operating environment and the patient, and may also include additional setup joints, as illustrated in figure 4 (b) for the latter and (a) for the former.

4   Verification

As the CIS systems become more complex and integrated, the risks that accompany such an evolution are inevitably increasing. In particular, both the logical behavior and the processing capabilities of the systems tend to become difficult to analyze. The main goal behind this verification step that precedes the intervention is to look for problematic states in which the system could be trapped. A preemptive approach based on a synchronous finite state machine representation is used. The major difficulty resides in finding a unified representation for robotic and surgical actions that will be used to rigorously describe the state of the patient-surgeon-environment. Preliminary analysis is being undertaken to adapt previous work in calssical robotics [12] and assess the needs for modifying the existing approach to better fit medical robotics. Figure 7 shows an example of the logical flow of the registration step (see section 6) implemented using the ESTEREL language [13]. Moreover, the same state machines can also be used as a safe supervision mechanism between the executing parts of the system (those in direct contact with the patient) and the rest of the interactive inputs (see section 7). Algorithmic aspects of critical parts of the system (e.g. collision detection) are formally proved using a logical assistant system [14], thus guaranteeing correct behavior both in planning and while execution.

5 Simulation

Simulation serves the two subtly different goals of training and rehearsal of surgical procedures. Simulation for training concentrates on teaching surgeons the different interventional strategies, as well as getting them accustomed to the surgical tools they will be using. Standard pathological cases and physiological complications can be included in instructive scenarios. On the other hand, simulation for rehearsal is a patient dependent validation and preparation of planned goals in settings that come as close as possible to those of the operating theater. This kind of simulation gives the surgeon the possibility to try out different strategies for his intervention, different tools, different positions of the patient, etc .. Naturally, patient dependent teaching is also possible. For the purpose of RMIS, rehearsal simulation is more interesting; however, it is more difficult to achieve. Indeed, the non-uniformity of the data requires a large amount of pre-processing to give results as good as those found in a pre-modeled and pre-calculated simulation system. Therefore, realism is often compromised for efficiency and accuracy.

Standard 3d input devices (space mice, PHANTOM^{TM} arms or the original input console of the system) are used to control the robots, whereas external and endoscopic views are provided through an OpenGL$^{®}$ rendering interface with possible stereoscopic output. Interference detection is possible between the robot and any modeled obstacle, which can include other parts of the robot (e.g. multiple arms) or modeled parts of the patient. Interaction between the tools and the segmented anatomical entities range from simple destruction (e.g. figure 5) to elastic deformation using techniques from [15]. Active constraints can also be added using scalar distance fields around the regions of interest. These operations require an increased level of data pre-processing.

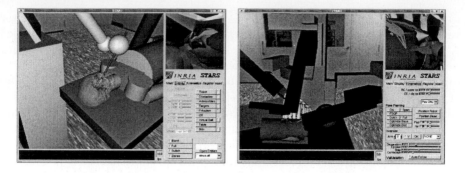

Fig. 5. (left) A simulation of removing a tumor in the pituitary gland using prototyped endoscopic instruments, (right) the Da Vinci™ robot in a coronary artery bypass graft simulation.

6   Transfer

Precision is one of the most important advantages robots bring into the operating room. However, what we are looking for is patient benefit; i.e., both precision and accuracy[2] in the accomplishment of either the preplanned tasks or the operated movements of the robot. This consolidation is made possible through registration between preoperative and intraoperative models, as well as between the robot, the patient and the environment. Moreover, during the intervention the accuracy should constantly be monitored through proper tracking.

A fiducial based least squares registration is used to register the robot to the patient. Precisions of $3mm$ have been observed while registering the Da Vinci™ robot to a pre-scanned plastic phantom. Animal experiments are currently being conducted to assess the amount error introduced between preoperative and intraoperative conditions, on which tracking method will be used to decrease the effect.

7   Execution and Monitoring

On-line interference evaluation and augmented reality are major safety and efficiency additions to MIS robotic systems. A minimum separation between critical parts of the robotic system is constantly monitored during the intervention, enabling proper preventive actions to be taken (e.g. alarm system). This simple safety test is being evolved to a logical supervision system using the techniques introduced in section 4. At the same time the surgeon is guided through intraoperative clues that help in endoscopic navigation and offer him an overlay of pertinent preoperative information.

---

[2] Precise not accurate: ⊕ , accurate not precise: ⊕ , precise & accurate: ⊕

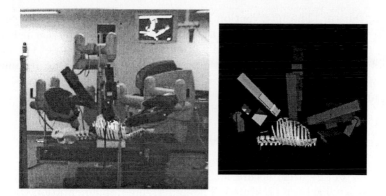

Fig. 6. Transferring planned results to the operating theater after proper registration steps.

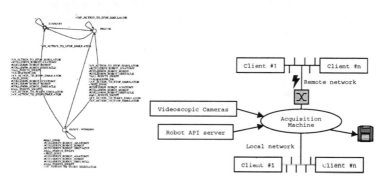

Fig. 7. (left) Part of a finite state machine for verification and monitoring, (right) Intraoperative data acquisition setup for local or remote processing.

Both the monitoring and execution help can be carried out locally or from a remote location provided appropriate throughput and delay times are respected.

Figure 7 shows the setup used for acquiring both robotic and image data during the intervention. The acquisition system serves as a transparency layer between low level API drivers and higher level data access commands from the clients. This setup has been implemented for the Da Vinci^{TM} system and used on the hospital LAN and between the hospital in Paris and the research center in Sophia-Antipolis (1000 km distance with 1 $Gbits/s$ throughput and a nominal delay of 10 ms).

8 Analysis

The settings and history of the intervention are conserved by recording the articular values of the robot, the endoscopic images and all the registration information between the patient, the robot and the rest of the modeled entities in the operating theater. The intervention can then be "replayed", shared, criticized, etc .. On the long run, the major advantage of such an analysis will appear. Namely, the planning results can be correlated to the outcome of the interventions and revisited in order to improve the optimization. The same argument also applies of the rest of the execution steps, where critical chains can be isolated and enhanced.

Conclusions and Perspectives

An overview of the architecture for a computer integrated minimally invasive robotic surgery has been presented. The underlying implementation (Simulation and Training Architecture for Robotic Surgery: STARS) is characterized by its versatility and modularity in what concerns both robotics and medical image processing. STARS is an integrated CIS system that is used for all the steps described in this paper, ranging from radiological image manipulation to intraoperative registration, going through planning and simulation performed with the surgeon.

Experimental validations on artificial data and phantoms have already shown positive results, and animal tests are currently being conducted to better asses the feasibility of the approach. Future work will evolve around experimental validation which will most surely lead to changes and improvements in all of the constituents of the proposed architecture.

References

1. Guthart, G., Salisbury Jr., J.K.: The intuitive telesurgery system: Overview and application. In: Proceedings of the 2000 IEEE International Conference on Robotics and Automation. (2000)
2. Tombropoulos, R.Z., Adler, J.R., Latombe, J.C.: Carabeamer: A treatment planner for a robotic radiosurgical system with general kinematics. Medical Image Analysis **3** (1999)
3. Chiu, A.M., Dey, D., Drangova, M., Boyd, W.D., Peters, T.M.: 3-d image guidance for minimally invasive robotic coronary artery bypass. Heart Surgery Forum (2000)
4. Tabaie, H., Reinbolt, J., Graper, P., Kelly, T., Connor, M.: Endoscopic coronary artery bypass graft (ECABG) procedure with robotic assistance. The Heart Surgery Forum **2** (1999)
5. Kühnapfel, U., Çakmak, H., Maaß, H.: 3D modeling for endoscopic surgery. In: Proc. IEEE Symposium on Simulation, Delft University, Delft, NL (1999)
6. Grimson, E., Leventon, M., Ettinger, G., Chabrerie, A., Ozlen, F., Nakajima, S., Atsumi, H., Kikinis, R., Black, P.: Clinical experience with a high precision image-guided neurosurgery system. Lecture Notes in Computer Science **1496** (1998)
7. Taylor, R.: Computer-integrated surgery: Coupling information to action in 21st century medicine. In: IEEE Int. Conf. on Robotics and Automation. (2001)
8. Adhami, L., Coste-Manière, È., Boissonnat, J.D.: Planning and simulation of robotically assisted minimal invasive surgery. In: Proc. Medical Image Computing and Computer Assisted Intervention (MICCAI'00). Volume 1935. (2000)

9. Coste-Manière, È., Adhami, L., Severac-Bastide, R., Lobontiu, Adrian Salisbury, K., Boissonnat, J.D., Swarup, N., Guthart, G., Mousseaux, É., Carpentier, A.: Optimized port placement for the totally endoscopic coronary artery bypass grafting using the da Vinci robotic system. In: Lecture Notes in Control and Information Sciences, Experimental Robotics VII. Volume 271. (2001)
10. Adhami, L., Coste-Manière, È.: Positioning tele-operated surgical robots for collision-free optimal operation. In: IEEE Int. Conf. on Robotics and Automation. (2002)
11. Duchemin, G., Dombre, E., Pierrot, F., Poignet, P.: Skin harvesting robotization with force control. In: Proc. 10th International Conference on Advanced Robotics. (2001)
12. Borrelly, J.J., Coste-Manière, E., Espiau, B., Kapellos, K., Pissard-Gibollet, R., Simon, D., Turro, N.: The Orccad architecture. International Journal of Robotics Research **17** (1998)
13. Berry, G.: The Esterel v5 language primer. CMA, Écoles des Mines de Paris and INRIA. (2000)
14. Huet, G., Kahn, G., Paulin-Mohring, C.: The Coq Proof Assistant : A Tutorial : Version 7.2. (2002)
15. Cotin, S., Delingette, H., Ayache, N.: Real-time elastic deformations of soft tissues for surgery simulation. IEEE Transactions On Visualization and Computer Graphics **5** (1999)

Measurements of Soft-Tissue Mechanical Properties to Support Development of a Physically Based Virtual Animal Model

Cynthia Bruyns[1,3] and Mark Ottensmeyer[2]

[1] BioVis Technology Center, NASA Ames Research Center
cbruyns@mail.arc.nasa.gov
[2] Simulation Group, CIMIT
mpo@alumni.mit.edu
[3] National Biocomputation Center, Stanford University
bruyns@biocomp.stanford.edu

Abstract. Though the course of ongoing development of a dynamic "Virtual Rat", the need for physically based simulation has been established. To support such physical modeling, data regarding the material properties of various tissues is required. We present the results of *in vitro* testing of rat organ tissues and discuss preliminary comparisons of the results with a Finite Element simulation of the test scenario and a method to extract parameters from test data.

1 Introduction

The goals of the Virtual Rat Project are to reduce the need for training on animals, create a system for training that allows for remote collaboration, and provide a system for training that is rich in content and flexible in user interaction.

The previous development of the system has focused on imaging and reconstruction of the anatomy of the Virtual Rat and development of the surgical manipulations commonly performed in an animal dissection.

The initial modeling efforts have created a combined surface and volumetric representation of the rat anatomy. These 3D models are simulated within a physically based modeling framework to allow the user to probe, cut and remove the various tissues [8],[4]. Within this framework, each organ is represented as surface and/or volumetric meshes and assigned dynamic properties that allow the tissue to respond to user interaction.

During the development of the simulation system, the need for more realistic soft-tissue deformations has been identified. Currently, we are using a mass-spring modeling paradigm. Therefore, surface representations of tissues deformations are commonly represented as bending of the surface. When a user interacts with the tissue locally, without "high spring constants," the deformations can look unrealistic. For volumetric objects however, interactions with the tissues become less localized and when coupled with volume preserving methods, can provide "more appealing" deformations.

T. Dohi and R. Kikinis (Eds.): MICCAI 2002, LNCS 2488, pp. 282–289, 2002.

However, it is more desirable to have the behavior of the object depend on the constitutive properties of the object being simulated and less dependent on the geometry used to represent it. Moreover, we want to avoid manipulating such low-level parameters such as spring constants and move toward modeling the organ as a continuous medium.

There are some issues, however to consider, if one wants to build a surgical simulation trainer that will provide the user with a meaningful learning experience. For example, the behavior of these tissues with which the user is learning to interact must be accurately recreated. Otherwise one runs the risk of training the user to perform a given task incorrectly.

Using a mass-spring model, there is very little real-world material parameter correlation. The only parameters that control the amount of deformation of the simulated soft tissue are the spring stiffness and damping coefficients. These parameters are often approximated for visual quality.

Alternative soft-tissue modeling paradigms, such as Finite Elements can use material parameters such as Poisson's ratio and Elastic Modulus directly in their computations. It is these properties along with geometry and loading and boundary conditions that can predict how a tissue will respond to a given interaction.

Mass-spring models however, have the advantage of being very simple to solve and are an order of magnitude faster than the more rigorous Finite Element Models [12]. In addition to computational efficiency, mass-spring systems have the benefit of allowing topological modifications to be made interactively.

Our goal is to combine the benefits of both modeling approaches to arrive at a simulation that is both fast and precise in its representation of tissue deformation.

Others have noted the need for incorporating material parameters into surgical simulations [7]. Moreover, others have expressed the need for a database of these parameters that can be easily accessed and shared throughout the surgical simulation community [5]. We aim to create a baseline protocol for obtaining soft-tissue properties and using this protocol we are beginning to develop an integrated anatomical atlas of baseline material properties for the Virtual Rat for use in the training system, and so that the effects of weightlessness, disease, and other abnormalities can be compared.

2   Methods

2.1   Necropsy

The testing protocol was approved by the NASA Ames Research Center IACUC Committee under Protocol Number 01-033-2. On separate occasions, four female rats (Rattus norvegicus) of approximately 250g were euthanized through inhalation of CO as accepted by the AVMA. For the *in situ* testing, the abdominal cavity was opened immediately after inhalalation and the instrument was placed over the tested organ. In this manner, blood was still inside the organ and the surrounding organs supported the tested organ, much as they would *in vivo*. One note however, is that the opening of the body cavity and rupture of the diaphragm did change the boundary conditions of the organ from exact *in vivo* conditions, but every effort was made to keep the variations to a minimum. For the *in vitro* testing the organs were removed and placed on a hard glass surface. The organs were kept moist and the time that had past *post-mortem* while testing the organs was noted so that the variation of material properties with time after death could be investigated.

2.2   TeMPeST 1-D Testing

To acquire tissue property data covering the range of frequencies relevant to simulation with haptic feedback, the TeMPeST 1-D instrument [9], [10] was used to deform the tissues and record the force/displacement response. The TeMPeST 1-D makes use of a voice coil motor to drive a right-circular punch with a 5mm diameter, normal to the tissue over a range of motion of $\pm500\mu$m with a force up to 300mN. The open loop bandwidth of the instrument is approximately 100Hz, and within these limits, an arbitrary trajectory can be generated. Absolute force and relative position are sampled at frequencies up to 2kHz.

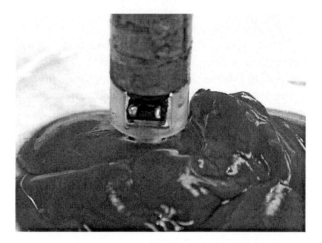

Fig. 1. *In vitro* testing of rat liver with TeMPeST 1-D instrument

A series of tests on the heart, liver, kidney and abdominal muscle layer were conducted with the organs/tissues *in situ* and *in vitro*; Figure 1 demonstrates the test apparatus. Previous use of the instrument includes testing on porcine solid organ tissue *in vivo*. Live testing complicates the boundary conditions of the tissue relative to *in vitro* testing, and more importantly, introduces disturbances in the position of the tissue due to either cardiac or pulmonary motion. Cardiac motion could not be suspended (for obvious reasons), but ventilation of the pig could be halted while data was acquired. Since the rat testing was conducted on sacrificed animals, longer duration sampling could be conducted, and the motion disturbances were not present. Table 1 summarizes the tests conducted (see also

[3]), however in this paper we focus on the data acquired from the latter two rats. As a result of a more restricted set of tissues and an improved measurement protocol, these tests were more informative and reliable.

Table 1. Summary of organ testing, including mode of testing, time post mortem and type of excitation.

rat ID #	organ/tissue	tests	time	test excitation
1	heart (3 tests)	*in situ*	4 - 7 min.	linear chirp
	liver (4)	”	11 - 21	”
	abdominal muscle (1)	”	25	”
	kidney (4)	*in vitro*	35 - 51	lin. & exponential chirp
	liver (3)	”	57 - 62	exp. chirp
2	lung (5)	*in vitro*	6 - 25	exp. chirp & sinusoidal
	liver (8)	”	29 - 52	exp. chirp
	kidney (6)	”	59 - 76	”
3	kidney (r&l) (18)	*in vitro*	0 - 52	exp. chirp
	liver (10)	”	56 - 79	”
	spleen (3)	”	86 - 95	”
4	kidney (r&l) (18)	*in vitro*	0 - 54	exp. chirp
	liver (9)	”	57 - 78	”

2.3   Finite Element Analysis

The imaging and 3D reconstruction of the Virtual Rat was performed as described in [2]. Figure 2 illustrates the high-resolution MDCT images and the resulting 3D reconstruction of the kidneys.

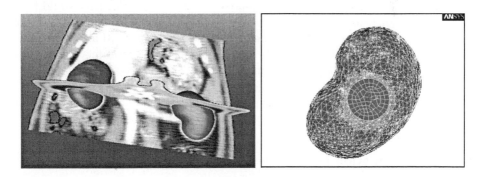

Fig. 2. MDCT imaging (left) and reconstructed FEM kidney with indenter contact zone defined (right)

For comparison with the actual testing, a reconstructed kidney was imported into TrueGrid (XYZ Scientific Applications, Inc, Livermore, Ca.) solid modeling software, and modified to obtain the Finite Element model of the organs. This software allows models obtained from common 3D reconstruction software, such as those obtained from General Marching Cubes algorithms to be converted to hexahedral finite elements. Then using the ANSYS (ANSYS Corporation, Cannonsburg, Pa.) Finite Element Analysis software, the test scenario was simulated using 95-node non-linear brick elements for the tissue and 45-node linear brick elements for the indenter tip. Contact elements were also placed between the tissue and indenter surface to simulate any possible loss of contact between the indenter and the tissue surface during testing. A pilot node was used to specify the position of the indenter as recorded during testing. Nodes were selected at the base of the tissue and fixed with respect to position, simulating their contact with the petri dish. Figure 2 demonstrates the initial triangulated kidney surface and the final solid model using the TrueGrid software.

Using this Finite Element model, an initial estimate for Young's Modulus was made and the corresponding force that resulted from the indenter-tissue contact was examined, and the initial guess was updated accordingly.

3   Results

3.1   Testing

Figures 3(a) and (b) show the mean and standard deviations of the ratios of the Fourier transforms of the position and force (i.e. non-parametric representation of compliance transfer function) for the kidney and liver (four and two organs, respectively, and 11–13 data sets for each of three loading conditions).

Additional tests on more different organs will be necessary to establish reliable mean and deviation estimates for the tissues. One result that can be immediately seen is that over the range of frequencies examined, the tissues have a small phase lag and a decrease in the magnitude of compliance. While this would indicate some viscous component, it is not as severe as a first order spring-dashpot model, so as a first approximation, the material could be treated as elastic. This result immediately simplifies the job of the simulation programmer, since time dependent effects can be omitted from the model. A more complex model could include non-linear elasticity, inhomogeneity and anisotropy, as well as terms to describe the frequency dependent properties. To date, insufficient data has been obtained to determine the post-mortem changes in material properties.

3.2   Implementation into a Mass-Spring System

[12] points out that assigning the same stiffness to all springs within a virtual organ fails to simulate a uniform elastic membrane for equilibrium calculations. Instead he proposes a derivation of stiffness that varies as triangle area over edge length squared. Using this derivation and the 2D Young's Modulus for surface-based representations and the 3D Young's Modulus for volumetric representations, we begin to see the effect that the choice of stiffness parameters has

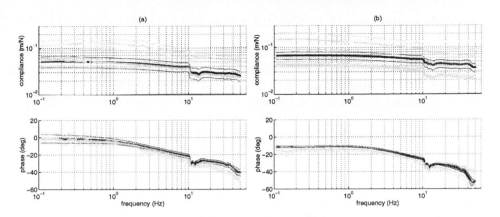

Fig. 3. Compliance of kidney (a) and liver (b) *in vitro* vs. frequency, mean±standard deviation for all *in vitro* measurements. Heavy lines indicate high preload force (42 vs. 21mN), dark colored lines indicate high amplitude (60 vs. 30mN)

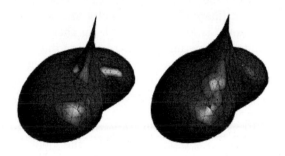

Fig. 4. (a) Uniform spring constant (b)Derived from material properties

on the simulation of these objects using springs. Figure 4 shows the effect that the choice of spring constants has on the static deformation on the simulated kidney.[1]

4   Discussion and Future Work

The figures above demonstrate the difference that the choice of material parameters has on the simulation of soft-tissues. As expected, mass-spring systems with estimated material parameters alone, does not go far enough to try to capture realistic tissue behavior. Instead by using the techniques described, one can approach the combination of the realism of finite element simulations with the speed and simplicity of mass-spring systems. As pointed out by [12] mass-spring

---

[1] Inertial effects due to distribution of mass throughout the object does not affect the static deformation. However, prior to beginning the simulation mass is redistributed in the object as a function of adjacent Voronoi area/volume for each node [4].

simulations cannot exactly simulate the stresses within a material under all stress conditions, however using physically derived stiffness constants, is a first attempt to incorporate the constitutive material of the object being simulated in such a modeling paradigm.

Although the imaging was performed on a different animal than was tested, we were careful to match the age and the size of the animals for a realistic representation of the kidney geometry. However, because the tissues were extracted, we were not able to recreate the loading scenario of the liver. In future experiments we will image the *ex vivo* tissues during loading to provide better approximations for the organ geometry and boundary conditions.

However, given the available results, certain notable features of the measured kidney compliance are apparent that will need to be reproduced in the finite element modeling. For example, with higher preloads, the contact region between the kidney and the dish is expected to be larger, and simultaneously, assuming a hyperelastic characteristic in the tissue itself, one would expect to, and does observe a lower compliance (higher stiffness) for this condition. At the same time, variations in amplitude of vibration (of those examined) do not result in significant changes in stiffness. The liver results are not as clear, most likely because the liver geometry is less constrained. Further tests with imaging will likely clarify the results, and permit the extraction of material properties.

In addition, although the Virtual Rat is currently being developed as a dissection trainer, one can foresee several uses for the simulation system including animal surgery and care. Therefore we are also planning on obtaining the material parameters of the same tissues *in vivo*.

We also plan to investigate how, by using other testing techniques, we can find the yield strength of these tissues. Currently the yield strength is approximated for visual realism during the simulation of manipulations such as cutting. However, it is desirable to be able to determine the point of plastic deformation and eventual fracture of the surface during puncture [11].

Acknowledgements

This work was supported by grants to the NASA Ames BioVis Technology Center and the National Biocomputation Center. Special thanks to Anil Menon, Marilyn Vasques, Kim Winges and Richard Boyle. Special thanks also to Robert Rainsberger and Matthew Koebbe of XYZ Scientific Applications, Inc. This work was also aided by discussions with Mark Rodamaker from ANSYS, Corporation. Portions of this work were also supported by the Department of the Army, under contract number DAMD17-99-2-9001. The views and opinions expressed do not necessary reflect the position or the policy of the government, and no official endorsement should be inferred.

References

1. Brown, J., Sorkin, S., Bruyns, C., Latombe, JC., Montgomery, K., Stephanides, M.: Real-time Simulation of Deformable Objects: Tools and Application, Computer Animation 2001, Seoul, Korea,(6-8 November 2001).
2. Bruyns, C; Montgomery, K; Wildermuth, S.: Advanced Astronaut Training/Simulation System for Rat Dissection, Medicine Meets Virtual Reality 02/10, J.D. Westwood, et al. (Eds.), Newport Beach, CA. IOS Press. (24-27 Jan 2001) 75-81. 2001.
3. Bruyns, C., Ottensmeyer, M.P.: The Development of a Physically Based Virtual Animal Model using Soft-Tissue Parameter Testing. 5th IASTED International Conference on Computer Graphics and Imaging, Kauai, HI, (12-14 Aug 2002) Accepted for publication. 2002.
4. Bruyns, C., Senger, S., Menon, A., Montgomery, K., Wildermuth, S., Boyle, R.: A survey of interactive mesh cutting techniques and a new method for implementing generalized interactive mesh cutting using virtual tools. The Journal of Visualization and Computer Animation. (In Press)
5. Open discussion at Common Anatomical Modeling Language Round Table, Utrecht, Netherlands, October 2001.
6. Fung, Y.C.: Biomechanics: Mechanical Properties of Living Tissues 2nd Edition. Springer Verlag, NY. 1993
7. Miller K., Chinzei K., Orssengo G. and Bednarz P.: Mechanical properties of brain tissue in-vivo: experiment and computer simulation. J. Biomechanics, Vol. 33, pp. 1369-1376, 2000.
8. Montgomery, K., Bruyns, C., Brown, J., Sorkin, S., Mazzella, F., Thonier, G., Tellier, A., Lerman, B., Menon A.: Spring: A General Framework for Collaborative, Real-time Surgical Simulation. Proceedings of Medicine Meets Virtual Reality 02/10, J.D. Westwood, et al. (Eds.), Newport Beach, CA. IOS Press. (23-26 Jan 2002) 296-303.
9. Ottensmeyer, M.P., Salisbury, J.K. Jr.: In Vivo Data Acquisition Instrument For Solid Organ Mechanical Property Measurement, Proceedings of the Medical Image Computing and Computer-Assisted Intervention – MICCAI'01. 4th International Conference, Utrecht, The Netherlands (14-17 Oct 2001) 975-982
10. Ottensmeyer, Mark P.: In vivo measurement of solid organ visco-elastic properties, Proceedings of Medicine Meets Virtual Reality 02/10, J.D. Westwood, et al. (Eds.), Newport Beach, CA. IOS Press. (23-26 Jan 2002) 328-333.
11. Terzopolous, D., Fleicher, K.: Modeling inelastic deformation: viscoelasticity, plasticity, fracture. Computer Graphics Proceedings of SIGGRAPH 1988; 269-278.
12. van Gelder, A.: Approximate simulation of elastic membranes by triangulated spring meshes. Journal of Graphics Tools, 3(2): 21-41, 1998.

Validation of Tissue Modelization and Classification Techniques in T1-Weighted MR Brain Images

M. Bach Cuadra[1], B. Platel[2], E. Solanas[1], T. Butz[1], and J.-Ph. Thiran[1]

[1] Signal Processing Institute (ITS),
Swiss Federal Institute of Technology (EPFL), Switzerland
{Meritxell.Bach,Eduardo.Solanas,Torsten.Butz,JP.Thiran}@epfl.ch
http://ltswww.epfl.ch/~brain
[2] Department of Biomedical Imaging
Eindhoven University of Technology (TUE), The Nehterlands
{b.platel}@stud.tue.nl

Abstract. We propose a deep study on tissue modelization and classification Techniques on T1-weighted MR images. Three approaches have been taken into account to perform this validation study. Two of them are based on Finite Gaussian Mixture (FGM) model. The first one consists only in pure Gaussian distributions (FGM-EM). The second one uses a different model for partial volume (PV) (FGM-GA). The third one is based on a Hidden Markov Random Field (HMRF) model. All methods have been tested on a Digital Brain Phantom image considered as the ground truth. Noise and intensity non-uniformities have been added to simulate real image conditions. Also the effect of an anisotropic filter is considered. Results demonstrate that methods relying in both intensity and spatial information are in general more robust to noise and inhomogeneities. However, in some cases there is no significant differences between all presented methods.

1   Introduction

The study of many brain disorders requires an accurate tissue segmentation from magnetic resonance (MR) images. Manual tracing of the three brain tissue types, white matter (WM), gray matter (GM) and cerebrospinal fluid (CSF) in MR images by an expert is too time consuming because most studies involve large amounts of data. Automated and reliable tissue classification is complicated due to different tissue intensities overlapping (partial volume effect, PVE), presence of noise and intensity non-uniformities caused by the inhomogeneities in the magnetic field of the MR scanner. Different approaches have been presented in recently to deal with this key topic. There is a need to explicitly take into account the pve but most used methods, as [1] only use a FGM representing three main tissue types. In other cases [2] pve is added as normal Gaussian distribution. In more evolved methods such as [3] mixing proportions are equally alike in PV voxels resulting in a density function. Recently, other methods that consider the

T. Dohi and R. Kikinis (Eds.): MICCAI 2002, LNCS 2488, pp. 290–297, 2002.

mixing proportions changing according to a MRF received an increasing interest
[4]. Finally, non-parametric techniques can be considered when no assumption
on the intensity distributions can be done [5]. Here we propose a detailed comparative study and validation of three different classification techniques, a fourth
technique using a statistical non-parametric method will be considered in a near
future. With this comparative study and taking into account the conditions of
our problem we will be able to propose the most suitable technique to solve the
classification problem.

2   Image Model

Theory behind voxel intensities is the same as the one used by Santago et al. in
[3]. In an ideal case, only three main tissues have to be considered: CSF, GM and
WM. But because of the finite resolution of an MR image the well-known partial
volume effect (PVE) appears. Voxel intensity (ν) is modeled as the weighted sum
of intensities of the tissues present in the voxel volume, plus an error term. It is
assumed that no particular combination of underlying tissues is more probable
than any other. If PVE is considered the probability density function $\rho_\nu(\nu)$ is
defined by:

$$\rho_\nu(\nu) = \sum_t Pr\,[t]\,\rho_{\nu_t}(\nu_t), \quad \text{where } t \in \{csf, gm, wm, cg, cw, gw, cgw\}, \qquad (1)$$

where $Pr\,[t]$ is the probability of tissue t and $\rho_{\nu_t}(\nu_t)$ is the probability density
function of ν given tissue t and cg, cw, gw, cgw, respresnts the mixtures for
csf/gm, csf/wm, gm/wm and csf/gm/wm respectivetly. Because $Pr\,[cgw]\,\rho_{\nu_{cgw}}$
(ν_{cgw}) and $Pr\,[cw]\,\rho_{\nu_{cw}}(\nu_{cw})$ are insignificant in $\rho_\nu(\nu)$, they will not be considered. $\rho_\nu(\nu)$ for single a tissue voxel and a mixed two-tissue (ab) voxel:

$$\rho_{\nu_i}(\nu_i) = \frac{1}{\sigma_\eta\sqrt{2\pi}}\,Exp\left[\frac{-(\nu - I_i)^2}{2\sigma_\eta^2}\right], \qquad (2)$$

and

$$\rho_{\nu_{ab}}(\nu_{ab}) = \int_0^1 \frac{1}{\sigma_\eta\sqrt{2\pi}}\,Exp\left[\frac{-(\nu - (\alpha I_a + (1-\alpha)I_b))^2}{2\sigma_\eta^2}\right]d\alpha, \qquad (3)$$

with mean and variance given by:

$$\mu_{\nu_{ab}} = \frac{1}{2}(I_a + I_b) \quad \text{and} \quad \sigma_{\nu_{ab}}^2 = \frac{1}{12}I_a^2 - \frac{1}{6}I_aI_b + \frac{1}{12}I_b^2 + \sigma_\eta^2. \qquad (4)$$

We can observe that PV function varies between a block function and a Gaussian
function depending on I_a (mean intensity of main tissue type a), I_b (mean intensity of main tissue type b) and σ_η^2 (noise variance of main tissues), see Fig. 1.
This means that for certain cases (for larger σ_η's, and when I_a and I_b are very
different) equation 3 can be replaced by a simple Gaussian. When validating
(see Fig. 2in section 6), this is a reasonable assumption, if the variance of the

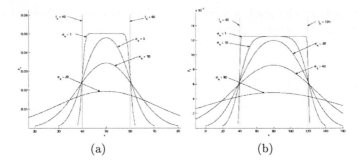

$$(a) \qquad\qquad\qquad (b)$$

Fig. 1. Plot of Equation 3 with (a) varying σ_η (where $I_a = 40$, $I_b = 60$) and (b) varying σ_η (where $I_a = 40$, $I_b = 120$)

Gaussian functions representing the tissue mixtures is considered independent of σ_η. Then, MR image histogram can be modeled solely by Gaussian distributions even for PV representation. As mentioned in [3], the continuous physical reality $\rho_\nu(\nu)$ is approximated by the normalized image histogram (h_i in Eq. 6). Finally, we have to find the set of parameters that solves the minimization problem:

$$\mathbf{p} = \{Pr\,[i]\,,\mu_j,\sigma_i\} \quad \text{for } i \in \{csf, gm, wm, cg, cw, gw\} \quad \text{and } j \in \{csf, gm, wm\}$$
$$(5)$$

$$\sum_{i=1}^{I}(h_i - \sum_t Pr\,[t]\,\rho_{\nu_j}(i))^2 \quad \text{for } t \in \{csf, gm, wm, cg, cw, gw\} \qquad (6)$$

The goal is to optimally classify an instance of ν, $\tilde{\nu}$, in one of the possible categories. It can be shown that the optimal classification of $\tilde{\nu}$, in terms of the probability error is the Bayes classification.

3   Method A: Pure Finite Gaussian Mixture Model

Here, the intensity histogram is modeled by 3, 4 or 5 Gaussian distributions. We deal with the mixture-density parameter estimation problem (see Eq. 6). A possible approach is to find the maximum of a mixture likelihood function. One of the most used methods is the Expectation Maximization (EM) algorithm. Here we follow the steps as explained by [6]. The following probabilistic model as defined in Eq. 2 is assumed:

$$p(\mathbf{x}|\Theta) = \sum_{i=1}^{M} w_i p_i(\mathbf{x}|\theta_i), \qquad (7)$$

where the parameters are $\Theta = (w_1,\dots,w_M,\theta_1,\dots,\theta_M)$ such that the sum of all the weights (w_i) is one and each p_i is a density function parameterized by θ_i. So it is assumed that there are M component densities mixed together with M mixing coefficients $P(w_l)$. In the case of the univariate normal mixture, the maximum likelihood estimates for the next iteration step $P(w_l)^{(t+1)}$ of the mixture coefficients, $\mu_l^{(t+1)}$ of the mean and $\sigma_l^{2(t+1)}$ of the variance are expressed as follows:

$$P(w_l)^{(t+1)} = \frac{1}{N} \sum_{i=1}^{N} p(w_l|x_i, \Theta)^{(t)} \quad \text{and} \quad \mu_l^{(t+1)} = \frac{\sum_{i=1}^{N} x_i p(w_l|x_i, \Theta)^{(t)}}{\sum_{i=1}^{N} p(w_l|x_i, \Theta)^{(t)}} \quad (8)$$

$$\sigma_l^{(t+1)} = \frac{\sum_{i=1}^{N} p(w_l|x_i, \Theta)^{(t)} (x_i - \mu_l^{(t)})(x_i - \mu_l^{(t)})^T}{\sum_{i=1}^{N} p(w_l|x_i, \Theta)^{(t)}} \quad (9)$$

where

$$p(w_l|x_i, \Theta)^{(t)} = \frac{p(x_i|w_l, \Theta_l) P(w_l)^{(t)}}{\sum_{j=1}^{M} p(x_i|w_j, \Theta_j) P(w_j)^{(t)}} \quad (10)$$

These four equations are used for the numerical approximation of the parameters of the mixture. Initial estimations of the parameters $P(w_l)$, μ_l and σ_l have to be specified and only pure Gaussian distributions are considered.

4   Method B: Finite Gaussian Mixture Model Considering a Partial Volume Model

In this case the main three tissue types are modeled by normal Gaussians (Eq. 2) and both CSF/GM and GM/WM partial volumes are modeled by the PVE presented in Eq. 3. PVE is numerically solve it with Newton's method and a *genetic algorithm* is used to find the mixture parameters as defined in 5. The genetic algorithm used here is the same presented in [1]. Genes are composed by the means of the three Gaussians (Eq. 2) μ_1, μ_2, μ_3, by the noise variance σ_η (considered the same for all tissues) and by a weight for either Gaussian or PV distributions w_1, w_2, w_3, w_4, w_5, where $\sum_{i=1}^{5} w_i = 1$.

5   Method C: Hidden Markov Random Field Model

A hidden Markov random field (HMRF) model [4] is used to improve the classification by using spatial information. The importance of the HMRF model derives from MRF theory, in which the spatial information in an image is encoded through contextual constraints of neighboring pixels. By imposing such constraints it is expected that neighboring pixels will have the same class labels. This is achieved by characterizing mutual influences among pixels using conditional MRF distributions. A Pure Gaussian Mixture model will be used for the HMRF method:

$$p(y_i|x_{\mathcal{N}_i}, \theta) = \sum_{l \in \mathcal{L}} g(y_i; \theta_l) p(l|X_{\mathcal{N}_i}), \quad (11)$$

where $\theta_l = (\mu_l, \sigma_l)$ and $g(y; \theta_l)$ is the guassian density function. This type of HMRF is often referred to as the *Gaussian hidden Markov random field*

(GHMRF) model. Note that finite mixture (FM) models is a particular case of HMRF where $p(l|X_{\mathcal{N}_i}) = w_l$ (note Eq. 7). The HMRF-EM algorithm will be used:

$$u_l^{(t+1)} = \frac{\sum_{i \in S} P^{(t)}(l|y_i)y_i}{\sum_{i \in S} P^{(t)}(l|y_i)} \quad \text{and} \quad \left(\sigma_l^{(t+1)}\right)^2 = \frac{\sum_{i \in S} P^{(t)}(l|y_i)(y_i - \mu_l)^2}{\sum_{i \in S} P^{(t)}(l|y_i)}, \quad (12)$$

which are the same update equations as for the finite Gaussian mixture model (Eq. 9), except for

$$P^{(t)}(l|y_i) = \frac{g^{(t)}(y_i; \theta_l) \cdot P^{(t)}(l|x_{\mathcal{N}_i})}{p(y_i)}. \quad (13)$$

$P^{(t)}(l|x_{\mathcal{N}_i})$ calculation involves the estimation of class labels, which are obtained through MRF-MAP estimation. Means, variances and label map estimation by EM algorithm is used to initialize the HMRF-EM algorithm.

6   Validation

Validation has been done using the *digital brain phantom* images [7]. Tissue classification (CSF, GM, WM and mixtures of these) of these phantoms are known *a priori*. This makes them suitable for segmentation algorithm assessment. The Brainweb web-site [7] provides several simulated MRI acquisitions of this phantom including RF non-uniformities and noise levels. It is possible to split phantom histogram into specific ones for each pure tissue type and its mixtures (see Fig. 2(a)). Note that three main tissues are pure Gaussians while mixture densities look a bit like a Gaussian, but with a larger variance. Quantitative results of Brainweb segmentation using Bayes classificator are shown in first row of table 4. The percentage of correctly classified voxels is computed with respect to this reference data. Pixels of the background are not considered. The overall percentage of the classification is calculated over all the voxels of the brain. The percentage of different tissue type volumes is also calculated. Classification has been done on MR images containing 5, 7 and 9% noise and of 0 or 20% RF non-uniformity. We also considered the effect of an anisotropic diffusion filter on the classification results. Test have been done in both filtered and not filered images.

7   Results

All tests have been done on Brainweb images (image size is 181x217x181 and isotropic voxel size of 1mm). Method A has been tested for 3, 4 and 5 Gaussians (see A3, A4, A5 in table 4). Results show that using 5 Gaussian distributions does not always yield better results and that the amount of PV is overestimated. This is due to the fact that the assumption of using a normal distribution for a PV is false in this cases (see Fig. 2(b)). The segmentation results of method B

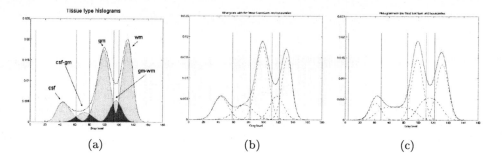

(a)   (b)   (c)

Fig. 2. (a) Segmentation from a Brainweb phantom with 5% noise and 0% RF, not filtered. Dark area represents errors made when using only histogram data. (b) FGM-EM technique, method A. (c) FGM-GA technique, method B

are not as good as expected since it models the PV more in line with physics. It actually highly overestimates PV (Fig. 2(c)). Restrictions on PV wheights when using genetic algorithm could probably improve final classifiaction. Method C yields in the best results even if it doesn't reach 100% correct classification. It performs the less noisy classification (see Fig. 3). Most of the errors performed by this method are locate in PV voxels. This can be easily explained: in a HMRF model the neighborhood of a voxel is considered. If we look at the neighborhood of a PV voxel its neighbours are mostly pure tissue voxels, in which case HMRF model will assign a pure tissue label to the PV voxel. This behaviour tends to eliminate PV voxels in label map (that's reflected on table 1 where PV volumes are the smallest). A possibility to solve this problem could be not to consider neighborhood pixels in the partial volume regions. Another possibility could be to adapt the way the *clique potentials* [4] are calculated, so that PV voxels are no longer assigned to a low probability.

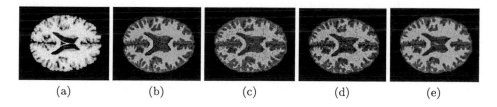

(a)   (b)   (c)   (d)   (e)

Fig. 3. Label map of image (a) with 7% noise found by different classification methods. (b) BW segmentation. (c) Method A. (d) Method B. (e) Method C.

8 Discussion

As we have seen in section 6, if the validation is done solely on intensity image spectra, the tissue classification can never be a 100% due to the noise (see

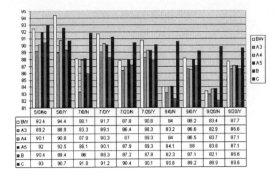

	5/0/No	5/0/Y	7/0/N	7/0/Y	7/20/N	7/20/Y	9/0/N	9/0/Y	9/20/N	9/20/Y
□ BW	92.4	94.4	88.1	91.7	87.8	90.8	84	88.2	83.4	87.7
▣ A3	89.2	88.9	83.3	89.1	86.4	88.3	83.2	86.6	82.9	86.6
□ A4	90.1	90.8	87.9	90.3	87	89.3	84	86.5	83.7	87.1
▪ A5	92	92.5	88.1	90.1	87.9	89.3	84.1	88	83.8	87.1
▪ B	90.4	89.4	86	88.3	87.2	87.8	82.3	87.1	82.1	86.6
▪ C	93	90.7	91.8	91.2	90.4	90.1	90.6	89.2	89.9	89.6

Fig. 4. Percentages of correctly classified pixels for different images: %noise/%RF/ filtered. Brainweb histogram segmentation (BW), FGM-EM segmentation using 3, 4 and 5 Gaussian (A3, A4 and A5, respectively), FGM-GA segmentation (B), and HMRF segmentation (C).

Table 1. The percentages of the volumes of the different tissue types.

	Image	csf	wm	gm	gm-wm	csf-gm
BW		11.8	34.7	36.8	10.5	6.17
A	5% noise, not filtered	13.0	26.5	36.1	12.8	11.6
	7% noise, not filtered	16.6	26.0	33.3	13.9	10.1
	7% noise, filtered	15.7	30.0	27.0	15.8	11.3
	9% noise, not filtered	15.0	30.3	28.0	14.6	12.1
	9% noise, filtered	19.2	15.9	31.7	27.2	6.00
B	5% noise, not filtered	7.62	24.3	26.8	23.2	18.3
	7% noise, not filtered	6.88	25.2	27.3	19.0	21.9
	7% noise, filtered	7.76	23.6	25.3	23.8	18.9
	9% noise, not filtered	8.20	26.6	29.1	15.8	20.5
	9% noise, filtered	5.96	25.1	26.1	18.8	24.2
C	5% noise, not filtered	12.1	28.7	47.2	7.07	9.441
	7% noise, not filtered	15.7	31.0	44.1	2.91	6.21
	7% noise, filtered	16.7	24.7	35.9	14.1	8.67
	9% noise, not filtered	17.2	31.2	43.4	2.60	5.64
	9% noise, filtered	19.6	24.3	36.9	13.8	5.39

Fig. 3). Actually, the less noise there is in the image the better the segmentation. When the noise variance is small, the overlap between the histograms of every tissue type and its mixtures is then also smaller. Results show (see Fig. 4) that the application of an anisotropic diffusion filter improves the classification techniques (2% mean error reduction for 5% of noise) and this improvement is more significative when dealing with more noisy images (until 4% mean error reduction for 9% noise). However, this filtering have no so much impact on intensity non-uniformities. We have seen also that FGM models (method A and B) are solely histogram-based methods. They don't consider any spatial information. Such a limitation causes these methods to work efficiently only on images with low level of noise. Unfortunately this is not often the case with MR images. Actually, method C shown to be more suited for MR brain image modelling in the sense that it has the ability to encode both statistical and spatial image properties. When the three methods are compared, method C is by far the best, not only because it scores the best in the percentage of correctly classified voxels and it gives the best volume estimation of the main tissue types. But mostly because the label map resulting from the classification hardly contains any noise

(Fig. 2). However, it presents also some weak points. It tends to eliminate PV and it approximates PV having a Gaussian distribution and that is not always realistic. Finally, it takes prohibitive computation time (it could take up to 8 hours with 181x217x181 image dimension) since it has been implemented in 3D. However, it would be very interesting to compare these methods with a statistical non-parametrical method such as the one we presented in[5] which is suposed to be better since it is a supervised method and uses spatial information.

9   Conclusion

We have presented here a validation study of MR brain images classification techniques. To perform this validation three different classification methods widely used for this application have been presented. All tests have been done in a ground truth image considering different noise and intensity non-uniformity levels. Also the effect of an anisotropic filter has been also considered when comparing between filtered and not filtered images. Results have shown that the techniques considering spatial information lead in better results when high noisy images are considered and that the application of an anisotropic filter lead in better a classification. However, it has been also demonstrated that in other cases histogram-based techniques lead to comparable results.

References

1. Schroeter, P., et al.: Robust parameter estimation of intensity distributions for brain magnetic resonance images. IEEE Transactions on Medical Imageing **17** (1998) 172–186
2. Ruan, S., Jaggi, C., Xue, J., Bloyet, J.: Brain tissue classification of magnetic resonance images using partial volume modeling. IEEE Transactions on Medical Imaging **19(12)** (2000) 172–186
3. Santago, P., Gage, H.D.: Quantification of mr brain images by mixture density and partial volume modeling. IEEE Trans. Medical Imaging **12** (1993) 566–574
4. Zhang, Y., et al.: Segmentation of brain mr images through a hidden markov random field model and the expectation-maximization algorithm. IEEE Trans. Medical Imaging **20** (2001) 45–57
5. E. Solanas, V. Duay, O.C., Thiran, J.P.: Relative anatomical location for statistical non-parametric brain tissue classification in mr images. Proc. of the 7th ICIP (2001)
6. Bilmes, J.A.: A gentle tutorial of the em algorithm and its application to parameter estimation for gaussian mixture and hidden markov models. Technical report, International Computer Science Institute, Berkeley California (1998)
7. McConell. World Wide Web, http://www.bic.mni.mcgill.ca/brainweb/ (1998)

Validation of Image Segmentation and Expert Quality with an Expectation-Maximization Algorithm

Simon K. Warfield, Kelly H. Zou, and William M. Wells

Computational Radiology Laboratory and Surgical Planning Laboratory, Harvard Medical School and Brigham and Women's Hospital, 75 Francis St., Boston, MA 02115 USA
{warfield,zou,sw}@bwh.harvard.edu

Abstract. Characterizing the performance of image segmentation approaches has been a persistent challenge. Performance analysis is important since segmentation algorithms often have limited accuracy and precision. Interactive drawing of the desired segmentation by domain experts has often been the only acceptable approach, and yet suffers from intra-expert and inter-expert variability. Automated algorithms have been sought in order to remove the variability introduced by experts, but no single methodology for the assessment and validation of such algorithms has yet been widely adopted. The accuracy of segmentations of medical images has been difficult to quantify in the absence of a "ground truth" segmentation for clinical data. Although physical or digital phantoms can help, they have so far been unable to reproduce the full range of imaging and anatomical characteristics observed in clinical data. An attractive alternative is comparison to a collection of segmentations by experts, but the most appropriate way to compare segmentations has been unclear.

We present here an Expectation-Maximization algorithm for computing a probabilistic estimate of the "ground truth" segmentation from a group of expert segmentations, and a simultaneous measure of the quality of each expert. This approach readily enables the assessment of an automated image segmentation algorithm, and direct comparison of expert and algorithm performance.

1 Introduction

Medical image segmentation has long been recognized as a challenging problem. Many different approaches have been proposed, and different approaches are often suitable for different clinical applications.

Characterizing the performance of image segmentation approaches has also been a persistent challenge. Interactive drawing of the desired segmentation by domain experts has often been the only acceptable approach, and yet suffers from intra-expert and inter-expert variability. Automated image segmentation algorithms have been sought in order to remove the variability introduced by experts.

The accuracy of automated image segmentation of medical images has been difficult to quantify in the absence of a "ground truth" segmentation for clinical data. Although physical or digital phantoms can provide a level of known "ground truth" [1, 2], they have so far been unable to reproduce the full range of imaging characteristics (partial volume artifact, intensity inhomogeneity artifact, noise) and normal and abnormal anatomical variability observed in clinical data. A common alternative to phantom studies, has been

T. Dohi and R. Kikinis (Eds.): MICCAI 2002, LNCS 2488, pp. 298–306, 2002.

a behavioural comparison: an automated algorithm is compared to the segmentations generated by a group of experts, and if the algorithm generates segmentations sufficiently similar to the experts it is regarded an acceptable substitute for the experts. Typically, good automated segmentation algorithms will also require less time to apply, and have better reproducibility, than interactive segmentation by an expert.

The most appropriate way to carry out the comparison of an automated segmentation to a group of expert segmentations is so far unclear. A number of metrics have been proposed to compare segmentations, including volume measures, spatial overlap measures (such as Dice [3] and Jaccard similarities [4]) and boundary measures (such as the Hausdorff measure). Agreement measures between different experts have also been explored for this purpose [5]. Studies of rules to combine segmentations to form an estimate of the underlying "true" segmentation have as yet not demonstrated any one scheme to be much favourable to another. Per-voxel voting schemes have been used in practice [6, 7].

We present here a new Expectation-Maximization (EM) algorithm for estimating simultaneously the "ground truth" segmentation from a group of expert segmentations, and a measure of the quality of each expert. Our algorithm is formulated as an instance of the Expectation-Maximization algorithm [8]. In our algorithm, the expert segmentation decision at each voxel is directly observable, the hidden ground truth is a binary variable for each voxel, and the quality of each expert is represented by sensitivity and specificity parameters. The complete data consists of the expert decisions, which are known, and the ground truth, which is not known. If we also knew the ground truth it would be straightforward to estimate the expert quality parameters. Since the complete data is not available, we replace the ground truth (hidden) variables with their expected values under the assumption of the previous estimate of the expert quality parameters. We can then re-estimate the expert quality parameters. We iterate this sequence of estimation of the quality parameters and ground truth variables until convergence is reached.

This approach readily enables the assessment of an automated image segmentation algorithm, and direct comparison of expert and algorithm performance.

We applied the estimation algorithm described here to several **digital phantoms** for which the ground truth is known. These experiments indicate the approach is robust to small parameter changes, and indicate how our algorithm resolves ambiguities between different experts in a natural way. We applied the method to the assessment of a previously published automated image segmentation algorithm [9] for the segmentation of **brain tumors** from magnetic resonance images [10]. We compared the performance of three experts to that of the segmentation algorithm on ten cases. Illustrative results are presented. We assessed multiple segmentations by a single expert for the task of identifying the **prostate peripheral zone** from magnetic resonance images.

2   Method

We describe an EM algorithm for estimating the hidden ground truth and expert segmentation quality parameters from a collection of segmentations by experts.

Let $\mathbf{T}$ be the hidden binary ground truth segmentation, $(\mathbf{p}, \mathbf{q})$ be the sensitivity and specificity parameters characterising the performance of each expert, and $\mathbf{D}$ be the segmentation decisions made by each expert. Hence, the probability mass function of the complete data is $f(\mathbf{D}, \mathbf{T} | \mathbf{p}, \mathbf{q})$.

We want to estimate the quality parameters of the experts as the parameters that maximize the log likelihood function

$$\hat{\mathbf{p}}, \hat{\mathbf{q}} = \arg \max_{\mathbf{p}, \mathbf{q}} \ln f(\mathbf{D}, \mathbf{T} | \mathbf{p}, \mathbf{q}). \tag{1}$$

If we knew the ground truth segmentation, we could construct a 2×2 conditional probability table, by comparing the decision D_{ij} of expert j (for $j = 1, ..., K$) as to presence or absence of a structure at voxel i with the ground truth. Let q_j represent the 'true negative fraction' or specificity (i.e. relative frequency of $D_{ij} = 0$ when $T_i = 0$) and p_j represent the 'true positive fraction' or sensitivity (relative frequency of $D_{ij} = 1$ when $T_i = 1$). These parameters $\{p_j; q_j\} \in [0, 1]$ are assumed to depend upon the expert, and may be equal but in general are not.

We assume that the experts decisions are all conditionally independent given the ground truth and the expert quality parameters, that is $(D_{ij} | T_i, p_j, q_j) \perp (D_{ij'} | T_i, p_{j'}, q_{j'})$, $\forall j \neq j'$.

Since we don't know the ground truth $\mathbf{T}$, we treat it as a random variable and instead solve for the parameters which maximize the function $Q(\theta | \hat{\theta})$, where

$$\theta = [\theta_1 \theta_2 \ldots \theta_k], \qquad \theta_j = (p_j, q_j)^T \quad \forall j \in [1, \ldots, K] \tag{2}$$

$$Q(\theta | \hat{\theta}) = E_{g(\mathbf{T} | \mathbf{D}, \hat{\theta})} [\ln f(\mathbf{D}, \mathbf{T} | \theta)] . \tag{3}$$

This can be written as

$$\hat{\mathbf{p}}, \hat{\mathbf{q}} = \arg \max_{\mathbf{p}, \mathbf{q}} E_{g(\mathbf{T} | \mathbf{D}, \hat{\mathbf{p}}^\circ, \hat{\mathbf{q}}^\circ)} [\ln f(\mathbf{D}, \mathbf{T} | \mathbf{p}, \mathbf{q})] \tag{4}$$

$$= \arg \max_{\mathbf{p}, \mathbf{q}} E_{g(\mathbf{T} | \mathbf{D}, \hat{\mathbf{p}}^\circ, \hat{\mathbf{q}}^\circ)} \left[\ln \frac{f(\mathbf{D}, \mathbf{T}, \mathbf{p}, \mathbf{q})}{f(\mathbf{p}, \mathbf{q})} \right] \tag{5}$$

$$= \arg \max_{\mathbf{p}, \mathbf{q}} E_{g(\mathbf{T} | \mathbf{D}, \hat{\mathbf{p}}^\circ, \hat{\mathbf{q}}^\circ)} \left[\ln \frac{f(\mathbf{D}, \mathbf{T}, \mathbf{p}, \mathbf{q}) f(\mathbf{T}, \mathbf{p}, \mathbf{q})}{f(\mathbf{T}, \mathbf{p}, \mathbf{q}) f(\mathbf{p}, \mathbf{q})} \right] \tag{6}$$

$$= \arg \max_{\mathbf{p}, \mathbf{q}} E_{g(\mathbf{T} | \mathbf{D}, \hat{\mathbf{p}}^\circ, \hat{\mathbf{q}}^\circ)} [\ln f(\mathbf{D} | \mathbf{T}, \mathbf{p}, \mathbf{q}) f(\mathbf{T})] \tag{7}$$

where $\hat{\mathbf{p}}^\circ, \hat{\mathbf{q}}^\circ$ are the previous estimates of the expert quality parameters, and the last follows under the assumption that $\mathbf{T}$ is independent of the expert quality parameters so that $f(\mathbf{T}, \mathbf{p}, \mathbf{q}) = f(\mathbf{T}) f(\mathbf{p}, \mathbf{q})$.

The process to identify the expert quality parameters and ground truth consists of iterating between 1) estimation of the hidden ground truth given a previous estimate of the expert quality parameters, and 2) estimation of the expert quality parameters based on how they performed given the new estimate of the ground truth. This algorithm can be recognized as an EM algorithm, in which the parameters that maximize the log likelihood function are estimated based upon the expected value of the hidden ground truth. The process can be initialized by assuming values for the expert specific sensitivity and specificity parameters, or by assuming an initial ground truth estimate. In most of our experiments we have initialized the algorithm by assuming that the experts are each equally good and have high sensitivity and specificity, but are not infallible. This is equivalent to initializing the algorithm by estimating an initial ground truth as an equal weight combination of each of the expert segmentations.

2.1 Estimation of Ground Truth Given Expert Parameters

In this section, the estimator for the hidden ground truth is derived.

$$g(\mathbf{T}|\mathbf{D}, \hat{\mathbf{p}}^o, \hat{\mathbf{q}}^o) = \frac{g(\mathbf{D}|\mathbf{T}, \hat{\mathbf{p}}^o, \hat{\mathbf{q}}^o)g(\mathbf{T})}{\sum_{\mathbf{T}} g(\mathbf{D}|\mathbf{T}, \hat{\mathbf{p}}^o, \hat{\mathbf{q}}^o)g(\mathbf{T})} \tag{8}$$

$$= \frac{\prod_i \left[\prod_j g(D_{ij}|T_i, \hat{p_j}^o, \hat{q_j}^o)g(T_i) \right]}{\sum_{T_1} \sum_{T_2} \cdots \sum_{T_N} \prod_i \left[\prod_j g(D_{ij}|T_i, \hat{p_j}^o, \hat{q_j}^o)g(T_i) \right]} \tag{9}$$

$$= \frac{\prod_i \left[\prod_j g(D_{ij}|T_i, \hat{p_j}^o, \hat{q_j}^o)g(T_i) \right]}{\prod_i \left[\sum_{T_i} \prod_j g(D_{ij}|T_i, \hat{p_j}^o, \hat{q_j}^o)g(T_i) \right]}. \tag{10}$$

$$g(T_i|\mathbf{D_i}, \hat{\mathbf{p}}^o, \hat{\mathbf{q}}^o) = \frac{\prod_j g(D_{ij}|T_i, \hat{p_j}^o, \hat{q_j}^o)g(T_i)}{\sum_{T_i} \prod_j g(D_{ij}|T_i, \hat{p_j}^o, \hat{q_j}^o)g(T_i)} \tag{11}$$

where $g(T_i)$ is the a priori probability of T_i, and a voxelwise independence assumption has been made.

We store for each voxel the estimate of the probability that the ground truth at each voxel is $T_i = 1$. Since the ground truth is treated as a binary random variable, the probability that $T_i = 0$ is simply $1 - g(T_i = 1|\mathbf{D_i}, \hat{\mathbf{p}}^o, \hat{\mathbf{q}}^o)$.

Let $\alpha = \prod_{j:D_{ij}=1} \hat{p_j}^o \prod_{j:D_{ij}=0}(1 - \hat{p_j}^o)$ and $\beta = \prod_{j:D_{ij}=0} \hat{q_j}^o \prod_{j:D_{ij}=1}(1 - \hat{q_j}^o)$ where $j : D_{ij} = 1$ denotes the values of the index j for which the expert decision at voxel i (i.e. D_{ij}) has the value 1. Using the notation common for EM algorithms, let W_i be the weight variable.

$$W_i \equiv g(T_i = 1|\mathbf{D_i}, \hat{\mathbf{p}}^o, \hat{\mathbf{q}}^o) \tag{12}$$

$$= \frac{g(T_i = 1)\alpha}{g(T_i = 1)\alpha + (1 - g(T_1 = 1))\beta}. \tag{13}$$

The weight W_i indicates the probability of the ground truth at voxel i being equal to one. It is a normalized product of the prior probability of $T_i = 1$, the sensitivity of each of the experts that decided ground truth was one and the product of (1 - sensitivity) of each of the experts that decided the ground truth was zero.

2.2 Estimation of the Quality Parameters of the Experts

Given the estimate of the value of the ground truth derived above, we can find the values of the expert quality parameters that maximize the expectation of the log likelihood function.

$$\hat{\mathbf{p}}, \hat{\mathbf{q}} = \arg\max_{\mathbf{p}, \mathbf{q}} E_{g(\mathbf{T}|\mathbf{D}, \hat{\mathbf{p}}^o, \hat{\mathbf{q}}^o)} \left[\ln\left(f(\mathbf{D}|\mathbf{T}, \mathbf{p}, \mathbf{q})f(\mathbf{T}) \right) \right] \tag{14}$$

$$= \arg\max_{\mathbf{p}, \mathbf{q}} E_{g(\mathbf{T}|\mathbf{D}, \hat{\mathbf{p}}^o, \hat{\mathbf{q}}^o)} \left[\ln \prod_{ij} f(D_{ij}|T_i, p_j, q_j) + \ln \prod_i f(T_i) \right] \tag{15}$$

Since $\ln \prod_i f(T_i)$ is not a function of $\mathbf{p}, \mathbf{q}$, it follows that

$$\hat{\mathbf{p}}, \hat{\mathbf{q}} = \arg \max_{\mathbf{p},\mathbf{q}} \sum_j \sum_i E_{g(\mathbf{T}|\mathbf{D},\hat{\mathbf{p}}^\circ,\hat{\mathbf{q}}^\circ)} \left[\ln f(D_{ij}|T_i, p_j, q_j) \right] \qquad (16)$$

$$\hat{p}_j, \hat{q}_j = \arg \max_{p_j,q_j} \sum_i E_{g(\mathbf{T}|\mathbf{D},\hat{\mathbf{p}}^\circ,\hat{\mathbf{q}}^\circ)} \left[\ln f(D_{ij}|T_i, p_j, q_j) \right] \qquad (17)$$

$$= \arg \max_{p_j,q_j} \sum_i \Big[W_i \ln f(D_{ij}|T_i = 1, p_j, q_j)$$

$$+ (1 - W_i) \ln f(D_{ij}|T_i = 0, p_j, q_j) \Big]$$

$$= \arg \max_{p_j,q_j} \sum_{i:D_{ij}=1} W_i \ln p_j + \sum_{i:D_{ij}=1} (1 - W_i) \ln(1 - q_j)$$

$$+ \sum_{i:D_{ij}=0} W_i \ln(1 - p_j) + \sum_{i:D_{ij}=0} (1 - W_i) \ln q_j \qquad (18)$$

A necessary condition at a maximum of the above with respect to parameter p_j is that the first derivative equal zero. On differentiating $Q(\theta|\hat{\theta})$ with respect to parameter p_j and solving for 0, we find (similarly for $\hat{q}_j$)

$$\hat{p}_j = \frac{\sum_{i:D_{ij}=1} W_i}{\sum_{i:D_{ij}=1} W_i + \sum_{i:D_{ij}=0} W_i}, \qquad (19)$$

$$\hat{q}_j = \frac{\sum_{i:D_{ij}=0} (1 - W_i)}{\sum_{i:D_{ij}=1} (1 - W_i) + \sum_{i:D_{ij}=0} (1 - W_i)}. \qquad (20)$$

We can interpret the weight estimate W_i as the strength of belief in the underlying ground truth being equal to 1. In the case of perfect knowledge about the ground truth, i.e. $W_i \in \{0.0, 1.0\}$, the estimator of sensitivity given by Equation 19 corresponds to the usual definition of sensitivity as the true positive fraction. When the ground truth is a continuous parameter, i.e. $W_i \in [0, 1]$ as considered here, the estimator can be interpreted as the ratio of the number of true positive detections to the total amount of ground truth $T_i = 1$ voxels believed to be in the data, with each voxel detection weighted by the strength of belief in $T_i = 1$. Similarly, the specificity estimator of Equation 20 is a natural formulation of an estimator for the specificity given a degree of belief in the underlying $T_i = 0$ state.

3   Results

We describe experiments to characterize our algorithm running on synthetic data for which the ground truth is known, for assessment of an algorithm and experts segmenting a brain tumor from MRI, and for assessing segmentations from MRI of the peripheral zone of the prostate.

Table 1. Digital phantom consisting of class 1 set to cover half the image, with each expert segmentation identical to the ground truth. In each case, thresholding the converged ground truth estimate at 0.5 recovered the known ground truth exactly. In each of the experiments with two experts, each generating a segmentation identical to the known ground truth but with imperfect initial estimates of expert quality, the final ground truth weights are identical to the known ground truth and the algorithm has discovered the experts are operating perfectly, even when the a priori probability for ground truth was varied.

# experts	initial p_j, q_j	$Pr(T_i = 1)$	final $\hat{p}_j, \hat{q}_j$	# iterations	$W_i\|T_i = 1,$ $W_i\|T_i = 0$
1	$\{0.9, 0.9\}$	0.5	$\{0.9, 0.9\}$	1	0.9, 0.1
1	$\{0.9, 0.9\}$	0.4	$\{0.95, 0.80\}$	22	0.76, 0.04
1	$\{0.9, 0.9\}$	0.6	$\{0.80, 0.95\}$	22	0.96, 0.24
2	$\{0.9, 0.9\}, \{0.9, 0.9\}$	0.5	$\{1.0, 1.0\}, \{1.0, 1.0\}$	4	1.0, 0.0
2	$\{0.9, 0.9\}, \{0.9, 0.9\}$	0.4	$\{1.0, 1.0\}, \{1.0, 1.0\}$	4	1.0, 0.0
2	$\{0.9, 0.9\}, \{0.9, 0.9\}$	0.6	$\{1.0, 1.0\}, \{1.0, 1.0\}$	5	1.0, 0.0

Table 2. Ground truth class 1 was set to be a small square occupying roughly 11% of the 256x256 pixel image. In each experiment, thresholding the converged ground truth weights at 0.5 recovers the known ground truth exactly. In each of the multi-expert experiments, the ground truth weights converged to $W_i = 1$ at the class 1 voxels and $W_i = 0$ at the class 0 voxels. In the final experiment, one of the experts segmentation was set equal to the ground truth, and one was set equal to the ground truth shifted left 10 columns, and one was set equal to the ground truth shifted right 10 columns. The algorithm was able to discover one of the experts was generating a segmentation identical to the ground truth, and that the other two experts were slightly incorrect. The correct ground truth was indicated by the final ground truth weights and the quality estimates for each expert accurately reflected the segmentations.

# experts	initial $p_j = q_j$	$Pr(T_i = 1)$	final $\hat{p}_j, \hat{q}_j$	# itns	$W_i\|T_i = 1,$ $W_i\|T_i = 0$
1	0.9	0.5	$\{0.217, 0.997\}$	9	0.98, 0.44
1	0.9	0.12	$\{0.696, 0.973\}$	21	0.78, 0.04
2	0.9, 0.9	0.5	$\{1.0, 1.0\}, \{1.0, 1.0\}$	8	1.0, 0.0
2	0.9, 0.9	0.12	$\{1.0, 1.0\}, \{1.0, 1.0\}$	4	1.0, 0.0
3	0.9, 0.9, 0.9	0.12	$\{0.88, 0.99\}, \{1.0, 1.0\}, \{0.88, 0.99\}$	11	1.0, 0.0

Results of Experiments with Digital Phantoms with Known Ground Truth Table 1 illustrates experiments with known ground truth and each class occupying half the image. Table 2 illustrates experiments with known ground truth class 1 set to be a small square occupying roughly 11% of the 256x256 pixel image.

Validation of Brain Tumor Segmentation from MRI Figure 1 illustrates our algorithm applied to the analysis of expert segmentations of a brain tumor [10]. The analysis indicates the program is generating segmentations similar to that of the experts, with higher sensitivity than one of the experts, but with lower sensitivity than two other experts.

(a) border of ground truth esti- (b) sum of manual segmenta- (c) expert quality assessment.
mate.   tions.

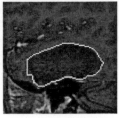 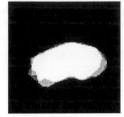

expert	$\hat{p}_j$	$\hat{q}_j$
1	0.8951	0.9999
2	0.9993	0.9857
3	0.9986	0.9982
program	0.9063	0.9990

Fig. 1. Part of MRI with a brain tumor visible and the border of the estimated ground truth overlayed, sum of expert segmentations, and quality assessment of three experts and a program. The results indicate the program is comparable to the experts, performing better than one expert and not as well as two other experts.

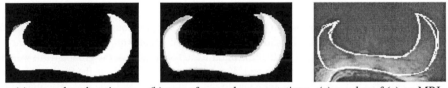

(a) ground truth estimate   (b) sum of manual segmentations   (c) overlay of (a) on MRI

Fig. 2. Ground truth segmentation estimate, sum of manual segmentations, and an overlay of borders of regions from the ground truth estimate on the MRI. The voxel intensity in (a) is proportional to the probability of the ground truth being 1 at each voxel. The overlayed borders of regions of different ground truth probability are readily appreciated in (c). The lowest probability is in regions where the expert segmentation is most difficult. The ground truth estimates rapidly reaches a near final configuration. The final result does not depend strongly upon the expert parameter initialization or the ground truth prior probability. **A binary estimate of the ground truth can be made by thresholding the ground truth estimate at 0.50, and in this case is equivalent to taking all the voxels indicated as prostate peripheral zone by at least three of the five segmentations, and then all the voxels indicated by two of the high quality segmentations but not those voxels indicated by only two of the lower quality segmentations.** Recall that our algorithm simultaneously estimates the quality of each of the segmentations together with the probabilistic ground truth estimate. This result cannot be achieved by a simple voting rule such as selecting voxels indicated by three out of five segmentations.

Validation of Prostate Peripheral Zone Segmentation from MRI Figure 2 illustrates our algorithm applied to the analysis of five segmentations by one expert of the peripheral zone of a prostate as seen in a conventional MRI scan (T2w acquisition, 0.468750 x 0.468750 x 3.0 mm^3). The ground truth estimates rapidly reaches a near final configuration, and more slowly refines the last few significant figures of the ground truth and expert parameter estimates. The final result does not depend strongly upon the expert parameter initialization or the ground truth prior probability. The final expert parameter estimates found are record in Table 3.

Table 3. Quality estimates for the five prostate segmentations generated by one expert, and Dice similarity coefficient (DSC), $DSC \equiv \frac{2|A \cap B|}{|A|+|B|}$ with $|A|$ the area of region A, comparing the expert segmentation with the ground truth estimate with $T_i \geq 0.5$. Results are shown for two different assumptions of the prior probability of prostate peripheral zone being present at each voxel and indicate the final estimates do not depend strongly on the ground truth prior probability assumption. The rank order of the experts is the same in each case. Note that our algorithm provides more information than DSC, for example, DSC of expert 2 and 4 is similar, but they have quite different sensitivities.

Expert segmentations	1	2	3	4	5
$g(T_i = 1) = 0.10$					
final $\hat{p}_j$	0.87509	0.987198	0.921549	0.907344	0.880789
final $\hat{q}_j$	0.999163	0.994918	0.999435	0.999739	0.999446
DSC	0.927660	0.957527	0.954471	0.949058	0.932096
$g(T_i = 1) = 0.02$					
final $\hat{p}_j$	0.878533	0.991261	0.936831	0.918336	0.894861
final $\hat{q}_j$	0.998328	0.993993	0.99932	0.999359	0.999301
DSC	0.913083	0.951027	0.967157	0.954827	0.944756

4   Discussion and Conclusion

We have presented an algorithm for simultaneously constructing an estimate of the "ground truth" segmentation from a collection of segmentations, and an estimate of the quality of each segmentation generator. This can be used to assess new segmentations by direct comparison to the ground truth estimate.

At least one digital brain phantom [2] was constructed from segmentations obtained from high signal-to-noise images by manual correction of the output of an automated segmentation algorithm. The approach described here provides a straightforward and principled way to combine manual segmentations to provide a "ground truth" estimate for the construction of such phantoms.

Acknowledgements

This investigation was supported by NIH grants P41 RR13218, P01 CA67165, R01 RR11747, R01 CA86879, R33 CA99015, R21 CA89449, by a research grant from the Whitaker Foundation, and by a New Concept Award from the Center for Integration of Medicine and Innovative Technology. We gratefully acknowledge the contributions of the experts who generated the segmentations of the clinical data, and of Dr. Clare Tempany for helpful discussions regarding the detection of the prostate peripheral zone, and its clinical significance.

References

1. M. Styner, C. Brechbühler, G. Székely, and G. Gerig, "Parametric estimate of intensity inhomogeneities applied to MRI," *IEEE Transactions On Medical Imaging*, vol. 19, pp. 153–165, March 2000.

2. D. Collins, A. Zijdenbos, V. Kollokian, J. Sled, N. Kabani, C. Holmes, and A. Evans, "Design and Construction of a Realistic Digital Brain Phantom," *IEEE Transactions on Medical Imaging*, vol. 17, pp. 463–468, June 1998.

3. L. R. Dice, "Measures of the amount of ecologic association between species," *Ecology*, vol. 26, no. 3, pp. 297–302, 1945.

4. P. Jaccard, "The distribution of flora in the alpine zone," *New Phytologist*, vol. 11, pp. 37–50, 1912.

5. A. P. Zijdenbos, B. M. Dawant, R. A. Margolin, and A. C. Palmer, "Morphometric Analysis of White Matter Lesions in MR Images: Method and Validation," *IEEE Transactions on Medical Imaging*, vol. 13, pp. 716–724, December 1994.

6. S. Warfield, J. Dengler, J. Zaers, C. R. Guttmann, W. M. Wells III, G. J. Ettinger, J. Hiller, and R. Kikinis, "Automatic Identification of Grey Matter Structures from MRI to Improve the Segmentation of White Matter Lesions," *J Image Guid Surg*, vol. 1, no. 6, pp. 326–338, 1995.

7. S. K. Warfield, R. V. Mulkern, C. S. Winalski, F. A. Jolesz, and R. Kikinis, "An Image Processing Strategy for the Quantification and Visualization of Exercise Induced Muscle MRI Signal Enhancement," *J Magn Reson Imaging*, vol. 11, pp. 525–531, May 2000.

8. A. Dempster, N. Laird, and D. Rubin, "Maximum-likelihood from incomplete data via the EM algorithm," *J. Royal Statist. Soc. Ser. B.*, vol. 39, pp. 34–37, 1977.

9. S. K. Warfield, M. Kaus, F. A. Jolesz, and R. Kikinis, "Adaptive, Template Moderated, Spatially Varying Statistical Classification," *Med Image Anal*, vol. 4, pp. 43–55, Mar 2000.

10. M. Kaus, S. K. Warfield, A. Nabavi, P. M. Black, F. A. Jolesz, and R. Kikinis, "Automated Segmentation of MRI of Brain Tumors," *Radiology*, vol. 218, pp. 586–591, Feb 2001.

Validation of Volume-Preserving Non-rigid Registration: Application to Contrast-Enhanced MR-Mammography

C. Tanner[1], J.A. Schnabel[1], A. Degenhard[2], A.D. Castellano-Smith[1],
C. Hayes[2], M.O. Leach[2], D.R. Hose[3], D.L.G. Hill[1], and D.J. Hawkes[1]

[1] Div. of Radiological Sciences & Medical Engineering, King's College London, UK
[2] Section of MR, Inst. of Cancer Research & Royal Marsden NHS Trust, Sutton, UK
[3] Dept. of Medical Physics and Clinical Engineering, University of Sheffield, UK
christine.tanner@kcl.ac.uk

Abstract. In this paper, we present a validation study for volume preserving non-rigid registration of 3D contrast-enhanced magnetic resonance mammograms. This study allows for the first time to assess the effectiveness of a volume preserving constraint to improve registration accuracy in this context. The validation is based on the simulation of physically plausible breast deformations with biomechanical breast models (BBMs) employing finite element methods. We constructed BBMs for four patients with four different deformation scenarios each. These deformations were applied to the post-contrast image to simulate patient motion occurring between pre- and post-contrast image acquisition. The original pre-contrast images were registered to the corresponding BBM-deformed post-contrast images. We assessed the accuracy of two optimisation schemes of a non-rigid registration algorithm. The first solely aims to improve the similarity of the images while the second includes the minimisation of volume changes as another objective. We observed reductions in residual registration error at every resolution when constraining the registration to preserve volume. Within the contrast enhancing lesion, the best results were obtained with a control point spacing of 20mm, resulting in target registration errors below 0.5mm on average. This study forms an important milestone in making the non-rigid registration framework applicable for clinical routine use.

1 Introduction

Contrast-enhanced magnetic resonance (CE MR) mammography is based on obtaining MR images before and after the injection of contrast agent into the bloodstream. Breast cancer malignancies can be detected in-vivo by their increased vascularity, increased vascular permeability and/or increased interstitial pressure [1, 2], causing a rapid rise in the intensity of CE MR-mammograms. However, a considerable proportion of benign lesions also enhance. The rate and amount of the enhancement as well as the characteristics of the intensity changes after the peak enhancement need to be taken into account if specificity is to be improved [3].

The detailed quantitative analysis of the intensity changes over time relies on the accurate alignment of all images. Patient movement will introduce correspondence errors that may invalidate such an analysis. Previously, an algorithm has been devised for

T. Dohi and R. Kikinis (Eds.): MICCAI 2002, LNCS 2488, pp. 307–314, 2002.
© Springer-Verlag Berlin Heidelberg 2002

the non-rigid registration of images [4] and applied to CE MR-mammograms. It was shown that this registration method significantly improved the quality of the pre- and post-contrast image difference [5].

Generally, non-rigid registration algorithms can change the volume of structures. This is for example necessary for inter-subject registration. Volume changes are, however, physically implausible during a CE MR-mammography acquisition since no external forces are applied to the breast and the gap between image acquisitions is short. In [6] we evaluated the volume change associated with non-rigid registration of 15 contrast enhancing breast lesions and found volume shrinkage and expansion of up to 20%. Previously, volume changes were reduced by the introduction of a volume preserving regularization term to the registration's optimisation scheme [7–9]. The question remains, however, how to measure the residual registration error since no ground truth exists.

In [10] we have proposed validation of non-rigid registration algorithms on the basis of applying it to misaligned images, generated from plausible deformations simulated by biomechanical models. This generic method has the advantage of providing a displacement vector at every position within the organ. We have employed this method for validating two non-rigid registration algorithms [4, 11] based on single and multi-level free-form deformations (FFDs) using B-splines and normalised mutual information [12] and found an improved accuracy for the multi-level FFD approach. In this validation study we will for the first time assess the influence of volume preserving constraints on the target registration error for a multi-resolution FFD non-rigid registration for the application of CE MR-mammography.

2   Materials

We selected from a large CE-MR mammography database four cases where almost no motion between image acquisitions was visible. The images have been acquired with a 3D gradient echo sequence on a Philips (case 1-3) or a Siemens (case 4) 1.5T MR system with TR=12ms, TE=5ms, flip angle=35° and a field of view of 350mm (case 1-3) or 340mm (case 4). The voxel dimensions are $1.37 \times 1.37 \times 4.2mm^3$ (case 1-2), $1.48 \times 1.48 \times 4.2mm^3$ (case 3) and $1.33 \times 1.33 \times 2.5mm^3$ (case 4). The slice orientation is axial (case 1-3) or coronal (case 4). Example slices of the difference of the original images are shown in Fig. 1a, where case 4 was reformatted to have an axial slice direction for better visual comparison.

3   Methods

3.1   Registration

In this study the non-rigid registration is based on the multi-resolution FFD approach based on accurate B-spline subdivision as described in [4]. In comparison to the multi-level FFD approach [11], this has the advantage that the analytical Jacobian of the transformation can be effectively determined at each resolution. Firstly, global motion is corrected by using a rigid transformation. Local motion is then modelled by FFDs based on B-splines where the object is deformed by manipulating an underlying mesh of control points. Starting from a coarser mesh to account for the larger deformations, the mesh is subdivided at each resolution to give the FFDs more local flexibility. At any stage, the transformation $\mathbf{T}$ between the images A and B can be described as the sum of the global 3D rigid transformation $\mathbf{T}_g$ and the local FFD transformation $\mathbf{T}_l$, i.e. $\mathbf{T}(\mathbf{x}) = \mathbf{T}_g(\mathbf{x}) + \mathbf{T}_l(\mathbf{x})$. This transformation maps the position $\mathbf{x} = (x_1\ x_2\ x_3)^T$ in A to the corresponding position $T(\mathbf{x})$ in B.

FFD transformation. Let $\Omega = \{\mathbf{x}\,|\,0 \le x_i < X_i,\ i \in \{1,2,3\}\}$ be the domain of the image volume and let $\Psi = \{\psi_{j_1,j_2,j_3}\,|\,j_i \in \{0,1,\dots,N_i-1\},\ i \in \{1,2,3\}\}$ be the mesh of control points with displacements $\phi^{(i)}_{j_1,j_2,j_3}$ and spacing $\delta_i = \frac{X_i}{N_i-1}$ for $i \in \{1,2,3\}$. $\mathbf{T}_l(\mathbf{x}) = (T_l^{(1)}(\mathbf{x})\ T_l^{(2)}(\mathbf{x})\ T_l^{(3)}(\mathbf{x}))^T$ can then be written as:

$$T_l^{(i)}(\mathbf{x}) = \sum_{m_1=0}^{3}\sum_{m_2=0}^{3}\sum_{m_3=0}^{3}\prod_{k=1}^{3} B_{m_k}(u_k)\phi^{(i)}_{j_1+m_1,j_2+m_2,j_3+m_3} \quad i \in \{1,2,3\} \quad (1)$$

where $j_i = \lfloor\frac{x_i}{\delta_i}\rfloor - 1$, $u_i = \frac{x_i}{\delta_i} - \lfloor\frac{x_i}{\delta_i}\rfloor$ for $i \in \{1,2,3\}$ and B_m is the m-th basis function of the B-spline defined by:
$$B_0(u) = (1-u)^3/6 \qquad\qquad B_2(u) = (-3u^3 + 3u^2 + 3u + 1)/6$$
$$B_1(u) = (3u^3 - 6u^2 + 4)/6 \qquad B_3(u) = u^3/6$$

Volume Preserving Regularization Term. In this validation we apply the volume preserving regularization term suggested by Rohlfing et al. [9]. The local volume change at position $\mathbf{x}$ after applying transformation $\mathbf{T}$ can be calculated by the determinant of the Jacobian:

$$J_{\mathbf{T}}(\mathbf{x}) = \det\begin{pmatrix} \frac{\partial}{\partial x_1}T_l^{(1)}(\mathbf{x}) & \frac{\partial}{\partial x_2}T_l^{(1)}(\mathbf{x}) & \frac{\partial}{\partial x_3}T_l^{(1)}(\mathbf{x}) \\ \frac{\partial}{\partial x_1}T_l^{(2)}(\mathbf{x}) & \frac{\partial}{\partial x_2}T_l^{(2)}(\mathbf{x}) & \frac{\partial}{\partial x_3}T_l^{(2)}(\mathbf{x}) \\ \frac{\partial}{\partial x_1}T_l^{(3)}(\mathbf{x}) & \frac{\partial}{\partial x_2}T_l^{(3)}(\mathbf{x}) & \frac{\partial}{\partial x_3}T_l^{(3)}(\mathbf{x}) \end{pmatrix} \quad (2)$$

where

$$\frac{\partial T_l^{(i)}(\mathbf{x})}{\partial x_n} = \frac{1}{\delta_n}\sum_{m_1=0}^{3}\sum_{m_2=0}^{3}\sum_{m_3=0}^{3}\frac{dB_{m_n}(u_n)}{du_n}\prod_{k\in\{1,2,3\}\cap n} B_{m_k}(u_k)\phi^{(i)}_{j_1+m_1,j_2+m_2,j_3+m_3}. \quad (3)$$

can be computed analytically. The regularization term for volume preservation from [9] is given by the mean absolute logarithm of the Jacobian at the control point positions:

$$C_{jacobian}(\mathbf{T}) = \frac{1}{N_1 N_2 N_3}\sum_{j_1=0}^{N_1-1}\sum_{j_2=0}^{N_2-1}\sum_{j_3=0}^{N_3-1} |\ln(J_{\mathbf{T}}(j_1\delta_1, j_2\delta_2, j_3\delta_3))|. \quad (4)$$

Volume shrinkage and expansion are equally penalised by (4). Transformation $\mathbf{T}$ is then found by minimising the cost function [9]:

$$C(\mathbf{T}) = -(1-\mu)C_{similarity}(A, \mathbf{T}(B)) + \mu C_{jacobian}(\mathbf{T}) \quad (5)$$

where μ is the weight of the volume preserving regularization term, that is balancing the two objectives of the cost function. Normalised mutual information (NMI) was used as the image similarity measure $C_{similarity}$.

3.2   Validation

The validation is based on the simulation of plausible breast deformation using biomechanical breast models based on finite element methods [10].

Biomechanical Breast Models. Four pre- and post-contrast image sets, which showed almost no motion, were selected from a large patient data base. The images were segmented into fat, glandular tissue and enhancing lesion. The outside surface of the fat and the enhancing lesion were then triangulated via vtk [13] and meshed into 10-noded tetrahedral elements with the ANSYS FEM package [14]. Elements within glandular tissue were assigned to have glandular material properties. All tissues were modelled as linear, isotropic and homogeneous. Elastic values (Young's modulus) of 1kPa, 1.5kPa, 3.6kPa were assigned to fat, glandular tissue and enhancing lesion, respectively, in accordance with [15]. Note that only the relative relationship of the Young's moduli are important since displacements rather than forces are applied. This model is therefore also very close to the values in [16] for 5% precompression. A Poisson's ratio of 0.495 was chosen to enforce incompressibility of the tissue. The average performance of this model is statistically (paired t-test) not significantly different at the 5% level to the best models from [17].

Simulation. Four different deformations were generated. 'Regional displacement' simulated a uniform displacement on one side of the breast, 'point puncture' imitated a deformation during biopsy, 'one-sided contact' simulated a deformation of the breast when pushed against the breast coil and 'two-sided contact' imitated the gentle fixation of the breast between two plates. All displacements were of maximal 10mm magnitude, which corresponds to the maximum offset observed during a normal CE MR-mammography session. For these boundary conditions, the BBMs were solved using ANSYS [14]. A continuous displacement field within the FEM mesh was produced by quadratic shape interpolation of the 10-noded tetrahedral elements. This field was applied to the post-contrast image to simulate deformations between pre- and post-contrast images. Locations outside the FEM-mesh had to be masked out for any further processing since no deformation information is available at these locations. We registered the pre-contrast images to the BBM-deformed post-contrast images to avoid any further interpolation of the latter.

Quantification. The accuracy of the registration can be quantified with respect to the gold standard displacements at each voxel position. The degree of alignment between two corresponding points after registration is described by the target registration error (TRE) [18]. Traditionally, TRE is calculated at anatomical landmarks. In the case of BBM-simulated deformations the correspondence is known at all position within the FEM mesh. We therefore calculate a more evenly distributed error by computing TRE at all voxel positions $\mathbf{x}$ within the FEM mesh:

$$TRE(\mathbf{x}) = ||\mathbf{T}_{2F} \circ \mathbf{T}_{F1}(\mathbf{x}) - \mathbf{x}|| \qquad (6)$$

where $\mathbf{T}_{F1}$ is the FEM-transformation mapping any voxel position in the post-contrast image I_1 into the BBM-deformed post-contrast image I_F. Transformation $\mathbf{T}_{2F}$ is obtained from the registration of the pre-contrast image I_2 to I_F. Equation (6) assumes that no motion has occurred between I_2 and I_1. We can try to estimate how much motion has occurred from a registration of I_2 to I_1 yielding transformation $\mathbf{T}_{12}(\mathbf{x})$ which in the ideal case is the identity transformation. This estimate can then be used to balance the TRE computation, providing a measure which we will call consistency registration error (CRE) [12]

$$CRE(\mathbf{x}) = ||\mathbf{T}_{12} \circ \mathbf{T}_{2F} \circ \mathbf{T}_{F1}(\mathbf{x}) - \mathbf{x}||. \tag{7}$$

4   Results

In this study, we investigated the registration performance of an unconstrained and a volume-preserving non-rigid registration scheme. All images were registered in a multi-resolution strategy, where an initial rigid registration was followed by non-rigid registrations of FFD resolutions of 20mm, 10mm and 5mm (see 3.1). The registration performance was assessed by calculating the target registration error (TRE) and consistency registration error (CRE) with respect to the simulated gold standard (see 3.2).

Regularization weight. A reasonable weight (μ_r) between image similarity and volume preservation was determined by calculating the volume change and the TRE for eight different values of μ within the range of 0.05 to 0.95 for two cases. In contrast to [9] we observed that a weight of 0.05 did not preserve volume. Mean volume shrinkage in these two cases was 13.2% without volume preservation and 13.0% with volume preservation. We chose μ_r=0.8, which reduced the shrinkage to 3.2% and provided the minimal median TRE over the whole breast tissue.

Validation. We conducted registrations of four patient cases and four BBM simulations each, for the volume preserving ($\mu=\mu_r$) and the unconstrained registration scheme ($\mu=0$). Fig. 1b shows examples of motion artifacts introduced by the BBM simulated deformations. These artifacts are greatly reduced after unconstrained multi-resolution registration (Fig. 1d). Visually similar results are achieved by the volume preserving non-rigid registration (Fig. 1f). Local registration failures at highly deformed regions can be observed for the 20mm FFD registrations (Fig. 1c,e).

The volume changes before and after registration were evaluated over the whole breast tissue and for the enhancing lesion region (Table 1). The BBM simulation introduced absolute volume changes below 0.6%. Within the lesion, the maximum absolute volume change increased to 17.6% for the unconstrained registration, while for the volume preserving scheme it only increased to 5.1%.

The volume preserving non-rigid registration, produced at every FFD resolution, lower target registration errors when compared with the unconstrained method (Fig. 2a,b). Registrations with finer control point spacing compensated better for severe local deformations. However, within the region of the enhancing lesion, the best results were obtained with a control point spacing of 20mm. The consistency registration errors followed a similar trend (Fig. 2c,d). The 20mm FFD registration results were obtained on average within 2.2 and 1.7 hours for the unconstrained and the volume preserving scheme, respectively, on a 1.8 GHz Athon processor with 1GByte 1.33 MHz SD RAM memory. The full multi-resolution results (20mm+10mm+5mm) of the unconstrained and the volume preserving registration were available after 5.1 and 5.4 hours, respectively.

5 Discussion

We have presented a validation of an unconstrained and a volume preserving non-rigid registration scheme on the example of CE MR-mammography. The validation was based on simulating biomechanical plausible breast deformations as a gold standard.

We found that the volume preserving non-rigid registration was more accurate than the unconstrained method. Severe local deformations were better compensated by finer control point spacing. However, the contrast enhancing lesions were more accurately aligned at a control point spacing of 20mm.

This validation study has measured for the first time the target registration error of a volume preserving non-rigid registration. Our application is the alignment of dynamically acquired volumes in CE MR-mammograms. This is an important step towards making the registration techniques applicable for clinical routine use.

6 Acknowledgements

CT, AD and ADCS acknowledge funding from EPSRC (MIAS-IRC, GR/M52779, GR/M52762, GR/M47294). JAS is supported by Philips Medical Systems, EasyVision Advanced Development. The authors wish to thank Torsten Rohlfing for valuable discussions. The image data were provided by Guy's and St.Thomas' Hospitals (case 1-3) and by the UK MR breast screening study (MARIBS) http://www.icr.ac.uk/cmagres/maribs/maribs.html (case 4).

References

1. C. H. Blood and B. R. Zetter, "Tumor Interactions with the Vasculature: Angiogensis and Tumor Metastasis," *Biochimica et Biophysica Acta*, vol. 1032, pp. 89–118, 1990.
2. P. W. Vaupel, *Blood Flow, Oxygenation, Tissue pH Distribution, and Bioenergetic Status of Tumors*. Berlin, Germany: Ernst Schering Research Foundation, 1st ed., 1994.
3. M. D. Schnall and D. M. Ikeda, "Lesion Diagnosis Working Group Report," *Journal of Magnetic Resonance Imaging*, vol. 10, pp. 982–990, 1999.
4. D. Rueckert, L. I. Sonoda, C. Hayes, D. L. Hill, M. O. Leach, and D. J. Hawkes, "Non-rigid Registration using Free-Form Deformations: Application to Breast MR Images," *IEEE Transactions on Medical Imaging*, vol. 7, pp. 1–10, August 1999.
5. E. R. E. Denton, L. I. Sonoda, D. Rueckert, S. C. Rankin, C. Hayes, M. O. Leach, and D. J. Hawkes, "Comparison and Evaluation of Rigid, Affine, and Nonrigid Registration of Breast MR Images," *Journal of Computer Assisted Tomography*, vol. 5, pp. 800–805, May 1999.
6. C. Tanner, J. A. Schnabel, D. Chung, M. J. Clarkson, D. Rueckert, D. L. G. Hill, and D. J. Hawkes, "Volume and Shape Preservation of Enhancing Lesions when Applying Non-rigid Registration to a Time Series of Contrast Enhanced MR Breast Images," in *Medical Image Computing and Computer-Assisted Intervention, Pittsburgh, USA*, pp. 327–337, 2000.
7. D. Terzopoulos and K. Waters, "Analysis and Synthesis of Facial Image Sequences using Physical and Anatomical Models," *IEEE Transactions on Pattern Analysis and Machine Intelligence*, vol. 15, pp. 569–579, 1993.
8. P. J. Edwards, D. L. G. Hill, J. A. Little, and D. J. Hawkes, "A Three-Component Deformation Model for Image-Guided Surgery," *Medical Image Analysis*, vol. 2, pp. 355–367, 1998.

9. T. Rohlfing and C. R. Maurer, "Intensity-Based Non-rigid Registration Using Adaptive Multilevel Free-Form Deformation with an Incompressibility Constraint," in *Medical Image Computing and Computer-Assisted Intervention, Utrecht, Netherlands*, pp. 111–119, 2001.

10. J. A. Schnabel, C. Tanner, A. D. Castellano-Smith, M. O. Leach, C. Hayes, A. Degenhard, R. Hose, D. L. G. Hill, and D. J. Hawkes, "Validation of Non-Rigid Registration using Finite Element Methods," in *Information Processing in Medical Imaging, Davis, CA, USA*, pp. 344–357, 2001.

11. J. A. Schnabel, D. Rueckert, M. Quist, J. M. Blackall, A. Castellano-Smith, T. Hartkens, G. P. Penney, W. A. Hall, C. L. Truwit, F. A. Gerritsen, D. L. G. Hill, and D. J. Hawkes, "A Generic Framework for Non-Rigid Registration based on Non-Uniform Multi-Level Free-Form Deformations," in *Medical Image Computing and Computer-Assisted Intervention, Utrecht, Netherlands*, pp. 573–581, 2001.

12. J. A. Schnabel, C. Tanner, A. D. Castellano-Smith, A. Degenhard, C. Hayes, M. O. Leach, D. R. Hose, and D. J. H. D. L. G. Hill, "Finite element based validation of non-rigid registration using single- and multi-level free-form deformations: Application to contrast-enhanced MR mammography," in *Proceedings SPIE Medical Imaging 2002, Image Processing, San Diego, CA*, pp. 550–581, 2002.

13. W. Schroeder, K. Martin, and B. Lorensen, *The Visualization Toolkit*. New Jersey, USA: Prentice Hall PTR, 2nd ed., 1998.

14. ANSYS. http://www.ansys.com.

15. A. Sarvazyan, D. Goukassian, E. Maevsky, and G. Oranskaja, "Elastic Imaging as a new Modality of Medical Imaging for Cancer Detection," in *Proceedings of the International Workshop on Interaction of Ultrasound with Biological Media, Valenciennes, France*, pp. 69–81, 1994.

16. T. A. Krouskop, T. M. Wheeler, F. Kallel, B. S. Garra, and T. Hall, "Elastic Moduli of Breast and Prostate Tissues Under Compression," *Ultrasonic Imaging*, vol. 20, pp. 260–274, 1998.

17. C. Tanner, A. Degenhard, J. A. Schnabel, A. Castellano-Smith, C. Hayes, L. I. Sonoda, M. O. Leach, D. R. Hose, D. L. G. Hill, and D. J. Hawkes, "A Comparison of Biomechanical Breast Models: A Case Study," in *Proceedings SPIE Medical Imaging 2002, Image Processing, San Diego, CA*, pp. 1807–1818, 2002.

18. J. M. Fitzpatrick, "Detecting failure, assessing success," in Hajnal *et al.* [19], ch. I-6, pp. 117–139.

19. J. V. Hajnal, D. L. G. Hill and D. J. Hawkes, eds., *Medical Image Registration*. CRC Press, 2001.

Volume change in %	whole breast tissue				enhancing lesion			
	mean	std	min	max	mean	std	min	max
BBM simulation	-0.10	0.13	-0.33	0.12	0.12	0.18	-0.03	0.57
20mm FFD, $\mu=0$	-0.53	0.71	-1.93	0.77	-2.04	5.03	-17.64	2.53
10mm FFD, $\mu=0$	-0.55	0.71	-1.95	0.76	-0.78	5.32	-13.53	5.95
5mm FFD, $\mu=0$	-0.55	0.69	-1.93	0.77	-0.71	5.84	-15.50	6.85
20mm FFD, $\mu=0.8$	-0.16	0.22	-0.75	0.08	0.08	0.90	-1.63	2.09
10mm FFD, $\mu=0.8$	-0.17	0.26	-0.70	0.16	-0.38	1.47	-5.07	1.56
5mm FFD, $\mu=0.8$	-0.18	0.31	-0.79	0.24	-0.16	1.05	-2.72	1.39

Table 1. Mean, standard deviation, minimal and maximal volume change of four patient cases and four BBM deformations each. Volume changes are evaluated over whole breast tissue (left) and over enhancing lesion (right) after BBM simulation and after multi-resolution FFD registration.

(a) original   (b) deformed   (c) 20mm, μ=0 (d) 5mm, μ=0   (e) 20mm,μ=.8 (f) 5mm, μ=.8

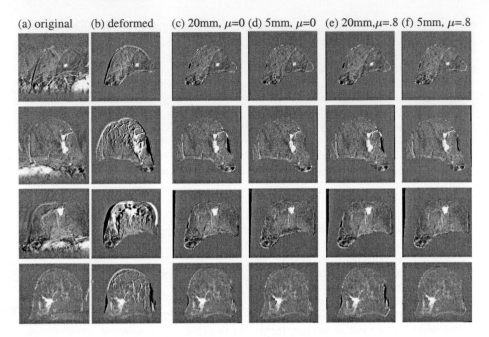

Fig. 1. Example slices for cases 1-4 (top to bottom) showing difference (a) of pre- and post-contrast images; (b) after deformation simulation; (c) after rigid + 20mm FFD registration without volume preveration constraint (μ=0); (d) after rigid + 20mm + 10mm + 5mm FFD registration with μ=0; (e) after rigid + 20mm FFD registration with μ=0.8; (f) after rigid + 20mm + 10mm + 5mm FFD registration with μ=0.8.

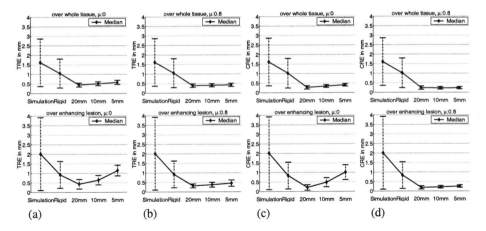

Fig. 2. Target registration error (TRE) for multi-resolution FFD registration (a) without volume preservation constraint (μ=0) and (b) for μ=0.8. Consistency registration error (CRE) for (c) μ=0 and (d) for μ=0.8. Top: Results evaluated over the whole breast tissue. Bottom: Results evaluated only over the region of the enhancing lesion. Error bars show the standard deviation from the mean over patients and simulations.

Statistical Validation of Automated Probabilistic Segmentation against Composite Latent Expert Ground Truth in MR Imaging of Brain Tumors

Kelly H. Zou, William M. Wells III, Michael R. Kaus, Ron Kikinis,
Ferenc A. Jolesz, and Simon K. Warfield

Surgical Planning Laboratory,
Harvard Medical School and Brigham and Women's Hospital,
75 Francis St., Boston, MA 02115 USA
{zou,sw,kaus,kikinis,jolesz,warfield}@bwh.harvard.edu

Abstract. The validity of segmentation is an important issue in image processing because it has a direct impact on surgical planning. Binary manual segmentation is not only time-consuming but also lacks the ability of differentiating subtle intensity variations among voxels, particularly for those on the border of a tumor and for different tumor types. Previously we have developed an automated segmentation method that yields voxel-wise continuous probabilistic measures, indicating a level of tumor presence. The goal of this work is to examine three accuracy metrics based on two-sample statistical methods, against the estimated composite latent ground truth derived from several experts' manual segmentation by a maximum likelihood algorithm. We estimated the distribution functions of the tumor and control voxel data parametrically by assuming a mixture of two beta distributions with different shape parameters. We derived the resulting receiver operating characteristic curves, Dice similarity coefficients, and mutual information, over all possible decision thresholds. Based on each validation metric, an optimal threshold was then computed via maximization. We illustrated these methods on MR imaging data from nine brain tumor cases, three with meningiomas, three astrocytomas, and three other low-grade gliomas. The automated segmentation yielded satisfactory accuracy, with varied optimal thresholds.

1   Introduction

Surgical planning and image-guided intervention procedures increasingly employ semi-automated segmentation algorithms. MR imaging of the brain provides useful information about its anatomical structure, enabling quantitative pathological or clinical studies. Brain segmentation frequently assigns unique labels to several classes, e.g., skin, brain tissue, ventricles and tumor, representing an anatomic structure to each voxel in an input gray-level image.

Binary (two-class) manual segmentation is a simple and yet time-consuming procedure. It also has the difficulty of differentiating subtle intensity variations among voxels, particularly for those on the border of a tumor. However, the results of such manual segmentations may ultimately influence the amount and degree of tumor removal.

Recently, Warfield et al. have proposed an automated segmenter that yields voxel-wise continuous probabilistic measures indicative of malignancy (see [1] for an example). Thus, methods for validating continuous segmentation data are required. The aim

T. Dohi and R. Kikinis (Eds.): MICCAI 2002, LNCS 2488, pp. 315–322, 2002.

of this study was to evaluate the performance of this segmenter by examining three validation metrics, compared against combined experts' manual segmentations as the ground truth.

The most important element in validating the accuracy of a segmentation algorithm is the ground truth, which is the classification truth of each voxel. For simplicity, we assume a two-class truth by labeling the non-tumor class as C_0 and tumor class as C_1.

For the purpose of comparing two sets of binary segmentation results, several accuracy and reliability metrics may be found in the literature [2]. For example, Jaccard (JSC) [3] and Dice (DSC) [4] similarity coefficients are typically used as a measure of overlap; DSC ranges from 0, indicating no similarity between these two sets of binary segmentation results, to 1, indicating complete agreement.

In order to evaluate the performance of a "continuous classifier", the distributions in the two distinct classes, C_0 and C_1, may be directly compared using two-sample statistics such as a Student's t-test or a nonparametric Mann-Whitney U-statistic. Alternatively, a Komogorov-Smirnov test may be used to directly compare the two underlying distributions. Other distance measures between the two sets may also be considered.

Several statistical methods may be adopted for assessing the performance of a continuous classifier. A popular method for assessing the overall classification accuracy is a receiver operating characteristic (ROC) curve, a function of sensitivity vs. (1-specificity). Zou et al. developed several methods, including nonparametric, semiparametric, and parametric, for estimating and comparing ROC curves derived from continuous data [5,6]. The goal of this work is to examine and illustrate three accuracy metrics, ROC curve, mutual information, and Dice similarity coefficient, to validate automated probabilistic brain tumor segmentations.

2   Notations and Assumptions

For simplicity, we assume that individual voxels belong to one of two distinct and independent populations (i.e., non-tumor control class, C_0 vs. tumor class, C_1), determined by the ground truth, T. Consider two random samples, X_i ($i = 1, ..., m$) and Y_j ($j = 1, ..., n$), drawn from C_0 and C_1, respectively. The observed continuous random variable is labeled Z of prosbabilistic segmentation measures. The continuous random variable Z generates our probabilistic segmentation data, while the ground truth T determines the true voxel-wise classes. Stratified by the truth, for each member of class C_0, there is a measurement $X \sim (Z|T = 0)$ assumed to have cumulative distribution function (c.d.f.) F, with probability density function (p.d.f.) f and survival function $\overline{F} = 1 - F$. Similarly, for each member of class C_1, there is a measurement $Y \sim (Z|T = 1)$ assumed to have c.d.f. G with p.d.f. g and survival function $\overline{G} = 1 - G$.

We assume that the ground truth, T, has a Bernoulli distribution, with a probability of $\Pr(T = 0) = \pi = m/(m + n)$ for class C_0 and the tumor probability of $\Pr(T = 1) = \overline{\pi} = 1 - \pi = n/(m+n)$ for class C_1. By Bayes' Theorem, the marginal distribution of Z is a mixture of F and G, with mixing proportions π and $\overline{\pi}$. That is, CDF $K = \pi \cdot F + \overline{\pi} \cdot G$ with pdf k, where the p.d.f. of Z is

$$k(z) = \pi f(z) + \overline{\pi} g(z), \quad \text{with} \quad \pi + \overline{\pi} = 1 \ (\forall z \in [0, 1]). \tag{1}$$

Specifying any arbitrary threshold, $\gamma \in (0, 1)$ for Z, yields a discretized version of a decision random variable, D_γ. This implies the equivalence of the following events: $\{D_\gamma = 0\} \equiv \{Z \le \gamma\}$ and $\{D_\gamma = 1\} \equiv \{Z > \gamma\}$. Thus, we may construct Table 1:

Table 1. A two-by-two table of the joint probabilities of the truth (T) vs. the corresponding segmentation decision (D_γ) at each possible threshold γ.

Decision vs. Truth	$T = 0$ (non-tumor)	$T = 1$ (tumor)
$D_\gamma = 0$ (non-tumor)	p_{11}	p_{12}
$D_\gamma = 1$ (tumor)	p_{21}	p_{22}
Marginal Total	π	$\overline{\pi}$

where

$$p_{11} = P(D_\gamma = 0, T = 0) = P(Z \le \gamma | T = 0)P(T = 0) = \pi F(\gamma),$$
$$p_{21} = P(D_\gamma = 1, T = 0) = P(Z > \gamma | T = 0)P(T = 0) = \pi \overline{F}(\gamma),$$
$$p_{12} = P(D_\gamma = 0, T = 1) = P(Z \le \gamma | T = 1)P(T = 1) = \overline{\pi} G(\gamma),$$
$$p_{22} = P(D_\gamma = 1, T = 1) = P(Z > \gamma | T = 1)P(T = 1) = \overline{\pi} \overline{G}(\gamma).$$

Note that the marginal totals, $p_{11} + p_{21} = \pi$ and $p_{12} + p_{22} = \overline{\pi}$, are related to the Bernoulli parameter of T. Let $p_\gamma = \overline{F}(\gamma)$ and $q_\gamma = \overline{G}(\gamma)$ (see Section 4.1) [5,6].

3   Estimation of the Composite Latent Binary Ground Truth and Modeling Assumptions for the Probabilistic Segmentations

3.1   Composite Latent Ground Truth Based on Experts' Manual Segmentations

Instead of directly observing the ground truth, T, we conduct manual segmentations by having R expert readers, each perform binary manual segmentation B_{lr} ($l = 1, ..., N = m + n$; $r = 1, ..., R$). Each expert gave a_{0r} and a_{1r} correct counts (agreements with the truth) for classes C_0 and C_1, respectively. Let Q_{0r} and Q_{1r} represent the true accuracy rates under these two classes. The experts' decisions are assumed to be conditionally independent, given the latent truth. We only observe binary classification decision B_{lr}, i.e., $(B_{lr} | T_l, Q_{0r}, q_{1r}) \perp (B_{lr'} | T_l, Q_{0r'}, Q_{1r'})$, for any two different experts, $r \ne r'$.

We wish to estimate the latent vector $\mathbf{T}$, of length N, by $\hat{\mathbf{T}} = \arg \max_T p(\mathbf{B} | \mathbf{T}, \mathbf{Q_0}, \mathbf{Q_1})$, for all $N = m + n$ voxels. However, these classification probabilities $\mathbf{Q_0}$ and $\mathbf{Q_1}$, each a vector of length R, are unknown quantities. An iterative maximum likelihood algorithm [7,8] has been developed by realizing that the quality fractions $(Q_{0r} | \mathbf{T})$ and $(Q_{1r} | \mathbf{T})$ have independent beta distributions with modes (a_{0r} / m) and (a_{1r} / n) as their estimates.

3.2   A Beta Mixture Model of Probabilistic Segmentation Data

Recall that the continuous random variables, X and Y, are the probabilistic segmentation results for classes C_0 and C_1, stratified by the ground truth T. Because both X and Y

take values between $[0, 1]$, it is conventional and flexible to assume independent beta distributions, i.e., $F(x) \sim \text{Beta}(\alpha_x, \beta_x)$ and $G(y) \sim \text{Beta}(\alpha_y, \beta_y)$. The expectation and variance of a $\text{Beta}(\alpha, \beta)$ distribution are known to be $\alpha/(\alpha+\beta)$ and $\alpha\beta/\{(\alpha+\beta)^2(\alpha+\beta+1)\}$, respectively. Thus, the estimates $(\hat{\alpha}_x, \hat{\beta}_x)$ of the shape parameters based on the x-sample of C_0 may be obtained by matching the first two moments (mean and variance). To match the sample mean $\overline{x}$ and standard deviation s_x of the x-sample, it can be shown that $\hat{\alpha}_x = \overline{x}\{\overline{x}(1-\overline{x})/s_x^2 - 1\}$, $\hat{\beta}_x = (1-\overline{x})\{\overline{x}(1-\overline{x})/s_x^2 - 1\}$. Similarly for $\hat{\alpha}_y$ and $\hat{\beta}_y$, computed based on the two moments, $\overline{y}$ and s_y, of the y-sample of C_1. Three validation metrics are presented with a higher value in $[0,1]$ indicating higher accuracy.

4 Three Validation Accuracy Metrics

4.1 Sensitivity, Specificity, and ROC Analysis

The accuracy of a diagnostic test can be summarized in terms of an ROC curve [5,6]. It is a plot of sensitivity (true tumor fraction) vs. (1-specificity) (true non-tumor fraction) based on Z and T, at all possible thresholds.

Conventionally, $p_\gamma = \overline{F}(\gamma)$ is labeled as false positive rate (FPR or $1 - $ specificity), on the x-axis of an ROC curve. True positive rate (TPR or sensitivity) is $q_\gamma = \overline{G}(\gamma)$ at the specified γ, or $q_p = \overline{G} \circ \overline{F}^{-1}(p)$ at any specified p, on the y-axis of an ROC curve. The ROC curve is $(\overline{F}(\gamma), \overline{G}(\gamma))$ for $\gamma \in [0, 1]$, or $(p, \overline{G} \circ \overline{F}^{-1}(p))$ for $p \in [0, 1]$. There is always a tradeoff between these two error rates, false positive and false negative rates, both taken values in $[0, 1]$.

An overall summary accuracy measure is the area under the ROC curve, AUC:

$$AUC = P(X < Y) = \int_{\gamma=0}^{1} \overline{G}(\gamma) \, d\overline{F}(\gamma) = \int_{p=1}^{1} q(p) \, dp. \tag{2}$$

4.2 Dice Similarity Coefficient

At any arbitrary threshold γ, Dice similarity coefficient (DSC), D_γ may be computed as a function of the sensitivity and specificity. Following the convention of an ROC plot, label the false positive rate $p_\gamma = P(Z > \gamma | T = 0) = P(D_\gamma = 1 | T = 0)$ and the true positive rate $q_\gamma = P(Z > \gamma | T = 1) = P(D_\gamma = 1 | T = 1)$. According to the definition of DSC_γ [4] for the tumor class and Bayes' Theorem, the Jaccard similarity coefficient at γ, JSC_γ, is defined as the voxel ratio of union and intersection between the two tumor classes determined separately by D_γ and by T [3]:

$$
\begin{aligned}
JSC_\gamma &\equiv \frac{\#\{(D_\gamma = 1) \cap (T = 1)\}}{\#\{(D_\gamma = 1) \cup (T = 1)\}} \\
&= \frac{P(D_\gamma = 1 | T = 1)P(T = 1)}{P(D_\gamma = 1) + P(T = 1) - P(D_\gamma = 1 | T = 1)P(T = 1)} \\
&= \frac{P(D_\gamma = 1 | T = 1)P(T = 1)}{P(D_\gamma = 1 | T = 0)P(T = 0) + P(T = 1)} = \frac{\overline{\pi} q_\gamma}{\pi p_\gamma + \overline{\pi}} = \frac{\overline{\pi} \overline{G}(\gamma)}{\pi \overline{F}(\gamma) + \overline{\pi}}.
\end{aligned}
$$

(Note that the DSC for the non-tumor may be computed similarly but may not be of interest.) An overall DSC, DSC, based on JSC_γ is defined by integrating over γ:

$$DSC = \int_{\gamma=0}^{1} 2JSC_\gamma/(JSC_\gamma + 1)\, d\gamma. \tag{3}$$

4.3   Entropy and Mutual Information

The mutual information between the binary decision D_γ at any threshold γ and the ground truth T can be computed as follows [9]:

$$MI_\gamma = MI(D_\gamma, T) = H(D_\gamma) + H(T) - H(D_\gamma, T), \tag{4}$$

where

$$
\begin{aligned}
H(D_\gamma) &= -(p_{11} + p_{12})\log_2(p_{11} + p_{12}) - (p_{21} + p_{22})\log_2(p_{21} + p_{22}) \\
&\quad - -(\pi\overline{p}_\gamma + \overline{\pi}\overline{q}_\gamma)\log_2(\pi\overline{p}_\gamma + \overline{\pi}\overline{q}_\gamma) - (\pi p_\gamma + \overline{\pi}q_\gamma)\log_2(\pi p_\gamma + \overline{\pi}q_\gamma), \\
H(T) &= -(p_{11} + p_{21})\log_2(p_{11} + p_{21}) - (p_{12} + p_{22})\log_2(p_{12} + p_{22}) \\
&= -\pi\log_2(\pi) - \overline{\pi}\log_2(\overline{\pi}), \\
H(D_\gamma, T) &= -p_{11}\log_2(p_{11}) - p_{12}\log_2(p_{12}) - p_{21}\log_2(p_{21}) - p_{22}\log_2(p_{22}) \\
&= -\pi\overline{p}_\gamma\log_2(\pi\overline{p}_\gamma) - \overline{\pi}\overline{p}_\gamma\log_2(\overline{\pi}\overline{p}_\gamma) - \pi p_\gamma\log_2(\pi p_\gamma) - \overline{\pi}q_\gamma\log_2(\overline{\pi}q_\gamma),
\end{aligned}
$$

with the joint probabilities, $(p_{11}, p_{12}, p_{21}, p_{22})$, given in Table 1.

The mutual information between the continuous random variable Z and T may also be computed using a conditioning entropy approach (with proof omitted):

$$
\begin{aligned}
MI(Z, T) &= H(Z) - H(Z|T) \\
&= -E_Z\left[\log_2\{k(Z)\}\right] - \pi E_Z\left[\log_2\{f(Z)\}\right] - \overline{\pi}E_Z\left[\log_2\{g(Z)\}\right] \\
&= -\int_{z=0}^{1}\left[k(z)\log_2\{k(z)\} - \pi f(z)\log_2\{f(z)\} - \overline{\pi}g(z)\log_2\{g(z)\}\right]dz,
\end{aligned}
$$

where $k(z) = \pi f(z) + \overline{\pi}g(z)$ as in (1).

4.4   Determination of an Optimal Threshold

Each of the above criteria, e.g., the square-root of the sum of squared sensitivity and specificity, $\sqrt{q_\gamma^2 + (1 - p_\gamma)^2}$, mutual information MI_γ, and Dice similarity coefficient (DSC_γ) may be maximized numerically over the entire range of γ in order to obtain an optimal threshold $\hat{\gamma}_{opt}$. Computations and optimizations were performed on a SunMicrosystem SunBlade 100 Workstation and in Matlab6, S-Plus6.0 and C languages.

5   A Clinical Example: MRI of Three Types of Brain Tumors

5.1   Materials and Methods

(1) The Cases: A total of nine patients were selected from a neurosurgical database of 260 brain tumor patients, of which three had meningiomas (M), three astrocytomas (A),

and three other low-grade gliomas (G)[10]. The meningiomas enhanced well but the gliomas did not.

(2) Imaging Protocol: Patient heads were imaged in the sagittal planes with a 1.5T MR imaging system (Signa, GE Medical Systems, Milwaukee, WI), with a postcontrast 3D sagittal spoiled gradient recalled (SPGR) acquisition with contiguous slices (flip angle, 45°); repetition time (TR), 35 ms; echo time (TE), 7 ms; field of view, 240 mm; slice-thickness, 1.5 mm; $256 \times 256 \times 124$ matrix). The acquired MR images were transferred onto a UNIX network via Ethernet.

(3) Automated Probabilistic Segmentation: The automated probabilistic segmentation was the relative tumor probability of lesion per voxel with signal intensity modeled as a Gaussian mixture of the two classes based on an initial semi-automated binary segmentation (left panel of Fig 1, in an example case) [10].

(4) Manual Binary Segmentation and Composite Ground Truth: An interactive segmentation tool (MRX, GE Medical Systems, Schenectady, NY) was employed and ran on an Ultra 10 Workstation (Sun Microsystems, Mountain View, CA). The structures were outlined slice-wise by expert operators using a mouse. The program connected consecutive points with lines. An anatomical object was defined by closed contour, and the program labeled every voxel of the enclosed volume. For the purpose of validation, we randomly selected one single 2D slice for each case from the subset of the MR volume with the tumor. Manual segmentation was performed independently by 3 expert operators (blinded to the machine segmentation results) to outline the brain and the tumor. An M.L.E of voxel-wise composite ground truth was determined. The remaining voxels were labeled as background. Stratified analyses are conducted by tumor type based on the estimated composite voxel-wise ground truth.

5.2   Results

We show semi-automated binary segmentations of a meningioma to derive the probabilistic results, with the empirical and approximated beta densities by truth (Fig 1).

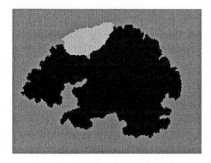
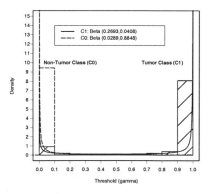

Fig. 1. Left Panel: Automated Binary segmentation of a slice of meningioma used as a basis for probablistic segmentation. Right Panel: The empirical (relative frequency histograms) and the approximated beta distributions (smooth lines) of the continuous segmentation data.

For all cases, we reported the voxel counts (m, n), stratified by the ground truth. The sample means and SD's of the non-tumor and tumor probability data were reported and were used to estimate the shape parameters of the beta distributions (Table 2).

Table 2. Sample Statistics and Estimated Beta Parameters for 9 Cases.

Tumor Type	Voxel Counts			Sample Means and SD's				Estimated Beta Parameters			
	m	n	$\bar{\pi} = n/N$	$\bar{x}$	s_x	$\bar{y}$	s_y	$\hat{\alpha}_x$	$\hat{\beta}_x$	$\hat{\alpha}_y$	$\hat{\beta}_y$
M	10534	1175	10%	0.0316	0.1264	0.8683	0.2954	0.0289	0.8848	0.2693	0.0408
	15363	1503	8.9%	0.0207	0.0890	0.8479	0.3344	0.0321	1.5227	0.1301	0.0233
	12891	1045	7.5%	0.1797	0.2746	0.7775	0.2619	0.1716	0.7832	1.1835	0.3387
A	10237	268	2.6%	0.3682	0.1548	0.6347	0.2703	3.2081	5.5044	1.3790	0.7937
	11579	1428	11.0%	0.1812	0.2496	0.7684	0.2773	0.2500	1.1303	1.0098	0.3043
	7148	1379	16.2%	0.0621	0.1229	0.9613	0.1742	0.1773	2.6790	0.2173	0.0087
G	8952	1417	13.7%	0.0112	0.0908	0.8693	0.3177	0.0038	0.3394	0.1090	0.0164
	12679	1177	8.5%	0.1564	0.2803	0.7398	0.2731	0.1063	0.5732	1.1691	0.4112
	9635	1873	16.3%	0.2275	0.2630	0.7369	0.2765	0.3505	1.1903	1.1314	0.4040

The overall validation accuracies were generally high but were variable, and generally the highest for meningiomas but lowest for astrocytomas. Furthermore, the recommended optimal thresholds varied by metric and case (Table 3).

Table 3. Estimated Accuracy metrics (ROC, MI and DSC) and Optimal Thresholds.

Tumor Type	Validation Metrics			Optimal Thresholds						
	AUC	MI	DSC	$\sqrt{(1-p)^2 + q^2}$	$\hat{\gamma}_{opt}$	MI	$\hat{\gamma}_{opt}$	DSC	$\hat{\gamma}_{opt}$
M	0.9842	0.2888	0.8154	1.3255	0.4709	0.3107	0.8625	0.8730	0.8734
	0.9684	0.3012	0.8415	1.2834	0.8448	0.3065	0.8521	0.8931	0.8268
	0.9242	0.1572	0.4220	1.1844	0.2622	0.1098	0.4657	0.5185	0.8414
A	0.7860	0.0557	0.1970	1.0050	0.7713	0.0415	0.7728	0.4871	0.7808
	0.9255	0.2319	0.5146	1.1881	0.4469	0.1598	0.6843	0.6321	0.8005
	0.9858	0.4649	0.8708	1.4142	1.0000	0.5669	0.8553	0.9724	0.8385
G	0.9829	0.4018	0.8961	1.3720	0.0120	0.4032	0.4905	0.8992	0.6736
	0.9157	0.1595	0.4396	1.1735	0.0773	0.1276	0.2232	0.4897	0.6511
	0.8956	0.2505	0.5276	1.1417	0.4547	0.1693	0.6191	0.6197	0.7113

6   Summary

In this work, we have presented systematic approaches to validating the accuracy of automated segmentation results that generates voxel-wise probabilistic interpretation of the tumor class. We developed an M.L.E. algorithm for estimating the latent ground truth. In addition, we modeled the probabilistic segmentation results using a mixture of two beta distributions with different shape parameters. Summary accuracy measures, including ROC curve, mutual information, and Dice similarity coefficient, are estimated. An optimal threshold was derived under each metric.

The example data showed satisfactory accuracy of our automated segmentation algorithm. The recommended optimal threshold, however, was significantly case- and task (metric)-dependent. The main advantage of our approaches is that the parametric modeling is simple and probabilistic. The estimation procedures are straightforward and are generalizable to similar statistical validation tasks of segmentation methods.

Acknowledgements

This work was supported by NIH grants P41 RR13218, P01 CA67165, R01 RR11747, R01 CA86879, R21 CA89449-01, a research grant from the Whitaker Foundation, and a New Concept Award from the Center for Integration of Medicine and Innovative Technology. We thank the three experts who performed manual segmentations of the brain tumor cases.

References

1. Warfield S. K., Westin C.-F., Guttmann, C. R. G., Albert, M., Jolesz, F. A., Kikinis, R.: Fractional segmentation of white matter. In Proceedings of Second International Conference on Medical Imaging Computing and Computer Assisted Interventions, Cambridge, UK (1999) 62-71.
2. Zijdenbos, A. P., Dawant, B.M., Margolin, R. A., Palmer, A. C.: Morphometric analysis of white matter lesions in MR images: method and validation. IEEE Transactions on Medical Imaging 13 (1994) 716-724.
3. Jaccard, P.: The distribution of flora in the alpine zone. New Phytologist 11 (1912) 37-50.
4. Dice, L. R.: Measures of the amount of ecologic association between species. Ecology, 26 (1945) 297-302.
5. Zou, K. H., Hall W. J., Shapiro, D. E.: Smooth nonparametric receiver operating characteristic curves for continuous diagnostic tests. Statistics in Medicine 16 (1997) 2143-2156.
6. Zou, K. H. , Hall W. J.: Two transformation models for estimating an ROC curve derived from continuous data. Journal of Applied Statistics 27 (2000) 621-631.
7. Dempster, A. P, Laird, N. M., Rubin, D. B.: Maximum-likelihood from incomplete data via the EM algorithm. J. Royal Statistical Society (Ser. B) 39 (1977) 34-37.
8. McLachlan G. J., Krishnan, T.: The EM Algorithm and Extensions. Wiley, New York (1997).
9. Cover, T. MM, Thomas J. A.: Elements of Information Theory. John Wiley & Sons, Inc., New York (1991).
10. Kaus, M., Warfield S. K., Nabavi A., Black, P. M., Jolesz, F. A., Kikinis, R.: Automated segmentation of MRI of brain tumors. Radiology 218 (2001) 586-591.

A Posteriori Validation of Pre-operative Planning in Functional Neurosurgery by Quantification of Brain Pneumocephalus

É. Bardinet[1], P. Cathier[1], A. Roche[2], N. Ayache[1], and D. Dormont[3]

[1] INRIA, Epidaure Project, Sophia Antipolis, France
[2] Robotics Research Laboratory, Dept. of Engineering, University of Oxford, UK
[3] Neuroradiology Dept and LENA UPR 640-CNRS, Salpêtrière Hospital, France

Abstract. Functional neurosurgery for Parkinson's disease is based on the stereotactic introduction of electrodes in a small, deeply located, nucleus of the brain. This nucleus is targeted on pre-operative stereotactic MR acquisitions. The procedure is time-consuming and can lead to the development of a pneumocephalus (presence of air in the intracanial cavity) because of CSF leak. This pneumocephalus leads to a brain shift which can yield a significative deformation of the entire brain and thus cause potential errors in the pre-operatively determined position of the stereotactic targets. In this paper, we conduct an a posteriori validation of the pre-operative planning, by quantifying brain pneumocephalus from the registration of pre and immediate post-operative MR acquisitions.

1 Introduction

MR image guided brain surgery is an actively developping field. In most of the cases, the techniques are based on the use of volumetric pre-operative MR acquisitions. These techniques implicitly assume that a pre-operative acquisition gives a faithful and precise representation of the brain anatomy during the intervention. A major limit of these techniques is the development of brain deformation during the surgical intervention, thus leading to anatomical differences, which can be significative, with the pre-operative MR images. To overcome this limit, there has been recent interest in quatifying brain deformation during neurosurgery [4, 11, 6, 12].

One interesting example of this type of procedures is functional neurosurgery for Parkinson's disease. This intervention is based on the stereotactic introduction of electrodes in a small, deeply located, nucleus of the brain, called the subthalamic nucleus. This nucleus is targeted on pre-operative stereotactic MR acquisitions. During the intervention, which is performed in the operating room, outside the MR unit, an electrophysiological and clinical study is performed with the electrodes to check the pre-operatively determined target position.

This exploration is time-consuming and can lead to the development of a pneumocephalus (presence of air in the intracanial cavity) because of CSF leak. This pneumocephalus leads to a brain shift which can yield a significative deformation of the entire brain and thus cause potential errors in the pre-operatively determined position of the stereotactic targets. Therefore, computing accurately the deformation induced by the pneumocephalus over the entire brain appears to be a key issue, as it will allow to quantify the deformation occurred around

T. Dohi and R. Kikinis (Eds.): MICCAI 2002, LNCS 2488, pp. 323–330, 2002.

the stereotactic targets and lead to a posteriori validation of the pre-operative planning.

We have developped a method to quantify brain deformation from pre and immediate post-operative MR acquisitions, based on rigid and non rigid registrations. Our method is related to the approach developped in [12] for estimating tissue deformation induced by intracranial electrode implantation in patients with epilepsy. Nevertheless, if [12] also used a registration based method, technical solutions provided here are different. The novel non rigid registration algorithm used in this paper is based on a true free form deformation modelisation coupled with a mixed regularization, unlike [12] who used cubic B-splines, thus implicitly limiting the search of the deformations to a specific and reduced transformation space. Therefore, the method presented below allows a finer analysis of the deformation.

2   Material and Methods

One patient with bilateral subthalamic lateral implantation was studied. The subthalamic targets were determined one day before the intervention using 3D stereotactic IR-FSPGR MR acquistion. Then, the patient had bilateral implantation of depth electrodes at the level of the subthalamic nuclei. MR control using the same acquistion as pre-operative was performed the day after the implantation. Voxel size of both acquisitions was $0.9375 \times 0.9375 \times 1.3$ mm, and image dimension was $256 \times 256 \times 124$. On the control acquisition, presence of air collection was clearly observed at the anterior part of the cranial cavity.

The methodology to quantify brain deformation from these pre and immediate post-operative MR acquisitions consisted in three steps:

1. Robust rigid registration of pre and post-operative MR acquisitions
2. Segmentation of the cortex on the registered images
3. Non-rigid registration of the resulting images

2.1   Rigid Registration

We first performed a rigid registration between the pre and post-operative MR acquisitions to correct differences in patient positioning. Notice that in the post-operative acquisition, some parts of the head have been deformed, namely an unknwon but limited part of brain tissue has deformed due to pneumocephalus, and skin and fat presented large deformations, mostly due to swelling. All these deformations could bias the rigid registration.

Therefore a robust variant of the correlation ratio based on the Geman-McClure scale estimator was used as the similarity measure [10]. The assumption underlying the correlation ratio is that there exists an unknown mapping between the MR intensities of the pre and post-operative images. This assumption actually did not hold in the whole image because of the deformed parts of the post-operative image. The use of a robust correlation measure prevented the registration from being biased by such outliers.

2.2   Cortex Segmentation

Brain deformation is caused by the pneumocephalus, but changes at the scalp level are not. Thus searching for a non rigid deformation accounting for these changes, that is searching for a deformation including discontinuities along the brain-scalp frontier, would be rather complex. Moreover, it could induce errors in the deformation estimate inside the brain. Therefore, before computing the non rigid residual deformation, brain was segmented from the rigidly registered MR images. This was done automatically: thresholding with the CSF grey value, morphological opening, erosion, maximal connected component extraction and dilation.

2.3   Non-rigid Registration

From the segmented and rigidly registered images, a non rigid registration was performed, using the PASHA algorithm, an iconic feature based algorithm.

Preliminaries. Most of the numerous non rigid registration techniques can be classified according to various criteria [1, 8, 7]. We focus here on one major axis: **the motion model** expressing the prior knowledge we have on the shape of the transformation, which is used to regularize the registration problem.

It is necessary to impose a motion model to a non rigid registration algorithm, otherwise the motion of a point would be estimated independently of the motion of neighboring points, and we would thus obtain a very discontinuous and unrealistic displacement field. In the field of image registration, we distinguish three kind of motion models: parametric, competitive, and fluid models.

The parametric approach constrains the estimate T of the transformation to belong to some low dimensional transformation space $\mathcal{T}$. Mathematically, if $D(I, J, T)$ is some registration distance between the images I and J registered by T, a parametric approach solves the following minimization problem: $\min_{T \in \mathcal{T}} D(I, J, T)$ Among the most popular choices of transformation space, we find rigid and affine groups, and kernels such as thin plate splines or B-splines.

Competitive models rely on the use of a regularization energy R (also called stabilizer) carrying on T. Whereas parametric regularization is a binary penalization — no transformation outside the transformation space is allowed, all the transformations inside are equiprobable — the competitive approach penalizes a transformation proportionally to its irregularity measured by the regularization energy R [13]. Competitive algorithms puts in competition (hence the name) D and R by solving the following problem: $\min_{\forall T} D(I, J, T) + R(T)$.

Fluid models also rely on the use of a regularization energy R. This time, however, this energy does not carry on the transformation itself, but on its *evolution*. In a discrete, or iterative, view of the process, the regularization energy carries on the difference between the current and the last estimate of the transformation: at iteration $n > 0$, the estimate T_n of the transformation is found by minimizing $\min_{\forall T_n} D(I, J, T_n) + R(T_n - T_{n-1})$. The typical example of a fluid approach is the viscoelastic algorithm of Christensen [3].

The PASHA Algorithm. We minimize the following energy: $E(C, T) = S(I, J, C) + ||C - T||^2 + R(T)$, where E depends on two variables, C and T, that are both vector fields (with one vector per pixel). C is a set of *pairings* between points: for each point of I, it gives a corresponding point in J that attracts this point. T is the estimate of the transformation: it is a smooth vector field (constrained by the regularization energy R) that is attracted by the set of correspondences C. In the energy, S is an intensity similarity measure, used to find the correspondences C, and R is a regularization energy, used to regularize T.

This algorithm is an iconic feature based algorithm, i.e. it is really intermediate between geometric feature based and standard intensity based algorithms. Indeed, on one hand, we search for correspondences C between iconic features in the images, and use a *geometric distance* to fit the transformation T to C. On the other hand, there is no segmentation of the images, as we use an intensity similarity measure to pair features. Note that other iconic feature based algorithms (e.g. the "demons" [14], adaptation of optical flow to registration [5], block matching [8,9]) generally do not minimize a global energy. Consequently, the analysis of the behavior of those algorithms is difficult.

We also propose a mixed competitive/fluid regularization for PASHA. Fluid algorithms are able to recover large displacements, but they often do not preserve image topology for real applications. We therefore use in PASHA a mix of fluid and competitive models in order to recover larger displacements, while still constraining the transformation, and thus avoiding dramatic topology changes. The energy minimized by PASHA at iteration n now becomes:

$$S(I, J, C_n) + \sigma||C_n - T_n||^2 + \sigma\lambda\left[\omega R(T_n - T_{n-1}) + (1 - \omega)R(T_n)\right] \qquad (1)$$

where $\omega \in [0, 1]$ fixes the relative importance of competitive and fluid regularization ($\omega = 0$ being a pure competitive regularization and $\omega = 1$ a pure fluid regularization). The λ parameter influences the smoothness of the deformation, and σ is related to the noise level in the images.

One could minimize the energy E with respect to C and T simultaneously. However, when the regularization energy R is quadratic, the alternate minimization w.r.t. C and T is appealing, because both partial minimizations are very fast: the minimization w.r.t. C can be done for each pixel separately most of the time, and the second step is easily solved by linear convolution. PASHA is designed on that principle. It minimizes the energy (1) alternatively w.r.t. C and T. We start from $T_0 = \mathrm{Id}$ at iteration 0; then, at iteration n, the alternated minimization scheme gives the following steps:

- Find C_n by minimizing $S(I, J, C_n) + \sigma||C_n - T_{n-1}||^2$. This is done in PASHA using gradient descent.
- Find T_n by minimizing $||C_n - T_n||^2 + \lambda\left[\omega R(T_n - T_{n-1}) + (1 - \omega)R(T_n)\right]$. This minimization step has a closed-form solution, using convolution.

Let us illustrate the advantage of this mixed regularization with an example: in Fig. 1, we have two noisy images presenting some large motion. Both the recovered deformation field and the intensity differences between the deformed and the original images show that: 1) fluid regularization is able to register the images, but being sensitive to noise, the recovered deformation field is aberrant; 2) competitive regularization is much more robust to noise, but it is more difficult to recover large deformations, as can be seen on the difference image; 3) mixed regularization combines the advantages of both approaches, i.e. good image match while having a regular deformation field.

Finally, the whole minimization process is embedded into a pyramidal framework. This classical technique has two advantages. First, the registration algo-

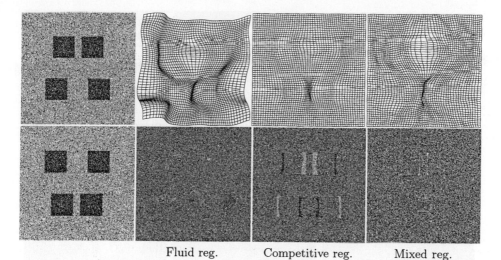

Fluid reg.   Competitive reg.   Mixed reg.

Fig. 1. Left most column: two noisy images to be registered. **Remaining right columns:** registration results using PASHA and different regularization techniques. **Upper row:** Recovered deformation field. **Lower row:** Intensity differences between the deformed and the original images.

rithm is much less sensitive to initial alignment and can go beyond local minima. Second, the cost of the pyramidal approach is relatively small, since the extra processed images are much smaller than the original one. The similarity measure used in PASHA relies on the computation of local statistics (namely the Gaussian-weighted local correlation coefficient). Local measures assume that the link between I and J is valid only locally. For local statistics, there exists a fast computation method based on convolution that makes it applicable for non rigid registration. For more details, we refer the reader to [2].

3   Results and Discussion

Robust rigid registration between the pre and post-operative MR acquisitions was performed first. Fig. 2 shows three independant slices (sagittal, coronal and axial) through both volumes after registration.

As can be seen with the cursor superimposed on the images, correspondences at the bone level are correct, as required because the bone is the only structure which didn't suffer deformation during surgery. Notice that these three slices are not related, as they were independantly selected to illustrate the quality of bone correspondence. Therefore, the cursor location is also independant in each slice. Starting from this rigid registration, the non rigid registration will only search for residual deformations due to pneumocephalus.

To avoid discontinuities along the brain-scalp frontier, brain was extracted from both volumes. Results of this segmentation can be seen in Figs. 3 and 4.

Then, non rigid registration was performed (8 minutes on a 450 Mhz Pentium III), with the PASHA algorithm, including the mixed fluid/competitive regularization, with $\omega = 0.6$, which enabled a total recovery of motion by a smooth

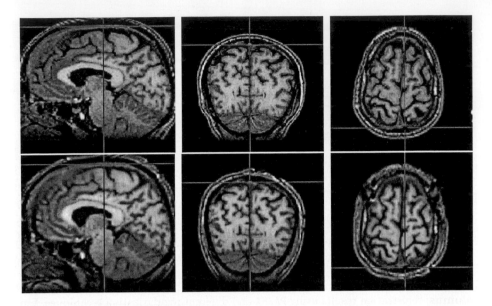

Fig. 2. Robust rigid registration of pre-operative (top row) and post-operative (bottom row) MR images of the same patient. Cursor location illustrates the accurate correspondences found at the bone level. From left to right: independant sagittal, coronal and axial views. Note that the three slices are not related . Therefore, the cursor location is also independant in each slice.

transformation. Fig. 3 shows slices of the post-operative and pre-operative (after rigid and non rigid registration) volumes, with post-operative contours superimposed in order to visually assess the quality of the registration. Notice in particular the consistent matching, both geometrical and textural, obtained around the pre-frontal lobe, where deformation caused by the pneumocephalus was largest. Once the deformation was computed (the maximal value of the deformation norm was 5.79 mm), it was possible to examine its spatial distribution, and especially to look at regions of brain that suffered deformations higher than a given value. Fig. 4 shows, on the first row, axial slices through the deformation field itself, the displacement of each voxel being represented by an arrow. Then, on the next two rows, isolines of the deformation norm are superimposed on the same axial slices of the pre-operative volume (after rigid registration and brain extraction) and of the post-operative volume (after brain extraction). The isovalues were set to 3, 2 and 1 mm (3 mm corresponding to the smallest region). As expected, the deformation maximal values coincided with the prefrontal lobe where the pneumocephalus was observed. Then, as can be seen, the deformation smoothly decreased, reaching values under 1 mm at the basal ganglia level. Also, deformation around the targets (identified by the dark holes located between the putamen and the thalamus on the post-operative images) was significantly lower than 1 mm (around 0.7 mm for the anterior part of the targets, and around 0.4 mm for the posterior part). Note that the localised deformation area (greater than 1 mm) at the level of the target on slice 134 was due to the electrode MR signal.

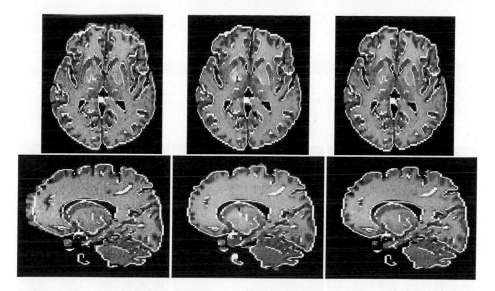

Fig. 3. Non rigid registration of pre-operative and post-operative MR images of the same patient. First row: axial slices; second row: sagittal slices. Left column: pre-operative volume after rigid registration; middle column: post-operative volume; right column: pre-operative volume after non rigid registration. Contours of the post-operative volume are superimposed on all the images.

4 Conclusion

We addressed the problem of validating *a posteriori* pre-operative planning in functional neurosurgery. Quantifying per-operative brain deformation around functional targets was done by registration of pre and immediate post-operative MR acquisitions. The non rigid registration algorithm used in this paper was based on a true free form deformation modelisation coupled with a mixed regularization, yielding a faithful deformation field. Analysis of the spatial distribution of brain deformation was then performed. On the patient under study, results confirmed surgeon intuition, i.e. pneumocephalus doesn't affect target pre-operative localisation. Indeed, the deformation was significantly inferior than 1 mm around the functional targets, knowing that the voxel size of the MR images was around 1 mm^3. To confirm the result obtained on this patient, a clinical study will now be conducted on a large series of Parkinsonian patients.

References

1. L. G. Brown. A Survey of Image Registration Techniques. *ACM Computing Surveys*, 24(4):325 − 276, 12 1992.
2. P. Cachier and X. Pennec. 3D Non-Rigid Registration by Gradient Descent on a Gaussian-Windowed Similarity Measure using Convolutions. In *Proc. of MMBIA'00, LNCS 1935*, pp. 182 − 189, June 2000.
3. G. E. Christensen, R. D. Rabitt, and M. I. Miller. Deformable Templates Using Large Deformation Kinematics. *IEEE TIP*, 5(10):1435–1447, October 1996.
4. N. Hata, A. Nabavi, S. Warfield, W. Wells, R. Kikinis, and F.A. Jolesz. A volumetric optical flow method for measurement of brain deformation from intraoperative magnetic resonance images. In *Proc. of MICCAI'99, LNCS 1679*, September 1999.

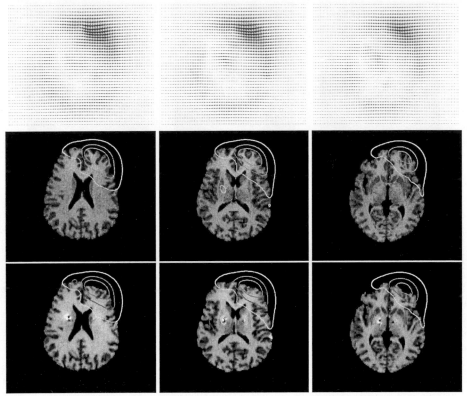

Slice 125   Slice 134   Slice 145

Fig. 4. Non rigid registration of pre and post-operative MR images of the same patient, starting from the rigidly registered images, after brain extraction. Three (columns 1, 2 and 3) axial slices. First row: deformation field; second row: pre-operative image; third row: post-operative image. On the last two rows, isolines of the deformation norm (3, 2, 1 mm) are superimposed on the images.

5. P. Hellier, C. Barillot, E. Mmin, and P. Prez. Medical Image Registration with Robust Multigrid Techniques. In *Proc. of MICCAI'99*, *LNCS* 1679, pp. 680 – 687, September 1999.
6. D.L.G. Hill, C.R. Maurer, A.J. Martin, S. Sabanathan, W.A. Hall, D.J. Hawkes, D. Rueckert, and C.L. Truwit. Assessment of Intraoperative Brain Deformation Using Interventional MR Imaging. In *Proc. of MICCAI'99*, *LNCS* 1679, pp. 910 – 919, September 1999.
7. H. Lester and S. R. Arridge. A Survey of Hierarchical Non-Linear Medical Image Registration. *Pattern Recognition*, 32:129 – 149, 1999.
8. J. B. A. Maintz and M. A. Viergever. A Survey of Medical Image Registration. *Medical Image Analysis*, 2(1):1–36, 1998.
9. S. Ourselin, A. Roche, G. Subsol, X. Pennec, and N. Ayache. Reconstructing a 3D Structure from Serial Histological Sections. *IVC*, 19(1-2):25–31, January 2001.
10. A. Roche, G. Malandain, and N. Ayache. Unifying Maximum Likelihood Approaches in Medical Image Registration. *Int.J.of Imaging Systems and Technology*, 11:71–80, 2000.
11. O.M. Skrinjar and J.S. Duncan. Real Time 3D Brain Shift Compensation. In *Proc. of IPMI'99*, *LNCS* 1613, pp. 42 – 55, June 1999.
12. C. Studholme, E. Novotny, I.G. Zubal, and J.S. Duncan. Estimating Tissue Deformation between Functional Images Induced by Intracranial Electrode Implantation Using Anatomical MRI. *NeuroImage*, 13:561 – 576, 2001.
13. R. Szeliski. Bayesian Modeling of Uncertainty in Low-Level Vision. *Int. J.of Comp. Vision*, 5(3):271 – 301, December 1990.
14. J.-P. Thirion. Image matching as a diffusion process: an analogy with Maxwell's demons. *Medical Image Analysis*, 2(3):243–260, 1998.

Affine Transformations and Atlases:
Assessing a New Navigation Tool for Knee Arthroplasty

B. Ma[1], J.F. Rudan[3], and R.E. Ellis[1,2,3]

[1] School of Computing   [2] Mechanical Engineering   [3] Surgery
Queen's University at Kingston, Canada
ellis@cs.queensu.ca

Abstract. We propose a new guidance paradigm for computer-assisted orthopædic surgery, based on nonrigid registration of a patient to a standard atlas model. Such a method would save costs and time compared to CT-based methods, while being more reliable than current imageless navigation tools. Here, we consider application of this paradigm to knee arthroplasty.

This work reports laboratory results of assessing the simplest nonrigid registration method, which is an affine transformation. Results from CT scans of 15 patients show the method is more repeatable than the standard mechanical guide rods in the frontal plane. The affine transformations also detected a potential difference between osteoarthritic patients and the normal population, which may have implications for the implantation of artificial knee components.

1 Introduction

Current computer-integrated surgical systems for knee arthroplasty provide navigational guidance relative to CT scans [7, 10, 12, 13, 19] or to anatomic features [4–6, 8, 15] that are identified intraoperatively (such as centers of rotation and anatomic axes). Both methods have notable limitations. The use of CT scans for knee arthroplasty is atypical and introduces extra costs, radiation exposure, and time to produce a patient-specific plan. Systems that require the identification of anatomic features are limited by the accuracy with which these features can be located, and it can be difficult to confirm that the guidance provided is accurate.

We propose that the use of a global deformable shape-based registration may be sufficiently accurate to align a patients' femur to a femur atlas. If our proposition is true, then it would be possible to intraoperatively digitize points from the surfaces of the femur to register the patient to the atlas. A plan defined on the atlas could be applied to the patient without the need for preoperative planning, which simplifies the logistics of delivering care in a clinical setting. Because the guidance is based on shape matching, it would be easy to visually confirm the accuracy of the registration by pointing to distinctive features with a tracked stylus.

Considerable research has been conducted on atlas generation and deformable registration [9], including the mapping of atlas data to patient data for diagnosis and visualization [17]. However, to the best of our knowledge, there have been no published results describing the validation of deformable registration to an atlas for guidance.

2 A Simple Affine Registration Algorithm

Our registration is a simple generalization of the ICP algorithm of Besl and McKay [1]. In the original algorithm, ICP repeatedly searches for the set X of model points nearest

T. Dohi and R. Kikinis (Eds.): MICCAI 2002, LNCS 2488, pp. 331–338, 2002.

to the transformed data points P. Using homogeneous notation and assuming X and P are matrices of column vectors, Horn's method is used to solve for the best rigid transformation $\mathbf{T}_{\text{rigid}}$:

$$\min \|\mathbf{T}_{\text{rigid}} P - X\|_2 \tag{1}$$

Since we desire the affine transformation $\mathbf{T}_{\text{affine}}$ we have:

$$\min \|\mathbf{T}_{\text{affine}} P - X\|_2 \tag{2}$$

which can be solved using any method for optimization of overdetermined linear systems. For the purposes of this study we have chosen to use a least-squares optimization with the QR decomposition.

Our algorithm has the same guaranteed convergence as the ICP algorithm. The proof of this statement is almost identical to the original proof [1] and is not provided here.

We have not yet explored the problem of how to reliably obtain an initial estimate for this affine registration algorithm. Details of how we proceeded for this study can be found in Section 3.

3   Materials and Methods

We conducted a retrospective study based on CT scans of patients who enrolled in an approved clinical study of computer-assisted orthopædic surgery and had consented to research use of medical data. Polygonal models of the hip and femur were computed, using an isosurface algorithm, from scans of 15 high tibial osteotomy (HTO) patients. An atlas model was created from the CT scan of a plastic phantom of a normal femur. On the models we identified: the mechanical axis, the anatomic axis, Whiteside and Arima's [18] anteroposterior (AP) axis, the knee center on the surface of the distal femur, and the approximate dimensions of the distal femur in the transverse plane. Studies of the distal femur [16, 20] have identified the transepicondylar line (TEL) as an important landmark but we were unable to reliably locate the TEL on some scans.

For each patient model and the atlas we defined the transverse plane to be perpendicular to the mechanical axis. The AP axis was projected into the transverse plane if it was not already perpendicular to the mechanical axis. The frontal plane was defined to be perpendicular to the AP axis, and the sagittal plane was defined to be perpendicular to both the frontal and transverse planes.

To test the baseline accuracy of affine registration for guidance we selected all of the vertices from the lateral, medial, and anterior surfaces of the distal femur, and the vertices from the patellar groove and small regions of the posterior condyles. We approximately matched each femur to the atlas by aligning the knee centers, mechanical axes, and AP axes, and then scaling in the AP and mediolateral (ML) directions. Starting from this initial alignment, we first used ICP to find a rigid registration and then used the modified ICP to find the affine registration. The affine transformation was applied to the patient femurs to assess the registration error relative to the atlas.

For shape-based registration algorithms the value of the registration objective function – usually the root-mean-square (RMS) error for ICP – is a commonly reported measure of error. For comparing a rigid registration to ground truth or a fiducial registration, it is more meaningful to report errors as a rotation and translation about a screw axis [2]. Unfortunately this approach is invalid for affine registration so, in addition to computing the RMS error, we also computed registration errors in a manner analogous to the target registration error described by Maurer *et al.* [11].

Our targets were the knee center and relevant axes of the knee. Reed and Gollish [14] have reported that the potential angular error in the distal femoral cut depends critically on the entry point of the intramedullary rod, and that the correct entry point is located where the anatomic axis exits the distal femur. Because some of our CT scans did not adequately image the distal shaft of the femur, we were unable to define the anatomic axis with reference to the ideal entry point. Instead, we computed the distances between the knee centers on the registered femurs and the atlas instead of the distances between the ideal entry points.

The mechanical axis is a natural target to use because knee arthroplasty attempts to recreate a neutral mechanical axis. We computed the angular alignment errors between the registered and atlas mechanical axes in the frontal and sagittal planes, and also computed the same errors for the respective anatomic axes.

It has been reported [18] that the AP axis is a reliable landmark for alignment in the valgus knee, so we computed the angular alignment errors between the registered and atlas AP axes in the transverse and sagittal planes. Errors were computed in the frame of the atlas. To analyze differences between the phantom and patient atlas results, we used the two-sample t-test with a significance level of $p < 0.01$ to test for differences in means and the F-test at a significance level of $p < 0.02$ to test for differences in variance.

Even though we used large data sets to perform the registrations, we were still concerned that our results may have been subject to "local-minima trapping", which is a well known drawback of ICP-like algorithms. We performed a stochastic analysis of the sensitivity of the affine-registration process to the initial estimate: starting from our manual alignment, we rotated the patient model by 15° about a random axis passing through the knee center, and translated by 10mm along this axis [1]. We used this new pose as the initial estimate for the registration process. This experiment was repeated 100 times for each patient and we computed the resulting target registration errors.

Finally, we randomly chose one patient to serve as the atlas and registered the remaining patients to the new atlas. We computed errors as for the phantom atlas.

4   Results

A visualization of a registered left femur and the atlas axes is shown in Figure 1 that illustrates our error conventions. Notice that if we followed a preoperative plan defined in the atlas coordinate frame, the arthroplasty would result in malalignments in the opposite directions e.g. a varus, hyperextended, internally rotated knee in the case of the illustration.

4.1   Phantom Atlas

The RMS error of registration was between 0.79 mm and 1.39 mm (mean 1.12 mm). The registration errors of the knee center and axes using the phantom atlas are shown in the left column of Figure 2. In the ML and AP directions, the mean knee-center

---

[1] The choice of these values is justified in Section 4.3

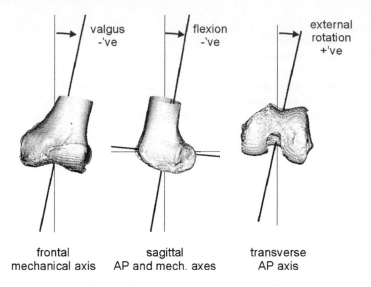

Fig. 1. A convention for measuring axis errors. A transformation that would make an arthroplasty component: in the frontal plane, more varus is positive and more valgus is negative; in the sagittal plane, more extended is positive and more flexed is negative; in the transverse plane, more externally rotated is positive and more internally rotated is negative.

alignment errors were -0.03mm and -0.18mm, respectively, with standard deviations (SD) of 1.53mm and 2.08mm. The results for the anatomic and mechanical axes were unusual in that there was a clear trend towards valgus and flexion alignment errors. In the frontal plane, the mean of the mechanical axis alignment errors was -2.45° (SD 2.53°). In the sagittal plane, the mean error was -4.98° (SD 4.60°). For the anatomic axis, the frontal and sagittal plane errors were -3.32° (SD 2.32°) and -5.29° (SD 4.89°). There was a slight trend towards external rotation of the registered femur as indicated by a mean AP axis alignment error in the transverse plane of 0.55° (SD 5.49 degrees).

4.2   Patient Atlas

The registration errors using patient 12 as the atlas are shown in the right column of Figure 2. For the knee center, the alignment errors were 0.31mm (SD 1.41mm) and 0.43mm (SD 2.23mm) in the ML and AP directions respectively. The F-test values were 1.18 and 0.83 for the ML and AP directions which suggested that there was no significant difference in the variances. The t-test values were -0.6193 and -0.7448 for the ML and AP directions which suggested that there was no significant difference in the means.

The registrations produced a mean neutral alignment of the mechanical axes in the frontal plane (mean -0.01°, SD 2.15°) with a slight trend towards extension alignment error (mean 0.81°, SD 3.81°). Variances were smaller than for the phantom atlas but the differences were not significant. (F-test values 1.38 and 1.46). Mean errors were smaller than for the phantom atlas and were significant (t-test values -2.78 and -3.68). Similar conclusions could be drawn for the anatomic axis errors (F-test values 1.53 and 1.39,

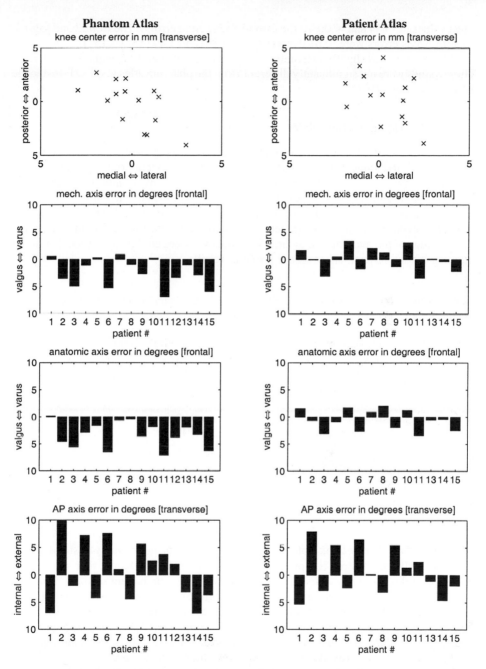

Fig. 2. Alignment errors for the phantom atlas (left) and patient atlas (right). Patient #12 was used as the atlas and is absent from the patient atlas results.

t-test values of -3.44 and -4.00 for the frontal and sagittal errors). The frontal and sagittal anatomic axis errors were -0.61 degrees (SD 1.88°) and 1.47° (SD 4.15°).

The AP axis was slightly externally rotated with a mean of 0.57 degrees (SD 4.33°). These values were not significantly different from the phantom atlas results (F-test value 1.60, t-test value -0.01).

4.3   Initial Alignment Sensitivity

Our results for the phantom atlas showed that the worst alignment errors for the axes were less than 12° and 5mm for the knee center. We arbitrarily increased these values to 15° and 10mm to displace the initial estimates. Since we were investigating the sensitivity to the initial alignment, we computed the standard deviations of the various alignment measurements over the 100 trials for each of the 15 patients. Table 1 shows the largest standard deviations over the 15 patients for each alignment measurement. Given the small values of the maximum standard deviations we were confident that local-minima trapping did not have an effect on our previous results.

Table 1. Initial alignment sensitivity results reported as maximum standard deviations over all patients for each alignment measurement.

Alignment Measurement	Maximum Standard Deviation
knee center, ML	0.02mm
knee center, AP	0.15mm
mechanical axis, frontal	0.07°
mechanical axis, sagittal	0.40°
anatomic axis, frontal	0.07°
anatomic axis, sagittal	0.40°
AP axis, frontal	0.01°
AP axis, sagittal	0.46°

5   Discussion

Our results show that the choice of atlas significantly affects the accuracy of shape-based registration. If the phantom is representative of the normal population, then our results suggest that the shape of the distal femur of an osteoarthritic patient deviates from the norm. This deviation has substantial surgical implications, because a surgeon attempts to align a femoral component so that it is perpendicular to the load-bearing mechanical axis: a malalignment can produce shear forces at the bone interface that can in turn lead to premature failure. If an osteoarthritic patient has a different anatomy than a normal subject, different standards of alignment may need to be considered.

By registering to the shape of the distal femur, we were unable to align the AP axes of the patients and the atlases with good consistency. This is not a surprising result since Whiteside and Arima advocate the use of the AP axis for rotational alignment of the valgus knee because such a knee typically has an abnormally small lateral condyle [18]. Furthermore, Feinstein et al. [3] have found that there is large variation in the alignment of the patellar groove relative to the transepicondylar line in the transverse plane. This suggests that affine registration to an atlas derived from a normal subject may not be suitable for determining the rotational alignment of an arthroplasty component.

Our alignment errors as measured in the frontal plane, with a standard deviation of about 2°, compare favorably with the alignment errors induced by intramedullary (IM) guides reported by Reed and Gollish [14]. In their study, the authors' mathematical model predicted up to 3° valgus malalignment if the insertion point of the IM rod was located at the center of the notch as in the typical textbook description of knee arthroplasty technique. Mechanical guides for unicompartmental arthroplasty are smaller in diameter and less than 1/3 the length of a guide for a total arthroplasty, so the expected alignment errors are much worse (we calculate up to 12°).

Limitations of our study include a relatively small number of patients, a very simple registration algorithm, and use of a large amount of data to perform the registration. An interesting extension to our work would be the determination of the minimal amount of data, from surgically accessible regions, needed to reliably perform a deformable registration. Finding a way to acquire or specify the initial registration is also desirable.

This work suggests that it may be practical to perform computer-assisted knee surgery in a completely new way. By comparison with navigation from patient-specific CT scans, deformable registration to an atlas is much less costly, requires no exceptional logistics or labor, and requires no additional radiation to the patient or to the surgical team. By comparison with navigation from anatomical features, deformable registration to an atlas offers the surgeon visual confirmation that (a) a good registration has been achieved, because the surgeon can see the correlation between navigation on the atlas and anatomical features being touched, and (b) visual confirmation that tracking devices attached to the patient or to surgical instruments have not inadvertently moved during surgery. Our results suggest that we can guide a surgeon accurately in the frontal plane, so that conventional instrumentation could be used to complete the procedure.

Affine transformations are a simple first step in exploring the use of deformable registrations for surgical guidance. They are global, and there is no difficulty in transforming simple guidance plans in the atlas (such as a single point, line or plane) to the patient. For guidance that uses more elaborate plans, care must be taken to ensure that all geometric constraints of the operative procedure are met when transforming guidance plans in the atlas to the patient. Future work includes the use of more complex deformable transformations and exploration of the clinical utility of deformable registrations for surgical guidance.

Acknowledgments

This research was supported in part by Communications and Information Technology Ontario, the Institute for Robotics and Intelligent Systems, the Ontario Research and Development Challenge Fund, and the Natural Sciences and Engineering Research Council of Canada.

References

1. Paul J. Besl and N. D. McKay. A method for registration of 3-d shapes. *IEEE Transactions on Pattern Analysis and Machine Intelligence*, 14(2):239–256, February 1992.
2. R. E. Ellis, D. J. Fleet, J. T. Bryant, J. Rudan, and P. Fenton. A method for evaluating ct-based surgical registration. In Jocelyne Troccaz, Eric Grimson, and Ralph Mösges, editors, *CVRMed-MRCAS'97*, pages 141–150. Springer-Verlag, March 1997.

3. William K. Feinstein, Philip C. Noble, Emir Kamaric, and Hugh S. Tullos. Anatomic alignment of the patellar groove. *Clinical Orthopaedics and Related Research*, 331:64–73, 1996.

4. K. B. Inkpen and A. J. Hodgson. Accuracy and repeatability of joint center location in computer-assisted knee surgery. In *Medical Image Computing and Computer-Assisted Intervention—MICCAI'99*, pages 1072–1079, 1999.

5. K. A. Krackow, L. Serpe, M. J. Phillips, M. Bayers-Thering, and W. M. Mihalkpo. A new technique for determining proper mechanical axis alignment during total knee arthroplasty: Progress toward computer-assisted tka. *Orthopedics*, 22(7):698–702, July 1999.

6. M. Kunz, F. Langlotz, M. Sati, J. M. Strauss, K. Bernsmann, W. Ruther, and L. P. Nolte. Advanced intraoperative registration of mechanical limb axes for total knee arthroplasty surgery. In *CAOS2000*, 2000.

7. J. Lea, D. Watkins, A. Mills, M. Peshkin, T. Kienzle III, and S. Stulberg. Registration and immobilization in robot-assisted surgery. *Journal of Image Guided Surgery*, 1995.

8. F. Leitner, F. Picard, R. Minfelde, H. Schulz, P. Cinquin, and D. Saragaglia. Computer-assisted knee surgical total replacement. In *CVRMed-MRCAS'97*, pages 629–636, 1997.

9. J. B. A. Maintz and M. A. Viergever. A survey of medical image registration. *Medical Image Analysis*, 2(1):1–36, 1998.

10. S. Mai, C. Lörke, and W. Siebert. Motivation, realization and first results of robot-assisted total knee arthroplasty. In *CAOS2001*, 2001.

11. C. Maurer, J. Fitzpatrick, R. Maciunas, and G. Allen. Registration of 3-d images using weighted geometrical features. *IEEE TMI*, 15(6):836–849, 1996.

12. P. F. La Palombara, M. Fadda, S. Martelli, L. Nofrini, and M. Marcacci. A minimally invasive 3-d data registration protocol for computer and robot assisted total knee arthroplasty. In *CVRMed-MRCAS'97*, pages 663–672, 1997.

13. F. Picard, A. M. DiGioia, D. Sell, J. E. Moody, B. Jaramaz, C. Nikou, R. S. LaBarca, and T. Levison. Computer-assisted navigation for knee arthroplasty: Intra-operative measurements of alignment and soft-tissue balancing. In *CAOS2001*, 2001.

14. Stephen C. Reed and Jeffrey Gollish. The accuracy of femoral intramedullary guides in total knee arthroplasty. *The Journal of Arthroplasty*, 12(6):677–682, 1997.

15. P. Ritschl, R. Fuiko, H. Broers, A. Wurzinger, and W. Berner. Computer-assisted navigation and robot-cutting system for total knee replacement. In *CAOS2001*, 2001.

16. J. Stiehl and B. Abbott. Morphology of the transepicondylar axis and its application in primary and revision total knee arthroplasty. *Journal of Arthrolasty*, 6(10):785–789, 1995.

17. P. St-Jean, A. F. Sadikot, L. Collins, D. Clonda, R. Kasrai, A. C. Evans, and T. M. Peters. Automated atlas integration and interactive three-dimensional visualization tools for planning and guidance in functional neurosurgery. *IEEE TMI*, 15(5):672–680, 1998.

18. Leo A. Whiteside and Junichi Arima. The anteroposterior axis for femoral rotational alignment in valgus total knee arthroplasty. *Clinical Orthopaedics*, 321:168–172, December 1995.

19. U. Wiesel, A. Lahmer, M. Tenbusch, and M. Boerner. Total knee replacement using the robodoc system. In *CAOS2001*, 2001.

20. Yuki Yoshioka, David Siu, and T. Derek V. Cooke. The anatomy and functional axes of the femur. *The Journal of Bone and Joint Surgery*, 69-A(6):873–880, July 1987.

Effectiveness of the ROBODOC System during Total Hip Arthroplasty in Preventing Intraoperative Pulmonary Embolism

Keisuke Hagio[1], Nobuhiko Sugano[2], Masaki Takashina[3],
Takashi Nishii[2], Hideki Yoshikawa[2], and Takahiro Ochi[1]

[1] Department of Computer Integrated Orthopaedics,
Osaka University Graduate School of Medicine, 2-2 Yamadaoka, Suita, Osaka, Japan
k-hagio@tc4.so-net.ne.jp
[2] Department of Orthopaedic Surgery, Osaka University Graduate School of Medicine,
2-2 Yamadaoka, Suita, Osaka, Japan
[3] Department of Anesthesiology, Osaka University Graduate School of Medicine
2-2 Yamadaoka, Suita, Osaka, Japan

Abstract. Intraoperative pulmonary embolism can occur not only during cemented total hip arthroplasty (THA) but also during cementless THA. In the present study, we demonstrated the usefulness of the ROBODOC femoral milling system in reducing intraoperative pulmonary embolism, as indicated by results of transesophageal echocardiography and hemodynamic monitoring. A prospective clinical trial was conducted with 58 patients (60 hips) who were randomly divided into 2 groups: group 1, 38 patients (40 hips) who underwent cementless THA with preparation of the femoral canal using ROBODOC; group 2, 20 patients (20 hips) who underwent conventional manual cementless THA surgery. During femoral preparation, severe embolic events were observed at a significantly lower frequency in group 1 (0%) than in group 2 (30%) ($p < 0.0001$). During stem insertion, incidence of severe embolic events was significantly lower in group 1 (0%) than in group 2 (20%) ($p < 0.0001$). Moreover, during hip relocation, incidence of severe embolic events was significantly lower in group 1 (8%) than in group 2 (45%) ($p < 0.0001$). The ROBODOC system decreased the incidence of severe embolic events during femoral preparation, resulting in low incidence of severe events during stem insertion and hip relocation. The present results suggest that the ROBODOC femoral milling system may reduce the risk of pulmonary embolism during cementless THA.

1   Introduction

Hypotension, hypoxemia, cardiopulmonary dysfunction and death are well-known complications of cemented total hip arthroplasty (THA) (1-3). These complications can be caused by increased intramedullary pressure of the femur as a result of cement infusion or stem insertion, and by introduction of fat and bone marrow cells into the venous system. These causes can activate the blood coagulation system. Formation of thrombi and migration of fat and bone marrow cells to the lungs produce pulmonary embolism (4-6). There have been reports that decompression in the medullary space

T. Dohi and R. Kikinis (Eds.): MICCAI 2002, LNCS 2488, pp. 339–346, 2002.
© Springer-Verlag Berlin Heidelberg 2002

of the femur can have a prophylactic effect against pulmonary embolism (7-11). However, there have even been reports of death from intraoperative pulmonary embolism in cases of cementless THA (12); risk of pulmonary embolism is thus not limited to cemented THA. Increases in intrafemoral pressure can be caused not only by application of cement and insertion of the femoral stem but also by preparation of the femoral canal (13)(14). Rasping the intramedullary canal of the femur can increase intrafemoral pressure, causing intravasation of fat and bone marrow. It is reasonable to hypothesize that the ROBODOC system (15), which precisely excavates the femoral canal automatically using a milling system that does not increase intrafemoral pressure, can reduce the risk of pulmonary embolism during cementless THA.

The purpose of this study was to estimate the effectiveness of the ROBODOC femoral milling system, compared with manual surgery, in preventing pulmonary embolism during cementless THA.

2   Materials and Methods

Between September 2000 and February 2002, we performed a prospective study of 58 patients (60 hips) with osteoarthritis of the hip joint who underwent cementless THA with or without the ROBODOC femoral milling system. The patients were randomly divided into 2 groups: group 1, 38 patients (40 hips) who underwent preparation of the femoral canal with ROBODOC; group 2, 20 patients (20 hips) who underwent manual surgery. Patients were matched for gender, age, height, weight at surgery, and preoperative physical status. Preoperative physical status was assessed according to the criteria of the American Society of Anesthesiologists (16).

Each patient was placed in the lateral decubitus position, and the hip joint was exposed through the postero-lateral approach. A press-fit acetabular component was inserted without cement in all cases.

In group 2, the femur was prepared with standard broaches and washed with pressurized lavage, followed by insertion of a tapered stem (VerSys Fiber Metal Taper, Zimmer, Warsaw, IN) in the largest size that provided a stable press-fit. In group 1, the femur was prepared using the milling tools of the ROBODOC system, which prepares the femoral canal by milling and lavaging the intramedullary space simultaneously, followed by insertion of a tapered stem (VerSys Fiber Metal Taper, Zimmer, Warsaw, IN) scheduled preoperatively.

In all cases, surgery was performed under general anesthesia with epidural anesthesia. Endotracheal intubation was performed, and mechanical ventilation was used for airway management. In all cases, inspired O2 concentration remained at a constant level (0.33%). After induction of anesthesia, a 5-MHz echocardiographic probe (Hewlett-Packard; Andover, MA) was inserted into the esophagus of each patient, and the heart was visualized. The frequency and grade of embolic events at each stage of the operation were assessed. Echocardiographic findings were classified into 4 grades, according to the classification system of Pitto et al (8), as follows: grade 0, no emboli; grade 1, a few fine emboli; grade 2, a cascade of fine emboli or embolic masses with a diameter <5 mm; grade 3, fine emboli mixed with embolic masses with a diameter $\geqq 5$ mm (Fig. 1 (a)-(d)).

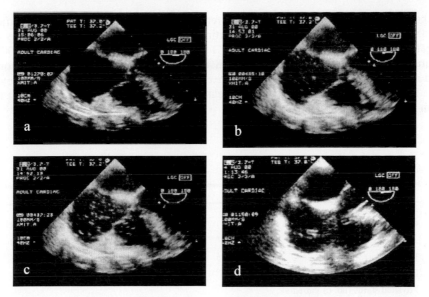

Fig. 1. (a)-(d): Right atrium during echocardiography
(a) Grade 0:No emboli. (b) Grade 1:A few fine emboli. (c) Grade 2:A cascade of fine emboli or embolic masses less than 5mm in diameter. (d) Grade 3:Large embolic masses more than 5mm in diameter.

Echocardiographic findings, blood gas (PaO2), arterial oxygen saturation (Sat), systolic blood pressure (SBP) and heart rate (HR) were recorded at the time of surgical incision, femoral preparation, stem insertion, hip relocation and the end of the operation. All data was expressed as percentage of the value at the time of skin incision. At each stage, the relationship between echocardiographic findings and change in measured data was evaluated, and the effectiveness of the ROBODOC femoral milling system in preventing pulmonary embolism during THA was estimated.

Statistical analysis was performed using the Mann-Whitney U test; and a P value of less than 0.05 was considered to indicate statistical significance.

3   Results

Mean age at surgery was higher in group 2 than in group 1, and average height and weight were lower in group 2 than in group 1. No patients in either group had severe systemic disease (class 3 or 4, according to the system of the American Society of Anesthesiologists (16)). There was no significant difference in gender, age, weight, height or preoperative physical status between the groups (Table 1).

In both groups, no embolic events were detected by transesophageal echocardiography during operative approach to the hip, dislocation of the joint or osteotomy of the femoral neck, or at the end of the operation.

In group 2, 6 hips (30%) had an embolic event of grade 2 or greater during preparation of the femur, but no patients in group 1 had an embolic event of grade 2 or greater during femoral preparation. The differences in frequency and intensity of embolic events during preparation of the femur between the 2 groups were significant (p<0.0001) (Table 2). During stem insertion, the incidence of events of grade 2 or greater was significantly lower in group 1 (0%) than in group 2 (20%) (p<0.0001). Moreover, during hip relocation, 3 hips (8%) in group 1 and 8 hips (40%) in group 2 had a grade-2 embolic event, and 1 hip (5%) in group 2 had a grade-3 embolic event. The incidence of events of grade 2 or greater was lower with ROBODOC (8%) than with manual surgery (45%).

Table 1. Data on the patients

	Group 1[a]	Guroup 2[b]	P-value[d]
Number of hips	40	20	
Gender (male/female)	7/33	3/17	0.808
Age (yrs.)	57.9±10.5[c]	61.0±8.0[c]	0.209
Weight (kg)	58.3±12.1[c]	55.5±10.0[c]	0.515
Height (cm)	155.9±6.5[c]	154.0±8.4[c]	0.380
Physical status (no. of patients)[e]			
class 1/2/3/4	25/15/0/0	14/6/0/0	0.851

[a]Patients had THAs with ROBODOC system.

[b]Patients had THAs with manual surgery.

[c]The values are given as the mean and the standard deviation.

[d]Mann-Whitney U test

[e]Physical status was assesed according to the system of American Society of Anesthesiologists

To evaluate changes in measured data at each stage, the data from the 2 groups were combined and then divided into 2 groups based on grade of embolic events: grade 1 or lower, and grade 2 or higher on echocardiography. At all stages, in the grade 2 or higher group, PaO2 and Sat values were significantly lower (p<0.05), and SBP values tended to be lower than in the grade 1 or lower group, but HR values showed no distinct tendency (Table 3).

Table 2.The frequency and grade of embolic events in each manipulation of the operation

	Group 1[a]			Guroup 2[b]			P-value[c]
	Grade 1	Grade 2	Grade 3	Grade 1	Grade 2	Grade 3	
Preparation of the femur							
No.(%) of hips	4(10)			14(70)	5(25)	1(5)	p<.0001
Implantation of stem							
No.(%) of hips	12(30)			14(70)	3(15)	1(5)	p<.0001
Relocation of hip joint							
No.(%) of hips	22(55)	3(8)		11(55)	8(40)	1(5)	p<.0001

[a]Patients had THAs with ROBODOC system.

[b]Patients had THAs with manual surgery.

[c]Mann-Whitney U test

4   Discussion

Intraoperative sudden death is the severest complication of THA. For cemented THA, intraoperative mortality reportedly ranges from 0.02 to 0.5%, and frequency of cardiac arrest reportedly ranges from 0.6 to 10% (17-20). The principal cause of these complications in cemented THA appears to be pulmonary embolism caused by femoral bone manipulation using cement, and prophylactic methods such as decompression of the femoral canal with venting holes (7-9, 10,11) or jet lavage (21) have also been reported. Death from intraoperative pulmonary embolism has even been reported in cases of cementless THA (12), and it is unclear what prophylactic methods can best prevent intraoperative pulmonary embolism during cementless THA.

Table 3.Hemodynamic change

		Preparation of the femur	Implantation of stem	Relocation of hip joint
	Grade 0 or 1	106.1±11.9	101.4±12.3	103.3±11.4
PaO2	Grade 2 or 3	87.5±9.1	87.1±8.0	92.0±9.0
	P-value[a]	0.0011	0.026	0.003
	Grade 0 or 1	98.2±11.6	97.1±11.8	99.2±14.0
SBP	Grade 2 or 3	90.7±11.7	90.6±5.9	91.9±5.6
	P-value[a]	0.273	0.211	0.046
	Grade 0 or 1	100.4±0.9	100.2±0.8	100.4±0.8
Sat	Grade 2 or 3	99.1±0.4	99.0±0.7	99.6±0.6
	P-value[a]	0.0004	0.0072	0.0013
	Grade 0 or 1	100.9±10.2	102.4±13.8	104.7±16.4
HR	Grade 2 or 3	98.3±5.1	98.0±11.2	102.2±8.2
	P-value[a]	0.488	0.442	0.747

The values are given as the mean and the standard deviation. Each data was expressed in percentage with the value at skin incision as reference.
[a]Mann-Whitney U test

Evaluation of embolic events using transesophageal echocardiography allows detection of passage of fat or bone marrow through the heart, which has been reported in a number of cases of orthopedic surgery (8,10,22-27). However, it is difficult to directly and clearly define the essential nature of echogenic particles. Pitto et al. (8) reported that grade-1 events also occurred when infusion of the central venous catheter was at maximum flow, and, in the present study, grade-1 events were observed when infusion of the peripheral venous catheter was at maximum flow. Also in the present study, events of grade 2 or greater were associated with a significant decrease in PaO2 and Sat and a tendency toward lower SBP, whereas grade-1 events were not associated with conspicuous differences in these values. This suggests that detection of events of grade 2 or higher by echocardiography is cause for concern. The association between severe embolic events (grade 2 or 3) and changes in hemodynamic and cardiorespiratory indicators observed in the present study is consistent with the findings of previous studies (8, 10, 23, 27,28).

Pitto et al. (8) used transesophageal echocardiography to study patients with osteo-arthrosis of the hip who underwent THA. Among their subjects who underwent ce-mented THA, they found severe embolic events (grade 2 or higher) in 10% during preparation of the femoral canal, 85% during stem insertion and 75% during reduc-tion. Among those who underwent cementless THA, they found severe embolic events in 15% during femoral preparation and 0% during stem insertion and reduc-tion. However, in group 2 of the present study, severe embolic events were found in 30% during femoral preparation, 20% during stem insertion, and 45% during hip relocation. Pitto et al. found a very low rate of embolic events in cases of cementless THA, but the stem design they used (CLS; Sultzer Medica) was different from the one used in the present study (VerSys Fiber Metal Taper; Zimmer, Warsaw, IN). Stem design and/or instruments used in femoral preparation may greatly affect generation of embolic particles.

Pitto et al. also found, among patients who underwent cementless THA, grade 1 embolic events in 10% and grade 2 embolic events in 15% during preparation of the femur, and they emphasized this finding despite the low frequency with which these events occurred. Schmidt et al. (29) also reported embolic events during preparation of the femur, and reported that embolic events could be reduced by using a cannulated awl and a cannulated rasp. In the present study, in group 2 (manual surgery), grade 1 events were found in 70% of hips, grade 2 in 25%, and grade 3 in 5% during femoral preparation, but severe embolic events (grade 2 or higher) were not found in group 1 (ROBODOC). This suggests that the ROBODOC femoral milling system is more effective than manual surgery in preventing pulmonary embolism during femoral preparation.

In the present study, in group 2, embolic events of grade 2 or higher occurred at higher frequency during hip relocation (45%) than during femoral preparation (30%) or stem insertion (20%). During femoral bone manipulation, the hip joint was main-tained at a flexion-adduction-internal rotation position until insertion of the stem. As a result, venous stasis occurred, and this may have interfered with observation of em-bolic events by echocardiography during preparation of the femur or stem insertion. Embolic events during reduction of the hip may be due to flow of fat and bone mar-row into the stagnated venous system as a result of femoral bone manipulation before reduction of the hip. This induces formation of thrombi. These embolic particles mi-grate to the lungs and pulmonary embolism then occurs when venous blood flow is resumed due to reduction (4-6). Apparently, it is important to avoid introducing fat and bone marrow into the venous system as a result of femoral bone manipulation. In contrast to our results for group 2, incidence of embolic events of grade 2 or higher in group 1 was 0% during femoral bone manipulation and 8% during hip relocation. The ROBODOC milling system decreased the amount of fat and bone marrow introduced into the venous system during femoral preparation, resulting in low incidence of se-vere events during stem insertion and hip relocation.

In the present study, severe embolic events were observed in patients who under-went cementless THA, but they occurred at a lower frequency than those reported for cemented THA in the literature. Despite this difference in frequency, it is clear that development of fatal embolic events during THA is an important concern whether or not cement is used. In order to prevent embolic events, it is important to avoid intro-ducing fat and bone marrow into the venous system during surgical manipulation. The present results indicate that the ROBODOC femoral milling system decreased the incidence of severe embolic events during femoral preparation, resulting in low incidence of severe events during stem insertion and hip relocation. This finding suggests that the ROBODOC femoral milling system may reduce the risk of pulmonary embolism during cementless THA.

References

1. Burgess DM: Cardiac arrest and bone cement (letter). Br Med J 3: 588, 1970
2. Jones R.H: Physiologic emboli changes observed during total hip replacement arthroplasty. A clinical prospective study. Clin Orthop 112: 192, 1975
3. Kallos T: Impaired arterial oxygenation associated with use of bone cement in the femoral shaft. Anesthesiology 42: 210, 1975
4. Modig J, Busch C, Olerud S, Saldeen T, Waernbaum G: Arterial hypotension and hypoxaemia during total hip replacement: the importance of thromboplastic products, fat embolism and acrylic monomers. Acta Anaesthesiol Scand 19: 28, 1975
5. Saldeen T: Intravascular coagulation in the lungs in experimental fat embolism. Acta Chir Scand 135: 653, 1969
6. Sharrock NE, Go G, Harpel PC, Ranawat CS, Sculco TP, Salvati EA: The John Charnley Award. Thrombogenesis during total hip arthroplasty. Clin Orthop 319:16, 1995
7. Kallos T, Enis JE, Gollan F, Davis JH: Intramedullary pressure and pulmonary embolism of femoral medullary contents in dogs during insertion of bone cement and a prosthesis. J Bone Joint Surg Am 56: 1363, 1974
8. Pitto RP, Koessler M, Kuehle JW: Comparison of fixation of the femoral component without cement and fixation with use of a bone-vacuum cementing technique for the prevention of fat embolism during total hip arthroplasty. A prospective, randomized clinical trial. J Bone Joint Surg Am 81: 831, 1999
9. Tronzo RG, Kallos T, Wyche MQ: Elevation of intramedullary pressure when methylmethacrylate is inserted in total hip arthroplasty. J Bone Joint Surg Am 56: 714, 1974
10. Wenda K, Degreif J, Runkel M, Ritter G: Pathogenesis and prophylaxis of circulatory reactions during total hip replacement. Arch Orthop Trauma Surg 112: 260, 1993
11. Herndon JH, Bechtol CO, Crickenberger DP: Fat embolism during total hip replacement. A prospective study. J Bone Joint Surg Am 56: 1350, 1974
12. Arroyo JS, Garvin KL, McGuire MH: Fatal marrow embolization following a porous-coated bipolar hip endoprosthesis. J Arthroplasty 9: 449, 1994
13. Modig J, Busch C, Olerud S, Saldeen T.:Pulmonary microembolism during intramedullary orthopaedic trauma. Acta Anaesthesiol Scand. 1974;18(2):133-43
14. Wenda K, Ritter G, Ahlers J, von Issendorff WD. [Detection and effects of bone marrow intravasations in operations in the area of the femoral marrow cavity] Unfallchirurg. 1990 Feb;93(2):56-61.
15. Bargar WL, Bauer A, Borner M: Primary and revision total hip replacement using the Robodoc system. Clin Orthop. Sep;(354):82-91, 1998
16. American Society of Anesthesiologists: New classification of physical status. Anesthesiology, 24:111-114,1963.
17. Coventry MB, Beckenbaugh RD, Nolan DR, Ilstrup DM: 2,012 total hip arthroplasties. A study of postoperative course and early complications. J Bone Joint Surg Am 56: 273, 1974
18. Duncan JA: Intra-operative collapse or death related to the use of acrylic cement in hip surgery. Anaesthesia 44: 149, 1989
19. Hyland J, Robins RH: Cardiac arrest and bone cement. Br Med J 4: 176, 1970
20. Patterson BM, Healey JH, Cornell CN, Sharrock NE: Cardiac arrest during hip arthroplasty with a cemented long-stem component. A report of seven cases. J Bone Joint Surg Am 73: 271, 1991

21. Christie J, Robinson CM, Singer B, Ray DC. :Medullary lavage reduces embolic phenomena and cardiopulmonary changes during cemented hemiarthroplasty. J Bone Joint Surg Br. 1995 May; 77(3):456-9.
22. Pitto RP, Blunk J, Kossler M: Transesophageal echocardiography and clinical features of fat embolism during cemented total hip arthroplasty. A randomized study in patients with a femoral neck fracture. Arch Orthop Trauma Surg 120: 53, 2000
23. Christie J, Burnett R, Potts HR, Pell AC: Echocardiography of transatrial embolism during cemented and uncemented hemiarthroplasty of the hip. J Bone Joint Surg Br 76: 409, 1994
24. Heinrich H, Kremer P, Winter H, Worsdorfer O, Ahnefeld FW, Wilder-Smith O: Embolic events during total hip replacement. An echocardiographic study. Acta Orthop Belg 54: 12, 1988
25. Woo R, Minster GJ, Fitzgerald RH Jr, Mason LD, Lucas DR, Smith FE: The Frank Stinchfield Award. Pulmonary fat embolism in revision hip arthroplasty. Clin Orthop 319:41, 1995
26. Christie J, Robinson CM, Pell AC, McBirnie J, Burnett R. Transcardiac echocardiography during invasive intramedullary procedures. J Bone Joint Surg Br. 1995 May;77(3):450-5.
27. Pitto RP, Koessler M, Draenert K. The John Charnley Award. Prophylaxis of fat and bone marrow embolism in cemented total hip arthroplasty. Clin Orthop. 1998 Oct;(355):23-34.
28. Ries MD, Lynch F, Rauscher LA, Richman J, Mick C, Gomez M. Pulmonary function during and after total hip replacement. Findings in patients who have insertion of a femoral component with and without cement. J Bone Joint Surg Am. 1993 Apr;75(4):581-7.
29. Schmidt J, Sulk C, Weigand C, LaRosee K: Reduction of fat embolic risks in total hip arthroplasty using cannulated awls and rasps for the preparation of the femoral canal. Arch Orthop Trauma Surg 2000; 120(1-2): 100-2.

Medical Image Synthesis via Monte Carlo Simulation

James Z. Chen, Stephen M. Pizer, Edward L. Chaney, and Sarang Joshi

Medical Image Display & Analysis Group, University of North Carolina, Chapel Hill, USA
{chenz,pizer}@cs.unc.edu, {chaney,sarang}@radonc.unc.edu

Abstract. A large number of test images and their "ground truth" segmentations are needed for performance characterization of the many image segmentation methods. In this work we developed a methodology to form a probability distribution of the diffeomorphism between a segmented template image and those from a population, and consequently we sample from these probability distributions to produce test images. This method will be illustrated by producing simulated 3D CT images of the abdomen for testing the segmentation of the human right kidney.

1 Introduction

This work explores a methodology for generating realistic, synthetic medical images for characterizing the performance of segmentation methods. It is intended to allow more effective validation and inter-comparison of algorithms that are designed to perform objective, reproducible segmentations of anatomical objects from medical images.

Test images intended for performance characterization should be able to represent the modality of interest and contain the "ground truth" segmentations, against which a particular segmentation method can be evaluated. Also, these images should represent statistical variations in the shape of target object across a population and span the range of image qualities found in a clinical setting. These properties mandate a large set of test images. In practice, however, it is a highly demanding task to define the ground truth segmentations for so many test images because 1) the manual segmentation by medical experts is a laborious and expensive process; 2) it has been shown that there exists a large variation even among the experts regarding the "correct" segmentations [1] due to subjective bias and the dependence on objectives.

A promising approach that could partially replace the costly performance evaluation procedures is to make use of synthetic images generated from simulations. Several statistical models of shape and appearance variability have been investigated and applied to perform various medical image analysis tasks. Examples are Active Shape Models (ASM) [2] and Statistical Deformation Models (SDM) [3]. These methods can also be adapted to generate synthetic images for performance characterization by sampling the distribution of variability. But in building an ASM, a set of segmentations of the shape of interest is required as well as a set of landmarks that can be unambiguously defined in each sample shape. The manual identification of the point correspondences is a time-consuming task and is prone to the subjective bias. In the SDM method, this difficulty is removed by applying an automated nonlinear image

T. Dohi and R. Kikinis (Eds.): MICCAI 2002, LNCS 2488, pp. 347–354, 2002.
© Springer-Verlag Berlin Heidelberg 2002

registration. However, since the sample points in this model are distributed in the entire image volume, the computational complexity is non-trivial. In our method, the shape of the target object is represented via a limited number of automatically determined fiducial points. The computational efficiency is thus dramatically improved. Similar to the SDM method, the point correspondence across a population is established by a nonlinear, diffeomorphic image registration.

This work focuses on simulating the shape variability of the target anatomical object as observed across a population. The methodology will be laid out first, which includes the scheme of fiducial-point shape representation, the training process, the shape analysis and the subsequent image synthesis. Then, this method will be applied to synthesize the CT images of the human abdomen as a demonstration. Although the illustration here is limited to a single-organ system, this method should be applicable for generating synthetic images of any anatomical structure in principle, including multi-organ complexes.

2   Methodology

Our method for generating realistic, synthetic medical images proceeds in two steps: training and sampling. In the training phase, the shape of the target object is studied, from which a distribution of its variation is derived. In the sampling phase, a large number of synthetic images can be produced by randomly sampling from the probability distribution.

For training purposes a set of clinical images containing the target object need to be collected, so as to capture the shape variations of the anatomical object of interest across the population. These images will be referred to as the training images $\{I_t\}$. One of $\{I_t\}$ will be chosen as the template image I_0, and other images will be registered to I_0 via a nonlinear, diffeomorphic warp function H_t: $I_t \cong H_t(I_0)$. Given a predefined segmentation S_0 of the target object in I_0, $\{H_t(S_0)\}$ can be analyzed to find its probability distribution (referred to as the "normal shape domain", or NSD). Artificial warp functions, and consequently the synthetic images and their segmentations, can then be generated by randomly sampling in the NSD. Details of this new method will be developed in the following sections.

2.1   Training Image Segmentation

Training defines the degrees of freedom that will characterize a typical object through observed shape variations across a population. The target object in a training image I_t can be recognized through an image segmentation S_t, which can be achieved via an automated image registration of I_t to the pre-labeled template image I_0. The large-scale fluid deformation method [4] is used in this work and I_0 is registered to I_t through a diffeomorphic function H_t:

$$I_t \cong H_t(I_0) \ . \tag{1}$$

It is assumed here that the correspondence between these images established by $\{H_t\}$ is the "true correspondence". With the target object in I_0 having been labeled *a priori* (denoted as S_0), that in I_t (denoted as S_t) can thus be defined by applying the same warp function H_t on S_0,

$$S_t = H_t(S_0) .$$ (2)

Here the "ground truth" S_0 is defined by the consensus of an expert panel.

2.2   Fiducial-Point Shape Representation

The shape of an object is defined as those aspects of its geometric conformation that are invariant under similarity transformations, for example, its topology. A fiducial-point shape representation made from a limited number of points on the surface will be developed next to represent an object's shape according to its variation in the training set. The shape analysis then becomes the study of the displacement distributions of these points.

Given a predefined template shape S_0, and a set $\{H_t\}$ that registers I_0 to $\{I_t\}$, the various shapes of the object of interest in $\{I_t\}$ can be represented by $(S_0, \{H_t\})$. Assume that each H_t can be encoded into the displacements of a limited number of points, from which another deformation field H'_t can be constructed to reproduce the deformation around $H_t(S_0)$. Then the representation of the various shapes is further simplified to the locations of these individual points and their corresponding displacements. The algorithm employed here to construct H'_t from a set of points and their displacements has been developed under the fluid deformation model and has been implemented as the "landmark fluid deformation" function in the fluid deformation program [5]. This function takes the initial and terminal locations of a set of points as the input, and generates a diffeomorphic deformation vector field that drives each point from its initial location to its destination.

This set of points on the surface of S_0 is named the "fiducial points", denoted by $\{F_m\}$, ($m \in [1, M]$, M being the total number of fiducial points in the representation). In the extreme case of including all points on the surface of S_0, we would have an enumerative representation of the surface. However, since the locations of these points are highly correlated due to the biological nature of the target object, some of these points are redundant in this representation and can be eliminated without losing significant information. The fiducial points predominantly reside at salient geometric and/or intensity features of an image.

An iterative procedure has been developed to find an optimal set of fiducial points in representing the shape of an anatomical object adequately and efficiently such that, on the average over all training samples, the difference between H_t and H'_t

$$\frac{1}{T \cdot N_0} \sum_{t=1}^{T} \sum_{x \in S_0} | H_t(x) - H'_t(x) |$$ (3)

is reduced below a predefined threshold on the surface of S_0, where N_0 is the number of voxels on the surface of S_0 and T is the total number of training samples. A surface curvature based geometric screening can be employed to initialize the seed point set – assuming large surface curvature implies important shape conformation, the first few points with the highest surface curvature are selected to define the initial fiducial point set $\{F_m\}$. Then the following algorithm can be applied to each I_t $(t \in [1, T])$ to find the optimal fiducial point selection.

1. Apply the training warp function H_t on $\{F_m\}$ to get the warped fiducial points: $F_{m,t}$ $= H_t(F_m)$;
2. Reconstruct the diffeomorphic warp field H'_t for the entire image volume based on the displacements $\{F_{m,t} - F_m\}$;
3. Locate the point p_t on the surface of S_0 that introduces the largest discrepancy between H_t and H'_t: $H_t(p_t) - H'_t(p_t) = \max\{ | H_t(x) - H'_t(x) | \}$, where p_t, $x \in$ the surface of S_0;
4. In the point set $\{p_t\}$ established from all training images, find the point p that introduces the largest discrepancy in $\{H_t(p_t) - H'_t(p_t)\}$ and add it to the fiducial point set: $\{\{F_m\}, p\} \Rightarrow \{F_m\}$;
5. Loop back to step 1 until an optimization criterion is reached.

The optimization criterion can take various forms and one example will be demonstrated in *Sect. 3*.

2.3   The Normal Shape Domain

Denote $\vec{f}_0 = ((x_{f_1}, y_{f_1}, z_{f_1}), (x_{f_2}, y_{f_2}, z_{f_2}), \dots (x_{f_M}, y_{f_M}, z_{f_M}))$ the collective coordinates of the fiducial point set $\{F_m\}$, and $\vec{f}_t$ the displaced fiducial points $\{F_{m,t}\}$ $(t = 1, 2, \dots T)$. So

$$\vec{f}_t = H_t(\vec{f}_0) . \tag{4}$$

The object's shape in I_t can be represented by $\vec{f}_t$ and the subsequent shape analysis will be on $\{\vec{f}_t\}$.

$\vec{f}_t$ is a single point in a $3M$ dimensional space (M being the total number of fiducial points in the shape representation). A set of T training shapes gives a cloud of T points in this $3M$-D space. Assume that these points lie within some region of the space, which is named the "normal shape domain" (NSD). Every $3M$-D point within this domain will give a shape definition $\vec{f}$ that complies with those in the original training set. Thus new shapes can be generated systematically by sampling in this NSD. Also assuming that the NSD is approximately ellipsoidal, we can calculate its center and its major axes to give an analytical definition.

For a set of T training samples represented by $\{\vec{f}_t\}$, the mean shape is $<\vec{f}>$. The principal axes of the ellipsoid can be calculated by applying a principal component analysis to the deviation in the data from the sample mean. Each principal axis gives a significant mode of variation, in which the fiducial points tend to move collectively as the shape varies. These principal axes are described by the unit eigenvector $\{\vec{p}_k\}$ ($k = 1, 2, \dots 3M$) of the covariance matrix S formed from the deviations:

$$S\vec{p}_k = \lambda_k \vec{p}_k .$$ (5)

Most of the variation can usually be explained by a small number of modes n, and the original ellipsoid has a relatively small width beyond these n dimensions.

2.4   Realistic Synthetic Image Generation

Each point in the NSD can be reached by taking the mean shape and adding a linear combination of the eigenvectors. Therefore, a new shape complying with those training samples is

$$\vec{f}_s = <\vec{f}> + \sum_{k=1}^{n} b_k \cdot \vec{p}_k , \quad -3\sqrt{\lambda_k} \leq b_k \leq 3\sqrt{\lambda_k}$$ (6)

where b_k is the component coefficient of $\vec{p}_k$ and suitable limits are typically of the order of three standard deviations. From the original and the displaced fiducial points ($\vec{f}_0, \vec{f}_s$), a deformation field (H_s) can be obtained by applying the landmark fluid deformation function. A synthetic image I_s and its "ground truth" segmentation will then be defined by

$$I_s = H_s(I_0)$$
$$S_s = H_s(S_0)$$ (7)

A large number of realistic, synthetic images with known ground truth segmentations can be thus produced and used for characterizing the performance of the image segmentation methods.

3   Application: Synthetic Images of the Human Right Kidney

A pool of 36 clinical CT images $\{I_t\}$ was prepared and one of them was selected as the template I_0, which has clear kidney region, low noise, minimal breathing artifacts and is close to the mean geometric conformation of all the training samples. The right kidney in I_0 was then carefully segmented by medical experts and was used as the ground truth S_0. For each training image I_t, its intensity was normalized to that of the template I_0, and its resolution was resampled to 2mm×2mm×2mm via trilinear interpolation. To improve the convergence of registration, the MIRIT program [6] was applied first to find the similarity transformation between each (I_0, I_t) pair. As image quality varies, parameters in the fluid deformation program were fine-tuned in each case to give the best registration between I_0 and I_t, as judged by visual inspection.

3.1   Fiducial Point Shape Representation

The algorithm developed in *Sect. 2.2* was applied to find the optimal point set for this data. The optimization criterion was taken from a previous independent study [7], in which a comparison was made between two human raters' manual segmentations on a subset of the human kidney CT images used in this work. It was found that the average volume overlap between these two manual segmentations was 94.0%, and the average surface distance was 1.2mm apart, as measured by VALMET [1]. Thus the iterative procedure was terminated when, on the average over all training samples, the similarity between $H_t(S_0)$ and $H'_t(S_0)$ surpassed the statistics from the human raters' comparison. In the fiducial point set initialization, a geometric screening selected the top 32 points with the highest surface curvature. The progress of optimization is graphed in *Fig. 1*.

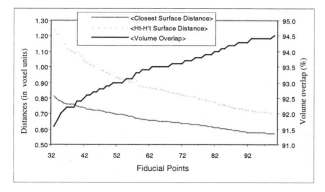

Fig. 1. Fiducial-point set optimization for the human right kidney

In this chart, each of the three statistical indices has been averaged over all training samples. Both surface distance measurements are the averaged magnitude over the surface voxels. The curve labeled "<H_t–H'_t Surface Distance>" shows the average point-wise (diffeomorphisms) error between H_t and H'_t on the surface of kidney. The curve labeled "<Closest Surface Distance>" shows the averaged nearest surface distance from every point on surface of $H_t(S_0)$ to that of $H'_t(S_0)$, so it is necessarily lower than the previous one. The curve in black gives the volume overlap between these two warped segmentations. The last two indices are calculated by the VALMET program, which compares and evaluates a pair of segmentations. Both distance measurements are in voxel units, and their ordinate is on the left. The volume overlap is measured in percentage, and its ordinate is on the right. It is seen that as more points are added into the fiducial-point set, the average volume overlap increases monotonically and the distance measurements decrease correspondingly.

In representing the human right kidney, the volume overlap index has already exceeded 90% when only about 30 fiducial points are selected. Intuitively, this few points can hardly represent a shape in detail even for a simple 3D object. In segmentation comparison, the volume overlap measurement alone is sometimes misleading and should be used with great caution. We therefore report the average surface distance index in combination with this volume overlap index, and we sometimes even include the quartile statistics for more detailed analysis.

Applying the optimization criteria, the fiducial point shape representation for the human right kidney was established to comprise 88 points on the surface of S_0, with <Volume Overlap> = 94.2%, <Closest Surface Distance> = 0.591, and < H_t–H'_t surface distance> = 0.743.

3.2   Synthetic Image Generation

MATLAB was used for the principal component analysis. Although the covariance matrix in this case was a 264-D (3×88=264) square matrix, only the first 35 modes were non-trivial and the NSD in this model case was defined by the first seven modes. They covered more than 88% of the total variance observed in the training samples. The validity of the NSD can be assessed by cross-validation, which shows that this NSD is able to explain the shape variations observed in these samples. Due to the page limit, the technique and the result will be reported in a separate publication.

An arbitrary large number of synthetic human kidney CT images can now be produced from the current system. One such image is shown in *Fig. 2*, in comparison with the template. Note that the kidney object in the synthetic image takes a different shape from that of the template, but their background conformations (structures like liver, lung, spinal cord, and soft tissues) are very similar. Also, the intensity contrast and the noise level in these images are almost identical.

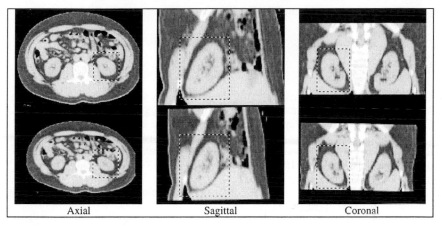

Fig. 2. The template (top) and one synthetic image (bottom)

4   Discussion & Conclusion

In the model system of the human right kidney, only the kidney organ is modeled as an object (defined by S_0) whereas all the other structures in the image are treated as the background intensity variation without any shape description. In order to produce truly realistic synthetic images for a large, multi-organ complex (for example, the entire abdominal region), the shape of each object in the complex needs to be studied to define an ensemble NSD of the system.

Also, because one single image I_0 is used as the template in this example, all the synthetic images will inevitably share a similar background and intensity profiles. To alleviate this situation, a template transformation procedure can be employed – in generating a synthetic image I_s, a transformed warp function $H_sH_t^{-1}$ can be used in place of H_s, with I_t as the template image instead of I_0. The characterization of this process is currently under investigation, and the result will be reported in a future publication.

In summary, a methodology has been developed to generate realistic, synthetic medical images via the Monte Carlo simulation for characterizing the performance of the image segmentation methods. As a demonstration, it has been applied to produce the synthetic CT images of the human right kidney. A test of the m-rep deformable model segmentation method [7] is currently in progress and its result will be reported in the next publication.

Acknowledgements

We sincerely appreciate the help and input from our colleagues during the development of this research work, with our special thanks to Dr. Keith Muller for the many insightful discussions on the statistical analysis and to Gregg Tracton for his superior technical support. The research reported here was carried out under the support of National Cancer Institute Grant P01 CA47982.

References

1. Gerig, G., M. Jomier, M. Chakos (2001). "Valmet: A new validation tool for assessing and improving 3D object segmentation." Proc. MICCAI 2001, Springer LNCS 2208: 516-523.
2. Cootes, T. F., A. Hill, C.J. Taylor, J. Haslam (1994). "The Use of Active Shape Models for Locating Structures in Medical Images." Image and Vision Computing 12(6): 355-366.
3. Rueckert, D., A.F. Frangi, and J.A. Schnabel (2001). "Automatic Construction of 3D Statistical Deformation Models Using Non-rigid Registration." MICCAI 2001, Springer LNCS 2208: 77-84.
4. Christensen, G. E., S.C. Joshi and M.I. Miller (1997). "Volumetric Transformation of Brain Anatomy." IEEE Transactions on Medical Imaging 16: 864-877.
5. Joshi, S., M.I. Miller (2000). "Landmark Matching Via Large Deformation Diffeomorphisms." IEEETransactions on Image Processing.
6. Maes, F., A. Collignon, D. Vandermeulen, G. Marchal, P. Suetens (1997). "Multi-Modality Image Registration by Maximization of Mutual Information." IEEE-TMI 16: 187-198.
7. Pizer, S.M., J.Z. Chen, T. Fletcher, Y. Fridman, D.S. Fritsch, G. Gash, J. Glotzer, S. Joshi, A. Thall, G. Tracton, P. Yushkevich, and E. Chaney (2001). "Deformable M-Reps for 3D Medical Image Segmentation." IJCV, submitted.

Performance Issues in Shape Classification

Samson J. Timoner[1], Pollina Golland[1], Ron Kikinis[2], Martha E. Shenton[3],
W. Eric L. Grimson[1], and William M. Wells III[1,2]

[1] MIT AI Laboratory, Cambridge MA, USA
{samson,polina,welg,sw}@ai.mit.edu
[2] Brigham and Women's Hospital, Harvard Medical School, Boston MA, USA
kikinis@bwh.harvard.edu
[3] Laboratory of Neuroscience, Clinical Neuroscience Division, Department of
Psychiatry, VAMC-Brockton, Harvard Medical School, Brockton, MA.
mshenton@warren.med.harvard.edu

Abstract. Shape comparisons of two groups of objects often have two
goals: to create a classifier to separate the groups and to provide information that shows differences between classes. We examine issues that are
important for shape analysis in a study comparing schizophrenic patients
to normal subjects. For this study, non-linear classifiers provide large accuracy gains over linear ones. Using volume information directly in the
classifier provides gains over a classifier that normalizes the data for volume. We compare two different representations of shape: displacement
fields and distance maps. We show that the classifier based on displacement fields outperforms the one based on distance maps. We also show
that displacement fields provide more information in visualizing shape
differences than distance maps.

1   Introduction

Statistical studies of shape generally compare the shape of a structure selected
from two different groups. They are used to form connections between shape
and the presence or absence of disease [1, 2], testing hypotheses in the differences
between men and women [1, 3, 4], as well as examining biological processes. The
goals of such studies are to classify new examples of a structure and to show a
doctor the differences between classes.

This paper examines a set of issues in classifying structures and presenting
information to doctors. Is it more important to use a good representation or
a particular classification method? Is the choice of alignment technique critical? We examine these issues in one study: segmented amygdala-hippocampus
complexes from fifteen normal and fifteen schizophrenic subjects [5].

1.1   Classification Methods

Until recently, most researchers classifying by shape used linear classifiers to
separate two groups. The technology has generally been motivated by the desire
to create deformable models of shape as the basis of automatic segmenters [6].
One creates a deformable model of shape using Principal Component Analysis

T. Dohi and R. Kikinis (Eds.): MICCAI 2002, LNCS 2488, pp. 355–362, 2002.

(PCA) on representations of example structures. A generative model can then be made by allowing the shape to deform along the most important modes of variation. To compare two groups, one forms such a model for each group, and separates the two models using a hyperplane. Visualization of differences between classes can be examined by moving perpendicular to the hyperplane.

Golland *et al.* demonstrated that non-linear classification can potentially improve the separation between groups of shapes. The gradient of the classifier can be used to show differences between groups.

1.2   Representation

There are numerous attractive representations of shape for classification. Most representations implicitly determine the points on a surface. For example, surfaces can be parameterized in a series of spherical harmonics [1]. Medial representations [7] are parameterizations of shapes based on a chain or sheet of atoms that project a surface. Distance maps embed a surface by labeling the voxels of a 3D-volume with the distance from the surface. Each of these parameterized models avoid establishing direct correspondences between surfaces.

Other representations, conversely, use explicit representations of correspondences. One can represent the surface of structures by a triangular mesh where the vertices of the mesh are at corresponding points on the different structures. One can also use volumetric displacement fields which establish correspondences on the surface as well as the interior of shapes.

Correspondence-based representations have the potential to yield more information than implicit representations. Displacement fields can show not only whether surfaces moved in or out, but can also show local rotation or compression of an organ. For this reason, we consider displacement fields in this paper.

Unfortunately, medical structures typically have large smooth surfaces so that finding correspondences is challenging. It is not intuitive where points in one smooth surface should lie on a second surface. One typically overcomes the challenge by matching two shapes while minimizing an additional constraint. For example, one can match structures by treating them as viscous fluids [8], though many have argued that this type of matching can form un-realistic correspondences. Finding corresponding surfaces that form a minimum description length of a dataset is a promising idea, though it is difficult to find in three spatial dimensions [9]. There have also been various types of surface matching by matching points of one surface to the closest points in another [10, 11].

Intuitively, in a good match, high curvature regions in one object match high curvature regions in a second object. Matching by minimizing an elastic energy should accomplish this feat. Matching a sharp portion of one surface against a sharp portion of another surface is lower energy than flattening the region to match against an less sharp adjacent region. Therefore, we align shapes using a linear elastic model.

2   Methods

We explore several issues that are important to shape-based classification. We examine two different representations of shape. We then compare the results of linear and non-linear classifiers. We explore the effects of normalizing the data by volume. Finally, we consider the effects of different alignment methods. Every combination is examined, though we report only a subset of the results.

The data consists of segmented amygdala-hippocampus complexes, fifteen from schizophrenic patients and fifteen from normal patients [5]. The objects are represented using both signed distance maps and displacement fields. Signed distance maps are formed by labeling each voxel with its distance from a surface [2]. The resulting representation is the vector of labels of the voxels.

To form the displacement field representations of the left complexes, one left amygdala-hippocampus complex is chosen randomly as a basis. It is meshed with tetrahedra to facilitate the matching process. The mesh is then treated as a linear elastic material and deformed to match the amygdala hippocampus complexes as described in [12]. A similar procedure is carried out for the right complexes starting with meshing a complex and then matching to the rest of the data. For each match, the displacement of the nodes of the tetrahedra form a roughly uniform sampling of the displacement field. The resulting representation vector is the concatenation of all the displacements of the nodes of the tetrahedra.

When both sides are considered together, the vectors of each side are simply concatenated. Each section of the paper indicates whether data has been normalized by volume, or not scaled at all. Except for Section 3.3, all results use a second order moment alignment of the data. In that section, we also aligned using the second order moments of the mesh nodes, the mesh tetrahedra moments, and absolute orientation [13] (removing global translations and rotations from a deformation field). We tested aligning left and right amygdalas together and seperately.

Let x be the representation vector of the complexes for either representation. The squared distance between two amygdalas, $||x - x'||^2$, is defined to be $(x - x')^T(x - x')$. For displacement fields, this distance is simply the square of the length of the displacement field between each complex. For distance maps, there is no simple interpretation of distance between shapes.

We train linear and non-linear classifiers of the data. The non-linear classifier is a support vector machine (SVM), described in [2]. We use the Radial Basis Function (RBF), $K(x, x_k) = -e^{||x-x_k||^2/\gamma}$, in the SVM where γ is proportional to the square of the width of the kernel. We pick γ to optimize the leave-one-out cross-validation accuracy of the classifier.

Our goal is not only to form the classifier, but to explicitly represent the shape differences between groups. Differentiating a pre-thresholded, SVM classifying function with respect to shape would seem to yield the answer. The derivative at x is $\sum_k \frac{2}{\gamma}\alpha_k y_k(x_k - x)e^{-||x-x_k||/\gamma}$, where the $\{\alpha_k\}$ are constants determined by the SVM and $\{y_k\}$ are -1 for on group and 1 for the other. Using distance maps this answer is not sufficient. A small change to a distance map does not yield another distance map. Therefore, one must project a derivative back onto the manifold of distance maps [2]. However, displacement fields form a vector space; a small change in a displacement field yields another displacement field. Thus for this case, differentiating the classifier is sufficient for our goals.

3   Results

We formed displacement fields between complexes using a linear elastic model [12]. Figure 1 shows a number of points found to correspond. The hand segmented complexes have notably different structure. The typical member of the data set has a nearly horizontal "tail" like the rightmost two complexes; a few have the tail at an angle (leftmost), or practically no such structure at all (second from the left). Even with the shape differences, in all examples, Point 1 stays slightly above the tip of the head and Point 2 stays on the side of the head. Examining the head of the complexes, some bases are nearly flat and level while others are curved and angled. A review of points near the base also shows that points are approximately in the same position relative to major structures.

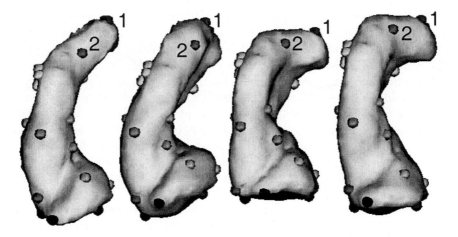

Fig. 1. Surfaces of four matched left complexes; the tail and head are at the top and bottom of the image respectively. To show correspondence across the shapes, points were randomly selected and represented by small spheres on each surface. Points 1 and 2 are referenced in the text.

3.1   Classifier Comparison

We compare the cross validation accuracy of linear and RBF-based [2] classifiers. Table 1 shows the classification accuracy using data normalized to remove relative volume. The table shows that support vector machines generally performed better than linear classifiers by 10 to 20 percentage points. We found this to be the case in all trials, with one exception. When deformation fields were aligned using absolute orientation [13], linear classifiers improved their classifying ability to as high as 70%. (See Section 3.3.)

For individual sides, deformation field-based classifiers perform slightly better than distance map-based classifiers. When considering both sides together, that performance improvement becomes much larger. For comparison to other methods, Table 1 shows results from Gerig et al. [1] who made a classifier comparing

Table 1. A comparison of cross-validation accuracy for RBF and linear classifiers. The data is normalized to the same volume. The range is the 95% confidence interval.

Normalized Structure	Cross Validation Accuracy using Linear Classifier		
	Displacement Field	Distance Map	
Left Complex	$60 \pm 18\%$	$57 \pm 18\%$	
Right Complex	$53 \pm 18\%$	$53 \pm 18\%$	
Both Complexes	$57 \pm 18\%$	$53 \pm 18\%$	
Normalized Structure	Cross Validation Accuracy using RBF		
	Displacement Field	Distance Map	Gerig *et al.*
Left Complex	$67 \pm 18\%$	$70 \pm 17\%$	
Right Complex	$73 \pm 17\%$	$77 \pm 17\%$	
Both Complexes	$80 \pm 16\%$	$67 \pm 18\%$	$73 \pm 17\%$

Table 2. Cross-validation accuracy for the different representations using RBF classifiers. For deformation fields and distance maps, the data is not normalized by volume. For the third column, volume was added separately to shape data [1].

Structure	Cross Validation Accuracy using RBF		
	Displacement Field	Distance Map	Gerig *et al.*
Left Complex	$77 \pm 17\%$	$73 \pm 17\%$	
Right Complex	$77 \pm 17\%$	$70 \pm 17\%$	
Both Complexes	$87 \pm 16\%$	$70 \pm 17\%$	$87 \pm 16\%$

the two sides in each subject using the same data. That classifier's accuracy is in between the two we tested.

3.2   Including Volume

Table 2 examines the effects of not normalizing for volume in the data, using RBFs. Comparing Tables 1 and 2, volume generates improvements for the displacement field based classifier of between 3 and 10 percentage points. For the classifier based on distance maps, volume improves or hurts a classifier, but the effect is roughly 3 percentage points each way. Gerig *et al.* [1] include volume as a separate feature in their classifier; doing so improves the performance of their classifier to the same as the deformation field-based classifier.

3.3   Alignment

We rigidly align shapes so that classifiers are not confused by variations in patient position during imaging. We tried the many alignment methods listed in Section 2. Choosing different alignment methods causes classifiers to have a range of between 3 and 10 percentage points, typically closer to 3%. The worst results are shown in Table 1, 67% accuracy. The best results are 87% achieved in three different ways. Most results are between 70 and 80%. Examining visualization of the differences between the classes as in Section 3.4, the different alignments had small impacts on the differences found between groups.

3.4   Visualization of Differences

An important goal of this study is to visualize differences between the classes. Figure 2 shows those differences, found from derivatives of the classifier evaluated at the examples as described in Section 2. For displacement field based classifiers, we found the gradients to be visually similar evaluated at nearly all the left complexes, and visually similar at nearly all of the right complexes. For distance map based classifiers, the gradients were visually similar across right complexes, but not across left complexes. Figure 2 also shows that for both classifiers, the deformations detected for the two groups are similar in nature but opposite in sign.

In the bottom of Figure 2, the derivatives of the classifier based on deformation fields are shown in the form of a vector field (because distance maps do not use correspondences, it is not possible to show motions tangential to the surface using distance maps). The vector fields show that there is motion along the surface in several places. Most notably, there is a clear rotation of the "tail" of the complex in the image. Conversely, most of the motion in the base is simply compression or expansion. There is also a rotation in the head of the left amygdala, though much smaller in magnitude than the rotation in the tail, and very difficult to see in the image.

4   Discussion

We examined which issues in shape classification have the largest impact on classification accuracy. It is clear from Table 1 that the non-linear RBF-based methods outperform linear classifiers by 10 to 20 percentage points. Volume information (Table 2) consistently improves results the deformation field-based classifier, by 4 to 10 percentage points, as well as the classifier of Gerig et al. [1]. Thus, for this case, including volume information was helpful, but not as helpful as using a non-linear classifier over a linear one. Alignment techniques generally had a smaller effect. Differences between alignment methods generally produced accuracy changes of only a few percentage points.

In this study, displacement fields outperformed distance maps. Classification rates were higher in almost every test performed. Interestingly, Tables 1 and 2 suggest that deformation field-based classifiers were able to find correlations between the deformations on different sides to improve the classification rate, while distance maps-based classifiers were not. Perhaps most importantly, displacement fields provided vector fields in visualizations which added an important tool for visualizing shape differences.

One concern with these results is that the non-linear classifiers created from such small numbers of examples may not generalize to new data. That the classifiers found a qualitatively similar class difference evaluated at many complexes is a good indicator of those classifiers ability to generalize to other data. Also, the observation that in several cases, displacement-field based classifiers worked somewhat well with a simple linear classifier (Section 3.1) may also be such an indication.

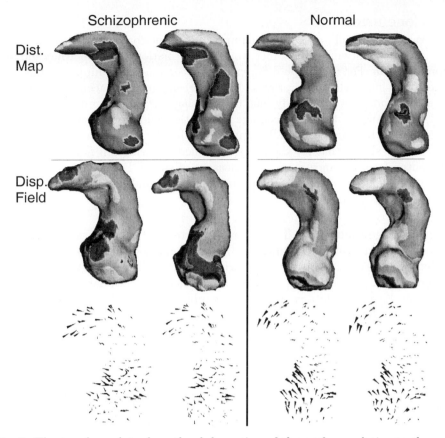

Fig. 2. The top four plots show the deformation of the surfaces relative to the surface normal for the left amygdala-hippocampus complex. For Schizophrenic subjects, "deformation" indicates changes to make the complexes more normal. For Normal subjects, "deformation" indicates changes to make the complexes more diseased. The 2x2 grid of surfaces shows deformations of Schizophrenic/Normal subjects using Distance Maps/Displacement Fields as representations. In each entry in the grid, the two largest deformations evaluated at the support vectors of the SVM classifier are shown; the larger one is on the left. The grayscale is used to indicate the direction and magnitude of the deformation, changing from white (inward) to grey (no motion) to black (outward). The bottom two plots are the deformations fields used to generate the plots directly above them. Note that motion along the surface does not affect the colors in the surfaces. For a color version of this figure, go to *http://www.ai.mit.edu/people/samson/papers/publications.html*

We are also concerned how well these conclusions generalize to other data sets. We believe that non-linear classification methods will almost always outperform linear classification methods. We also believe that the gains due to the inclusion of volume, or various alignment techniques exist, but will be much smaller. When correspondences can be found, correspondence-based methods do provide an advantage over non-correspondence-based methods because they provide additional information for visualizing class differences.

5   Conclusion

We examined several issues that are important for performing shape comparison studies: complexity of the classifier, volume information, alignment method, and representation. For the shape differences between amygdala-hippocampus complexes, non-linear classifiers provide 10-20 percentage point accuracy gains over linear methods. For this study, not normalizing for volume provides a smaller gain, in the range of 4 to 10 percentage points. Using different alignment methods generally produce an even smaller impact on classification accuracy.

We have shown that for the cases examined, deformation field-based classifiers outperform distance maps as a measure of shape. Deformation fields form classifiers of higher accuracy and produce more information for the visualization of shape differences.

Acknowledgements: S.J. Timoner is supported by the Fannie and John Hertz Foundation and NSF ERC grant, J.H.U Agreement #8810274. W. Wells is supported by the same NSF grant and NIH grant 1P41RR13218. P Golland is supported by NSF IIS 9610249 grant and a Martinos Center collaborative research grant. Dr. Shenton's data collection was supported by NIMH grants R01 50740 and K02 01110, and a Veterans Administration Merit Award.

References

1. G. Gerig, M. Styner, et al., "Shape versus size: Improved understanding of the morphology of brain structures," in *MICCAI*, (Utrecht), pp. 24–32, October 2001.
2. P. Golland, W. E. L. Grimson, M. E. Shenton, and R. Kikinis, "Deformation analysis for shape based classification," in *IPMI*, (Davis, CA), pp. 517–530, June 2001.
3. C. Davatzikos, et al., "A computerized approach for morphological analysis of the corpus callosum," *Journal Computer Assisted Tomography*, 20(1):88–97, 1996.
4. A. M. C. Machado and J. C. Gee, "Atlas warping for brain morphometry," in *SPIE Medical Imaging, Image Processing*, pp. 642–651, 1998.
5. M. E. Shenton et al., "Abnormalities in the left temporal lobe and thought disorder in schizophrenia: A quantitative magnetic resonance imaging study," *New England Journal of Medicine*, 327:604–612, 1992.
6. T. F. Cootes et al., "The use of active shape models for locating structures in medical images," *Image and Vision Computing*, 12(6):9–18, 1992.
7. S. Pizer et al., "Segmentation, registration and measurement of shape variation via image object shape," *IEEE Trans. on Medical Imaging*, 18(10):851–865, 1996.
8. G. Christensen, R. Rabbit, and M. Miller, "Deformable templates using large deformation kinematics," *Transactions on Image Processing*, 5(10):1435–1447, 1996.
9. R. H. Davies, T. F. Cootes, and C. J. Taylor, "A minimum description length approach to statistical shape modeling," in *IPMI*, (Davis), pp. 50–63, June 2001.
10. L. Cohen and I. Cohen, "Finite-element methods for active contour models and balloons for 2-d and 3-d images," *PAMI*, 15:1131–1147, November 1993.
11. L. Staib and J. Duncan, "Boundary finding with parametrically deformable models," *PAMI*, 14:1061–1075, November 1992.
12. S. J. Timoner, W. E. L. Grimson, R. Kikinis, and W. M. Wells, "Fast linear elastic matching without landmarks," in *MICCAI*, (Utretcht), pp. 1358–60, October 2001.
13. B. K. P. Horn, "Closed-form solution of absolute orientation using unit quaternions," *Journal of the Optical Socienty of America A*, vol. 4, pp. 629–642, 1987.

Statistical Analysis of Longitudinal MRI Data: Applications for Detection of Disease Activity in MS

Sylvain Prima[1], Nicholas Ayache[2], Andrew Janke[1], Simon J. Francis[1], Douglas L. Arnold[1], and D. Louis Collins[1]

[1] McConnell Brain Imaging Centre, Montreal Neurological Institute
3801 University Street, Montreal, Quebec, Canada
{prima,rotor,simon,doug,louis}@bic.mni.mcgill.ca
[2] INRIA Sophia Antipolis, EPIDAURE Project
2004, route des Lucioles, BP 93, 06902 Sophia Antipolis Cedex, France
ayache@sophia.inria.fr

Abstract. We present a method to detect intensity changes in longitudinal volumetric MRI data from patients with multiple sclerosis (MS). Preprocessing includes spatial and intensity normalization. The intrasubject intensity normalization is achieved using a polynomial least trimmed squares method to match the histograms of all images in the series. Viewing the detection of disease activity in MRI as a *change-point problem*, we present two statistical tests and apply them to a patient's series of grey-level images on a voxel-by-voxel basis. Results are compared with manual lesion segmentation for one MS patient scanned approximately every 5 months for 5 years. Results are also shown for 12 MS patients with 30 monthly scans.

1 Introduction

Motivation: It has been difficult to evaluate the effect of therapy for patients with multiple sclerosis (MS) in clinical trials, since it is a complex disease with a high degree of variability in clinical signs and symptoms that vary over time and between individuals. The most standard clinical tool used to measure impairment and disability in MS is the Expanded Disability Status Scale (EDSS). The EDSS is highly weighted towards motor disability and is notoriously subject to high inter-rater variability [12, 23]. The search for better measures of disease burden has turned to MRI, since it was the first method to allow direct visualization of MS plaques *in vivo*. MRI has had a major impact on the diagnosis [5, 16, 1] and understanding of MS [28, 14]. Perhaps most importantly, MRI has shown that clinical measures (attacks) tend to grossly underestimate disease activity, since new lesions on MRI occur with roughly 10 times the frequency of clinical attacks [10]. Since T_2-weighted lesion volume has been used as a surrogate for disease burden in MS, and new lesions are indicative of disease activity, we have been interested in automated techniques for segmentation of active MS lesions.

T. Dohi and R. Kikinis (Eds.): MICCAI 2002, LNCS 2488, pp. 363–371, 2002.

Previous work: In the image processing literature, much effort has been dedicated to the development of techniques for the automatic segmentation of brain structures and lesions in individual MR scans [32, 11, 27]. For a given patient, a follow-up of this segmented data through time gives an insight into the course of the disease, and allows to monitor its evolution [3]. More specifically, focusing on the evaluation of disease activity, some authors have proposed to use non-rigid matching techniques and deformation field analysis to discriminate static tissues from evolving ones between two consecutive time points [26, 19]. An alternative approach has been proposed by Gerig *et al.*, which takes into account the whole time series simultaneously, with a voxel-by-voxel analysis of the intensity profiles through time [8]. Scalar operators are devised and applied to these profiles, indicating the voxels where significant intensity changes occur, conveying an underlying biological process. Dempster-Shafer's theory is then used to fuse the information brought by each operator, leading to a 3D probability map of evolving regions. More recently, other authors have proposed to detect active lesions using an *a priori* knowledge about the evolution process, and taking into account the neighbourhood of each voxel for better rejection of false positives [29, 18].

Overview of the paper: Following the idea of a voxel-by-voxel analysis of the intensity profiles, and viewing the detection of activity in time series of MR brain images as a *change point problem*, we introduce two statistical tests to discriminate voxels where an actual biological change occurs. One is very generic, whereas the other is more specific, detecting voxels where the intensity significantly *increases* through time. The latter is particularily suited for the follow-up of MS lesions and brain atrophy in T_2-weighted images, since both lesions and ventricles appear brighter than the surrounding brain structures. Before applying these tests, preprocessing of the MRI data is required to make the voxel intensities comparable over time. This includes bias field correction, registration and intensity normalization (Section 2.1). Subsequently, we devise the statistical tests in Section 2.2. In Section 3, we apply the whole analysis procedure to time series of real MR data of MS patients before concluding in Section 4.

2   Methods

2.1   Preprocessing Steps

Before longitudinal statistical analysis of intensity change, each subject-timepoint data volume must be spatially and intensity normalized to ensure that the intensities used in the statistical test come from the same anatomical point and that intensity variations due to imaging artefacts are minimized. There are a number of steps for both spatial and intensity normalization:

Intensity non-uniform correction: Intensity non-uniformity in MR images, or the so-called MR *shading artefact*, is due to a number of causes during the acquisition of the data. If left uncorrected, such an artifact precludes direct comparison of voxel intensities. The intensity artefact can be modelled as a slowly varying multiplicative bias field. We begin preprocessing by applying the

N3 correction algorithm of Sled *et al.* [24] to reduce the effect of this artefact. The N3 algorithm iteratively proceeds by computing the image histogram and estimating a smooth intensity mapping function that tends to sharpen peaks in the histogram.

Intensity normalization: In preparation for registration and subsequent analysis, each image is intensity normalized using a two pass procedure. In order to remove outlier intensity values, the middle 0.1 to 99.9% of the image histogram is mapped to the arbitrary range of 0 to 100, respectively. This procedure eliminates bright voxel values corresponding to blood flow artefacts that reduce the dynamic range of the tissues in the data. The second intensity normalization procedure is described below, after spatial normalization.

Spatial normalization: Each data set is transformed into a standard brain-based coordinate system so that no single data set have a preferred position in processing and so that similar anatomical structures from different data sets are mapped to same spatial position. We have selected the Talairach brain-based coordinate system known as *stereotaxic space* since it has become the defacto standard in the brain mapping community [6,13]. The registration algorithm proceeds with a coarse-to-fine approach by registering subsampled and blurred MRI volumes with an average MRI image, already registered in the stereotaxic coordinate system by optimizing a 9 parameters transform (3 translations, 3 rotations, 3 scalings) [4]. While this procedure is quite robust, we have found that there can be small (sub-millimeter) mis-registrations between the different time-points for a given subject. To address this problem, a second-phase registration is run using the average of all the subject's stereotaxically resampled time-points as a target. The use of the *patient-specific* stereotaxic target reduces the misregistration described above.

Refined intensity normalization: At this point, each data volume has been spatially normalized and an initial intensity normalization has been completed. This first pass intensity normalization is insufficient for comparison between different time points. Actually, even with the same protocol and the same scanner, the intensities within a given brain area are generally different between two acquisitions of the same patient, notably due to drift in receiver coil sensitivity. This is particularily true when the time frequency of the acquisitions is in the range of months or years, as in the case of MS patients. Thus, even though it is classical to assume affine dependence between the intensities of monomodal MR images of the same patient (as often done in registration algorithms [20]), a more complex relationship sometimes holds, making a simple affine mapping of the intensities fail (Figure 1).

Here, we propose to correct the intensities of each image J of the MRI time series with respect to a reference image I: the *patient-specific* stereotaxic target built in the spatial normalization step. As I is the average of all the images of the time series, its signal-to-noise ratio is higher than that of each of the individual MR image used for its computation. Rather than assuming that $J = f(I)$ with f affine ($f = a_1 x + a_0$), we suppose that f is a polynomial of a higher order $d > 1$ ($f = \sum_{k=0}^{d} a_k x^k$) and look for the Least Trimmed Squares (LTS) fit between J

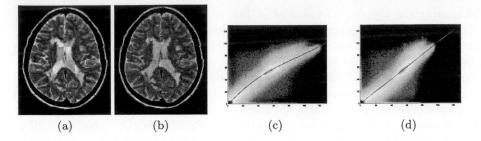

(a)   (b)   (c)   (d)

Fig. 1. Example of intensity normalization using LTS polynomial fitting. (a) Screen-door visualization of two transverse images from two successive time points at the level of the ventricles after the first pass intensity normalization (note the differing intensities in the lateral ventricles). (b) Same images after correction. Note contrast in ventricles is similar, but now the true shape change is evident between the two time points. (c) Joint intensity histogram of the images before correction with the estimated polynomial ($d = 3$). (d) Joint histogram of the two images after correction; it is now close to the line x=y, indicating that the intensities are now matched.

and $f(I)$. This has been previously proposed by Guimond *et al.* for multimodal registration [9]. Routinely, we have found that $d = 3$ yields satisfying results.

The LTS regression [21] is far more robust to outliers than the classical Least Squares (LS) method. This is critical here, where biological changes are likely to occur (lesions and/or brain atrophy); these voxels do not fit the polynomial model and must be eliminated from its computation. No explicit solution exists for the computation of the LTS estimate of f. An iterative scheme described by Rousseeuw and Van Driessen [22] locates a (at least local) minimum of the LTS criterion, which amounts to numerous successive LS regressions (that can be solved by standard matrix algebra) on subsets of the image voxels. An example of the procedure is presented in Figure 1.

2.2   Statistical Analysis

In the following, we note $(x_1, \ldots, x_n)$ the series of values at a given voxel after the whole preprocessing has been completed. Among the operators proposed by Gerig *et al.* [8], some do not relate to the temporal pattern of the data, like the variance, or the difference between extremes values in the time series. Some others do, like those based on the fluctuations around the mean value $\bar{x}$ of the time series: high frequency fluctuations are likely to be noise, whereas low frequency variations probably convey actual biological changes. These operators closely relate to classical statistics such as the number of runs, the length of the longest run, the number of runs up and down, *etc.* The distributions of these statistics under the null hypothesis of no intensity change can be computed exactly [25, 15], leading to a set of statistical tests termed as *randomness tests*, which are often used in cryptography.

Here, we propose an alternative approach, which consists in considering the problem of activity detection as a *change-point problem*. There is an extensive literature about these problems [31], particularily met in the field of quality control. In the following, after stating some reasonable hypotheses about the time series, we show how to derive two simple statistics to test a null hypothesis of "no intensity change" against the alternative of "intensity change".

When there is no biological change underlying the considered voxel (null hypothesis H_0), the fluctuations of its intensity through time only relate to the acquisition noise, that can be supposed to be additive, stationary, spatially white and Gaussian with standard deviation σ, as usually stated. The values x_i can then be seen as realizations of n independent normal random variables X_i with distributions $N(\mu_i, \sigma^2)$, where $\mu_1 = \ldots = \mu_n = \mu$. In this framework, detecting an intensity change amounts to detecting a change in the mean value μ. A simple alternative hypothesis H_1 is to consider that there is only one change in the time series, between time points m and $m + 1$, with m unknown. The problem can then be stated as follows:

- $H_0 : \mu_1 = \ldots = \mu_n$
- $H_1 : \mu_1 = \ldots = \mu_m, \mu_{m+1} = \ldots = \mu_n, 1 \le m \le n - 1, \mu_m \ne \mu_{m+1}$

A natural way to derive a statistic to test H_0 against H_1 is to compute the ratio of the likelihoods of the data under these two hypotheses respectively. Noting f_0 (resp. f_1) the density of $(X_1, \ldots, X_n)$ under the null (resp. the alternative hypothesis), this ratio is:

$$L(X_1, \ldots, X_n) = \frac{f_1(X_1, \ldots, X_n)}{f_0(X_1, \ldots, X_n)}$$

Further modelings of the unknown nuisance parameters m and $\delta = \mu_{m+1} - \mu_m$ (the amount of change) allow to simplify this expression. First, the possible biological change is *a priori* equally likely to happen at any time; we model m as the realization of a discrete random variable with uniform distribution. Second, we model δ as the realization of a normal distribution $N(0, \tau^2)$. If τ is small, it can be demonstrated that L is an increasing function of a statistic S with a very simple expression:

$$S = \sum_{k=1}^{n} \left(\sum_{i=k+1}^{n} (X_i - \bar{X}) \right)^2$$

Under H_0, and up to a multiplicative constant depending on σ, S converges in distribution to the limiting distribution of Smirnov's ω_n^2 criterion [7]. It is then straightforward to build a test for H_0 against H_1 based on S, high values of S indicating a statistically significant change. This statistic S is very generic, and is tailored to detect increasing as well as decreasing intensities. In the case of T_2-weighted MR images of MS patients, the changes in intensities are more likely to be unilateral ($\delta > 0$), since lesions appear brighter than the white matter where they are generally located. In the same way, brain atrophy implies the growing of the ventricles, which appear also brighter than the surrounding white matter. Thus, one could want to test H_0 against the more restrictive hypothesis H_2 defined as:

$- H_2 : \mu_1 = \ldots = \mu_m, \mu_{m+1} = \ldots = \mu_n, 1 \leq m \leq n - 1, \mu_m < \mu_{m+1}$

Still using the ratio of the likelihoods, a more specific and thus statistically more powerful test can be built for the purpose of detecting this unilateral change by modifying the hypotheses on the nuisance parameter δ. Modeling δ as the realization of a semi-normal (instead of normal) distribution, we can derive another statistic T:

$$T = \sum_{k=1}^{n} \sum_{i=k+1}^{n} (X_i - \bar{X})$$

Under H_0 and up to a multiplicative constant depending on σ, T follows a Gaussian law $N(0,1)$. Thus, a statistical test can be built based on T for H_0 against H_2, high values of T indicating a statistically significant increase in intensity [2]. In the preliminary set of experiments described in the next section, we give a qualitative comparison of the two tests based on S and T.

3   Experiments

Data for the first experiment consisted of a T_2-weighted sequence of MR images from a transverse dual-echo, turbo spin-echo sequence (256x256 matrix, 1 signal average, TR/TE1/TE2=2075/32/90 ms, 250mm field of view, 3mm slice thickness). Eleven image volumes over a four year period were acquired of a patient with very active disease. The *patient-specific stereotaxic target (i.e.,* the average of the first phase stereotaxic registration procedure of the 11 volumes) is shown in Fig. 2-a. Lesions were labelled manually in each image volume. A lesion difference map, created by subtracting lesions from time $n - 1$ from n was used to approximate new lesion activity. The sum of the ten difference maps is shown in Fig. 2-d and represents disease activity over the 4 year period. The tests based on the statistics T and S were applied and the results are shown in Fig. 2-b and 2-c, respectively. (Note that while only 2D images are shown, all processing is completed in 3D.)

Data for the second experiment comes from the PRISMS Study Group [17]. This data consists in monthly MRI scanning for 30 months for 12 patients from placebo group. The T_2-weighted data was acquired with parameters similar to those above, but with a 5mm slice thickness and a 0.5mm slice gap. Both T and S tests were run for each subject after prepocessing all data as described above. Fig. 3 shows the result of the statistical test associated with S (*i.e.,* detection of a change in any direction). One can see that there are bright pixels due to lesions, brain atrophy and possible mis-registration. These patients have much less disease activity compared to that of experiment one, as demonstrated by fewer and smaller detected regions.

4   Discussion and Future Work

In this paper, we derive two statistics (one-sided, T and two-sided, S) for testing the hypothesis of no change against the hypothesis of one and only one change at

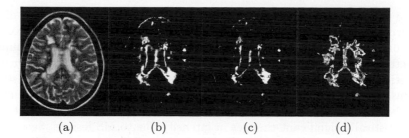

(a)   (b)   (c)   (d)

Fig. 2. Results: (a) Transverse MR image of patient with MS at the level of the lateral ventricles. The image is from the *patient-specific stereotaxic target, i.e.,* the average of all time-points for the patient. We display the results of the test based on the statistic T (b), S (c), and the manual label difference image (d). The one-sided statistic T yields more evolving points than the two-sided statistic S. The power of the test based on T is higher, because most of the observed changes are unilateral (lesions intensities are higher than those of the white matter where they are generally located). Both results are qualitatively similar to that of the manual segmentation of the evolving voxels.

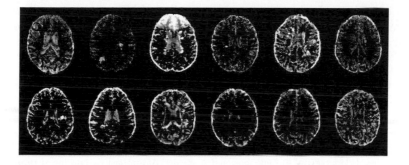

Fig. 3. Results: the images above show transverse slices (z=28mm) through the test result (statistic S) for 12 placebo patients from the PRISMS Study Group [17]. Small focal lesions are apparent in the 3rd, 4rth and 5th images of the first row and in the 1st, 2nd, 3rd and 6th images of the second row. One can also see false positives due to brain atrophy and possible image mis-registration. Note that the bright anterior region in the 3rd image of row 1 is due to a failed image intensity normalization in one of the 30 individual time-points, making these images appropriate for quality control in automated processing.

an unknown point in the time series. For the detection of activity in T_2-weighted images of MS patients, the test based on T is more specific. Other tests could be derived in the same way, to be more specific to the problem which is tackled. The more realistic the alternative hypothesis, the more powerful the corresponding test. In particular, due to the relapsing-remitting course of the disease for most MS patients, tests based on alternative hypotheses including the possibility of more than one change should be statistically more powerful. Non-parametric tests could be also investigated.

We envision four avenues for future work in longitudinal analysis of MRI data from MS patients. First, the statistical tests are applied only on a voxel by voxel basis. While a p-value can be computed from the test results, it must be corrected for multiple comparisons across all voxels of the volume. Bonferroni correction may be too strict; individual voxels are not independent in a statistical sense since their value is likely to depend on their neighbours. We plan to use Gaussian Random Field theory [30] to compute the proper corrections to identify statistically significant changes in intensity due to MS lesions. Second, The tests presented here have been applied to single modality data (*i.e.*, T_2-weighted images only). Since T_2-weighted data is often acquired in a dual echo sequence that also yields registered PD-weighted data, we plan to extend the tests to combine information from multiple modalities. Third, we plan to look into the sensitivity of the one-sided test based on T to detect brain atrophy around the ventricles, where T_2-weighted voxels will change from a medium intensity (tissue) to bright (CSF). Finally, we wish to investigate additional metrics of disease activity. Combination of global or local atrophy metrics with the lesion activity measure described here may result in a better surrogate of disease activity. Such a metric may lead to better understanding of MS pathology and will have important implications for disease prognosis, and monitoring treatment effect in clinical trials.

References

1. F. Barkhof, M. Filippi, D. H. Miller, P. Tofts, L. Kappos, and A. J. Thompson. Strategies for optimizing mri techniques aimed at monitoring disease activity in multiple sclerosis treatment trials. *J Neurol*, 244(2):76–84, Feb 1997.
2. H. Chernoff and S. Zacks. Estimating the current mean of a normal distribution which is subject to changes in time. *Ann. of Math. Stat.*, 35:999–1018, 1964.
3. D. Collins, J. Montagnat, A. Zijdenbos, and A. Evans. Automated Estimation of Brain Volume in Multiple Sclerosis with BICCR. In *IPMI'01*, volume 2082 of *LNCS*, pages 141–147, Davis, USA, June 2001. Springer.
4. D. L. Collins, P. Neelin, T. M. Peters, and A. C. Evans. Automatic 3D inter-subject registration of MR volumetric data in standardized Talairach space. *JCAT*, 18(2):192–205, March/April 1994.
5. F. Fazekas, H. Offenbacher, S. Fuchs, R. Schmidt, K. Niederkorn, S. Horner, and H. Lechner. Criteria for an increased specificity of MRI interpretation in elderly subjects with suspected multiple sclerosis. *Neurology*, 38(12):1822–5, Dec 1988.
6. P. T. Fox, J. S. Perlmutter, and M. E. Raichle. A stereotactic method of anatomical localization for positron emission tomography. *JCAT*, 9(1):141–153, 1985.
7. L. Gardner. On detecting changes in the mean of normal variates. *Ann. Math. Stat.*, 40:116–126, 1969.
8. G. Gerig, D. Welti, C. Guttmann, A. Colchester, and G. Székely. Exploring the discrimination power of the time domain for segmentation and characterization of active lesions in serial MR data. *MedIA*, 4(1):31–42, 2000.
9. A. Guimond, A. Roche, N. Ayache, and J. Meunier. Multimodal Brain Warping Using the Demons Algorithm and Adaptative Intensity Corrections. *IEEE TMI*, 20(1), 2001.
10. C. Isaac, D. K. Li, M. Genton, C. Jardine, E. Grochowski, M. Palmer, L. F. Oger, and D. W. Paty. Multiple sclerosis: A serial study using MRI in relapsing patients. *Neurology*, 38(10):1511–1515, 1988.
11. R. Kikinis, C. Guttmann, D. Metcalf, W. Wells III, G. Ettinger, H. Weiner, and F. Jolesz. Quantitative follow-up of patients with multiple sclerosis using MRI: Technical aspects. *JMRI*, 9(4):519–530, 1999.
12. J. F. Kurtzke. Rating neurologic impairment in multiple sclerosis: An expanded disability status scale. *Neurology*, 33:1444–1452, 1983.
13. J. Mazziotta, A. Toga, A. Evans, P. Fox, and J. Lancaster. A probabilistic atlas of the human brain: theory and rationale for its development. the international consortium for brain mapping. *NeuroImage*, 2(2):89–101, 1995.

14. D. H. Miller, R. I. Grossman, S. C. Reingold, and H. F. McFarland. The role of magnetic resonance techniques in understanding and managing multiple sclerosis. *Brain*, 121(Pt 1):3–24, Jan 1998.
15. A. Mood. The distribution theory of runs. *Ann. Math. Stat.*, 11:367–392, 1940.
16. D. W. Paty. Magnetic resonance imaging in the assessment of disease activity in multiple sclerosis. *Canadian Journal of Neurological Sciences*, 15(3):266–72, Aug 1988.
17. PRISMS-4. Long-term efficacy of interferon-beta-1a in relapsing ms. *Neurology.*, 56(12):1628–1636, 2001.
18. D. Rey, J. Stoeckel, G. Malandain, and N. Ayache. Spatio-temporal Model-based Statistical Approach to Detect Evolving Multiple Sclerosis. In *IEEE Workshop on Mathematical Methods in Biomedical Image Analysis, MMBIA'01*, Kauia, USA, Dec. 2001.
19. D. Rey, G. Subsol, H. Delingette, and N. Ayache. Automatic Detection and Segmentation of Evolving Processes in 3D Medical Images: Application to Multiple Sclerosis. In *IPMI'99*, LNCS, Visegrád, Hungary, June 1999. Springer.
20. A. Roche, G. Malandain, and N. Ayache. Unifying Maximum Likelihood Approaches in Medical Image Registration. *International Journal of Imaging Systems and Technology: Special Issue on 3D Imaging*, 11:71–80, 2000.
21. P. Rousseeuw and A. Leroy. *Robust Regression and Outlier Detection*. Wiley Series in Probability and Mathematical Statistics, 1987.
22. P. Rousseeuw and K. Van Driessen. Computing LTS Regression for Large Data Sets. Technical report, Statistics Group, University of Antwerp, 1999.
23. R. Rudick, A. J, C. Confavreux, G. Cutter, G. Ellison, J. Fischer, F. Lublin, A. Miller, J. Petkau, S. Rao, S. Reingold, K. Syndulko, A. Thompson, J. Wallenberg, B. Weinshenker, and E. Willoughby. Clinical outcomes assessment in multiple sclerosis. *Ann. Neurol.*, 40(3):469–79, Sep 1996.
24. J. G. Sled and G. B. Pike. Standing-wave and rf penetration artifacts caused by elliptic geometry: an electrodynamic analysis of mri. *IEEE TMI*, 17(1):87–97, 1998.
25. W. Stevens. Distributions of groups in a sequence of alternatives. *Ann. Eugen.*, 9:10–17, 1939.
26. J.-P. Thirion and G. Calmon. Deformation Analysis to Detect and Quantify Active Lesions in Three-Dimensional Medical Image Sequences. *IEEE TMI*, 18(5), May 1999.
27. K. Van Leemput, F. Maes, D. Vandermeulen, A. Colchester, and P. Suetens. Automated segmentation of multiple sclerosis lesions by model outlier detection. *IEEE TMI*, 20(8):677–688, Aug. 2001.
28. C. J. Wallace, T. P. Seland, and T. C. Fong. Multiple sclerosis: The impact of MR imaging. *AJR Am. J. Roentgenol.*, 158:849–857, 1992.
29. D. Welti, G. Gerig, E.-W. Radue, L. Kappos, and G. Szekely. Spatio-temporal Segmentation of Active Multiple Scleroris Lesions in Serial MRI Data. In *IPMI'01*, volume 2082 of *LNCS*, pages 438–445, Davis, USA, June 2001. Springer.
30. K. Worsley, S. Marrett, P. Neelin, A. Vandal, K. Friston, and A. Evans. A unified statistical approach for determining significant signals in images of cerebral activation. *Human Brain Mapping*, 4:58–73, 1996.
31. S. Zacks. Survey of classical and Bayesian approaches to the change-point problem: fixed sample and sequential procedures of testing and estimation. In M. Rizvi, J. Rustagi, and D. Siegmund, editors, *Recent advances in statistics, Herman Chernoff Festschrift*, pages 245–269, New York, USA, 1983. Academic Press.
32. A. Zijdenbos, A. Jimenez, and A. Evans. Pipelines: Large scale automatic analysis of 3d brain data sets. In A. Evans, editor, *4th International Conference on Functional Mapping of the Human Brain*, Montreal, June 1998. Organization for Human Brain Mapping. abstract no. 783.

Automatic Brain and Tumor Segmentation

Nathan Moon[1], Elizabeth Bullitt[2], Koen van Leemput[4,5], and Guido Gerig[1,3]

[1] Dept. of Computer Science,
[2] Dept. of Surgery,
[3] Dept. of Psychiatry, University of North Carolina, Chapel Hill, NC 27599, USA
[4] Radiology-ESAT/PSI, University Hospital Gasthuisberg, B-3000 Leuven, Belgium
[5] Department of Radiology, Helsinki University Central Hospital, Helsinki, Finland

Abstract. Combining image segmentation based on statistical classification with a geometric prior has been shown to significantly increase robustness and reproducibility. Using a probabilistic geometric model of sought structures and image registration serves both initialization of probability density functions and definition of spatial constraints. A strong spatial prior, however, prevents segmentation of structures that are not part of the model. In practical applications, we encounter either the presentation of new objects that cannot be modeled with a spatial prior or regional intensity changes of existing structures not explained by the model.
Our driving application is the segmentation of brain tissue and tumors from three-dimensional magnetic resonance imaging (MRI). Our goal is a high-quality segmentation of healthy tissue and a precise delineation of tumor boundaries. We present an extension to an existing expectation maximization (EM) segmentation algorithm that modifies a probabilistic brain atlas with an individual subject's information about tumor location obtained from subtraction of post- and pre-contrast MRI. The new method handles various types of pathology, space-occupying mass tumors and infiltrating changes like edema. Preliminary results on five cases presenting tumor types with very different characteristics demonstrate the potential of the new technique for clinical routine use for planning and monitoring in neurosurgery, radiation oncology, and radiology.

1 Introduction

The segmentation of medical images, as opposed to natural scenes, has the significant advantage that structural and intensity characteristics are well known up to a natural biological variability or the presence of pathology. Most common is pixel- or voxel-based statistical classification using multiparameter images [1, 2]. These methods do not consider global shape and boundary information. Applied to brain tumor segmentation, classification approaches have met with only limited success [3,4] due to overlapping intensity distributions of healthy tissue, tumor, and surrounding edema. Often, lesions or tumors were considered as outliers of a mixture Gaussian model for the global intensity distribution, [5,6], assuming that lesion voxels are distinctly different from normal tissue characteristics. Other approaches involve interactive segmentation tools [7], mathematical

T. Dohi and R. Kikinis (Eds.): MICCAI 2002, LNCS 2488, pp. 372–379, 2002.

morphology [8], or calculation of texture differences between normal and pathological tissue [9].

A geometric prior can be used by atlas-based segmentation, which regards segmentation as a registration problem in which a fully labeled, template MR volume is registered to an unknown dataset. High-dimensional warping results in a one-to-one correspondence between the template and subject images, resulting in a new, automatic segmentation. These methods require elastic registration of images to account for geometrical distortions produced by pathological processes. Such registration remains challenging and is not yet solved for the general case.

Warfield et al. [10, 11] combined elastic atlas registration with statistical classification. Elastic registration of a brain atlas helped to mask the brain from surrounding structures. A further step uses "distance from brain boundary" as an additional feature to improve separation of clusters in multi-dimensional feature space. Initialization of probability density functions still requires a supervised selection of training regions. The core idea, namely to augment statistical classification with spatial information to account for the overlap of distributions in intensity feature space, is part of the new method presented in this paper.

Wells et al. [12] introduced expectation maximization (EM) as an iterative method that interleaves classification with bias field correction.

Leemput et al. [13, 14] developed automatic segmentation of MR images of normal brains by statistical classification, using an atlas prior for initialization and also for geometric constraints. A most recent extension detects brain lesions as outliers [15] and was successfully applied for detection of multiple sclerosis lesions. Brain tumors, however, can't be simply modeled as intensity outliers due to overlapping intensities with normal tissue and/or significant size.

We propose a fully automatic method for segmenting MR images presenting tumor and edema, both mass-effect and infiltrating structures. This method builds on the previously published work done by [13, 14]. Additionally, tumor and edema classes are added to the segmentation. The spatial atlas that is used as a prior in the classification is modified to include prior probabilities for tumor and edema. As with the work done by other groups, we focus on a subset of tumors to make the problem tractable. Our method provides a full classification of brain tissue into white matter, grey matter, cerebrospinal fluid (csf), tumor, and edema. Because the method is fully automatic, its reliability is optimal.

2   Expectation Maximization Segmentation

An algorithm for fully automatic segmentation of normal brain tissue using an expectation maximization (EM) algorithm has been previously developed by [13, 14]. This algorithm interleaves probability density function (pdf) estimation for each tissue class (gray matter, white matter, and csf), classification, and bias field correction using the classic EM approach. The equation for the classification step is

$$p(\Gamma_i = j|y_i, \theta) = \frac{p(y_i|\Gamma_i = j, \theta_j)p(\Gamma_i = j)}{\sum_k p(y_i|\Gamma_i = k, \theta_k)p(\Gamma_i = k)} \tag{1}$$

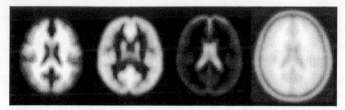

Fig. 1. SPM atlas providing spatial probabilities. From left to right: white matter, gray matter, csf, template T1 image for registration.

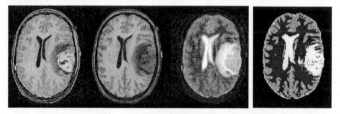

Fig. 2. Left: Registered dataset showing a malignant glioma. From left to right: T1 post-contrast, T1 pre-contrast, T2. The tumor (mostly) enhances with contrast agent in the post-contrast image. Also note the edema surrounding the tumor. Right: Segmentation of dataset using EMS algorithm for healthy brains.

where y_i is the intensity at voxel i, and Γ_i is the class of voxel i.

The EM segmentation algorithm (EMS) uses a spatial atlas from the Statistical Parametric Mapping (SPM) package for initialization and classification. The SPM atlas contains spatial probability information for brain tissues. It was created by averaging segmentations of normal subjects that had been registered by an affine transformation (Fig. 1).

This spatial atlas is registered to the patient data, with an affine transformation, providing spatial prior probabilities for the tissue classes. The pdfs are then initialized based on the atlas probabilities. This allows the algorithm to be fully automatic. The atlas is also used as the prior probability $p(\Gamma_i = j)$ during the classification step (Eq. 1).

3   Application of EMS to Tumors

When a dataset contains a tumor (see Fig. 2 left), there are several problems with the EMS algorithm described in section 2. First, the atlas used does not contain a spatial prior for tumor tissue. The atlas is a normal brain atlas, and cannot be used directly in the presence of pathology. When the atlas is used as a spatial prior for tissue classification, all brain tissue must be classified as one of the available tissue types, either white matter, gray matter, or csf (see Fig. 2 right). Second, tumors are often accompanied by edema, which is a swelling of normal tissue surrounding the tumor, and which changes the tissue properties in that area. The amount and regional extent of edema that accompanies a tumor is variable. Edema or infiltrating phenomena in general are also not explained by the SPM atlas.

As one would expect, making certain assumptions and using prior knowledge can help greatly in the problem of segmenting brain tumors. We make some important simplifying assumptions for our segmentation framework.

Tumor Characteristics: We assume that tumors are ring-enhancing or fully enhancing with contrast agent. The major tumor classes that fall in this category are meningiomas and malignant gliomas. The basic characteristics of *meningiomas* are a) smooth boundaries b) normally space occupying and c) smoothly and fully enhancing with contrast agent. The basic characteristics of *malignant gliomas* are a) ragged boundaries, b) initially only in white matter, possibly later spreading outside white matter, c) only margins enhance with contrast agent, and d) accompanied by edema.

MR Sequences: We assume that all datasets analyzed include a T1 pre-contrast image, a T1 post-contrast image (both with $1 \times 1 \times 1.5mm^3$ voxel dimensions), and a T2 image ($1 \times 1 \times 3mm^3$ voxel dimensions) (Fig. 2). This inter-slice spacing is the standard protocol at the hospitals where our datasets were acquired. All of our data are acquired on Siemens 1.5T and 3T scanners.

4   Extension of the EMS Algorithm

We have extended the EMS algorithm in three significant ways. The first modification is the addition of a tumor class and an edema class. Second, while the original EMS algorithm is not dependent on the number or type of input channels, our algorithm depends on T1 pre- and post-contrast images. The T1 images are necessary because information is extracted from their difference image. The T2 image simply makes the segmentation more robust. The gadolinium enhanced T1 image is not used as a channel for classification but only provides information through the difference image. This strategy is reasonable because, in theory, the gadolinium enhanced T1 image does not provide any extra information in addition to the pre-contrast T1 image except what the difference image provides. Other modalities can be used in addition to the T1 and T2 images. Finally, we modify the spatial atlas to allow for the tumor and edema classes.

Tumor Class: In addition to the three tissue classes assumed in the EMS segmentation (white matter, grey matter, csf), we add a new class for tumor tissue. Whereas the (spatial) prior probabilities for the normal tissue classes are defined by the atlas, the spatial tumor prior is calculated from the T1 pre- and post-contrast difference image. We assume that the (multiplicative) bias field is the same in both the pre- and post-contrast images. Using the log transform of the T1 pre- and post-contrast image intensities then gives a bias-free difference image, since the bias fields (now additive) in the two images cancel out.

Difference Image Histogram: The histogram of the difference image shows a peak around 0, corresponding to noise and subtle misregistration, and a positive response corresponding to contrast enhancement (see Fig. 3 left). We would like to determine a weighting function, essentially a soft threshold, that corresponds to our belief that a voxel is contrast enhanced. We calculate a mixture model fit to the histogram. Two Gaussian distributions are used to model the normal

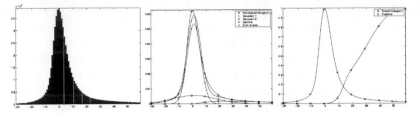

Fig. 3. Left: A T1 pre- and post-contrast difference histogram. Center: The histogram is fit with two Gaussian distributions and a gamma distribution. The gamma distribution represents the enhanced voxels in the post-contrast image. Right: The posterior probability of the gamma distribution (shown along with the scaled histogram) gives the probability that a voxel in the post-contrast image is enhanced. This probability is used to create a spatial prior for tumor tissue.

difference image noise, and a gamma distribution is used to model the enhanced tissue. The means of the Gaussian distributions and the location parameter of the gamma distribution are constrained to be equal (see Fig. 3 center).

Tumor Class Spatial Prior: The posterior probability of the gamma distribution representing contrast enhancement (Fig. 3 right) is used to map the difference image to a spatial prior probability image for tumor. This choice of spatial prior for tumor causes tissue that enhances with contrast to be included in the tumor class, and prevents enhancing tissue from cluttering the normal tissue classes. We also maintain a low base probability (5%) for the tumor class across the whole brain region. In many of the cases we have examined, the tumor voxel intensities are fairly well separated from normal tissue in the T1 pre-contrast and T2 channels. Even when contrast agent only causes partial enhancement in the post-contrast image, the tumor voxels often have similar intensity values in the other two images (see Fig. 2 left). Including a small base probability for the tumor class allows non-enhancing tumor to still be classified as tumor, as long as it is similar to enhancing tumor in the T1 and T2 channels. The normal tissue priors are scaled appropriately to allow for this new tumor prior, so that the probabilities still sum to 1.

Edema Class: We also add a separate class for edema. Unlike tumor structures, there is no spatial prior for the edema. As a consequence, the probability density function for edema cannot be initialized automatically. We approach this problem as follows: First, we have found that edema, when present, is most evident in white matter. Also, we noticed from tests with supervised classification that the edema probability density appears to be roughly between csf and white matter in the T1/T2 intensity space (see Fig. 4). We create an edema class prior that is a fraction of the white matter spatial prior (20%, obtained experimentally). The other atlas priors are scaled to allow for the edema prior, just as for the tumor prior. The edema and the white matter classes share the same region spatially, but are a bimodal probability density composed of white matter and edema.

During initialization of the class parameters in a subject image, we calculate the estimates for gray matter, white matter, csf, tumor and edema using the

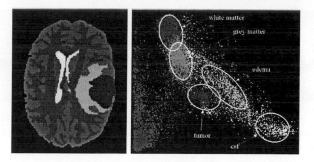

Fig. 4. Feature-space analysis of the T1 and T2 slices from Fig. 2. Left: Segmentation. Right: Scatterplot of the two slices, with colors corresponding to the segmentation. X axis is T2 intensity, Y axis is T1 intensity.

modified atlas prior. Thus, white matter and edema would result in similar probability density functions. The bimodal distribution is then initialized by modifying the mean value for edema to be between white matter and csf, using prior knowledge about properties of edema.

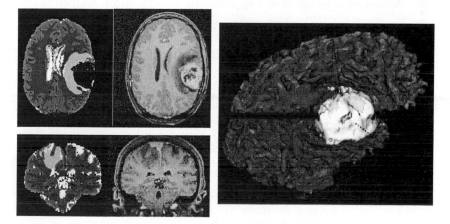

Fig. 5. Left: Two segmented datasets containing malignant glioma (top) and meningioma (bottom), with T1 post-contrast images for reference. Blue = white matter, green = grey matter, yellow = csf, orange = edema, red = tumor. Right: Three-dimensional rendering of segmented tumor (yellow), white matter tissue (red) and surrounding cortical gray matter (light gray).

5   Results

We have applied our tumor segmentation framework to five different datasets, including a wide range of tumor types and sizes. All datasets were registered to the SPM atlas using mutual information registration as described by [16]. Fig. 5 shows results for two datasets. Because the tumor class has a strong spatial prior, many small structures, mainly blood vessels, are classified as tumor because they enhance with contrast. Post-processing is necessary to get a final

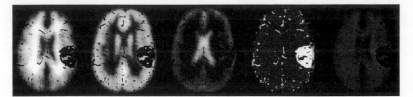

Fig. 6. Spatial prior for the dataset in Fig. 2, created from the SPM atlas and the T1 pre- and post-contrast difference image. From left to right: white matter, grey matter, csf, tumor, edema.

segmentation for the tumor, based on the assumption of large blobs (e.g. using level set evolution [17]). Also note that a small rim around the ventricles is classified as edema, due to partial voluming. This effect would be reduced with higher resolution images. Fig. 6 shows the final spatial priors used for classification of the dataset in Fig. 2 with the additional tumor and edema channels.

6   Conclusions

We have developed a model-based segmentation method for segmenting head MR image datasets with tumors and infiltrating edema. This is achieved by extending the spatial prior of a statistical normal human brain atlas with individual information derived from the patient's dataset. Thus, we combine the statistical geometric prior with image-specific information for both geometry of newly appearing objects, and probability density functions for healthy tissue and pathology. Applications to five tumor patients with variable tumor appearance demonstrated that the procedure can handle large variation of tumor size, interior texture, and locality. The method provides a good quality of healthy tissue structures and of the pathology, a requirement for surgical planning or image-guided surgery (see Fig. 5 right). Thus, it goes beyond previous work that focuses on tumor segmentation only.

Currently, we are testing the validity of the segmentation system in a validation study that compares resulting tumor structures with repeated manual experts' segmentations, both within and between multiple experts. A preliminary machine versus human rater validation showed an average overlap ratio of > 90% and an average MAD (mean average surface distance) of 0.8mm, which is smaller than the original voxel resolution.

In our future work, we will study the issue of deformation of normal anatomy in the presence of space-occupying tumors. Within the range of tumors studied so far, the soft boundaries of the statistical atlas could handle spatial deformation. However, we will develop a scheme for high dimensional warping of multichannel probability data to get an improved match between atlas and patient images.

Acknowledgments

This work was supported by NIH-NCI R01CA67812. We acknowledge KU Leuven for providing the MIRIT image registration package.

References

1. Just, M., Thelen, M.: Tissue characterization with T1, T2, and proton density values: Results in 160 patients with brain tumors. Radiology (1988) 779–785
2. Gerig, G., Martin, J., Kikinis, R., Kubler, O., Shenton, M., Jolesz, F.: Automating segmentation of dual-echo MR head data. In: IPMI. Volume 511. (1991) 175–185
3. Velthuizen, R., Clarke, L., Phuphianich, S., Hall, L., Bensaid, A., Arrington, J., Greenberg, H., Siblinger, M.: Unsupervised measurement of brain tumor volume on MR images. JMRI (1995) 594–605
4. Vinitski, S., Gonzales, C., Mohamed, F., Iwanaga, T., Knobler, R., Khalili, K., Mack, J.: Improved intracranial lesion characterization by tissue segmentation based on a 3D feature map. Mag Re Med (1997) 457–469
5. Kamber, M., Shingal, R., Collins, D., Francis, D., Evans, A.: Model-based, 3-D segmentation of multiple sclerosis lesions in magnetic resonance brain images. IEEE-TMI (1995) 442–453
6. Zijdenbos, A., Forghani, R., Evans, A.: Automatic quantification of MS lesions in 3d MRI brain data sets: Validation of INSECT. In: MICCAI. Volume 1496 of LNCS., Springer (1998) 439–448
7. Vehkomaki, T., Gerig, G., Szekely, G.: A user-guided tool for efficient segmentation of medical image data. In: CVRMED. Volume 1205 of LNCS. (1997) 685–694
8. Gibbs, P., Buckley, D., Blackband, S., Horsman, A.: Tumour volume determination from MR images by morphological segmentation. Phys Med Biol (1996) 2437–2446
9. Kjaer, L., Ring, P., Thomson, C., Henriksen, O.: Texture analysis in quantitative MR imaging: Tissue characterization of normal brain and intracranial tumors at 1.5 T. Acta Radiologic (1995)
10. Warfield, S., Dengler, J., Zaers, J., Guttman, C., Wells, W., Ettinger, G., Hiller, J., Kikinis, R.: Automatic identification of gray matter structures from MRI to improve the segmentation of white matter lesions. Journal of Image Guided Surgery 1 (1995) 326–338
11. Warfield, S., Kaus, M., Jolesz, F., Kikinis, R.: Adaptive template moderated spatially varying statistical classification. In: MICCAI. Volume 1496 of LNCS., Springer (1998) 431–438
12. Wells, W.M., Kikinis, R., Grimson, W.E.L., Jolesz, F.: Adaptive segmentation of MRI data. IEEE TMI 18 (1996) 429–442
13. van Leemput, K., Maes, F., Vandermeulen, D., Suetens, P.: Automated model-based tissue classification of MR images of the brain. IEEE TMI 18 (1999) 897–908
14. van Leemput, K., Maes, F., Vandermeulen, D., Suetens, P.: Automated model-based bias field correction of MR images of the brain. IEEE TMI 18 (1999) 885–896
15. van Leemput, K., Maes, F., Vandermeulen, D., Colchester, A., Suetens, P.: Automated segmentation of multiple sclerosis lesions by model outlier detection. IEEE TMI 20 (2001) 677–688
16. Maes, F., Collignon, A., Vandermeulen, D., Marchal, G., Seutens, P.: Multimodality image registration by maximization of mutual information. IEEE-TMI (1997) 187–198
17. Ho, S., Bullitt, E., Gerig, G.: Level set evolution with region competition: Automatic 3-D segmentation of brain tumors. to appear in Proc. ICPR 2002 (2002)

Atlas-Based Segmentation of Pathological Brains Using a Model of Tumor Growth

M. Bach Cuadra[1], J. Gomez[1], P. Hagmann[1],
C. Pollo[2], J.-G. Villemure[2], B.M. Dawant[3], and J.-Ph. Thiran[1]

[1] Signal Processing Institute (ITS),
Swiss Federal Institute of Technology (EPFL), Lausanne, Switzerland
{Meritxell.Bach,JP.Thiran}@epfl.ch, http://ltswww.epfl.ch/~brain
[2] Department of Neurosurgery,
Lausanne University Hospital (CHUV), Lausanne, Switzerland
[3] Department of Electrical and Computer Engineering,
Vanderbilt University, Nashville, Tennessee, USA

Abstract. We propose a method for brain atlas deformation in presence of large space-occupying tumors or lesions, based on an *a priori* model of lesion growth that assumes radial expansion of the lesion from its central point. Atlas-based methods have been of limited use for segmenting brains that have been drastically altered by the presence of large space-occupying lesions. Our approach involves four steps. First, an affine registration brings the atlas and the patient into global correspondence. Secondly, a local registration warps the atlas onto the patient volume. Then, the seeding of a synthetic tumor into the brain atlas provides a template for the lesion. The last step is the deformation of the seeded atlas, combining a method derived from optical flow principles and a model of lesion growth. Results show that a good registration is performed and that method can be applied to automatic segmentation of structures and substructures in brains with gross deformation, with important medical applications in neurosurgery, radiosurgery and radiotherapy.

1 Introduction

The use of deformable models to segment and project structures from a brain atlas onto a patient's MRI image is a widely used technique. Potential applications for those methods include segmentation of structures and substructures of the patient's brain for radiation therapy or pre-surgical planning.

But when large space-occupying tumors or lesions drastically alter the shape and position of brain structures and substructures, atlas-based methods have been of limited use. The purpose of this work is to deform a brain atlas onto a patient's MRI image in the presence of large space-occupying tumors. Our work is based on the previous works of Dawant, Hartmann and Gadamsetty [1]. In this method a brain atlas is first affinely registered to the patient's image. Then a non-linear deformation is performed in order to bring the atlas and the patient into local correspondence. After that, the brain atlas is "seeded" with a

T. Dohi and R. Kikinis (Eds.): MICCAI 2002, LNCS 2488, pp. 380–387, 2002.

synthetic lesion centered on the centroid of the patient's lesion, and finally the seeded atlas is deformed to completely match the patient image. In our work, instead of relying on the deformation calculation of the non-linear registration algorithm on the whole image, we apply an *a priori* model of tumor growth inside the tumor area, which assumes that the tumor has grown from its centroid in a radial way. As it will be shown, this model allows the placing of a smaller lesion seed (in comparison with [1]) into the brain atlas, therefore, minimizes the amount of atlas information that is masked by the voxels of the tumor seed, and thus improves the quality of the results. As for the validation, we present results obtained on real patient images together with the assessment by an expert. These results show that an atlas registration onto a patient with large space-occupying lesions is well performed even when small lesion seed is placed into the brain atlas.

2   Material and Method

2.1   Data Sets

The patient images have been retrieved from the Surgical Planning Laboratory (SPL) of the Harvard Medical School & NSG Brain Tumor Database [1]. They consist in volumes of 128 coronal slices of 256 x 256 pixels and 0.9375 x 0.9375 x 1.5 mm^3 of voxel size. The digital atlas used in this work also comes from the SPL [2]. It is made of MR data from a single normal subject scanned with high resolution $256 \times 256 \times 160$ volume data set in coronal orientation with $0.9375 \times 0.9375 \times 1.5$ voxel size.

2.2   Seeded Atlas Deformation Method

The approach that we propose is based on the *seeded atlas deformation* (SAD) method presented by Dawant et al.[1]. This method involves the following steps:

 - A nine degrees of freedom transformation is computed to globally register the atlas and the patient volume.
 - A first non-rigid registration is applied. It performs a first atlas deformation to warp the image patient and, since the atlas doesn't have any tumor, nothing happens in the lesion area.
 - The tumor is segmented manually.
 - The intensity inside the tumor contour is highlighted using an intensity level different from that of the surrounding tissues.
 - Successive erosions is applied to the tumor mask (using morphological operations) to create the seed mask. This seed is then placed in the first non-rigidly deformed atlas.
 - A second non-rigid registration is then applied, this time allowing a more elastic deformation.

---

[1] http://spl.bwh.harvard.edu:8000/~warfield/tumorbase/tumorbase.html

The *demons* algorithm of J.-Ph. Thirion is used for the non-rigid registration [3]. For each voxel a displacement vector is found. The regularity of the displacement field is imposed by a Gaussian filtering to regularize the free form deformation. The standard deviation (σ parameter) of the filter is used to change the characteristics of the matching transformation: the larger the sigma, the less elastic the deformation. A deep study on the effect of sigma parameter can be found in [4].

The SAD method leads to good results (as it could be seen in section 3), but it also presents some weak points. Specifically there is an important compromise to be found between the seed size and the elasticity of the model, governed by σ. To obtain a realistic deformation of the brain a large σ has to be chosen but that means not too much deformability of the model [4]. In this case, a relatively big seed must be introduced to obtain a good seed deformation. Therefore a large region of original atlas information has to be masked. Finally, seed deformation is also strongly dependent of the number of iterations of the algorithm (more iterations are needed since large morphological differences still exist). In the next section we detail the method we propose, modifying the work of [1] to improve the robustness of the seeded atlas deformation method.

2.3   Model of Tumor Growth

Our approach introduces a major improvement with respect to the SAD: we introduce an a priori model of tumor growth inside the lesion area, which assumes that the tumor has grown from its centroid in a radial way. This improvement introduces significant advantages. The most important one is that there is no more dependency on the seed size, neither on the elasticity parameter, nor on the number of iterations. Our Model of Tumor Growth (MTG) method is chronologically described in the following subsections.

Affine Transformation. Before performing the non-rigid deformation algorithm, it is necessary to bring the atlas and patient volumes into global correspondence. This is achieved by applying an affine transformation to the brain atlas with the objective of minimizing the Euclidian distance between the atlas cortical surface to the correspondent cortical surface in the target image, as proposed by Cuisenaire, Thiran et al. in [5].

Non-rigid Deformation Algorithm. After the global transformation, a first non-linear registration is performed with the objective of bringing the atlas and the patient volumes in local correspondence. Relying on our previous experience, we also use here the *demons* algorithm proposed by J.-Ph. Thirion [6] [3]. For a detailed description of our algorithmic implementation please refer to [7] [4]. At this point, the non-rigid registration technique is applied between the atlas and the patient with *sigma* = 2.0 as proposed in [1].

Lesion Segmentation. In order to apply the deformation method, a segmentation of the patient's lesion is needed. This segmentation is necessary first for the generation of the synthetic lesion seed and, secondly, for the construction of the model of tumor growth. The automated segmentation algorithm that has been used in this study is the *Adaptive Template Moderated Spatially Varying Statistical Classification (ATM SVC)* algorithm proposed by Warfield, Kaus, Jolesz and Kikinis [8].

Atlas Seeding. After the first two steps of the proposed algorithm the atlas and the patient volumes are in correspondence except in regions that have been drastically deformed by the tumor. Now, the seed mask is generated by eroding the lesion mask. At the points marked by the seed mask, atlas voxels are replaced by patient tumor voxels. This way, a synthetic tumor seed is inserted into the atlas volume. Contrary to [1], neither the seed nor the tumor is highlighted. It should be noted also that the size of the seed, in terms of loss of atlas information, should be as small as possible.

Non-rigid Deformation Using a Model of Tumor Growth. At this point, there is a template of lesion in the brain atlas, and there is an overlap between it and the patient's lesion. The *demons algorithm* is applied outside the lesion area and a model of tumor growth is applied inside. This model consists in assuming a radial growth of the tumor from the tumor seed. The model of tumor growth is implemented in two steps. First, the distance map is calculated to measure the distance from the seed border to the tumor border. So, it indicates how far the voxels inside the tumor region are with respect to the seed. These values will be used as the module of the deformation vector inside the tumor area. Second, the distance map gradient is computed. This gradient will indicate the direction of the shortest path leading to the lesion seed, and it will be used as the direction of the deformation force inside the tumor area. Note that radial term is not use here in terms of a direction normal to the contour but as the shortest path. Therefore, the formal expression of the displacement vector at every voxel inside the tumor area is

$$\overrightarrow{v}_{lesion} = -\frac{D_{seed} \cdot \overrightarrow{\nabla} D_{seed}}{N_{iterations}}, \tag{1}$$

where D_{seed} is the distance map computed from the seed border to the outside of the seed, and $N_{iterations}$ is the number of iterations of the deformation algorithm that have to be performed. So, a displacement vector is computed at every voxel using either the demons algorithm or the tumor growth algorithm. Then, the entire field is regularized with $\sigma = 1$ to avoid possible discontinuities. By using the model of lesion growth, dependence on the number of iterations of the non-rigid deformation algorithm is eliminated (see Eq. 1).

3   Results and Validation

3.1   Deformed Atlas Images and Deformation Field

The algorithm has been tested and validated on 6 different patients having either meningioma or low grade glioma. Because of limited space we present here just one case. The initial images (patient and seeded atlas) and the resulting deformed atlas for a patient with left parasellar meningioma are shown in Fig. 1. The performance of our method (MTG) and the *seeded atlas deformation* (SAD) method are compared for two different sizes of the tumor seed that is inserted into the brain atlas. Lesion segmentation results (see Fig. 1(a)) have been obtained by applying the *ATM SVC* algorithm with $k = 7$ for the k-NN classification, and using 100 prototypes for each one of the classes. Two lesion contours are shown in Fig. 1(b): the red one corresponds to an expert manual segmentation and green one to the ATM SVC segmentation. Patient's tumor size is 41.25x42.1875x52.5 mm^3. The biggest seed has size 16.875x16.875x24.0 mm^3 and the smallest has size 10.3125x10.3125x12.0 mm^3 (Fig. 1(c)) and Fig. 1(d)). As the results show, the SAD method achieves results that are comparable to those of our method, when using the big seed (note that norm of deformation field is almost the same for both methods, see Fig. 1(i) and 1(j)). But when using the small one, for the SAD method, the deformation inside the tumor area does not reach the target while the method using the model of tumor growth (MTG) does (Fig. 1(g) and 1(h)). In the SAD method, the force on the lesion contour is actually misguided. It should also be noted that the MTG method performs in a very similar way for both seed sizes (compare Fig. 1(j) and Fig. 1(l)). This different behavior can be explained as follows. While the SAD method relies on the intensity gradient for the deformation inside the tumor area, the MTG method uses a model that applies the deformation independently from the intensity gradient and using only *a priori* information (i.e. a model of tumor growth). In the first case, there is a strong gradient on the tumor and seed contour due to the highlighting. But between them, just the atlas gradient is used to lead the direction of the deformation inside tumor area. This gradient information is not enough when using a small seed since a large deformation is need. That explains the dependency of SAD method on the seed size and iteration number. On the contrary, MTG can compensate these large differences thanks to the growing model.

3.2   Segmentation Results Study

In this section, structures and substructures from the deformed brain atlas have been projected to the patient's image. The seed has deformed onto the lesion mask with a voxel overlapping of 91%. The structures that were initially inside the region area have been pushed out of the lesion contour (see Fig. 2(a) and (b)). We can see in Fig. 2(c) that these structures not always reach perfectly their target. Actually, there is a little imprecision due to the regularization step. The use of a regularization parameter such as $\sigma = 1.0$ can cause some misguiding in the lesion contour because of the interaction between deformation field

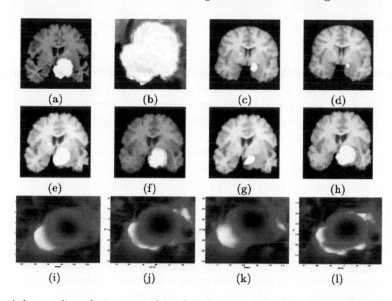

Fig. 1. Atlas seeding, lesion growth and deformation field analysis. (a) Patient with left parasellar meningioma. (c) Warped atlas, big seed. (d) Warped atlas, small seed. (e) Deformation of seeded atlas with the big seed using SAD. (f) Deformation of seeded atlas with the big seed using MTG. (g) Deformation of seeded atlas with the small seed using SAD. (h) Deformation of seeded atlas with the small seed using MTG. (i) SAD: deformation module using a big seed. (j) MTG: deformation module using a big seed. (k) SAD: deformation module using a small seed. (l) MTG: deformation module using a small seed. NOTE: highest module deformation corresponds to white and yellow areas.

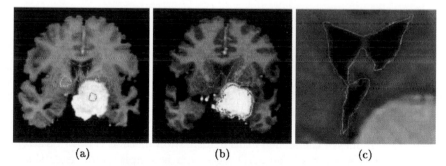

Fig. 2. Segmentation analysis: model of lesion growth method applied to small seed. (a) Initial structures: ventricles and globus pallidus are inside lesion area. (b) Lesion, ventricles and central nuclei resulting segmentation contours are superposed to patient image. One colour segmentation contour for each initial seed position. (b) Zoom of the ventricules.

inside and outside lesion area. So we have to consider that we have a significant contribution of the radial force outside and in the lesion contour since we are filtering the total deformation field. It might be possible that the lesion area pulls in some way the rest of the structures to the seed position. Another important point to consider is how sensible the final result is with respect to the initial seed position. We have no *a priori* knowledge about lesion size or position. Actually, for some kinds of lesions such as the meningioma it would be more realistic from a biomedical point of view to consider a seed placed at the external border of the tumor since this kind of lesions starts at the dura mater (in brain surface) instead of a central seed growing. We present the segmentation results obtained from different initial seed positions in Fig. 2. Lesion, ventricles and central nuclei system have been considered. Variation have been performed with seed translations from 4mm to 9mm in the three main directions and calculations have been done in a region of interest of 3cm around the tumor. Quantitative measures such as the maximum displacement, the mean and variance of the vector field norm are shown in Table 1. For all displacements the mean transformation field remains approximately the same. The mean overlap of all contours is about 90% voxels. Validation has been done visually by an expert c onsidering segmentation contours superposed on the original patient image (C.P.).

Table 1. Variability study with small seed. All values are in millimeters and per voxel. Maximum value, mean and variance of the vector field norm are shown.

Displacement	center	+4X	-4X	-6X	+4Y	-4Y	+6Y	+6Z	-6Z	-9Z
Max	19.18	16.83	21.62	22.83	20.59	19.56	22.61	18.05	23.32	19.63
Mean	4.17	3.75	3.80	3.96	3.79	3.76	3.93	3.71	4.01	3.89
Variance	8.16	9.41	10.7	12.58	9.98	10.67	11.65	9.53	13.44	11.89

4   Discussion

The work presented here is not the first attempt at atlas-based segmentation when large occupying tumors exists. We are of course referring to [1] but also to [9]. We completely agree with [1] in the idea that lack of an explicit underlying mathematical model in the seeded atlas deformation method is both its strength and its potential weakness. The SAD algorithm is simpler and faster than [9]. But this simplicity (the consistency of the deformation field relies only in the regularization parameter) is at the same moment the weak point since the size of the smoothing filter becomes a critical choice to get good results or not. The method we propose tries to increase the robustness of the SAD method, leading to an algorithm that is largely independent to the seed size and to the number of iterations and, the most important, much less sensitive to the regularization parameter. Of course the use a such a simple model of tumor growth can be questionable. Even if no study clearly discuss this, it is reasonable to believe that some lesions grow radially if they have no constraint (bone, dura circumvolution, etc.) Meningioma, low grade glioma, but also metastasis or abscesses, can follow this model when they produce brain deformation.

5   Conclusion

We proposed a new approach for brain atlas deformation in the presence of large space-occupying tumors, which makes use of a simple model of tumor growth. The use of an *a priori* model for the brain atlas deformation inside the tumor area enables a good matching, even when brain structures have been drastically altered by the presence of a tumor. Results show that our method overcomes the limitation such as the "seed" size dependence and convergence to the target that the most similar article in the literature had. Finally, the model of lesion growth method improves the robustness of the seeded atlas deformation method since it is not so sensitive to the choice of the regularization parameter.

Acknowledgement

This work is supported by the Swiss National Science Foundation grants numbers 21-55580-98 and 20-64947.01.

References

1. Dawant, B.M., Hartmann, S.L., Gadamsetty, S.: Brain Atlas Deformation in the Presence of Large Space-occupying Tumors. In: MICCAI. (1999) 589–596
2. Kikinis, R., et al.: A digital brain atlas for surgical planning, model driven segmentation and teaching. IEEE Transactions on Visualization and Computer Graphics **2** (1996) http://splweb.bwh.harvard.edu:8000.
3. Thirion, J.P.: Image matching as a diffusion process: an analogy with Maxwell's demons. Medical Image Analysis **2** (1998) 243–260
4. Bach, M., et al: Atlas-based Segmentation of Pathological Brains using a Model of Tumor Growth. Technical report, ITS-EPFL (2002)
   http://ltswww.epflch/~brain/publications/meri/techreports/report.ps.gz.
5. Cuisenaire, O., Thiran, J.P., Macq, B., Michel, C., Volder, A.D., Marques, F.: Automatic Registration of 3D MR images with a Computerized Brain Atlas. In: SPIE Medical Imaging. Volume 1719. (1996) 438–449
6. Thirion, J.P.: Fast Non-Rigid Matching of 3D Medical Images. Technical Report 2547, INRIA (1995)
7. Bach, M., Cuisenaire, O., Meuli, R., Thiran, J.P.: Automatic segmentation of internal structures of the brain in MRI using a tandem of affine and non-rigid registration of an anatomical atlas. In: ICIP. (2001)
8. Warfield, S.K., Kaus, M., Jolesz, F.A., Kikinis, R.: Adaptive, Template Moderated, Spatially Varying Statistical Classification. Medical Image Analysis **4** (2000) 43–55
9. Kyriacou, S., Davatzikos, C.: Nonlinear elastic registration of brain images with tumor pathology using a biomechanical model. IEEE Trans. Med. Imaging **18** (1999) 580–592

Recognizing Deviations from Normalcy
for Brain Tumor Segmentation

David T. Gering[1], W. Eric L. Grimson[1], and R. Kikinis[2]

[1] Artificial Intelligence Laboratory, Massachusetts Institute of Technology,
Cambridge, MA, 02139 USA
{gering,welg}@ai.mit.edu
http://www.ai.mit.edu/people/gering
[2] Brigham and Women's Hospital, Harvard Medical School, Boston MA, USA
kikins@bwh.harvard.edu

Abstract. A framework is proposed for the segmentation of brain tumors from MRI. Instead of training on pathology, the proposed method trains exclusively on healthy tissue. The algorithm attempts to recognize deviations from normalcy in order to compute a fitness map over the image associated with the presence of pathology. The resulting fitness map may then be used by conventional image segmentation techniques for honing in on boundary delineation. Such an approach is applicable to structures that are too irregular, in both shape and texture, to permit construction of comprehensive training sets. The technique is an extension of EM segmentation that considers information on five layers: voxel intensities, neighborhood coherence, intra-structure properties, inter-structure relationships, and user input. Information flows between the layers via multi-level Markov random fields and Bayesian classification. A simple instantiation of the framework has been implemented to perform preliminary experiments on synthetic and MRI data.

1 Introduction

The literature is rich with techniques for segmenting healthy brains – a task simplified by the predictable appearance, size, and shape of healthy structures. Many of these methods fail in the presence of pathology – the very focus of segmentation for image-guided surgery [1]. Furthermore, the techniques that are intended for tumors leave significant room for increased automation and applicability. Specifically, we consider the task of segmenting large brain tumors such as gliomas, meningiomas, astrocytomas, glioblastoma multiforme, cavernomas, and Arteriovenous Malformations (AVM). In practice, segmentation of this class of tumors continues to rely on manual tracing and low-level computer vision tools such as thresholds, morphological operations, and connective component analysis. Automatic techniques tend to be either region- or contour-based.

Region-based methods usually reduce operator interaction by automating some aspects of applying the low-level operations [2]. Threshold selection can be assisted through histogram analysis, and logic can be applied to the application of low-level vision techniques through a set of rules to form a knowledge-based system [3]. Since

T. Dohi and R. Kikinis (Eds.): MICCAI 2002, LNCS 2488, pp. 388–395, 2002.
© Springer-Verlag Berlin Heidelberg 2002

statistical classification alone may not allow differentiation between non-enhancing tumor and normal tissue, anatomic information derived from a digital atlas has been used to identify normal anatomic structures. Of these approaches, the most successful has been the iteration of statistical classification and template matching as developed in [4,5,6]. However, the use of morphological operations has the drawback of making assumptions about the radius parameter that are both application-dependent (anatomy) and scan-dependent (voxel size). Such operations destroy fine details and commit to irreversible decisions at too low of a level to benefit from all available information – thus violating Marr's principle of least commitment.

Contour-based methods evolve a curve based on internal forces (e.g.: curvature) and external forces (e.g.: image gradients) to delineate the boundary of a tumor. Since they experience similar drawbacks as the region-based approaches, they tend to apply only to tumors that are easily separable from their surroundings [7,8]. Level-set based curve evolution [9, 10] has the advantage over region-based approaches in that the connectivity constraint is imposed implicitly rather than through morphological operations. However, 3D level-sets find limited use in medical practice due to their reliance on the operator to set the sensitive parameters that govern the evolution's stopping criteria. The more heterogeneous the tumor, the more user interaction is required.

Both region- and contour-based segmentation methods have largely ignored the bias field, or patient-specific, signal inhomogeneities present in MRI. The bias field is slowly varying, and therefore its computation from the regions of healthy tissue could be extrapolated over tumor tissue to provide some degree of benefit. Methods for segmenting healthy brains have incorporated the EM algorithm [11] to simultaneously arrive at both a bias field and segmentation into healthy tissue classes [12]. There have been several extensions, such as collecting all non-brain tissue into a single class [13], handling thermal noise with a Markov random field [14], using a mean-field solution to the Markov random field [15], incorporating geometric constraints [15], using a digital brain atlas as a spatially-varying prior [16], automating the determination of the tissue class parameters [17], and identifying MS lesions as hyper-intense outliers from white matter [18].

In contrast to existing methods for tumor segmentation, the hypothesis underlying our work is that we can segment brain tumors by focusing not on what typically represents tumor, but on what typically represents healthy tissue. Our method extends EM-based segmentation to compute a fitness map over the image to be associated with the probability of pathology. In this paper, we present our proposed framework and the preliminary results that we achieved with a simple implementation. We hope that more detailed, future implementations of this framework will be able to address many of the drawbacks to the existing region- and contour-based methods.

2   Method

Inherent ambiguity necessitates the incorporation of contextual information into the brain segmentation process. Consider the example of non-enhancing tumor tissue that garners the same intensity classification of healthy gray matter, but is too thick to be gray matter. An algorithm's low-level computer vision techniques could first classify the tissue as gray matter, and a higher-level stage – through its broader understanding of context – could correct the classifications of the first-pass. This example motivates the introduction of hierarchical context into the segmentation process. A voxel's classification could be considered on several levels: the voxel itself, the voxel's immediate (Markov) neighborhood, the voxel's region (entire connected structure), the global setting (position of the voxel's structure relative to other structures), and user guidance. Just as a voxel-wise classification must be computed prior to a neighborhood-wise refinement, a voxel's region must be classified before features regarding the size and shape (or other intrinsic properties) of that region can be computed.

One way to approach the above example would be to employ a combination of morphological operations and a high-level expert system (such as [3]) to simultaneously switch the classification of every voxel in the mistaken connected mass from gray matter to tumor. However, in keeping with our goal of adhering to the principle of least commitment, we propose an alternative approach where voxels toward the center of the mass could be first classified as tumor based on their unusually high distance from their structure's boundary. This tumor classification would subsequently flow outward throughout the mass over several iterations in a *probabilistic flow*. The flow is driven by our introduction of novel multi-layer Markov random fields. A given voxel would change its high-level classification in the evolving presence of tumor if the attributes of lower-level layers shared strong similarities.

Table 1. The Layered Vision framework features no decisions made by certain layers that permanently (and perhaps adversely) affect other layers. Information flows between the layers (bidirectionally depending on implementation details) while converging toward a solution

#	Layer	Definition	Computation
5	User *(oracle)*	Spatially specific points clicked on by the user either at initialization, or on the fly between iterations as a corrective action.	Quickly and crudely drawn line during initialization.
4	Inter-structure *(global)*	Relative position of a voxel's structure to other structures.	Distance from scalp
3	Intra-structure *(region)*	Relative position of a voxel within its own structure.	Distance from boundary.
2	Neighborhood *(local)*	Classification of a voxel's immediate neighbors.	Mean Field MRF
1	Voxel *(point)*	Classification based on voxel's intensity.	EM, ML or MAP

2.1   Layer 1: EM Segmentation

EM segmentation models the image intensities as visible variables, Y, tissue classifications as hidden variables, Γ, and the bias field as governed by model parameters, β. We would like to choose the parameters that maximize the log likelihood of the data, log $p(Y, \Gamma | \beta)$, but we do not know this likelihood because Γ's invisibility renders $p(Y, \Gamma | \beta)$ to be a random variable. Thus, although we cannot maximize it, we can *maximize* its *expectation*. This results in the following two iterative steps until convergence to a local minimum. In our implementation, we followed [12].

E-Step: Compute the expectation $\Sigma_\Gamma p(\Gamma|Y,\beta)\log p(\Gamma,Y|\beta)$ using the current β.

M-Step: Find new $\beta^{(t+1)}$ to maximize the expectation, assuming $p(\Gamma|Y,\beta^t)$ is correct.

2.2   Layer 2: Spatial Coherence with Markov Random Field

Following [15], the prior knowledge of spatial coherence over a configuration, W, of segmented voxels is modeled with a Gibbs distribution, P(W). The energy function, U(W) is an Ising model generalized to the case of discrete, multi-valued labels [19]:

$$P(W) = \frac{\exp(-U(W))}{\sum_{W'} \exp(-U(W'))} \tag{1}$$

Given M possible label values, let W_s be an M-length binary vector of classification at the voxel indexed by s. Let N_s be the set of voxels in the neighborhood of s (which, in our case, are the 6 closest voxels in 3D). Let the superscripts refer to the layer of processing from Table 1.

$$U^2(W) = V_1(W_s^2) + \sum_{n \in N_s} V_2(W_s^2, W_n^2) \tag{2}$$

Then V_1 is the clique potential of all cliques of size 1. In other words, V_1 encodes our prior knowledge about an isolated voxel prior to viewing the image data (the tissue class prior probability). V_2 is the potential over all cliques of size 2, and represents the tendency of two classified voxels to be neighbors. That tendency is encoded in the MxM Class Interaction Matrix, J^2, and is computed from a segmented scan offered as training data.

$$V_1(W_s^2) = -\sum_{s \in S} p(\Gamma)W_s^2 \tag{3}$$

$$V_2(W_s^2) = -\sum_{s \in S} \sum_{n \in N_s} (W_s^2)^T J^2 W_n^2 \tag{4}$$

For tractable computation, our implementation follows the Mean-Field approximation as derived in [15]. Thus, Layer 2 effectively relaxes Layer 1's E-Step weights.

2.3   Layer 3: Region Properties Propagated with a Multi-level MRF

We now derive our simple implementation of Layer 3 where the feature computed over the output of Layer 2 is the radius to each structure's own boundary. The per-class probability distributions, $p(r|\Gamma)$ are readily computed from a sample segmented scan presented as training data. We perform a Maximum A Posteriori (MAP) classification of the features (just radius at present) computed over Layer 2's output. Recall that the EM algorithm of Layer 1 must compute $p(\Gamma|Y,\beta)$ at each E-Step. It can be shown that $p(\Gamma|Y,\beta,r)$ can be computed with the same update equation except for an extra multiplicative term, $p(r|\Gamma)$. Therefore, the posterior probabilities for the Layer 3 MAP classification are equal to the relaxed weights of Layer 2 multiplied by this new likelihood. That is, the Layer 2 weights provide the spatially varying prior for the Layer 3 MAP classification.

Next, we desire the MAP result (corrections to Layer 2's classifications) to propagate over regions that are homogenous at Layer 2, as demonstrated in Figure 2. We introduce a multi-level Markov random field, and define the Gibb's energy function to encode our prior knowledge of its behavior. Compare equations 5-7 with their Layer 2 counterparts:

$$U^3(W) = V_1(W_s^2, W_s^3) + \sum_{n \in N_s} V_2(W_s^2, W_s^3, W_n^2, W_n^3) \tag{5}$$

$$V_1(W_s^2, W_s^3) = -\sum_{s \in S} \overline{W}_s^2 W_s^3 \tag{6}$$

$$V_2(W_s^2, W_s^3, W_n^2, W_n^3) = -\sum_{s \in S} \sum_{n \in N_s} (W_s^3)^T J^3 \overline{W}_n^2 \tag{7}$$

The MxM square similarity matrix, J^3 is chosen to drive voxels classified to structures with large radii to propagate over voxels associated with structures with small radii. The bar over W denotes the Mean Field approximation, thus a vector of probabilities.

2.4   Layer 4: Global, Inter-structure Relationships

Broader context regarding relationships between structures can be incorporated in several ways. The stationary prior used in the calculation of the posterior probabilities by Layer 1 can be replaced by a spatially varying prior. [15] uses joint distances from ventricles and skin, while [16-18] use a rigidly registered digital atlas. Another approach, experimented with in Figure 1, is to associate a probability distribution in a similar manner as the distance to structure boundaries in Layer 3.

2.5   Layer 5: User Interaction

User time (such as in [6]) can be spent either initializing the segmentation, or correcting it to resolve ambiguities reached by the algorithm. Moreover, very small tumors in early stages of growth may require input from the 5th Layer (oracle) to disambiguate them from their surroundings. For our initial experiments, we have used Layer 5 for quick initialization of the Gaussian models for healthy tissue classes.

2.6   Expressing Tumors as Deviations from Normalcy

While the algorithm employs models of healthy tissue classes, pathology is only modeled by its deviation from normalcy. The degree to which each voxel belongs is its minimum class distance expressed in standard deviations, which is commonly known as the Mahalanobis-distance. Besides providing the basis for the fitness map, this computation also weights the evaluation of the bias field in Layer 1.

$$\min_{\Gamma} \sqrt{\frac{(I - \mu_\Gamma)^2}{\sigma_\Gamma^2}} \tag{8}$$

3   Preliminary Experiments

Figure 1 depicts results of determining outliers with respect to each layer separately, and in total combination. Observe that a single layer is insufficient for recognition. Figure 2 explores a "toy" example to clearly illustrate the effects of layered vision.

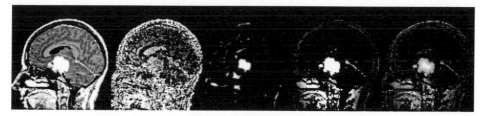

Fig. 1. From left to right: Input MRI, Map of outliers based on intensity only, Map of outliers based on structure size only, Map of outliers based on relative position only, Combined map of outliers based on voxel intensity, structural size, and relative position to other structures. (Note: neck structures become removed upon rigid registration to a digital atlas)

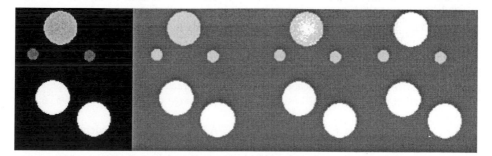

Fig. 2. The "toy" volume consists of 2 small, dark spheres and 2 large bright ones corrupted with Gaussian noise. The top, somewhat dark, and large sphere is ambiguous, and it is classified incorrectly by the lower-level layers of MAP and MRF. The 3rd layer then identifies that the center voxels are too distant from the boundary, and corrects their classification. The multi-level MRF propagates this information across the structure because its lower-level segmentation is mostly homogenous. From left to right: Original, Result after Layer 2, Result after 15 iterations of Layer 3's multi-level MRF, Result after 50 iterations of Layer 3's multi-level MRF

4   Discussion

The contributions of this paper are two-fold. First, we proposed segmenting large brain tumors by training exclusively on healthy brains to recognize deviations from normalcy. Second, we designed a framework for layered vision that incorporates context at various levels. We extended EM-based segmentation with region-level properties, and we derived the novel multi-level MRF. While preliminary experiments are encouraging, there is future development to be performed before a clinical validation can be run. For example, Layer 3 is sensitive to noise in the lower layers, which is why the algorithm depends on the MRF relaxation of Layer 2. Additionally, voxels that contain tissue belonging to more than one tissue class display an intensity value along the linear combination of the classes' distributions. While partial volume artifacts always present somewhat of an obstacle to segmentation, their effect becomes much more pronounced in our algorithm because the entire interface between structures incorrectly appears abnormal. We believe these issues can be solved, and that this approach, in general, represents a step in a new direction towards automated tumor segmentation.

References

1. D. Gering, A. Nabavi, R. Kikinis, N. Hata, L. Odonnell, W. Eric L. Grimson, F. Jolesz, P. Black, W. Wells III. "An Integrated Visualization System for Surgical Planning and Guidance Using Image Fusion and an Open MR". *Journal of Magnetic Resonance Imaging* June 2001; 13:967-975.
2. B.N. Joe, M.B. Fukui, C.C. Meltzer, Q. Huang, R.S. Day, P.J. Greer, M.E. Bozik. "Brain Tumor Volume Measurement: Comparison of Manual and Semiautomated Methods". *Radiology* 1999; 212:811-816.
3. M.C. Clark, L.O. Hall, D.B. Goldgof, R. Velthuizen, F.R. Murtagh, M.S. Silbiger. "Automatic Tumor Segmentation Using Knowledge-Based Techniques". *IEEE Transactions on Medical Imaging* April 1998; 17:238-251.
4. S. Warfield, J. Dengler, J. Zaers, C.R.G. Guttmann, W.M. Wells III, G.J. Ettinger, J. Hiller, R. Kikinis. "Automatic Identification of Grey Matter Structures from MRI to Improve the Segmentation of White Matter Lesions". *Journal of Image Guided Surgery* 1995; 6:326-338.
5. S.K. Warfield, M. Kaus, F.A. Jolesz, R. Kikinis. "Adaptive, Template Moderated, Spatially Varying Statistical Classification". *Medical Image Analysis* October 2000; 4:43-55.
6. M.R. Kaus, S.K. Warfield, A. Nabavi, P.M. Black, F.A. Jolesz, R. Kikinis. "Automated Segmentation of MR Images of Brain Tumors". *Radiology* 2001; 218:586-591.
7. Y. Zhu, H. Yan. "Computerized Tumor Boundary Detection Using a Hopfield Neural Network". *IEEE Transactions on Medical Imaging* February 1997; 16:55-67.
8. A.X. Falcao, J.K. Udupa, S. Samarasekera, S. Sharma. "User-Steered Image Segmentation Paradigms: Live Wire and Live Lane". *Graphical Models and Image Processing* 1998; 60:233-260.

9. Yezzi, S. Kichenassaym, A. Kumar, P. Olver, A. Tannenbaum. "A Geometric Snake Model for Segmentation of Medical Imagery". *IEEE Transactions on Medical Imaging* April 1997; 16:199-209.
10. S. Kichenassamy, A. Kumar, P. Olver, A. Tannenbaum, A. Yezzi. "Gradient Flows and Geometric Active Contour Models". In: *International Conference on Computer Vision*. Boston: ; 810-815.
11. A.P. Dempster, N.M. Laird, D.B. Rubin. "Maximum Likelihood from Incomplete Data via the EM Algorithm". *Journal Royal Statistical Society* 1977; 39:1-38.
12. W.M. Wells III, W.E.L. Grimson, R. Kikinis, F.A. Jolesz. "Adaptive Segmentation of MRI Data". *IEEE Transactions on Medical Imaging* 1996; 15(4):429-443.
13. R. Guillemaud, M. Brady. "Estimating the Bias Field of MR Images". *IEEE Transactions on Medical Imaging* June 1997; 16:238-251.
14. K. Held, E.R. Kops, B.J. Krause, W.M. Wells III, R. Kikinis, H.-W. Muller-Gartner. "Markov Random Field Segmentation of Brain MR Images". *IEEE Transactions on Medical Imaging* December 1997; 16:878-886.
15. T. Kapur. "Model Based Three Dimensional Medical Image Segmentation". Ph.D. Thesis, Massachusetts Institute of Technology, 1999.
16. K.V. Leemput, F. Maes, D. Vandermeulen, P. Suetens. "Automated Model-Based Bias Field Correction of MR Images of the Brain". *IEEE Transactions on Medical Imaging* October 1999; 18:885-896.
17. K.V. Leemput, F. Maes, D. Vandermeulen, P. Suetens. "Automated Model-Based Tissue Classification of MR Images of the Brain". *IEEE Transactions on Medical Imaging* October 1999; 18:897-908.
18. K.V. Leemput, F. Maes, D. Vandermeulen, P. Suetens. "Automated Segmentation of Multiple Sclerosis Lesions by Model Outlier Detection". *IEEE Transactions on Medical Imaging* August 2001; 20:677-688.
19. S.Z.Li. *Markov Random Field Modeling in Image Analysis.* Springer-Verlag, 2001.

3D-Visualization and Registration for Neurovascular Compression Syndrome Analysis

P. Hastreiter[1,2], R. Naraghi[1], B. Tomandl[3], M. Bauer[2], and R. Fahlbusch[1]

[1] Neurocenter, Dept. of Neurosurgery, Schwabachanlage 6, 91054 Erlangen, Germany
hastreiter@neurocenter.imed.uni-erlangen.de
[2] Computer Graphics Group, University of Erlangen-Nuremberg, Germany
[3] Division of Neuroradiology, Schwabachanlage 6, 91054 Erlangen, Germany

Abstract. Neurovascular compression syndromes are caused by a pathological contact between vessels and the root entry or exit zone of cranial nerves. Associated with a number of neurological diseases such as trigeminal neuralgia, hemifacial spasm or vertigo, there is also strong evidence for a direct relation with essential arterial hypertension. To treat the related conditions, operative microvascular decompression has proven to be very effective. So far, as a drawback for the examination, 2D representations of tomographic volumes served as exclusive source of information. Aiming at an improved spatial understanding, we introduce a noninvasive and fast approach providing clear delineation and interactive 3D visualization of all relevant structures. It is based on strongly T2 weighted MR volumes with sufficiently high resolution. Due to the size of the nerves and vessels at the brainstem, an explicit segmentation is extremely difficult. Therefore, we propose to segment only coarse structures with a sequence of filtering and volume growing. Consecutively, implicit segmentation with pre-defined transfer functions is applied to delineate the tiny target structures included in the area of cerebrospinal fluid. Additionally, we suggest registration with MR angiography to differentiate between vessels and nerves on one side and between arteries and veins on the other side. Overall, our approach contributes significantly to an optimized 3D analysis of vascular compression syndromes. The high value for the planning of surgery is demonstrated with several clinical examples.

Keywords: Visualization, Registration, Neurovascular Compression

1   Introduction

Neurovascular compression syndromes (NVC) such as trigeminal neuralgia or hemifacial spasm characterized by hyperactive cranial nerve dysfunction result from compression of the root entry or exit zone of cranial nerves by small vessels [1] (see Fig. 1). Although the pathophysiology of neurovascular compression is still unknown, microvascular decompression has been proven to be effective and is regarded as the treatment of choice. Since the neurovascular structures are very small, imaging and consecutive visualization of neurovascular compression is extremely difficult [2].

Intraoperative observations in cases with trigeminal neuralgia or hemifacial spasm with additional arterial hypertension showed a distinct neurovascular compression of the ventrolateral medulla on the left at the level of the root entry zone of the cranial nerves IX and X [1]. Microvascular decompression of the ventrolateral medulla was

T. Dohi and R. Kikinis (Eds.): MICCAI 2002, LNCS 2488, pp. 396–403, 2002.

able to reduce high blood pressure permanently in about 70 % of the operated cases [3]. These observations were supported by comparative microanatomical dissections [4]. As a result, three distinct types of neurovascular compression at the ventrolateral medulla were described and the posterior inferior cerebellar artery (PICA) was identified as the predominant offending vessel. Further studies showed that operative microvascular decompression effectively contributes to reduce an abnormal elevated blood pressure[5].

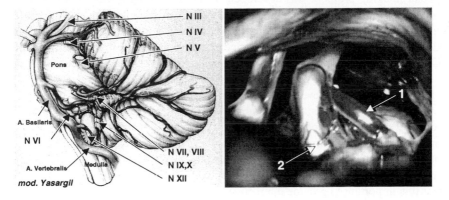

Fig. 1. Anatomical illustration *(left)* showing the neurovascular relations at the brainstem including the cranial nerves (III-XII) and vessels. — Intraoperative view *(right)* showing neurovascular compression (1 →) and trigeminal nerve with distortion of the root entry zone (2 →)

A comprehensive analysis of neurovascular compression syndromes in preparation of surgery requires detailed understanding of all relevant structures. Therefore, it is important to display the relationship of the cranial nerves to the vascular structures and the brainstem. A delineation of these structures is obtained with magnetic resonance imaging *(MRI)*. In this context the strongly T2 weighted CISS *(Constructive Interference in the Steady State)* sequence turned out to be most appropriate since it reveals high contrast between the vascular structures and the cerebrospinal fluid *(CSF)*. Thereby, even small structures of less than 1 mm in diameter are visible. However, the 2D visualization of slice images is insufficient to precisely identify the location and relation of cranial nerves and vessels. To overcome this situation a clear and interactive 3D visualization is necessary contributing to an improved spatial understand.

After an overview about the image data in section 2, the applied segmentation is explained in section 3 integrating experience presented in [6]. Since an explicit segmentation of the tiny vessels and nerves is too time-consuming and error-prone, we suggest to use implicit segmentation based on direct volume rendering. Using standard PC graphics hardware [7] transfer functions for color and opacity values are interactively adjusted starting with pre-defined lookup tables. As a prerequisite this approach requires only a coarse segmentation of the image data which is conveniently obtained with a fast semi-automatic strategy. Then, section 4 outlines the evolved transfer functions and the actual visualization. Further on, voxel based registration with MR angiography (MRA) is suggested. Thereby, the differentiation between vessels and nerves in MR-CISS data is made easier and faster. Finally, section 6 discusses our approach and presents clinical examples demonstrating its value for practical application.

2   Image Data

Using different scanning parameters, MRI provides enormous potential in order to differentiate a great variety of tissues non–invasively. It is the only imaging modality to scan neuronal tissue, cranial nerves and vascular structures within the posterior fossa with sufficiently high resolution. For the analysis of neurovascular compression syndromes a special imaging protocol was developed. In the beginning a MR-FLAIR *(Fluid Attenuated Inversion Recovery)* sequence is used which produces water suppressed T2 weighted images. Thereby, other lesions such as infarction or tumerous lesions are excluded. Consequently, a MR-CISS sequence is applied providing images with high signal of CSF and low intensity for nerves and vascular structures. Since the target structures are within the space of the CSF surrounding the brainstem, they are clearly defined as can be seen in Fig. 3. However, they are in the same range of data values as the remaining soft tissues which prohibit simple maximum intensity projection *(MIP)*. In the same way, the explicit segmentation of tiny structures is very time-consuming and, on top of this, error-prone due to the extremely low resolution and partial volume effects. However, using locally applied color and opacity lookup tables exclusively, it is possible to clearly delineate all vascular structures and nerves with direct volume rendering. In addition to that it is important to provide interactive manipulation of transfer functions ensuring time-saving and accurate implicit segmentation.

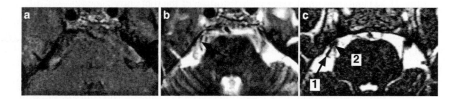

Fig. 2. Imaging of a right trigeminal neuralgia with different MR sequences: (a) no detailed anatomical structures with MR-FLAIR, (b) unreliable delineation of neurovascular relations (→) with MR-T2 due to CSF pulsation artifacts, (c) clear detection of vessels (1 →) and nerves (2 →) in CSF with MR-CISS

3   Segmentation

An important issue of the presented approach is the high difference of signal contrast produced for CSF and non-liquid structures using the MR-CISS sequence. As shown in section 2, the CSF is mapped to high intensity values while the enclosed target vessels and nerves are reproduced with low signal. However, applying implicit segmentation with a single lookup table for color and opacity values leads to unsatisfying visualization results. This results from identical ranges of intensity values for the target structures, the brainstem and further surrounding tissues. As a solution to this problem, we suggest to explicitly segment the essential CSF area containing all vessels and nerves. In consequence, local transfer functions provide a clear visualization if they are applied to this segmented object.

The process of segmentation as a necessary prerequisite for a consecutive meaningful visualization subdivides into the following steps:

Noise Reduction: Due to the noisy character of the data (compare Fig. 2) it is helpful to perform a noise reduction in the beginning. For this purpose anisotropic diffusion [8] is performed providing more homogeneous areas while preserving boundaries.

Morphological Filtering: In order to simplify the actual segmentation of the CSF volume, morphological filtering with a 3D greyvalue closing operation is applied. Thereby, the vessels and nerves are removed which are represented by low intensity values within the CSF volume. Afterwards, the "closed" CSF volume forms a compact object with a clear boundary which is easily extracted. To ensure good results the applied spherical filter kernel should be smaller than surrounding structures and greater than the target vessels and nerves. For this purpose a radius of $r = 2$ turned out to be optimal.

Volume Growing: The actual extraction of the CSF volume is then performed with volume growing. To make this process more robust, it is important to use bounding boxes and to proceed stepwise. Thereby, restricting the growing process to user-defined subvolumes, the integration of irrelevant neighboring structures is prevented. The segmented "closed" CSF volume is consecutively used as a mask to label the original MR-CISS data for volume rendering.

Manual Labeling: For the differentiation of vessel structures and cranial nerves within the segmented CSF volume, labeling of the nerves must be performed. This is so far achieved manually since it requires a comprehensive anatomical knowledge. Additionally, the brainstem is labeled to obtain an improved 3D representation. Since the ventral side of the brainstem is of interest, the already existing mask of the CSF volume serves as an explicit boundary for a further manual but fast labeling.

Attributing: As a final step of segmentation the original MR-CISS data is attributed (compare Fig. 3) with different tags for the background (tag 0), the CSF volume including the vessels (tag 1), the cranial nerves (tag 2) and the brainstem (tag 3).

The suggested semi-automatic segmentation approach leads to fast pre-processing, due to the immediate visual control and the low computational expense required for the single steps. Further on, integrating the experts knowledge directly for this highly specialized task ensures robust results.

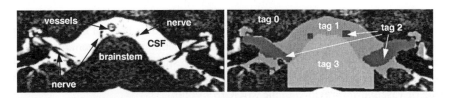

Fig. 3. MR-CISS slice showing with CSF containing tiny vascular structures and nerves *(left)* and coarse segmentation *(right)* of background (tag 0), CSF containing vessels (tag 1), CSF including nerves (tag 2), and brainstem (tag 3)

4   Visualization

Having segmented and labeled the MR-CISS volume as explained in section 3, the actual delineation of the vessels and nerves is performed implicitly based on direct volume rendering using 3D texture mapping with standard PC graphics hardware. For this purpose pre-defined lookup tables for colors and opacity values are used for every subvolume (see Fig 4). They are interactively adjusted to match an individual dataset. The intensity histogram displayed within the color editor serves as supporting information. The actual volume rendering is performed with 3D texture mapping using standard PC graphics hardware [7].

In general, the background (tag 0) is made completely transparent since the most relevant information is contained in the remaining subvolumes. Only for further anatomical orientation it is made visible by using a linear ramp for the color values combined with low opacity values. The visualization of the vessels and nerves as part of the CSF subvolumes (tag 1, tag 2) is implicitly achieved using the suggested transfer functions. Considering the target structures with MR-CISS volumes low data values are mapped to high opacity and color values. Further on, a clear delineation of the tiny vessels and nerves requires to adjust a decline for the opacity. Thereby, high data values are made transparent which guarantees a smooth transition to CSF. The respective color components obtain a higher slope to intensify the impression of depth. Additionally, full opacity and cyan color is applied to the brainstem (tag 3) supporting the anatomical orientation.

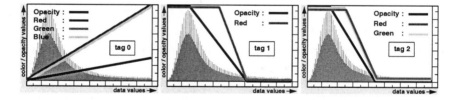

Fig. 4. Transfer functions: background (tag 0), CSF & vessels (tag 1) and CSF & nerves (tag 2)

5   Fusion with MR-Angiography

The segmented MR-CISS data allow visualizing all structures relevant for neurovascular compression syndromes in a robust way. However, as a drawback of the approach presented in section 3 manual labeling has to be performed to separate cranial nerves from vessels requiring extensive anatomical expertise. To simplify this process we introduce the integration of MR-angiography (MRA, "time of flight" (TOF)) data as additional source of vascular information in the MR-CISS volume.

An important prerequisite is the correct transformation of the MRA data to the MR-CISS coordinate system by means of registration. For this purpose, a rigid voxel based registration with mutual information [9, 10] was used. To ensure fast alignment a hardware accelerate strategy was applied which was introduced in [11]. Thereby, capabilities of 3D texture mapping subsystems are used to cope with the huge amount of trilinear interpolation operations dominating the overall calculation time.

In order to extract the vascular information we applied anisotropic diffusion for initial noise suppression and consecutive thresholding. Attempts using line filters improved our results only marginally. Thereafter, the segmented structures were copied into the MR-CISS data and served as a mask to label the respective subvolumes. Thereby, vessels are conveniently separated from nerves and arteries are differentiated from veins. Furthermore, vascular structures at the boundary layer of the CSF are delineated in a more robust way.

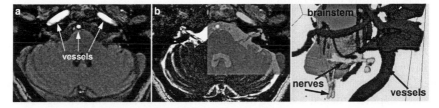

Fig. 5. Fusion of MR-CISS and MRA-TOF: (1) vessels within MRA, (2) overlay of MR-CISS and MRA using magic lens, (3) 3D visualization from MR-CISS using vessel mask from MRA

6   Results and Discussion

The presented approach was so far applied to 27 patients. Out of this group, 19 suffered from trigeminal neuralgia, 4 from hemifacial spasm and 4 from hypertension. Surgery was conducted in 23 cases. In all cases, MR-FLAIR, -T2, -TOF and -CISS data were acquired. All volumes were scanned with a Siemens MR Magnetom Sonata 1.5 Tesla scanner. In all cases the MR-CISS and -TOF data consisted of $384 \times 512 \times 62$–128 voxels with an average size of $0.39 \times 0.39 \times 0.7$ mm^3. In case of MR-FAIR and MR-T2 volumes of $408 \times 512 \times 23$ voxels with a size of $0.45 \times 0.45 \times 6.0$ mm^3 were obtained.

A standard PC (AMD Athlon 1.2 GHz) with NVidia GeForce3 graphics card providing 64 MB texture memory was used for the interactive direct volume rendering based on 3D texture mapping. In order to find the optimal setting for the transfer functions only a few and simple operations were necessary. The same platform was also applied for the registration requiring 4.5 min for the alignment. Thereby, a single interpolation of the volume including the evaluation of mutual information requires only 0.73 sec using a viewport of 150×150 pixels.

To our knowledge the presented approach produced for the first time meaningful 3D visualizations for the analysis of neurovascular compression syndrome based on MR-CISS data. In all cases, the brainstem, the small vessels (PICA, AICA, SCA) and the cranial nerves were identified. Two selected cases demonstrate the clinical value of our strategy.

Case 1: In Fig. 6 the situation of a trigeminal neuralgia is illustrated. The 3D representations clearly show the relation of the relevant vessels and nerves confirmed by operative findings. For the same case the masking of vascular structures was also performed with MRA-TOF as shown in Fig. 5. In this way the bigger vessels are clearly delineated while the small vessels are problematic due to reduced flow signal. Consequently, MR-CISS remains indispensable to detect all relevant structures but MRA-TOF is a good supplement to simplify labeling.

Case 2: Fig. 7 presents the neurovascular anatomy in arterial hypertension. In this case a close relationship of the PICA-loop to the left ventrolateral medulla at the root entry zone of the cranial nerves IX and X as type 1 [4] is visible.

At the current stage, the overall time for a 3D analysis of neurovascular compression syndromes requires about 2 hours. It consists of MR imaging (25 min), complete explicit segmentation (1 hours), registration (4.5 min) and visualization (5 min). Thereby, most of the time is still consumed for labeling the MR-CISS data. However, this step provides further potential for optimization.

7   Conclusion

A non-invasive approach was introduced allowing for a comprehensive 3D analysis of neurovascular compression syndromes. It clearly shows the relation of all relevant structures implicitly delineated from MR data after only a coarse explicit segmentation. Overall, this strategy is robust and comparatively fast. For the future a fully automatic strategy for the differentiation of vessels and nerves is envisaged. Resulting from comparisons with operative findings our method is of high value for preoperative evaluation and contributes to optimize clinical practice.

References

1. P. Jannetta. Neurovascular compression in cranial nerve and systemic disease. *Ann. Surg.*, 192:518–525, 1980.
2. R. Naraghi, H. Geiger, J. Crnac, W. Huk, R. Fahlbusch, G. Engels, and F. Luft. Posterior fossa neurovascular anomalies in essential hypertension. *The Lancet*, 344:1466–1470, 1994.
3. P. Jannetta, R. Segal, and S. Jr. Wolfson. Neurogenic hypertension: etiology and surgical treatment. I. Observations in 53 patients. *Ann. Surg.*, 201:391–398, 1985.
4. R. Naraghi, M. Gaab, G. Walter, and B. Kleineberg. Arterial hypertension and neurovascular compression at the ventrolateral medulla. A comparative microana-tomical and pathological study. *J. Neurosurg.*, 77:103–112, 1992.
5. H. Geiger, R. Naraghi, H.P. Schobel, H. Frank, R.B. Sterzel, and R. Fahlbusch. Decrease of blood pressure by ventrolateral medullary decompression in essential hypertension. *The Lancet*, 352:446–449, 1998.
6. C. Rezk-Salama, P. Hastreiter, K. Eberhardt, B. Tomandl, and T. Ertl. Interactive Direct Volume Rendering of Dural Arteriovenous Fistulae. In *Proc. MICCAI*, Lect. Notes in Comp. Sc., pages 42–51. Springer, 1999.
7. C. Rezk-Salama, K. Engel, M. Bauer, G. Greiner, and T. Ertl. Interactive Volume Rendering on Standard PC Graphics Hardware Using Multi-Textures and Multi-Stage Rasterization. In *Proc. Eurographics/SIGGRAPH Workshop on Graphics Hardware*, 2000.
8. G. Gerig, O. Kübler, R. Kikinis, and F. Jolesz. Nonlinear Anisotropic Filtering of MRI Data. *IEEE Trans. on Med. Imag.*, 11(2):221–232, 1992.
9. P. Viola and W. Wells. Alignment by Maximization of Mutual Information. In *Proc. Vth Int. Conf. Comp. Vision*, pages 16–23, Cambridge, MA, 1995.
10. A. Collignon, D. Vandermeulen, P. Suetens, and G. Marchal. Automated Multi-Modality Image Registration Based on Information Theory. *Kluwen Acad. Publ's: Comput. Imag. and Vis.*, 3:263–274, 1995.
11. P. Hastreiter and T. Ertl. Integrated Registration and Visualization of Medical Image Data. In *Proc. CGI*, pages 78–85, Hannover, Germany, 1998.

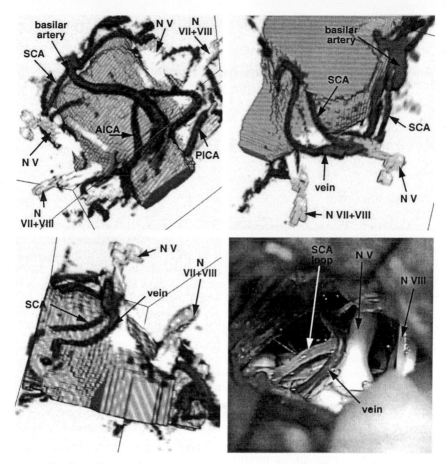

Fig. 6. Visualization of NVC in trigeminal neuralgia showing relations between vessels and nerves (top row). Visualization compared to operative finding (bottom row)

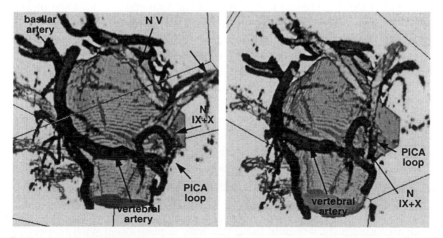

Fig. 7. Visualization of NVC at the ventrolateral medulla in essential hypertension, looping PICA

3D Guide Wire Reconstruction
from Biplane Image Sequences for 3D Navigation
in Endovascular Interventions

S.A.M. Baert, E.B. van der Kraats, and W.J. Niessen

Image Sciences Institute, University Medical Center Utrecht
Rm E 01.334, P.O.Box 85500, 3508 GA Utrecht, The Netherlands
{shirley,everine,wiro}@isi.uu.nl

Abstract. Using 3D rotational X-ray angiography (3DRA), 3D information of the vasculature can be obtained prior to endovascular interventions. However, during interventions, the radiologist has to rely on fluoroscopy images to manipulate the guide wire. In order to take full advantage of the 3D information from 3DRA data during endovascular interventions, a method is presented which yields an integrated display of the position of the guide wire and vasculature in 3D. The method relies on an automated method developed by the authors that simultaneously tracks the guide wire in biplane fluoroscopy images. Based on the known geometry, the 3D guide wire position is reconstructed and visualized in the 3D coordinate system of the vasculature. The method is illustrated in an intracranial anthropomorphic vascular phantom.

1 Introduction

In response to the demand for minimally invasive interventions, the number of endovascular interventions has increased rapidly over the last years. During these interventions, a guide wire is inserted into the groin and advanced under fluoroscopic guidance. Due to the complexity of the vasculature, and the narowness of the blood vessels, accurate positioning of the guide wire is difficult, especially during neuro-interventions. This results in prolonged examination times and hence prolonged exposure to X-rays for patients and medical staff.

The recent introduction of motorized calibrated X-ray angiography systems allows 3D reconstruction of the vasculature by performing a 180 degree rotation around the patient. During a rotation a large number of images is taken from known positions. For all positions the geometric distortions have been estimated in a calibration procedure and hence they can be corrected for. Whereas the 3D reconstruction can be used before starting endovascular interventions, the acquisition time is too long to acquire images during an intervention. In this paper a method is developed which, based on the position of the guide wire in calibrated biplane fluoroscopic projection images, reconstructs the 3D guide wire position and subsequently projects this position on the 3D volume reconstruction of the vasculature. This indicates how the guide wire is positioned with respect to the vasculature and can be used as a 3D navigation tool for radiologists.

T. Dohi and R. Kikinis (Eds.): MICCAI 2002, LNCS 2488, pp. 404–410, 2002.

Whereas a number of researchers have used biplane acquisitions in order to reconstruct the centerlines of the vascular tree [5, 8, 9], or to determine other objects in 3D [4], dynamically relating the guide wire position to prior obtained 3D vasculature is new.

This paper is organized as follows: In Section 2 the 2D tracking procedure is presented, which is based on the energy minimization of a spline parameterization of the guide wire in a feature image where line-like structures are enhanced. In Section 3 the calibration procedure to correct for distortion and to determine the geometrical projection parameters of the biplane fluoroscopic images is discussed. Section 4 presents the determination of the correspondence of the splines in the biplane images and the reconstruction of the guide wire in 3D based on the knowledge of the projection geometry. In Section 5 the results are presented and Section 6 concludes with a discussion.

2   Guide Wire Tracking in 2D

The 2D guide wire tracking procedure used in this paper is an extension to a method previously presented [1]. The main steps of the algorithm are briefly summarized here. The guide wire is simultaneously tracked in images acquired using a biplane system. In order to represent the guide wire, a third order spline parameterization is used. In the tracking method, first the spline is positioned on the guide wire and subsequently the spline is moved towards the tip of the guide wire for more accurate tip localization.

In order to find the spline in frame $n + 1$ if the position in frame n is known, first a rough displacement of the guide wire is estimated. Hereto a template is constructed which is rigidly registered to a feature image using cross-correlation. In the feature image line-like structures are enhanced by analyzing the eigenvalues of the Hessian matrix, which is computed with scaled Gaussian derivative operators. The largest absolute eigenvalue of the Hessian matrix has a high output on line-like structures. The sign of this eigenvalue determines whether it concerns a dark (positive) or a bright (negative) structure. Since a guide wire is a dark elongated structure on a brighter background, the feature image is set to the largest eigenvalue if positive and to zero otherwise.

Subsequently, the spline is fitted on the feature image using an energy minimization approach (Powell's direction set method), using internal constraints which are related to the geometry of the curve (curvedness) and external constraints which depend on greyvalue and directional information contained in the feature image. In this step the inner product between the spline and the orientation of the feature is used. This assures that the spline achieves a similar orientation as the guide wire in the image.

After this step, the endpoint is not necessarily positioned on the endpoint of the guide wire, especially in case of guide wires with a straight tip. In order to the determine the endpoint, the length of the guide wire is increased at the tip, while fixing the tail position. Tip localization is then achieved using a discriminant function based on the gradient of the feature image along the spline and the distance to the endpoint position of the guide wire in the previous frame.

2.1   Acquisition

For the experiments an intracranial anthropomorphic vascular phantom which is filled with contrast material (Ultravist-300 (Schering, Weesp, the Netherlands), diluted to 50% with Natriumchloride 0.9% (Fresenius, 's-Hertogenbosch, the Netherlands)) is used. The rotational angiography facility of a Philips Integris BV5000 C-arm imaging system was used to acquire 100 X-ray images at different views by automatic rotation of the C-arm over 180 degrees in about eight seconds. All projection images have a matrix size of 512x512 pixels. Finally a filtered back-projection algorithm [3], which is a modification of Feldkamp's cone-beam algorithm [2] was applied to generate a 3D reconstruction with a resolution of 128x128x128 voxels. A biplane image sequence of 25 images was obtained, while advancing the guide wire in the phantom.

3   Calibration

In order to relate the coordinates in the 2D projection images to world coordinates, the acquired biplane projection data have to be corrected for various types of distortion. Pincushion distortion (curved input screen) and the earth magnetic field variations (s-shaped distortion) which are different for each projection direction have to be corrected for, in order to guarantee correlation of corresponding pixels (see [6, 7]). These distortions are measured using a Cartesian-grid phantom of which a 3D acquisition is made. For all projection angles, the distortion is modelled using bivariate polynomials. The distortion correction is performed with subpixel accuracy. Additionally the focal spot position is determined. Furthermore, the projection geometry is measured, since the mechanical bending of the C-arm causes the isocentre not being constant during the rotation.

4   3D Reconstruction from Biplane Images

In order to reconstruct the guide wire in 3D world coordinates, pairs of corresponding points have to be determined in the two splines that have been calculated using 2D tracking in the biplane images. Since the projection parameters and the locations and orientations of the focal spot are known, the correspondence can be solved using the epipolar constraint.

Figure 1 illustrates the three independent coordinate systems: the volume system $\{v_x, v_y, v_z\}$, the detector system $\{d_x, d_y, d_z\}$ which moves relative to the other systems due to the rotation of the image intensifier, and a global system $\{g_x, g_y, g_z\}$, represented by the global origin O.

Given a point on the spline in the first image, we are now looking for the corresponding point on the spline in the other image. Therefore first the epipolar

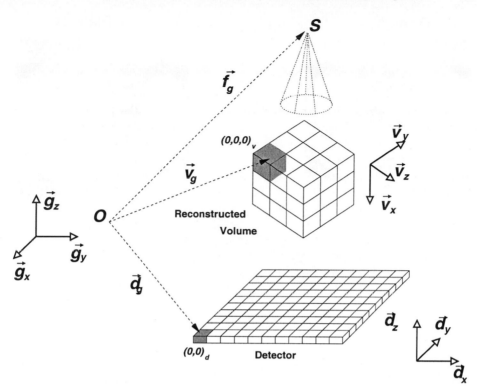

Fig. 1. *Illustration of the geometric framework, in which three independent coordinate systems coexist: the volume system* **v**, *the detector system* **d**, *and a global system* **g**. *S is the position of the X-ray source.*

line is calculated. Given a point P_a on the spline representing the guide wire in image A:

$$P_a = \begin{pmatrix} x \\ y \end{pmatrix} \qquad (1)$$

then the transformation to global coordinates is given by

$$P_{a,global} = d_{a,global} + x p_{dx} \cdot d_{a,x} + y p_{dy} \cdot d_{a,y} \qquad (2)$$

where $d_{a,global}$ is the vector pointing from the global origin to the lower left corner of the detector plane (see Figure 1) and $d_{a,x}$ and $d_{a,y}$ are the detector normals of image A in the x- and y-direction. The epipolar line is obtained by the intersection of plane H, which is defined by the point $P_{a,global}$ and the two focal spots f_a and f_b, and the image plane B, see Figure 2.

The corresponding point P_b in image B can be generated by calculating the intersection of the epipolar line and the spline, representing the guide wire, in image B. If there is more than one intersection, the point of the intersection nearest to the previous intersection point is taken as the corresponding point. Intersection of the line defined by $P_{a,global}$ and f_a, and the line defined by

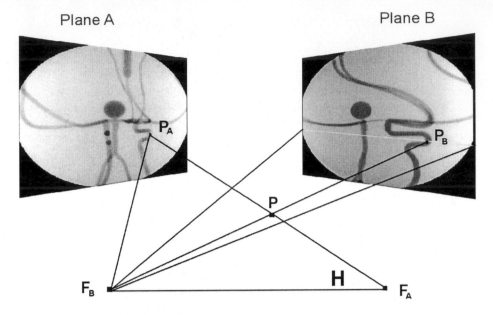

Fig. 2. *Schematic example of the epipolar concept.*

$P_{b,global}$ and f_b, gives point P in 3D. This approach is iteratively applied for all points in the spline from tip to tail, so as to construct full correspondence of the splines in the fluorosopic images and the guide wire position in 3D world coordinates.

5   Results

In this paper experiments were carried out, involving a phantom for which a 3D reconstruction of the vasculature and biplane image sequences in which a guide wire is advanced, are available. Independent 2D guide wire tracking in each of the two projection planes is applied using a method previously presented [1]. In this method the guide wire could accurately be tracked in 96% of the frames. Subsequently corresponding points are determined using the epipolar constraint. 3D reconstruction is then performed and the 3D position of the guide wire is obtained in the same coordinate system as the 3D reconstruction of the vasculature. Therefore, the position of the guide wire in the vasculature can be visualized. Figure 3 shows the calculated position of the guide wire projected into the 3DRA data for four timepoints in the image sequence. It can be observed that the estimated position is within the vasculature.

6   Discussion

A method has been presented which, based on simultaneously tracking a guide wire in biplane fluoroscopic images, reconstructs the guide wire position in 3D

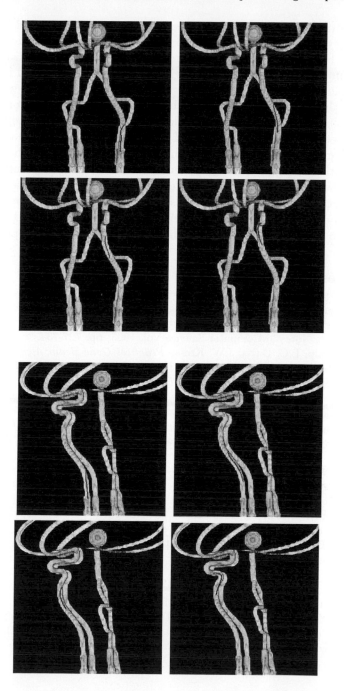

Fig. 3. *Four non-subsequent frames, 1, 10, 15 and 20 of the image sequences with the frontal images (upper four) and lateral images (lower four). It can be observed that the estimated guide wire position is inside the vasculature at all timepoints. For color images, see the digital version of this paper.*

during endovascular interventions. Since this position is expressed in the same coordinate system as in which the pre-intervention 3D reconstructions of the vasculature have been made, this approach enables a 3D visualization of the guide wire in the vasculature which provides a 3D navigational tool for interventional radiologists. In order to improve the accuracy of 3D guide wire position estimation, the 2D biplane images have been corrected for pincushion distortion, distortions due to the earth magnetic field, and the projection geometry has been measured to compensate for mechanical bending of the C-arm. In an anthropomorphic phantom it was shown that the estimated position of the guide wire coincides with the position of the vasculature in the pre-intervention images. In order to validate the estimated guide wire position, and to assess the influence of correcting for the distortions, a series of experiments will be initiated in which 3D reconstructions of the guide wire will be made next to 2D fluoroscopic sequences, so as to provide a gold standard for the 3D guide wire position.

References

1. S.A.M. Baert, W.J. Niessen, A.F. Frangi, E.H.W. Meijering and M.A. Viergever, *Guide Wire Tracking during Endovascular Interventions*, Proceedings of MICCAI 2000, Lecture Notes in Computer Science Vol. 1935, pp. 727-734.
2. L.A. Feldkamp, L.C. Davis, J.W. Kress, *Practical Cone-Beam Algorithm*, Journal of the Optical Society of America A. 1984, Vol. 1, No. 6, pp. 612-619.
3. M. Grass, R. Koppe, E. Klotz et al., *3D Reconstruction of High Contrast Objects using C-Arm Image Intensifier Projection Data*, Computerized Medical Imaging and Graphics 1999, Vol. 23 pp. 311-321.
4. K.R. Hoffmann, B.B. Williams, J. Esthappan et al., *Determination of 3D Positions of Pacemaker Leads from Biplane Angiographic Sequences*, Medical Physics 1997, Vol. 24, No. 12, pp. 1854-1862.
5. K.R. Hoffmann, A. Sen, L. Lan et al., *A System for Determination of 3D Vessel Tree Centerlines form Biplane Images*, International Journal of Cardiac Imaging 2000, Vol.16, No.5: pp. 315-330.
6. R. Koppe, E. Klotz, J. Op de Beek and H. Aerts, *3D Vessel Reconstruction based on Rotational Angiography*, Proceedings of CAR 1995, pp. 103.
7. R. Koppe, E. Klotz, J. Op de Beek and H. Aerts, *Digital stereotaxy/stereotactic procedures with C-arm based Rotational Angiography*, Proceedings of CAR 1996, pp. 17-22.
8. B. Movassaghi *3D Reconstruction by Modeling of Coronary Arteriograms*, Diploma Thesis, Heinrich-Heine University, Düsseldorf, June 2001.
9. L. Sarry, J.Y. Boire, *Three-dimensional Tracking of Coronary Arteries from Biplane Angiographic Sequences using Parametrically Deformable Models*, IEEE Transactions on Medical Imaging 2001, Vol.20, No. 12, pp. 1341-1351.

Standardized Analysis of Intracranial Aneurysms Using Digital Video Sequences

S. Iserhardt-Bauer[1], P. Hastreiter[2], B. Tomandl[3],
N. Köstner[3], M. Schempershofe[3], U. Nissen[2], and T. Ertl[1]

[1] Visualization and Interactive Systems Group, University of Stuttgart, Germany
iserhardt-bauer@informatik.uni-erlangen.de
[2] Neurocenter, Dept. of Neurosurgery, University of Erlangen-Nuremberg, Germany
[3] Division of Neuroradiology, University of Erlangen-Nuremberg, Germany

Abstract. CT-angiography is a well established medical imaging technique for the detection, evaluation and therapy planning of intracranial aneurysms. Different 3D visualization algorithms such as maximum intensity projection, shaded surface display and direct volume rendering support the analysis of the resulting volumes. Despite the available flexibility, this general approach leads to almost unreproducible and patient specific results. They depend completely on the applied algorithm and the parameter setting chosen in a wide range. Therefore, the results are inapplicable for inter-patient or inter-study comparisons. As a solution to this problem, we suggest to make the visualization fully independent of any user interaction. In consequence the main focus of the presented work lies on standardization and automation which guarantees comparable 3D representations for the analysis of intracranial aneurysms. For this purpose, we introduce a web-based system providing digital video sequences based on automatically performed hardware accelerated direct volume rendering. Any preprocessing such as the setting of transfer functions and the placement of clip planes is performed according to a predefined protocol. In addition to an overview using the whole volume, every dataset is divided into four subvolumes supporting a detailed inspection of the vessels and their branches. Overall, the value of the system is demonstrated with several clinical examples.

Keywords: Visualization, Standardization, Automation

1 Introduction

Over the last decade CT-angiography (CTA) was established as one of the most important imaging techniques for the analysis of various vascular pathologies. For the immediate examination and fast detection of intracranial aneurysms CTA is a common approach. Depending on the size of the aneurysm the detection rate with CTA results to 85–95 % [1, 2]. However, digital subtraction angiography (DSA) still represents the golden standard providing the highest spatial and temporal resolution.

In addition to the actual image acquisition strategy the subsequent post-processing of the datasets is of crucial importance for a valuable medical evaluation [3]. A common strategy in clinical routine is maximum intensity projection (MIP) as demonstrated in Fig. 1a. Along each ray of integration it considers only the voxel with the highest intensity value and projects its value onto the viewing plane. Contrary to its popularity based on

T. Dohi and R. Kikinis (Eds.): MICCAI 2002, LNCS 2488, pp. 411–418, 2002.

its inherent robustness, MIP leads to inconsistent images missing any depth information. Another well established technique is shaded surface display (SSD) shown in Fig. 1b which generates iso-surface representations. Since only the first layer of voxels defined by a threshold is rendered along each ray of integration, efficient software based algorithms are applied. As a drawback of this approach any density information of the original data is lost.

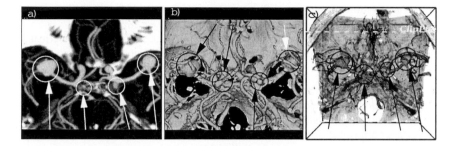

Fig. 1. Different visualization techniques of the same CTA dataset showing 4 aneurysms ($\rightarrow$): a) maximum intensity projection b) shaded surface display and c) direct volume rendering

The most comprehensive 3D visualization technique is direct volume rendering (dVR) (see Fig. 1c). Following the image based strategy it considers the entire volume data by summing over all values along every ray of integration. Or, it projects every voxel onto the image plane applying the object based strategy. As a result, various software solutions have been suggested including ray casting [4] and shear warp factorization [5]. However, hardware supported approaches gained increasing attention achieving most impressive results [6, 7]. Taking into account the size of medical image data and the required visualization quality, direct volume rendering based on 3D texture mapping [8–10] on reasonably scaled graphics computers represents an optimal approach for the analysis of intracranial aneurysms.

In general, modern interactive visualization environments provide a great variety of degrees of freedom ensuring high interactivity and flexibility. Among various rendering parameters this comprises mostly the definition of thresholds, the precise adjustment of transfer functions for color and opacity values, or simply the choice of a suitable visualization strategy. Aiming at optimized 3D representations supporting the evaluation of difficult cases, this process is very time-consuming. Overall, it requires comprehensive expertise even if predefined settings are provided. Furthermore, analyzing the data by rotating or zooming the volume in an efficient and time saving way is critical with respect to application in clinical routine. As a result, any inter-patient or inter-study comparisons are extremely difficult. To overcome these drawbacks, standardization of 3D visualization is an important issue. For this purpose we present a web-based fully automatic approach addressing the meaningful delineation and volume rendering of aneurysms based on CTA data and the generation of digital video sequences.

In section 2 the developed web-based approach is presented outlining technical features such as the web interface and security issues. To obtain standardized digital video sequences from automatic direct volume rendering of high quality and reproducibility, several procedures had to be developed. This comprises the placement of clip planes and the extraction of specified subvolumes for a closer inspection of risked locations. All these procedures are described in section 3. Further on, the scenario for the evaluation of our approach is presented in section 4 which also discusses the potential for clinical environments.

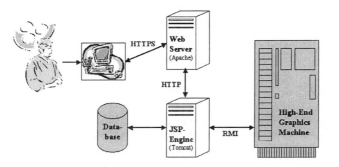

Fig. 2. Overview about the system architecture

2   System Architecture

The suggested approach was implemented as a web service. It supports clinical 3D analysis in generating standardized digital video sequences automatically via the Internet. In this section the underlying architecture as illustrated in Fig. 2 is briefly outlined which is described in detail in [11].

For the communication with the remote system a web-based user interface is provided which presents patient related data to the physician. At the beginning of a session it allows sending DICOM data via the Internet onto a high-end graphics computer. At the end of the automatic volume rendering it presents the generated videos for down load. JSP (Java Server Pages) technology is employed to transfer data and to create each HTML page dynamically. This technology offers easy handling, and is available for virtually any platform. Since the graphics server should only be responsible for the rendering, a different computer is employed to manage the web service. In order to communicate between these two computers and to launch different processes from one computer on the other one, Java RMI (Remote Method Invocation) is used.

Since medical data contain patient related information, it is of crucial importance to provide high security. Therefore, our system permits access only to registered users after login based on password verification. Furthermore, one is automatically logged out after a specific time period, if there was no communication in order to prohibit access of unauthorized persons. Ensuring safe transfer of the image data and any information to or from the web service encoding via HTTPS is used.

3   Algorithms

Our system includes several specialized algorithms which are essential for the automatic preprocessing and volume rendering of the applied CTA datasets. Thereby, these procedures perform three important tasks which physicians have to do in interactive environments. Firstly, the appropriate adjustment of transfer functions for color and opacity values to clearly delineate the target structures. Secondly, the detection of intracranial aneurysms. Thirdly, the transformation of the volume to visually access all relevant locations in a convenient way. Specifically, this refers to the definition of a patient specific flight path according to a predefined setting. In this context, the main focus lies in the creation of several subvolumes extracted from the original data. These subvolumes allow inspecting typical locations for the existence of aneurysms.

Subvolumes. The detection of intracranial aneurysms, especially small aneurysms, is a very difficult task. It depends on various factors such as the visualization technique, the experience of a physician and the amount of information inherent to the data. Important indications about single structures can be hidden by other structures like bones (in our case mainly the skull base) or other blood vessels. For this reason, it is important to restrict the volume of inspection. Additionally, one can focus on the specific locations since intracranial aneurysms often grow at branches of blood vessels. Nevertheless, it is important not to omit parts of the image data. Mainly, aneurysms can be found at the tip of the basilar artery, the left and right cerebral artery and at the communicating artery. The presented system supports a semi-automatic approach to define the position of these critical points. For this purpose, one has to specify the position of the clivus which is a bony structure lying centrally within the volume. It serves as a reference point. As a result of measurements performed by our clinical partners, the distance between the clivus and every single critical point was determined for several datasets and the mean value was calculated. These four values are used to specify the critical points. They also represent the centers of the subvolumes. Since the size of the subvolumes (60 mm in each dimension) is uniformly scaled for safety reasons in such a way that they overlap in any case it is not necessary to specify the exact position of the critical points.

Clip Planes. In case of the applied CTA scans important information about arteries is often hidden by veins located in the occipital part. Therefore, it is most helpful to virtually cut off these disturbing vessels from rendering by defining a clip plane which suppresses one half space form rendering. It is used within the original volume which gives an overview visualization about the whole situation and within the subvolume around the basilar artery. For the two remaining subvolumes its application is not necessary. According to our experiments the position of the plane is optimal if located 30 mm dorsal and parallel to the clivus (compare Fig.3).

Transfer Functions. After a reduction of the topological information using subvolumes and a clip plane, it is also necessary to reduce the structural information. In addition to the data inherent noise the information about various soft tissues enclosing the target structures prohibits a clear 3D representation of vascular structures. Using a transfer function for opacity values these structures are easily made transparent considering respective lower Hounsfield units. Further transfer functions for color values allow the effective accentuation of vessels and bone even if a light model is missing during rendering with 3D texture mapping [9]. In consequence, the locations of intracranial aneurysms are easily detected. In order to adjust a predefined setting of these transfer functions a lot

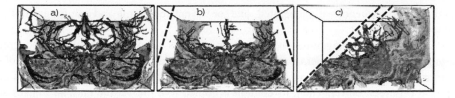

Fig. 3. The predefined clip plane: a) The whole volume data without any clip plane. It is not possible to look into the critical regions. b) The clip plane is 30mm in front of the clivus and rotated by 45°. c) Using the clip plane the critical locations are visible

of expertise is required. Besides, this process remains time-consuming although the required effort was already reduced to a minimum using simple manipulation operations. As a solution to this drawback an approach was previously presented [12] which allows an automatic calculation. A reference dataset and a related optimized function are used to adapt the setting on-the-fly to a submitted volume.

Standardized Camera Path. An important part of the presented approach is the generation of standardized rendering sequences recorded to digital video files. In general, standardization is an essential issue for the diagnosis of intracranial aneurysms in order to achieve comparable results for medical studies. For this purpose, 50 patients were analyzed at the Division of Neuroradiology, University of Erlangen-Nuremberg and the typical approach of the data was studied. Thereby, the most common locations of intracranial aneurysms were defined which are the anterior communication arteries (ACA), the bifurcations of the medial cerebral arteries (MCA) and the internal carotid arteries (ICA). Based on this experience a camera path was developed taking into account essential directions of view as following:

1. Posterior overview — provides the best view for the vertebro-basilar system.
2. Lateral views — important for the analysis of the internal carotid arteries.
3. Multiple views — necessary in order to examine the medial cerebral arteries.

Concerning the entire dataset, the camera moves initially from posterior to anterior and then to left and right lateral. For a closer inspection, the volume is zoomed and the preceding movement to lateral views is repeated. Consecutively, the subvolumes are rendered with a circular flight of 360 degrees.

Rendering Process. Using the predefined camera paths, the actual visualization process is launched. Thereby, the volume rendering is performed with an application developed at the Universities of Erlangen-Nuremberg and Stuttgart. It is integrated in the OpenInventor class hierarchy and takes advantage of 3D texture mapping capabilities of graphics subsystems providing high frame rates and rendering quality [9].

In the beginning, details of the volume data extracted from the DICOM headers and the calculated coordinates of the clip plane described in section 3 are loaded. Then, the predefined setting of transfer functions are adapted to the volume data. Finally, five digital video sequences are generated, one for the entire volume and one for each of the four subvolumes.

During the rendering process the camera position is sampled in steps of small degrees along the predefined camera path. Following a circular path this results in a smooth movement. At each step the visualization tool renders the scene into pbuffer which is a special offscreen buffer. Then, its content is copied to a file. At the end, all images are automatically converted to a digital video of a user-defined format (e.g.: MPEG, AVI).

4   Results and Discussion

For the volume rendering a SGI Onyx Infinite Reality3 ($2 \times$ R12000, 400 MHz) equipped with 1 GB of 3D texture memory was used. It provides large scale and fast trilinear interpolation capabilities. The actual web service was established on a standard Linux PC (AMD Athlon 1.2 GHz).

The described system was developed in cooperation with the Div. of Neuroradiology, Dept. of Neurosurgery of the University of Erlangen-Nuremberg. Two physician evaluated the system in terms of quality, speed and reliability. During the evaluation process datasets of 15 patients were examined. The important issue of theses tests was the visual detection of the intracranial aneurysms based on the resulted digital video sequences. All image data contained a total of 19 aneurysms which were detected previously with DSA by a different physician. In addition to the detection, it was also of major interest to obtain information about the shape and neck of the aneurysms.

As a result 18 of the 19 aneurysms were detected. One aneurysm of the internal cerebral artery was not detected since it was covered by bone structures. Another large aneurysm close to the skull base was detected but the definition of the neck was not possible. The remaining aneurysms located above the skull-base were analyzed recognized correctly with a better definition of the shape and neck in five cases when compared to DSA. Overall, the video sequences were of good diagnostic quality. The mean time of calculation including the transfer of the data and the automatic generation of video-sequences was about 60 minutes.

For the first time our approach allows for a reproducible 3D-visualization of intracranial vasculature making the time-consuming and individual manipulation of interactive visualization environments superfluous. Thus, the physician must not be familiar with specific manipulators and techniques of volume rendering in order to use this approach for the investigation of intracranial vessels. As a general result, the web service allows a user-independent and standardized visualization of constant quality. Beyond this, high-end graphics computers are now accessible for a much wider range of clinical institutions performing CTA examinations.

Our initial results indicate that aneurysms lying above the skull-base are accurately depicted while the visualization of aneurysms lying within the area of the skull-base is still problematic. Thus, further algorithms have to be developed in order to separate the blood vessels exactly from bone.

5   Conclusion and Future Work

The results of the investigations and the consequential conclusions confirm that the proposed approach is applicable in medical practice. The support for the physicians is fully acceptable. Also the depiction of the intracranial aneurysms were mostly of a higher quality than in the case of DSA. But the results show also the problems of our approach. In case of aneurysms which were above the skull base the results were satisfying. The problems are visible in case of aneurysms which involve the skull base. One technical solution for this problem is to remove the bone and to separate the blood vessels. Due to the partial volume effect a simple threshold-based elimination is insufficient. In this case more complicated approaches, e.g. combinations of region-based segmentation approaches and Watershed transformation to remove the partial volume effect are necessary. These approaches are subject to future work.

References

1. N. Young, N. Dorsch, R. Kingston, G. Markson, and J. McMahon J. Intracranial aneurysms: evaluation in 200 patients with spiral CT angiography. *Eur Radiol*, 11:123–30, 2001.
2. Y. Korogi, M. Takahashi, K. Katada, Y. Ogura, K. Hasuo, M. Ochi, H. Utsunomiya H, T. Abe, and S. Imakita. Intracranial aneurysms: detection with three-dimensional CT angiography with volume rendering–comparison with conventional angiographic and surgical findings. *Radiology*, 211:497–506, 1999.
3. B. Tomandl, P. Hastreiter, Ch. Rezk-Salama, K. Engel, T. Ertl, W. Huk, O. Ganslandt, Ch. Nimsky, and K. Eberhardt. Local and Remote Visualization Techniques for Interactive Direct Volume Rendering in Neuroradiology. *RadioGraphics*, 21:1561–1572, 2001.
4. D. Laur and P. Hanrahan. Hierarchical Splatting: A Progressive Refinement Algorithm for Volume Rendering. *Comp. Graphics*, 25(4):285–288, July 1991.
5. P. Lacroute and M. Levoy. Fast Volume Rendering Using a Shear-Warp Factorization of the Viewing Transform. In *Computer Graphics, Proc. SIGGRAPH '94*, volume 28, pages 451–458, 1994.
6. H. Pfister, J. Hardenbergh, J. Knittel, H. Lauer, and L. Seiler. The VolumePro Real-Time Ray-Casting System. In *Proc. of ACM SIGGRAPH*, page 251260, 1999.
7. C. Rezk-Salama, K. Engel, M. Bauer, G. Greiner, and T. Ertl. Interactive Volume Rendering on Standard PC Graphics Hardware Using Multi-Textures and Multi-Stage Rasterization. In *Proc. Eurographics/SIGGRAPH Workshop on Graphics Hardware*, 2000.
8. B. Cabral, N. Cam, and J. Foran. Accelerated Volume Rendering and Tomographic Reconstruction Using Texture Mapping Hardware. In *ACM Symp. on Vol. Vis*, pages 91–98, 1994.
9. P. Hastreiter, C. Rezk-Salama, B. Tomandl, K. Eberhardt, and T. Ertl. Fast Analysis of Intracranial Aneurysms based on Interactive Direct Volume Rendering and CT–Angiography. In *Proc. MICCAI*, Lect. Notes in Comp. Sc., pages 660–669. Springer, 1998.
10. R. Westermann and T. Ertl. Efficiently Using Graphics Hardware in Volume Rendering Applications. In *Computer Graphics (SIGGRAPH '98)*, Comp. Graph. Conf. Series, pages 169–177, 1998.
11. S. Iserhardt-Bauer, T. Ertl, C. Rezk-Salama, and P. Hastreiter. Webservice für die automatische Generierung von Videodokumenten von Aneurysmen. In T. Schulze, S. Schlechtweg, and V. Hinze, editors, *Simulation und Visualisierung*, pages 163–173. European Publishing House, 2001.
12. C. Rezk-Salama, P. Hastreiter, J. Scherer, and G. Greiner. Automatic Adjustment of Transfer Functions for 3D Volume Visualization. In *Proc. Workshop Vision, Modeling, and Visualization (VMV)*, pages 357–364. in cooperation with IEEE Sig. Proc. Soc. and Gesell. f. Informatik (GI), Infix Verlag St. Augustin, 2000.

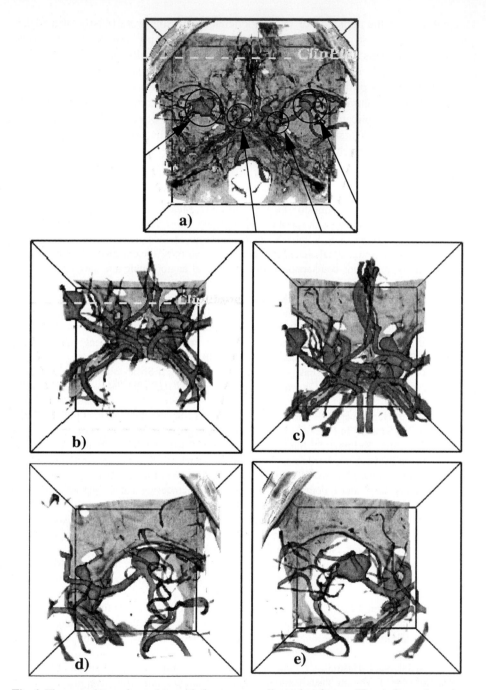

Fig. 4. The complete volume data with the corresponding sub volumes: Fig. a) shows the volume data, the marked positions demonstrates the recognizable intracranial aneurysms. The 4 subvolumes represents the regions around b) the internal carotid c) the anterior communication artery d) the left and e) the right medial cerebral artery.

Demarcation of Aneurysms
Using the Seed and Cull Algorithm

Robert A. McLaughlin and J. Alison Noble

Medical Vision Laboratory, Dept. Engineering Science, University of Oxford,
Oxford, England
{ram,noble}@robots.ox.ac.uk

Abstract. This paper presents a method to demarcate the extent of
an intracranial aneurysm given a 3-D model of the vasculature. Local
shape descriptors are grouped using a novel region-splitting algorithm.
The method is used to automatically estimate aneurysm volume. Results
are presented for four clinical data sets.

1 Introduction

An intracranial aneurysm is a localised persistent dilation of the wall of a blood
vessel in the brain. There are several possible treatments, including coiling and
clipping. The treatment appropriate depends upon factors such as aneurysm
volume and neck size. It is common to image the aneurysm using a 3-D modality
such as 3-D X-ray angiography or magnetic resonance angiography (MRA). Such
scans can be segmented to derive a 3-D model of the vasculature [1] [2]. Given
such a 3-D model, it would be useful to automatically demarcate the aneurysm,
identifying where it connects to the vessel. This could allow automatic estimation
of volume and neck size, aiding the clinician to choose the appropriate treatment.

Several researchers have suggested methods to demarcate aneurysms by locating the aneurysm neck. Van Der Weide et al. [3] computed distances to the
surface of the vasculature from a point selected inside the aneurysm, detecting the neck as a discontinuity in these distances. Wilson et al. [4] developed a
variant of this idea, using a series of such distance functions from points along
a user-defined spline. As noted in [4], such methods experience difficulties in
aneurysms with wide necks. We propose a different approach, defining shape descriptors over a surface mesh and using region-splitting to identify the section of
the mesh covering the aneurysm. The region-splitting algorithm has been termed
the *Seed and Cull algorithm*. The method is applied to four clinical data sets.

2 Method

2.1 Local Shape Descriptors

The method begins with a surface mesh defined over a 3-D model of the vasculature. At each vertex in the mesh, a local description of vessel shape is computed,

T. Dohi and R. Kikinis (Eds.): MICCAI 2002, LNCS 2488, pp. 419–426, 2002.

illustrated in figure 1. Taking the unit surface normal n_i to the mesh at a particular vertex d_i, a ray is extended from d_i into the vessel, measuring the distance to the opposite side of the vessel. Halving this value gives an estimate of vessel radius r_i at d_i. Next, the algorithm estimates the vessel centre p_i as $p_i = d_i + r_i.n_i$, and the direction of maximum absolute curvature c_i^{max}. A vector is extended from p_i in the directions c_i^{max} and $-c_i^{max}$, and the distance to the vessel surface is measured in each direction. Adding these two distances together gives an estimate of the vessel width w_i in a direction perpendicular to n_i. The two values (r_i, w_i) characterise the data point d_i, and are computed for every vertex in the mesh. The task is now to group points that lie on the aneurysm, and distinguish these from points on adjoining vessels.

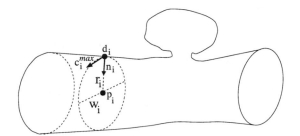

Fig. 1. Local shape descriptors: vessel radius r_i and the perpendicular width w_i.

2.2   Seed and Cull Algorithm

Region-growing [5] and region-splitting [6] algorithms typically require the number of regions to be known a priori. Such methods are insufficient for aneurysm demarcation. When considering the entire vasculature, variation in size and shape between different sections of blood vessel tend to be greater than the variation between vessel and aneurysm, in all but the extreme cases of giant aneurysms. Hence it is unrealistic to group all vessel points into a single region. Thus we require an algorithm to segment points on the surface mesh into an unknown number of regions, where each region will correspond to a section of vessel or an aneurysm. One solution is to use an augmented Markov Random Field, where an extra region label is defined for new regions, and a parameter is pre-set to define the probability assigned to this extra state. Such a method was proposed in [7] for texture segmentation. We have adopted an alternative approach which adaptively uses Parzen windows [8] to estimate region statistics.

The Seed and Cull algorithm begins by assigning all points to a single region. A point is then selected somewhere on the mesh and a new region seeded, growing it as described in the next section. If the region does not grow, then it is culled and a different seed is chosen. The novelty of this algorithm lies in the mechanism by which regions are grown when appropriate, while being retarded when they will not improve the segmentation.

2.3   Growing Regions

Consider classifying the point d_0 shown in figure 2. We add the restriction that it must be of the same class as one of the other five data points that lie within the neighbourhood of radius $r_{classify}$. Each point d_i has a vector $v_i = (r_i, w_i)$ associated with it, where (r_i, w_i) are the local shape descriptors described in Section 2.1. For each class C_i, we can compute a probability distribution over these numeric values $P(v_0|d_0 \in C_i)$. Using this, we classify the point d_0 using a Bayesian framework by computing the maximum a posteriori estimate for C_i.

$$P(d_0 \in C_i|v_0, D, C) \propto P(v_0|d_0 \in C_i, D, C).P(d_0 \in C_i|D, C) \qquad (1)$$

where $D = \{d_1, d_2, d_3, d_4, d_5\}$ denotes the set of nearby data points and $C = \{d_1, d_2 \in C_1; d_3, d_4 \in C_2; d_5 \in C_3\}$ denotes which class each point is currently assigned to. By assuming that the probability assigned to the numeric value is statistically independent of data points in a particular neighbourhood (the D and C terms), we can replace $P(v_0|d_0 \in C_i, D, C)$ with $P(v_0|d_0 \in C_i)$. The term $P(d_0 \in C_i|D, C)$ is a prior probability that d_0 belongs to class C_i. We have chosen a prior directly proportional to the number of data points of each class within the neighbourhood, although others are possible.

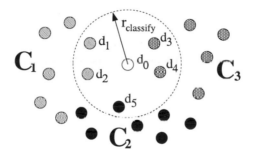

Fig. 2. Point and neighbourhood for classification.

2.4   Seeding New Regions

We will illustrate the seeding of new classes with the synthetic example shown in figure 3a, where each point d_i in the data set has an intensity value v_i. The method described here is directly applicable to the case of aneurysms and blood vessels, where we are segmenting points on a surface mesh, and where each point has a 2-D numeric value (r_i, w_i). However, it is conceptually easier to understand the algorithm using the synthetic example shown in figure 3a.

The method begins by assigning all pixels to a single class C_0 and evaluates the probability distribution over the intensity values $P(v_j|d_j \in C_0)$, as shown in figure 3b. Note that there is a peak in the distribution corresponding to each class. To generate this probability distribution, a histogram of the numeric

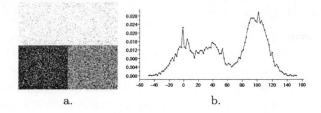

a.   b.

Fig. 3. a.) Three groups synthetic data. b.) Initial probability $P(v_j|d_j \in C_0)$.

values is computed and then smoothed using Parzen windows [8]. This involves smoothing the histogram by convolving the values with a kernel function. A common choice of kernel function is the Gaussian, although others are possible.

An important issue arises in the selection of variance for the Gaussian kernel function. This will greatly affect the probability distribution produced. When the histogram comprises few values, it is appropriate to use a large variance, resulting in heavy smoothing. If the histogram consists of a large number of values, then less smoothing is desirable and a small variance is appropriate.

In the Seed and Cull algorithm, the variance is a function of the number of values in the histogram, which equals the size of the class. A large variance is used for small classes, and a small variance for large classes. We have chosen the variance to equal the inverse square of an affine function of class size, although other functions are possible. As a new class C_i grows in size, progressively smaller variances are used in evaluating the probability $P(v_j|d_j \in C_i)$. It is this change in variance that will allow us to promote the growth of a class under certain conditions, and retard the growth of unnecessary regions.

Returning to the data shown in figure 3a, a new class is seeded by choosing a point, defining a neighbourhood of radius r_{seed} around it and assigning all points within the neighbourhood to the new class C_1, as shown in figure 4a. In figure 4b, we show $P(v_j|d_j \in C_1)$, the distribution over intensity values for this new class. Note that the probability distribution is much smoother than that shown in figure 3b, as a much large variance was used for this new, small class.

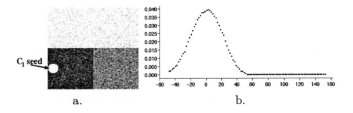

a.   b.

Fig. 4. a.) Seed for class C_1. b.) Initial probability $P(v_j|d_j \in C_1)$.

As the new class only contains points from one distribution, the probabilities assigned to this distribution are larger than those in C_0, which divides its probabilities between three distributions. Note that the maximum in figure 4b for $P(d_j \in C_1|v_j, D, C)$ is 0.040, while the corresponding value at $v_j = 0$ for $P(d_j \in C_0|v_j, D, C)$ is only 0.024, as shown in figure 3b. Choosing a data point $d_j \in C_0$ that comes from this distribution and re-evaluating its classification will re-assign it to C_1, provided the prior probabilities are approximately equal.

The algorithm now proceeds to 'grow' this distribution. Recall from Section 2.3, the assumption that the class of a data point was only directly affected by points within a neighbourhood of radius $r_{classify}$. Thus all points $\{d_j\}$ within a radius $r_{classify}$ of the new class C_1 are tested to decide whether they should be re-classified. This is recursively repeated for each point d_j that is re-classified to class C_1. Note that only points currently assigned to class C_0 will be tested. Once a point is re-classified as belonging to C_1, it will not be changed. This process is continued until no more points are added to class C_1, and no more remain that need to be tested. The result at convergence is shown in figure 5a.

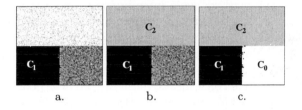

a.   b.   c.

Fig. 5. a.) Classification after C_1 converges. b.) Classification after C_2 converges. c.) Final classification.

As each point is removed from C_0 and added to C_1, the probability distributions are re-evaluated. The variance used when computing $P(v_j|d_j \in C_0)$ increases as the class shrinks, and decreases for $P(v_j|d_j \in C_1)$ as the class grows. Thus C_1 will improve its model of the distribution of numeric values v_j, and this distribution will be removed from the three distributions shown in figure 3b for class C_0. This process is then repeated, seeding a new class C_2. Once C_2 has converged, the data will be classified into classes C_0, C_1 and C_2 as shown in figure 5b. It is important that the segmentation algorithm recognise that no further classes should be introduced. The algorithm achieves this because of its adaptive choice of variance as a function of class size.

The algorithm will seed a new class C_3 as shown in figure 6a, and the initial points in the neighbourhood will give a distribution for $P(v_j|d_j \in C_3)$ as shown in figure 6b. However, this class will fail to grow in the way that C_1 and C_2 did. First note that because C_3 contains less points than C_0, the probability distribution was generated by convolving with a Gaussian with a larger variance than was used for C_0. Hence $P(v_j|d_j \in C_3)$ is more smoothed, resulting in lower probabilities for values from the distribution. Note that the maximum for $P(v_j|d_j \in C_3)$ shown in figure 6b is 0.045, while the maximum for class C_0 is greater than 0.06, as shown in figure 6c. This in turn reduces the probabilities $P(d_j \in C_3|v_j, D, C)$. As the algorithm attempts to grow C_3, most data points

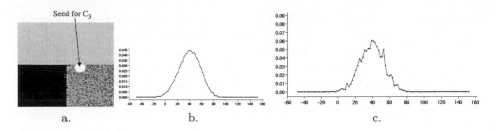

Fig. 6. a.) Seed for class C_3. b.) Initial probability $P(v_j|d_j \in C_3)$. c.) Probability $P(v_j|d_j \in C_0)$ when C_3 is seeded.

will not be re-classified from C_0 to C_3, instead remaining in C_0. In this implementation, we set a threshold that requires a class to grow to at least three times its original seed size. Classes that fail to meet this criterion are 'culled' and discarded. In this way, we avoid introducing excess classes. The algorithm will continue attempting to seed new classes on each point left in C_0, but each new class will be culled. The final segmentation is left as shown in Fig 5c.

The above algorithm extends, without conceptual change, to the case of segmentation using local shape descriptors (r_i, w_i) instead of intensities, and where the points are defined on a surface mesh instead of as pixels in an image. At completion, the mesh will be separated into regions, with the aneurysm separated from its adjoining vessels.

3   Experiment

We applied the method to four clinical examples shown in figure 7. The data sets for Patients 1 and 2 were segmented from phase contrast MRA data with voxel size 0.78 x 0.78 x 1.5mm. They were segmented using both flow speed and direction information, as detailed in [1], The data sets for Patients 3 and 4 were generated from 3-D X-ray angiographic data with voxel resolution 0.25 x 0.25 x 0.25mm, and segmented using thresholding. For each data set, a surface mesh was generated and segmented by applying the Seed and Cull algorithm to local shape descriptors. Each voxel within the vasculature was then assigned to the same group as the closest mesh point. The group covering the aneurysm was identified by a user and the volume of that group computed. These results were compared against aneurysm volumes obtained from a manual segmentation, where each slice was segmented by hand.

4   Results

Results of the aneurysm demarcation algorithm are shown in figure 7, where the voxels forming each aneurysm have been highlighted. Two different views are given of each example. Table 1 compares the automatic volume estimates with those from manual segmentation. In each of the four data sets, the aneurysm was identified as a single region. Note that with Patient 4, the edge of the giant aneurysm was identified as approximately halfway through the intersection of the five adjoining vessels. The poorly defined neck of this aneurysm made this example particularly difficult. Wilson et al. [4] noted that neck-based demarcation methods will exhibit similar problems with such examples.

The parameter $r_{classify}$ was chosen empirically, with one value being set for the MRA data sets, and a second value appropriate for the two 3-D X-ray angiographic data sets. The value was found to depend upon both the resolution of the data, and the scale of the features being demarcated. Results were found to be robust under minor perturbations of the value of $r_{classify}$.

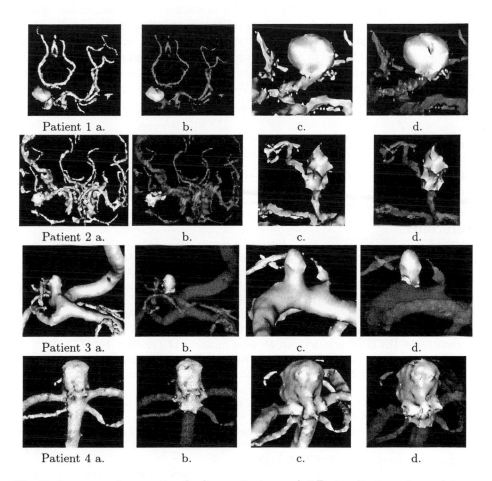

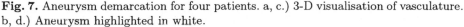

Fig. 7. Aneurysm demarcation for four patients. a, c.) 3-D visualisation of vasculature. b, d.) Aneurysm highlighted in white.

Table 1. Results of volume estimation, with error as a percentage of the manual volume estimate.

Patient #	Automatic volume (mm^3)	Manual volume (mm^3)	% error
1	2120	2180	2.8
2	915	991	7.7
3	13.7	14.5	5.5
4	305	270	13.0

5   Conclusion

We have outlined a method to demarcate intracranial aneurysms. Using a surface mesh defined over a 3-D segmentation of the vasculature, local shape descriptors were computed and grouped using a novel region-splitting method referred to as the Seed and Cull algorithm. Results for four clinical data sets have been presented, generated from both 3-D X-ray angiographic data and phase-contrast MRA data. The results have demonstrated the applicability of this method to aneurysms of different sizes and shapes. Volume estimates from this method were compared against those obtained manually, with an average error of 7.2%.

Acknowledgements

The 3-D X-ray angiographic data was kindly provided by GE Medical Systems. This work was supported by EPSRC grant GR/M55008.

References

1. Chung, A., Noble, J.: Fusing magnitude and phase information for vascular segmentation in phase contrast mr angiograms. In: Proc. MICCAI. (2000) 166–175
2. Chung, A.C.S., Noble, J.A.: Statistical 3D vessel segmentation using a Rician distribution. In: Proc. MICCAI. (1999) 82–89
3. van der Weide, R., Zuiderveld, K., Mali, W., Viergever, M.: CTA-based angle selection for diagnostic and interventional angiography of saccular intracranial aneurysms. IEEE Transactions on Medical Imaging **17** (1998) 831–841
4. Wilson, D., Royston, D., Noble, J., Byrne, J.: Determining x-ray projections for coil treatments of intracranial aneurysms. IEEE Transactions on Medical Imaging **18** (1999) 973–980
5. Adams, R., Bischof, L.: Seeded region growing. IEEE Transactions on Pattern Analysis and Machine Intelligence **16** (1994) 641–647
6. Horowitz, S.L., Pavlidis, T.: Picture segmentation by a directed split-and-merge procedure. In: Second International Joint Conference On Pattern Recognition, Copenhagen, Denmark, IEEE (1974) 424–433
7. Kervrann, C., Heitz, F.: A markov random field model-based approach to unsupervised texture segmentation using local and global spatial statistics. Technical Report 2062, INRIA, France. Available from http://www.inria.fr (1993)
8. Bishop, C.M.: Neural Networks for Pattern Recognition. Oxford University Press, Oxford, England (1999)

Gyral Parcellation of the Cortical Surface Using Geodesic Voronoï Diagrams

A. Cachia[1,2,3,4], J.-F. Mangin[1,2,4], D. Rivière[1,4],
D. Papadopoulos-Orfanos[1,4], I. Bloch[3,4], and J. Régis[5]

[1] Service Hospitalier Frédéric Joliot, CEA, 91401 Orsay, France
mangin@shfj.cea.fr, cachia@shfj.cea.fr, http://www-dsv.cea.fr/
[2] INSERM ERITM Psychiatrie et Imagerie, Orsay, France
[3] Département Traitement du Signal et des Images, CNRS URA 820, ENST, Paris
[4] Institut Fédératif de Recherche 49 (Imagerie Neurofonctionnelle), Paris
[5] Service de Neurochirurgie Fonctionnelle et Stereotaxique, Marseille, France

Abstract. In this paper, we propose a generic automatic approach for the parcellation of the cortical surface into labelled gyri. These gyri are defined from a set of pairs of sulci selected by the user. The selected sulci are first automatically identified in the data, then projected onto the cortical surface. The parcellation stems from two nested Voronoï diagrams computed geodesically to the cortical surface. The first diagram provides the zones of influence of the sulci. The boundary between the two zones of influence of each selected pair of sulcus stands for a gyrus seed. A second diagram yields the gyrus parcellation. The distance underlying the Voronoï diagram allows the method to extrapolate the gyrus limits where the sulci are interrupted. The method is applied on three different brains.

1 Introduction

The recent advent of automatic methods dedicated to brain morphometry has raised a large interest in the neuroscience community. These tools, indeed, provide a new way of addressing issues related to the links between anatomy and function. While none of these tools can be considered as the perfect one, simply because of the huge complexity of brain anatomy, it is assumed that analyzing hundreds of brains overcome the failures observed for a few ones.

Most of the approaches applied at a large scale rely on a coordinate system, which may be either three dimensional for **voxel based morphometry** [1], or two dimensional for studies of cortical thickness [8, 14]. In each case, various warping operations are used to match as far as possible the different brains under study with a template endowed with the coordinate system. We will denote this warping principle **"iconic spatial normalisation"**. Morphometry is performed on a point by point statistical basis, either on data related features or on deformation related features [4].

While the coordinate based paradigm has a lot of success in the neuroimaging community, an alternative approach consists of mimicing the classical anatomical morphometry, namely defining some anatomical structures by a segmentation method and deriving some shape descriptors that will be compared across brains. This alternative is sufficiently attractive to be applied manually, although tedious work has to be performed, which prevents large scale studies [22, 10]. The motivation behind this **"structure based**

T. Dohi and R. Kikinis (Eds.): MICCAI 2002, LNCS 2488, pp. 427–434, 2002.
© Springer-Verlag Berlin Heidelberg 2002

morphometry" is the idea that some neuroscience results deeply related to the brain architectural organisation may be either lost during the non perfect iconic spatial normalisation or inaccessible via a coordinate based point of view. Finally, it should be noted that some morphometry approaches are hybrid because local coordinate systems are used to compute some shape descriptors [9].

Two directions of algorithmic research aim at providing automatic methods to perform structure based morphometry. The first one stems directly from the iconic spatial normalisation scheme: a manual segmentation of the template is warped toward any new brain in order to obtain an automatic segmentation [5]. While this approach gives good result for stable brain areas like the deep nuclei, it is more questionable for the cortex [17] because the warping algorithms are disturbed by the high variability of the folding patterns [18, 21]. Therefore, a concurrent strategy for the cortex consists of linking blind geometric parcellations of the cortex with pattern recognition methods [12, 13, 21, 3, 20], in order to achieve a better definition of sulco-gyral shapes to be compared across brains. A lot of other dedicated segmentation schemes have been defined for various other brain areas [6].

The methods dedicated to the cortex always focus on geometrical properties allowing to devise a definition of cortical folds (depth, curvature, medial axes, etc...). The usual neuroscience point of view about the cortical surface segregation, however, is gyrus based. A gyrus, indeed, is usually considered to be a module of the cortex endowed with dense axonal connexions throughout local white matter [23]. Unfortunately, cortical gyri are relatively difficult to define from a pure geometrical point of view, even if they are supposed to be delimited by two parallel sulci.

In this paper, we propose a two stage strategy for the parcellation of the cortical surface into gyri. First, the main cortical sulci are automatically extracted and identified using a contextual pattern recognition method that may be viewed as a structural alternative to the brain warping approach [21]. Second, the dual gyri are defined as patches of the cortical surface yielded by the computation of two nested Voronoï diagrams, whose initial seeds are inferred from the the identified sulcus bottom lines. This definition of the main gyri is a mixture between geometrical information related to the geodesic distance used to define the diagrams, and a high level cortex model for the recognition of the main sulci which provide the seed lines. The method proposed in this paper, which converts a set of sulci into the set of dual gyri, is generic and may be applied with an alternative different identification of the sulci.

2   Method

2.1   The Sulcus Identification

The first stage of the method, which has been described by Rivière in [21], provides automatically the set of the main sulci, each sulcus being represented by a set of voxels obtained from a skeleton segmentation (see Fig. 1). For each sulcus, discrete topology properties allows us to obtain the subset of connected voxels corresponding to bottom lines (main part and branches, see Fig. 2) [15, 16], called *sulcal lines*. Another outcome of this preprocessing stage is two smooth meshes of the cortex hemispheres endowed with a spherical topology [16]. The sulcus bottoms will be projected on this representation of the cortical surface to define some limits between the dual gyri. Therefore, to have access to the method described in this paper, the user has to provide a list of pairs of sulcus names. Each pair will usually correspond to two parallel sulci possibly interrupted.

2.2   Projection of the Sulcal Bottom Lines onto the Triangulation

The main problem disturbing the definition of gyri is the interruption of the delimiting sulci, because these interruptions are highly variables. The idea proposed in this paper overcomes this difficulty using the Voronoï diagram principle. If a set of lines approximatively located at the level of the crowns of the gyri of interest can be provided as gyrus seeds, the whole gyral parcellation can be defined from a distance computed geodesically to the cortical surface. Each gyrus will be the zone of influence of its own seed, namely the subset of the cortical surface closest to its seed than to the other seeds. To try to impose the sulcus bottoms as parts of the boundaries between these influence zones, the idea consists of removing the projected bottom lines from the mesh to prevent the distance to be propagated across these lines. Hence the resulting diagram is inferred from an iterative dilation of the gyrus seeds that is stopped either at the level of the sulcus bottoms, or when two zones of influence get in touch with each other. All the geodesic distance computations used in this paper stem from the thick front propagation idea proposed in [24]. Such distances are also used to apply isotropic geodesic morphological treatments (closing, dilation, etc...)

To make the projected bottom lines behave like walls for the geodesic distance propagation, their connectivity has to be preserved during the projection onto the cortical surface. This is not straightforward because the smooth mesh stems from a decimation algorithm which leads to a non stationary triangle sampling. Morphological closing operations are performed to reach this goal. Another important constraint is the localisation of the projection that has to correspond to the deepest part of the fold on the cortical surface (see Fig. 2). The sequence of processing used to achieve these goals is the following. The ith Sulcal bottom Line (defined with voxels) is noted SL_i^v; its projection on the triangulation (defined with nodes) is noted SL_i^t. The label of the ith sulcal line is l_i. The projection is done for each sulcal line (i.e. for each connected component of the sulcal bottom lines) independently.

1. The first step of the projection is an adaptation of the well-known ICP algorithm [2, 7] which allows to find an affine transformation which preserves the global structure of the bottom line. This prevents the creation of large gaps in the middle of the projected points.
    - Definition of a set $MATCH_i$ of matched point pairs. The construction is the following: for each point M_i^v of the sulcal line SL_i^v, a pair (M_i^v, M_i^t) is added to $MATCH_i$, where M_i^t is the node of the cortical mesh minimising the function $d(M_i^v, M) = d_E(M_i^v, M) + \alpha Depth(M)$ (see Fig. 2), where M is a mesh node, α ia positive weighting constant, $d_E(M_i^v, M)$ is the 3D Euclidean distance and $Depth(M)$ is the geodesic depth. This geodesic depth computation follows the following steps: 1) apply a 3D morphological closing to the white matter binary mask. 2) apply a 3D erosion of 5mm to the closed mask. 3) Define all the mesh nodes outside this mask as gyrus crowns. The geodesic depth of all these nodes is then null. 4) Compute the geodesic distance to these crowns (a similar approach may be found in [20]).

- For each sulcus i, perform a least square evaluation of the best affine transformation, which map the sulcus bottom line on the cortical mesh. Each point of SL_i^v is then projected onto the closest mesh node after affine transformation.

2. The second step consists of closing and thinning the previous projected sulcal lines (see Fig. 3). This operation is applied independently on the projection of each connected component of SL_i^v. The sulcal lines are imposed to be *actual* lines on the mesh (i.e. a chain of node). The set of projected points is first iteratively dilated geodesically to the triangulation until reaching exactly one connected component. The second stage is a skeletonization like algorithm. The underlying idea is a heuristic computing connected set diameter. A first point is randomly selected in the connected dilated line. A distance (geodesic to the connected set) is computed from this point. The more distant point is selected as the first set extremity. A second (geodesic distance) is computed from this first extremity. The more distant point is selected as the second extremity. The set skeleton (i.e. set diameter) is inferred by a step by step backtracking along the geodesic distance propagation.

2.3 Gyral Parcellation

Once the sulci have been projected onto the cortical surface, the remaining processing is embedded into the spherical topology of the cortical surface. The following sequence of stages leads first to the definition of gyral seeds from each pair of sulci given by the user. The second stage leads to the gyral parcellation (see Fig. 3). The two stages of computation rely on the well known Voronoï diagram notion, which is widely used in computer vision. Such a diagram can be computed into any space domain for a given set of seeds. The diagram is a parcellation of the space into the seed influence zones, where each point is given to the closest seed according to a distance. In the following, this distance is an approximation of the geodesic Euclidean distance [24] (the geodesic distance between two mesh nodes is estimated as the shortest path, through the mesh nodes, linking the two nodes). The diagram is efficiently computed from the previous thick front propagation[24].

A detailed sketch of the process is the following:

1. Computation of the Voronoï diagram of the labelled sulcal lines (see Fig. 3.B) . The nodes that have the label l_i correspond to the nodes whose closest seed (i.e. sulcal line), from a geodesic point of view, has the label l_i. The goal of this diagram is the detection of the boundaries between the zone of influences of the pair of sulci given by the user (see Fig. 3.C). Such a boundary will represent further the seed of the corresponding gyrus. The set of boundaries of the diagram is sometimes called a skeleton by influence zone (SKIZ) [11]. The boundaries are the nodes with at least two different labels in their direct neighborhood. Hence, the boundaries of interest are set of nodes with exactly two labels in their neighborhood corresponding to one of the user specified sulcus pairs. This definition of the gyral seed leads to the ideal localisation for these seeds. The boundary between two neighboring sulcus zones of influence, indeed, is equidistant to the wished gyrus limits. Therefore, during the second diagram computation, the extrapolation of the limits given by the sulcus bottoms will really be equidistant between the crowns of the gyri in competition.

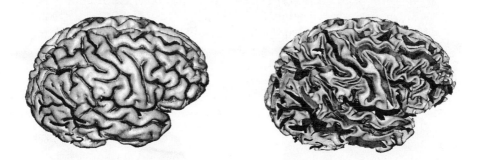

Fig. 1. An example of the result of the sulcus extraction and identification (on right: the white matter mesh used as a spherical model of the cortex). The colors correspond to the various names used by our neuroanatomist to train the recognition system [21]. These names belong to a hierarchy of neuroanatomy names. The sulcus list on which is applied the parcellation is chosen by the system user. Hence several different parcellations can be computed according to the user needs.

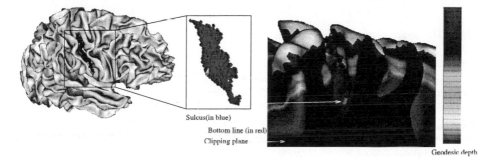

Fig. 2. Each sulcal bottom line is projected onto the cortical surface along the line of maximal geodesic distance to the gyrus crowns.

2. Computation of the second voronoï diagram using the gyrus seeds (see Fig. 3.D). The main difference with the previous diagram is the removal of the sulcal seeds from the mesh, to prevent the distance from crossing the sulcus bottom.

3 Results and Discussion

The method has been applied on three different brains. The list of sulcus pairs selected by the user was corresponding to long neighboring parallel sulci, in order to obtain as far as possible the usual anatomical parcellation. While the results provided in Fig. 4 share striking similarities across the three brains and with standard anatomical drawing, some more work has to be done on the sulcus pair selection to reach the more intuitive parcellation.

The huge folding variability highlighted by the figure illustrates the difficulties preventing a pure geometrical definition of gyri. Some frontal sulci that are often long non

432   A. Cachia et al.

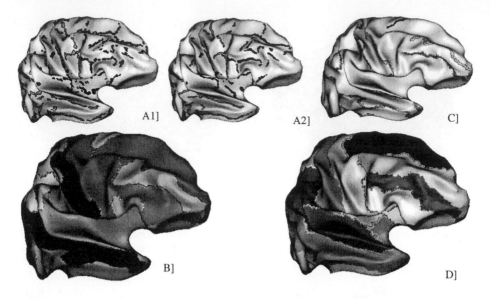

Fig. 3. This figure proposes a sketch of the method mapped on an inflated version of the cortical surface for the sake of understanding. Most of the remaining surface curvature is related to the gyral parcellation targeted by the algorithm. Each sulcus bottom line connected component is first projected (A1). Then the projection is closed using geodesic mathematical morphology, and skeletonised using a geodesic diameter strategy in order to obtain a continuous line (A2). A first Voronoï diagram is computed for the seeds corresponding to these projected lines using a geodesic distance (B). This diagram provides a sulcal based parcellation of the surface. The seeds that will stand for the gyri are boundaries of this first diagram related to the pairs of sulci initially defined by the user (C). Finally a second diagram is computed for these gyral seeds after removal of the sulcal seeds from the mesh in order to prevent the geodesic distance to cross a sulcus bottom (D).

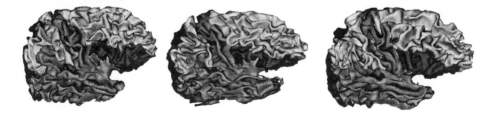

Fig. 4. A typical result obtained from three different brains and some of the main gyri. For instance, the external part of the frontal lobe is split into four parallel horizontal gyri. Back, two vertical gyri correspond to motor and somesthesic areas, etc... Other kind of parcellations can be obtained if the user selects a different list of sulcus pairs.

interrupted furrows can be split into several pieces in some brains. This phenomenum disturbs both the sulcus recognition and the gyrus definition. Nevertheless, our method can extrapolate the standard parcellation to this complex intriguing configurations. Hence, any brain can be processed in a rather consistent automatic way, which opens the door to large scale comparisons between pathological and standard subjects. According to the user interest, different sulcus pair list may be provided to the method in order to compare gyral areas and shapes from various definitions.

Another interest of this generic cortical parcellations into gyral patches stems from the recent development of MR diffusion imaging for fiber tracking [19]. The methods used to detect the fiber bundles linking two different cortical areas are still in their infancy, but this new possibility leads now to develop dedicated mapping methods. One possibility is the inference of the matrix of connectivity of the main cortical gyri. For each individual, using gyral patches as input and output may allow the sorting of the huge number of tracked bundles. Then individual matrices of connectivity could be compared on a statistical basis. This approach could provide new research and diagnostic tools for the pathologogies related to the brain connectivity.

References

1. J. Ashburner and K. J. Friston. Voxel-based morphometry–the methods. *NeuroImage*, 11:805–821, 2000.
2. P. Besl and N. McKay. A method for registration of 3d shapes. *IEEE Transaction on Pattern Analysis and Machine Intelligence*, 14(2):239–256, Feb 1992.
3. A. Cachia, J.-F. Mangin, D. Rivière, N. Boddaert, A. Andrade, F. Kherif, P. Sonigo, D. Papadopoulos-Orfanos, M. Zilbovicius, J-B. Poline, I. Bloch, F. Brunelle, and J. Régis. A mean curvature based primal sketch to study the cortical folding process from antenatal to adult brain. In Springer Verlag, editor, *MICCAI '01, Utrecht*, LNCS, pages 897–904, 2001.
4. M. K. Chung, K. J. Worsley, T. Paus, C. Cherif, D. L. Collins, J. N. Giedd, J. L. Rapoport, and A. C. Evans. A unified statistical approach to deformation-based morphometry. *NeuroImage*, 14(3):595–606, 2001.
5. D. L. Collins, C. J. Holmes, T. M .Peters, and A. C. Evans. Automated 3D model-based neuroanatomical segmentation. *Human Brain Mapping*, 3:190–208, 1995.
6. J. Duncan and N. Ayache. Medical image analysis: Progress over two decades and the challenges ahead. *IEEE Transactions on Pattern Analysis and Machine Intelligence*, 22(1):85–106, 2000.
7. J. Feldmar and N. Ayache. Rigid, affine and locally affine registration of free-form surfaces. *The International Journal of Computer Vision*, 18(2), May 1996.
8. B. Fischl, M. I. Sereno, R. B. Tootle, and A. M. Dale. High-resolution intersubject averaging and a coordinate system for the cortical surface. *Hum Brain Mapp.*, 8(4):272–84, 1999.
9. G.Gerig, M Styner, ME Shenton, and JA Lieberman. Shape versus size: Improved understanding of the morphology of brain structures. In *MICCAI 2001, LNCS 2208, Springer Verlag*, pages 24–32, 2001.
10. Kim J.J., Crespo-Facorro B., Andreasen N.C., O'Leary D.S., Zhang B., Harris G., and Magnotta V.A. An mri-based parcellation method for the temporal lobe. *Neuroimage*, 11(4):271–88, Apr 2000.
11. C. Lantuejoul and S. Beucher. On the use of the geodesic metric in image analysis. *J.of Microscopy*, 121:39–49, 1981.
12. G. Le Goualher, E. Procyk, D. L. Collins, R. Venugopal, C. Barillot, and A. C. Evans. Automated extraction and variability analysis of sulcal neuroanatomy. *IEEE Medical Imaging*, 18(3):206–217, 1999.
13. G. Lohmann and D. Y. von Cramon. Automatic labelling of the human cortical surface using sulcal basins. *Medical Image analysis*, 4(3):179–188, 2000.

14. D. Mac Donald, N. Kabani, D. Avis, and A. C. Evans. Automated 3-d extraction of inner and outer surfaces of cerebral cortex from mri. *Neuroimage*, 12(3):340–56, 2000.

15. G. Malandain, G. Bertrand, and N. Ayache. Topological segmentation of discrete surfaces. *International Journal of Computer Vision*, 10(2):158–183, 1993.

16. J.-F. Mangin, V. Frouin, I. Bloch, J. Regis, and J. López-Krahe. From 3D MR images to structural representations of the cortex topography using topology preserving deformations. *J. Mathematical Imaging and Vision*, 5(4):297–318, 1995.

17. Tzourio-Mazoyer N., Landeau B., Papathanassiou D., Crivello F., Etard O., Delcroix N., Mazoyer B., and Joliot M. Automated anatomical labeling of activations in spm using a macroscopic anatomical parcellation of the mni mri single-subject brain. *Neuroimage*, 15(1):273–89, Jan 2002.

18. M. Ono, S. Kubik, and C. D. Abernethey. *Atlas of the Cerebral Sulci*. Georg Thieme Verlag, 1990.

19. C. Poupon, J.-F. Mangin, C. A. Clark, V. Frouin, J. Régis, D. Le Bihan, and I. Bloch. Towards inference of human brain connectivity from MR diffusion tensor data. *Medical Image Analysis*, 5:1–15, 2001.

20. M.E. Rettman, Xiao Han, Chenyang Xu, and J.L. Prince. Automated sulcal segmentation using watersheds on the cortical surface. *NeuroImage*, 15:329–344, 2002.

21. D. Rivière, J.-F. Mangin, D. Papadopoulos, J.-M. Martinez, V. Frouin, and J. Régis. Automatic recognition of cortical sulci using a congregation of neural networks. In *MICCAI, Pittsburgh*, LNCS-1935, pages 40–49. Springer Verlag, 2000, to appear in Medical Image Analysis.

22. E.R. Sowell, P.M. Thompson, D. Rex, D. Kornsand, K.D. Tessner, T.L. Jernigan, and A.W. Toga. Mapping sulcal pattern asymmetry and local cortical surface gray matter distribution in vivo : maturation in perisylvian cortices. *Cerebral Cortex*, 12:17–26, Jan 2002.

23. D. C. Van Essen. A tension-based theory of morphogenesis and compact wiring in the central nervous system. *Nature*, 385:313–318, 1997.

24. B. J. H. Verwer, P. W. Verbeek, and S. T. Dekker. An efficient uniform cost algorithm applied to distance transforms. *IEEE PAMI*, 11(4):425–428, 1989.

Regularized Stochastic White Matter Tractography Using Diffusion Tensor MRI

Mats Björnemo[1,2], Anders Brun[1,2], Ron Kikinis[1], and Carl-Fredrik Westin[1]

[1] Laboratory of Mathematics in Imaging, Brigham and Women's Hospital,
Harvard Medical School, Boston MA, USA
{mats,anders,kikinis,westin}@bwh.harvard.edu
[2] Linköping University, Linköping, Sweden

Abstract. The development of Diffusion Tensor MRI has raised hopes in the neuro-science community for *in vivo* methods to track fiber paths in the white matter. A number of approaches have been presented, but there are still several essential problems that need to be solved. In this paper a novel fiber propagation model is proposed, based on stochastics and regularization, allowing paths originating in one point to branch and return a probability distribution of possible paths. The proposed method utilizes the principles of a statistical Monte Carlo method called Sequential Importance Sampling and Resampling (SISR).

1 Introduction

The development of Magnetic Resonance Imaging (MRI) has led to the design of numerous imaging techniques. One of these is Diffusion Tensor MRI (DT-MRI), which measures the motion of hydrogen atoms within water in all three dimensions. In tissue containing a large number of fibers, like skeletal muscle or white brain matter, water tends to diffuse only along the direction of the fibers. The DT-MRI technique has raised hopes in the neuro-science community for a better understanding of the fiber tract anatomy of the human brain. Various methods have been proposed to use DT-MRI data to track nerve fibers and derive connectivity between different parts of the brain *in vivo* [1, 2, 11–13, 15, 16].

A simple and effective method for tracking nerve fibers using DT-MRI is to follow the direction of the maximum diffusion in each voxel, equivalent to the direction of the main eigenvector in each tensor. This method is usually referred to as tracking using the Principal Diffusion Direction (PDD). Although this method is widely spread and used in various ways [4, 5], it suffers from some major disadvantages. The connectivity is restricted to a one-to-one mapping between points, not allowing the branching that real fiber tracts may undergo. The PDD tracking also gives the impression of being precise, not taking uncertainty of fiber paths into account in the tracking procedure. Further, the direction of the eigenvector corresponding to the largest eigenvalue is very unstable when in proximity to the generic cases of planar and spherical diffusion [14, 16].

While there are strong indications that DT-MRI reveals information of the fiber pathways in the brain, it is important to stress the fact that the explicit quantity measured is water diffusion and not fibers. As DT-MRI is a fairly new field of research, many

T. Dohi and R. Kikinis (Eds.): MICCAI 2002, LNCS 2488, pp. 435–442, 2002.

studies are yet to be made to compare the measured diffusion tensors to detailed tissue properties important for fiber path inference. However, in contrast to approaches such as solving the diffusion equation [6], it might be important to separate the physical phenomenon of water diffusion from the solution of the tracking problem through the use of a fiber model. In this way *a priori* knowledge about nerve fibers such as fiber stiffness could be taken into account [12].

In this paper we propose a fiber propagation method that is based on stochastics and regularization, allowing paths originating in one point to branch and return a probability distribution of possible paths. The proposed method utilizes the principles of Sequential Importance Sampling and Resampling (SISR) that belongs to the class of Monte Carlo methods.

2   Fiber Models

Inspired by the nomenclature used by Liu et al. [10], single fiber paths will be represented by a sequence $\mathbf{X} = (\mathbf{x}_0, \mathbf{x}_1, \ldots, \mathbf{x}_N)$, where $\mathbf{x}_i$ usually refers to positions in space. Fiber path probability distributions are denoted $\pi(\mathbf{X})$ and the tracking of a fiber path originating from a point $\mathbf{x}_0$ give raise to the conditional fiber path distribution $\pi(\mathbf{X}|\mathbf{x}_0)$. The distribution $\pi(\mathbf{X}|\mathbf{x}_0)$ assigns a probability to all possible fiber paths originating in $\mathbf{x}_0$, which in theory can depend on both the shape of the path, its alignment to the measured diffusion tensor field $\mathbf{D}$ and other prior knowledge. The distribution $\pi_t(\mathbf{X}_t)$ will be used to describe the fiber path distribution after t steps of tracking and $\pi_t(\mathbf{X}_{t-1})$ will denote the probability of the first part of a path $\mathbf{X}_{t-1}$, after t steps of tracking. The tracking is assumed to be finished after N steps and the final distribution is denoted $\pi_N(\mathbf{X})$.

The build-up of fiber paths will be sequential, and the direction from the current point, $\mathbf{x}_t$, to the next point in the fiber path, $\mathbf{x}_{t+1}$, will be denoted $\dot{\mathbf{x}}_t$. The actual distance to the next point on the path will depend on the size of the step, Δt.

$$\mathbf{x}_{t+1} = \mathbf{x}_t + \dot{\mathbf{x}}_t \Delta t \tag{1}$$

3   Sequential Importance Sampling and Resampling

A Monte Carlo method called Sequential Importance Sampling and Resampling (SISR), can be used to calculate an approximation of a probability distribution.

3.1   Properly Weighted Sample

In order to work with a distribution $\pi(\mathbf{X})$, it should be represented in some convenient way. One choice of representation is by a set of properly weighted samples [10]. A set of weighted random samples $\{(\mathbf{X}^{(j)}, w^{(j)})\}_{j=1}^m$ is called proper with respect to the distribution $\pi(\mathbf{X})$ if for any square integrable function $h(\cdot)$,

$$E[h(w^{(j)}\mathbf{X}^{(j)})] = cE_\pi[h(\mathbf{X})], \text{ for } j = 1, \ldots, m, \tag{2}$$

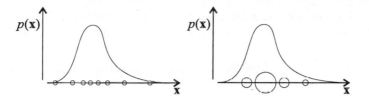

Fig. 1. Left: An unweighted sample representing $p(\mathbf{x})$. Note how the density of samples reflects the distribution. **Right:** A weighted sample representing $p(\mathbf{x})$. Note how fewer samples can be used to represent the distribution.

where c is a normalizing constant common to all the m samples [10]. Using this definition, it is straight forward to confirm that the expectation $\theta = E_\pi[h(\mathbf{X})]$ can be estimated as

$$\hat{\theta} = \frac{1}{W} \sum_{j=1}^{m} w^{(j)} h(\mathbf{X}^{(j)}), \tag{3}$$

where W is a normalizing factor. Drawing for example $\mathbf{X}^{(j)}$ directly from $\pi(\mathbf{X})$ with $w^{(j)} = 1$ gives a proper set of samples [10].

The ability to estimate expectations is an important quality for the approximation of a distribution. In fact, every probability distribution, no matter how complicated it is, can be represented to an acceptable degree of accuracy by a set of properly weighted samples from it [10]. However, it might be difficult to perform the actual sampling. One frequently used method to draw random samples from complicated distributions is the Metropolis-Hastings algorithm [7].

By the use of weighted samples the representation can be made more efficient. Figure 1 gives an intuitive understanding of the difference between weighted and unweighted sets of samples. In general, a set of weighted samples can represent a distribution with higher accuracy than a set of equally many non-weighted samples.

3.2 Importance Sampling

An often effective way to draw a properly weighted sample $\{(\mathbf{X}^{(j)}, w^{(j)})\}$ from a distribution $\pi(\mathbf{X})$, is to use so called importance sampling. A sample is drawn from a trial distribution $q(\mathbf{X})$ and then assigned a weight $w^{(j)} = \pi(\mathbf{X})/q(\mathbf{X})$ to make it proper [10].

3.3 Sequential Build-Up

In Sequential Importance Sampling a set of properly weighted samples of $\pi(\mathbf{X})$ is built up sequentially, through a series of sample sets of increasing dimension,

$$\pi_0(\mathbf{X}_0), \pi_1(\mathbf{X}_1), \ldots, \pi_N(\mathbf{X}_N),$$

smoothly approaching the final distribution so that $\pi_N(\mathbf{X_N}) = \pi(\mathbf{X})$ [10]. Suppose now that we have a set of properly weighted samples $\{(\mathbf{X}_{t-1}^{(j)}, w_{t-1}^{(j)})\}$ representing

$\pi_{t-1}(\mathbf{X}_{t-1})$ and we use a $q_t(\mathbf{x}_t|\mathbf{X}_{t-1})$ close or equal to the true $\pi_t(\mathbf{x}_t|\mathbf{X}_{t-1})$ to draw a new set of samples $\{(\mathbf{X}_t^{(j)}, w_t^{(j)})\}$. The weights should then be adjusted according to

$$w_t = w_{t-1} \frac{\pi_t(\mathbf{X}_t)}{\pi_{t-1}(\mathbf{X}_{t-1})q_t(\mathbf{x}_t|\mathbf{X}_{t-1})} = w_{t-1} \frac{\pi_t(\mathbf{X}_{t-1})}{\pi_{t-1}(\mathbf{X}_{t-1})} \frac{\pi_t(\mathbf{x}_t|\mathbf{X}_{t-1})}{q_t(\mathbf{x}_t|\mathbf{X}_{t-1})} \qquad (4)$$

to represent $\pi_t(\mathbf{X}_t)$ [10].

3.4   Resampling and Reallocating

Sometimes a representation of a distribution becomes inefficient by having many small weights compared to other dominating large weights. In those cases a more efficient representation can be obtained by pruning away samples with small weights and duplicating samples with large weights by doing a resampling of the distribution. One way of doing this is to generate a new set of properly weighted samples by *resampling with replacement* from the set, using the weight as a probability for a sample being resampled [10].

3.5   Related Methods

Sequential Importance Sampling and Resampling is a method that belongs to the class of population Monte Carlo algorithms [8]. Similar methods are found in for instance control theory and are then often called particle filters. The name has been chosen because samples can be seen as particles in a state space, and the sampling from $q_t(\mathbf{x}_t|\mathbf{X}_{t-1})$ can be seen as making the particles walk stochastically along a path in state space. Population Monte Carlo algorithms have also proved to be useful tools in a number of other scientific fields such as statistical physics, quantum mechanics and polymer science [8].

4   Tracking Using SISR

Tracking of nerve fibers can benefit from a statistical framework [3]. We will present a model for fiber propagation and relate it to the SISR framework.

4.1   A Rough Model for Fiber Propagation

In an attempt to build a more realistic model for fiber propagation, it is assumed that fibers 1) are aligned according to the tensors, 2) do not change direction abruptly in case of spherical and planar tensors, and 3) the uncertainty of fiber propagation increases in planar and spherical tensors.

   In the following section, $\mathbf{D}$ will refer to the current tensor $\mathbf{D}(\mathbf{x}_t)$. Also, as the size of the tensor will not matter, the tensor is normed according to its largest eigenvalue, λ_1.

$$\hat{\mathbf{D}} = \frac{\mathbf{D}}{\lambda_1} \qquad (5)$$

The first condition listed above is already accounted for in the PDD tracking method, where the tracking always proceed in the direction of the main eigenvector, $\hat{e}_1$, of the current tensor:

$$\dot{x}_{t,\text{PDD}} = \hat{e}_1(D). \tag{6}$$

To fulfill the second condition, regularization is added to the tracking model. A simple way of doing this is to add a small bias towards the previous tracking direction.

$$D_{\text{reg}} = (\hat{D} + \alpha \dot{x}_{t-1} \dot{x}_{t-1}^T) \tag{7}$$

$$\dot{x}_t = \hat{e}_1(D_{\text{reg}}) \tag{8}$$

By varying α, the bias towards the previous direction can be controlled. This will help stabilize the fiber propagation in case of a spherical tensor, where the main eigenvector might point in any direction before regularization. A larger value of α will smooth the proposed fiber paths to a greater extent.

To incorporate uncertainty in the fiber model, a stochastic part is added perpendicular to the regularized fiber propagation direction. The distribution of the stochastic part is derived from Gaussian noise and transformed using the current tensor to reflect assumption 3), listed before. Thus a linear tensor will result in a small spread.

$$e \in N(\mu, C), \ \mu = (0\,0\,0)^T, \ C = I \tag{9}$$

$$r = D_{\text{reg}} e - (D_{\text{reg}} e \cdot \dot{x}_t) \dot{x} \tag{10}$$

Finally the stochastic part is added to form the complete fiber propagation model.

$$\dot{x}_t = \hat{e}_1(D_{\text{reg}}) + r_{proj}\beta = \tag{11}$$

$$\hat{e}_1(\hat{D} + \alpha \dot{x}_{t-1} \dot{x}_{t-1}^T) + r_{proj}\beta \tag{12}$$

In short, a stabilized propagation direction is calculated and a stochastic part is added. By using different values of α and β both the regularization of direction and the stochastic contribution can be varied.

Simulations on synthetic data are shown in figure 2 below. The tensors used in this tracking experiment were disturbed by noise and the overlayed grid is schematic. These simulations show the effect of choosing different values on alpha and beta. For realistic tracking, suitable values on alpha and beta should be estimated and validated.

4.2   Connections to SISR

The rough model presented above can be interpreted in the SISR framework, giving it meaning and further guide the search for a good fiber path model. The propagation step of the rough model is viewed as the sequential build-up presented in 3.3.

- The propagation step of the rough model can be interpreted as sampling from a trial distribution $q_t(x_t|X_{t-1}) = \pi(x_t|X_{t-1})$ and assuming that $\pi_t(X_{t-1}) = \pi_{t-1}(X_{t-1})$. In this way, the rough model fully describes fiber propagation and no further weighting is needed.

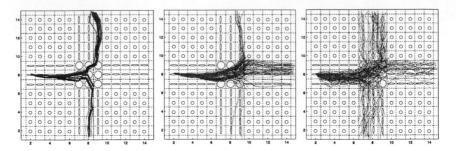

Fig. 2. Left: Normal eigentracking used as a reference (from multiple starting points). **Middle:** Tracking using a higher value of α, resulting in more regularized fiber paths. This supports propagation through spherical tensors. **Right:** Tractography using a higher value of β, achieving an increased stochastic spread and a representation of tracking uncertainty in fiber crossings.

- The rough model can be extended by assigning weights to paths by assuming $\pi_t(\mathbf{X}_{t-1}) \neq \pi_{t-1}(\mathbf{X}_{t-1})$. Still the conditional path propagation is considered to be fully described by the rough model propagation step as described above, but some compensation is done to for instance to punish some paths. One example is setting the weight to zero or close to zero for a fiber path entering or touching a forbidden area of the brain such as the ventricles.
- To make full use of the SISR framework the propagation step of the rough model should only be considered as the conditional trial distribution close to the real fiber path distribution. This is true importance sampling of the paths and the weight should be adjusted according to equation 4, compensating for the slightly incorrect conditional trial distribution $q_t(\mathbf{x}_t|\mathbf{X}_{t-1})$. This is the most general approach, giving a large freedom to choose a realistic fiber model by selecting the weight appropriately.

5   Results

The methods mentioned can be simulated using a sequential build-up or sequential sampling algorithm. To ensure a satisfying representation, as many as 100 000 samples (particles) were used.

A white matter mask was used to determine when the particles had reached the border between the white and the gray matter, i.e. when to stop the tracking. The mask was created using the EM-MFA segmentation method presented by Kapur et al. [9].

In figure 3 below, the paths of only 200 particles are shown. Notice that the visualized paths should be interpreted as a representation of the probability distribution for 'true' paths, and not as individual 'true' paths themselves.

6   Discussion

The method of Sequential Importance Sampling and Resampling has the ability of simulating rich fiber path models. It can take advantage of the full tensor data as opposed to

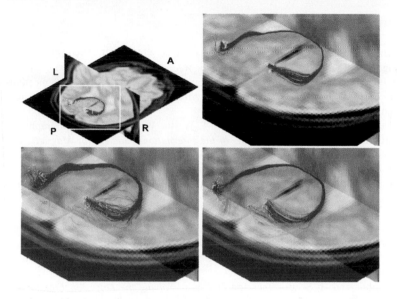

Fig. 3. Top left: Axial and coronal slices indicating the area of the brain where the white matter tractography was performed. **Top right:** Regularized stochastic tractography, showing one single starting point (at the center of corpus callosum) resulting in multiple end points. **Bottom left:** Tractography using a higher value of β, achieving an increased stochastic spread. **Bottom right:** Tracking using a higher value of α, resulting in more regularized fiber paths.

methods based solely on the principal diffusion direction. Though our proposed model depends heavily on the tensor as such, the SISR method is not dependent of the tensor representation. The SISR framework should be easy to adapt to more accurate diffusion measures in the future, a property it is expected to share with other Monte Carlo methods as well. A rich set of fiber models can be used and the theoretical framework provide means for approximately solving a well defined problem up to a chosen level of accuracy.

Despite using a simple model, it has been demonstrated how uncertainty can be taken into account during the tracking procedure. Using a Monte Carlo approach, the tracking paradigm has been extended from a one-to-one mapping to a one-to-many mapping, connecting one starting point to multiple end points in the brain. This could give a different and possibly better view of connectivity in the brain, taking branching of nerve fibers into account.

Acknowledgments

This work was supported by CIMIT and NIH grant P41-RR13218.

References

1. P.J. Basser, S. Pajevic, C. Pierpaoli, J. Duda and A. Aldroubi In Vivo Fiber Tractography Using DT-MRI Data *Magnetic Resonance in Medicine*, 44:625–632, 2000.
2. P.G. Batchelor, D.L.G. Hill, F. Calamante, and D. Atkinson Study of Connectivity in the Brain Using the Full Diffusion Tensor from MRI IPMI 2001, pp 121–133, Springer-Verlag Berlin Heidelberg, 2001.
3. A. Brun, M. Björnemo, R. Kikinis and C.-F. Westin White Matter Tractography Using Sequential Importance Sampling *Proc. of the International Society for Magnetic Resonance Medicine (ISMRM)*, Honolulu, Hawaii, USA, May 2002.
4. T.E. Conturo, N.F. Lori, T.S. Cull, E. Akbudak, A.Z. Snyder, J. S. Shimony, R. C. McKinstry, H. Burton and M. E. Raichle Tracking neuronal fiber pathways in the living human brain *Proceedings of the National Academy of Sciences of the United States of America*, 96:10422–10427, August, 1999.
5. Z. Ding, J. C. Gore and A. W. Anderson Tracking, Bundling and Quantitatively Characterizing in vivo Neuronal Fiber Pathways Using Diffusion Tensor Magnetic Resonance Imaging *Proc. of the International Society for Magnetic Resonance Medicine (ISMRM)*, 9:1530, Glasgow, Scotland, April 2001.
6. D. Gembris and H. Schumacher and D. Suter *Solving the Diffusion Equation for Fiber Tracking in the Living Human Brain Proc. of the International Society for Magnetic Resonance Medicine (ISMRM)*, 9:1529, Glasgow, Scotland, April 2001.
7. W.R. Gilks, S. Richardson and D.J. Spiegelhalter. *Markov Chain Monte Carlo in Practice*, Chapman & Hall, 1996.
8. Y. Iba Population Monte Carlo algorithms *Transactions of the Japanese Society for Artificial Intelligence*, 2:279:286, 2001.
9. T. Kapur, W.E.L. Grimson, W. M. Wells III and R. Kikinis Enhanced Spatial Priors for Segmentation of Magnetic Resonance Imagery *Proceedings of Second International Conference on Medical Image Computing and Computer-assisted Interventions (MICCAI)*, Cambridge MA, USA, October 1996.
10. J.S. Liu, R. Chen and T. Logvienko. A Theoretical Framework For Sequential Importance Sampling and Resampling *Sequential Monte Carlo Methods in Practice*, New York, 2001.
11. G.J.M. Parker, C.A.M. Wheeler-Kingshott, and G.J. Barker Distributed Anatomical Brain Connectivity Derived from Diffusion Tensor Imaging IPMI 2001, pp 106–120, Springer-Verlag Berlin Heidelberg, 2001.
12. C. Poupon, C.A. Clark, V. Frouin, J. Regis, I. Bloch, D. Le Bihan, and J.-F. Mangin Regularization of Diffusion-Based Direction Maps for the Tracking of Brain White Matter Fascicles NeuroImage, 12:184-195, 2000.
13. D.S. Tuch, M.R. Wiegell, T.G. Reese, J.W. Belliveau and V.J. Weeden Measuring Cortico-Cortical Connectivity Matrices with Diffusion Spectrum Imaging *Proc. of the International Society for Magnetic Resonance Medicine (ISMRM)*, 9:502, Glasgow, Scotland, April 2001.
14. C.-F. Westin, S. Peled, H. Gudbjartsson, R. Kikinis and F. A. Jolesz Geometrical Diffusion Measures for MRI from Tensor Basis Analysis *Proc. of the International Society for Magnetic Resonance Medicine (ISMRM)*, Vancouver Canada, April 1997.
15. C.-F. Westin, S. E. Maier, B. Khidir, P. Everett, F. A. Jolesz and R. Kikinis Image Processing for Diffusion Tensor Magnetic Resonance Imaging *Proceedings of Second International Conference on Medical Image Computing and Computer-assisted Interventions (MICCAI)*, 441–452, Cambridge, England, July 1999.
16. C.-F. Westin, S.E. Maier, H. Mamata, A. Nabavi, F.A. Jolesz, R. Kikinis R. Processing and Visualization for Diffusion Tensor MRI Medical Image Analysis, 6(2):93–108, 2002.

Sulcal Segmentation for Cortical Thickness Measurements

Chloe Hutton, Enrico De Vita, and Robert Turner

The Wellcome Department of Imaging Neuroscience, 12 Queen Square, ION, UCL, London
WC1N 3BG, UK
{chutton,edevita,rturner}@fil.ion.ucl.ac.uk
http://www.fil.ion.ucl.ac.uk

Abstract. Thickness of the cerebral cortex may provide valuable information about normal and abnormal neuroanatomy. For accurate cortical thickness measurements in brain MRI, precise segmentation of the grey matter border is necessary. In this paper we specifically address the problem of extracting the deep cortical folds or sulci, which can be difficult to resolve or totally obscured due to limited MRI resolution and contrast. We propose a method that iteratively solves Laplace's equation for adjacent sub-layers of the cortex. This approach preserves the laminar structure of the cortex and provides clear definition of deep sulci. The implementation is computationally efficient. We present inter-subject and intra-subject results that are consistent with the literature.

1   Introduction

The human cortex is comprised of a sheet of grey matter surrounding white matter. The thickness of the grey matter sheet is of great interest in studies of normal and abnormal neuroanatomy. Within individual brains cortical thickness varies from region to region, reflecting changes in the underlying cytoarchitecture. These changes relate to differences in cell types [1] and may also be associated with functionally distinct areas [2]. Although cortical thickness varies between individuals, abnormally thick or thin cortex may correlate with specific neuropathology and neurological conditions (e.g. [3, 4]) suggesting that thickness may be useful as a diagnostic tool.

Until recently, studies of cortical thickness have mostly involved postmortem measurements. With high resolution neuroanatomical MRI it is possible to make measurements *in vivo*. However, making these measurements manually necessitates displaying the brain as 2-D slices when in fact the cortex is a highly convoluted 3-D structure. Therefore accurate measurements of cortical thickness can only be made if the image plane is orthogonal to the cortical surface in the region of interest. As the direction of the cortical surface is constantly varying, manual measurements are susceptible to errors. Many methods have been proposed for segmenting brain MRI (e.g. [5]). In this paper we present a method that focuses on the segmentation of deep folds of grey matter (sulci) for the automated measurement of cortical thickness. Our approach divides the cortex into sub-layers of a specified thickness. We use Laplace's equation to calculate the thickness of adjacent layers and determine whether it is equal to the specified layer thickness. Sulci are identified where this equality breaks down. Our approach exploits the laminar structure of the cortex to segment sulci that

T. Dohi and R. Kikinis (Eds.): MICCAI 2002, LNCS 2488, pp. 443–450, 2002.
© Springer-Verlag Berlin Heidelberg 2002

cannot be identified in the MR image because of limited spatial resolution and contrast.

2   Issues Related to Measuring Cortical Thickness

A basic requirement for accurate brain morphometry is good quality, high contrast and resolution ($\leq 1\text{mm}^3$) MRI. For cortical thickness measurements, the finest details of interest are the deep sulci between folds of grey matter that are surrounded by cerebrospinal fluid (CSF). In T1-weighted images, most commonly used for neuro-anatomical investigations, grey and white matter have similar intensities so it is crucial to optimize the contrast between them for successful tissue segmentation [6]. CSF has a much lower intensity, but small CSF spaces can be difficult to resolve because of partial volume effects (where more than one tissue type co-exists in a voxel). The following sections highlight the main issues related to measuring cortical thickness.

Extraction of Grey Matter Boundaries: For measuring cortical thickness, the grey matter boundaries following deep sulcal folds must be accurately segmented. Methods have been proposed that fit deformable models to the cortical surface [7-10]. A disadvantage of such methods is the long processing times. Here, we present a computationally efficient method that extracts grey matter boundaries, segments deep sulci and calculates cortical thickness in less than an hour for 1mm resolution whole brain images.

Segmenting Deep Sulci: If the narrow CSF spaces between sulci are not well resolved, regions of cortex can become 'hidden' and thickness measurements can be overestimated as illustrated in figure 1. The deformable model methods in [8] and [9] address this 'hidden cortex' problem using topological constraints that explicitly prevent points on the same surfaces from coming too close together and points on opposing surfaces from being too far apart. The disadvantage of this approach is that the long processing times required for deformable model methods are further increased by these additional constraints. In [10], sulcal locations are estimated using image averaging and subtraction to amplify regions with high frequency changes. The resulting decrease in CSF intensity is then identified using 'thinning' routines.

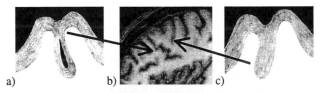

a)   b)   c)

Fig. 1. 'Hidden cortex' where cortical thickness may be overestimated. a) Incorrectly resolved banks of cortex. b) Examples of a) and c) on MRI. c) Incorrectly resolved bottom of sulcus

We address the 'hidden cortex' problem by modeling the cortical sheet as a series of adjacent sub-layers of a specified thickness. We then calculate the thickness of each sub-layer and compare it with the specified layer thickness. Sulcal locations are identified where the calculated thickness of a sub-layer is greater than the specified thickness. To calculate the thickness of each layer, we use the definition of thickness proposed in [10] and described in the following section.

Definition of Cortical Thickness as a Robust Metric: The thickness of the cortical sheet can be thought of as the distance between the two surfaces bordering the grey matter sheet. However, the cortical sheet is a highly folded three-dimensional structure with variable thickness so the definition of thickness as a metric must be carefully considered. For example, if thickness is defined as the straight-line distance between the two surfaces, this distance could be the perpendicular projection from one surface to the other (Fig. 2a) or the minimum distance from one surface to the other (Fig 2b). The problem with these straight-line definitions is that if the two surfaces are not parallel, the thickness will be different depending on which surface the measurement is made from (as illustrated in Figures 2a and b). We therefore use the non-straight line definition of thickness outlined in [10]. This approach models the cortex as a series of nested sub-layers that are bounded by the inner and outer grey matter surfaces. The thickness at any point in the cortex is calculated by integrating along the direction perpendicular to each sub-layer between the two surfaces.

The sub-layers are modeled by assigning different boundary conditions to the two surfaces and solving Laplace's equation at each point between them. Laplace's equation is a second order partial differential equation for a scalar field Ψ that can be enclosed between two boundaries and has the following form:

$$\nabla^2\Psi = \frac{\partial^2\Psi}{\partial x^2} + \frac{\partial^2\Psi}{\partial y^2} + \frac{\partial^2\Psi}{\partial z^2} = 0. \tag{1}$$

Equation 1 can be solved iteratively using a standard relaxation method such as the one described in [10]. The resulting scalar field makes a smooth transition from one surface to the other describing the nested sub-layers (dashed lines in Fig. 2c). The perpendicular direction of each point in each sub-layer is determined by calculating the gradients of the scalar field which are normalized to produce a tangential vector field (solid lines with arrows in Fig. 2c). Integrating along the direction of the tangential vector field at any point in the cortex provides the cortical thickness.

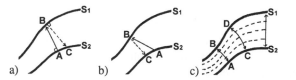

Fig. 2. Definitions of thickness between surfaces S_1 and S_2. a) The perpendicular projection from A to B $\neq$ B to C. b) The minimum distance from A to B $\neq$ B to C. c) Thickness defined using Laplace's equation (solid lines) from A to B and C to D

3   Sulcal Segmentation and Cortical Thickness Measurement

3.1   Tissue Segmentation and Preparation of Grey Matter Boundaries

Initial tissue segmentation is carried out using the method implemented in SPM'99 [11], which combines tissue classification with correction for image inhomogeneities. For this work, the segmentation procedure was adapted to include a cutting plane through the brain stem separating cortical white matter from the cerebellum. The resulting probability maps of CSF, grey and white matter plus the cutting plane (matched with the image) are used in the following steps: **1) Label white matter** when white matter probability is greater than that for grey matter. A 'connected component' analysis determines the final map of cortical white matter voxels (separated from the brain stem using the cutting plane). **2) Label grey matter** when grey matter probability is greater than that for CSF. The largest grey matter connected component is selected as the initial map of grey matter voxels.

3.2   Segmentation of Sulci

Next, we must identify sulcal spaces that were incorrectly labeled as grey matter in the previous step. We do this by successively adding grey matter layers of an arbitrarily specified thickness to surround the white matter (Fig. 3a-b). Using Laplace's equation we calculate vector normals and thickness for the sub-layer. Voxels for which the calculated thickness is greater than the specified thickness are identified as belonging to sulci because they must be in contact with grey matter voxels within the same layer but from an opposing sulcal bank (Fig. 3c).

The initial grey matter map also includes the cerebellum and some extra-cortical tissue attached to cortical grey matter. We must therefore determine the limits of the cortical grey matter using image intensity (which is low for CSF) and intensity gradient information (high at the grey matter CSF boundary). This border prevents grey matter layers from going beyond the cortex.

The processing steps are illustrated in Fig. 3. and described below.

Repeat the following steps while there are voxels to process within the grey matter limits:
1: Add a layer of grey matter of specified thickness T to surround previous layer. **1st layer:** add layer to white matter in direction of pre-computed normals of white matter surface (Fig 3a). **Nth layer:** add layer to previous layer in direction of normals of previous layer (Fig 3b).
2: Solve Laplace's equation for layer to determine the normal direction of each voxel.
3: Calculate the thickness at each voxel. Label voxels with a thickness > T as sulci (Fig 3c).

Sulcal voxels must be connected to the CSF voxels outside the cortex so that the grey matter sheet is bounded by two complete surfaces. This is achieved with the following morphological operations:

1: Combine CSF voxels with sulcal voxels and dilate the result.
2: Find the largest connected component of dilated CSF+sulci map (resulting from step 1).
3: Erode the CSF-sulci connected component.
4: Find largest connected component of the eroded CSF+sulci = final CSF+sulci (Fig 3d).

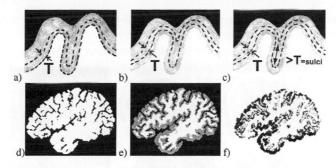

Fig. 3. Sulcal segmentation. a) **1st layer:** add layer (dashed lines) of grey matter, thickness T to white matter. b) **Nth layer:** add layer (dashed lines) of grey matter, thickness T to previous layer. c) Label voxels with thickness > T as sulci. d) Map of CSF and sulci. e) Grey matter borders f) Averaged thickness map (darker = greater thickness)

The final grey matter CSF border that includes the sulci (Fig 3d) is combined with the white matter surface so that two complete boundaries surround the grey matter (Fig 3e). Laplace's equation is solved for the resulting surfaces and the cortical thickness at each point is calculated using integration as described in [10] (Fig. 3f).

In this work we have used an arbitrary thickness of T=1 mm, a 1mm sampling size for solving Laplace's equation and for calculating thickness. However, using interpolation, the method can be adapted to use sub-voxel thickness and image sampling sizes. Averaged cortical thickness maps are calculated by replacing each thickness value with the mean of the thicknesses along each path between the two surfaces.

3.3   Implementation and Image Acquisition

The routines described above are implemented in Matlab 5 [12]. Using a pseudo-parallel implementation, a full volumetric image of the brain can be processed in less than an hour on a standard desktop computer. Anatomical MRI of 1mm^3 resolution were acquired on a Siemens Vision 2T scanner with an MP-RAGE sequence optimised for grey and white matter contrast and minimal inhomogeneities [6].

4   Results

We applied the above methods to MR brain volumes of 3 subjects. For subject 1, 3 volumes were acquired during different scanning sessions. We calculated averaged cortical thickness maps and thickness histograms for each subject with and without sulcal segmentation. For subject 1, we matched the 3 images together using SPM'99, applied the resulting transformations to the thickness maps then calculated the mean and standard deviation of the averaged thickness maps. We generated isosurface renderings of the final thickness maps using Matlab 6 [12].

Identification of Deep Sulci. Figure 4 shows a slice from each of the three subjects with the border between grey matter and CSF overlaid in black. The grey scale of the images has been inverted and the borders thickened to improve visualization of the results. The original images are shown in the right column. The grey matter CSF border without sulcal segmentation is shown in the left column and with sulcal segmentation in the middle column. The figure clearly shows that many sulci, especially deep ones are only detected using the sulcal segmentation method.

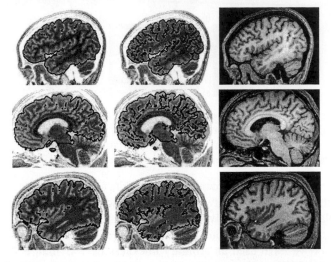

Fig. 4. Example slices from each subject overlaid with grey matter-CSF border without (left column) or with (middle column) sulcal segmentation. Original images shown in right column

Histograms of Averaged Cortical Thickness Maps. Figure 5 shows the histograms of averaged cortical thickness maps for each brain volume (3 for subject 1 and 1 each for subjects 2 and 3). With sulcal segmentation (solid lines), all of the histograms show a peak between 2-3 mm, which is consistent with results in the literature [7-10]. The within subject results (Fig. 5a) show good agreement with each other. The literature states that cortical thickness measures up to 5mm, but our histograms show some values greater than this. We attribute these large values to sub-cortical grey matter structures. Without sulcal segmentation (dashed lines in Fig 5), thickness values are significantly greater.

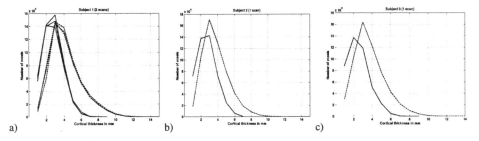

Fig. 5. Histograms of whole brain cortical thickness measurements (in mm) for three subjects (a-c), with (solid lines) and without (dashed lines) sulcal segmentation. Subject 1 (a) has 3 sets of results

Surface Rendering of Cortical Thickness Maps. Figure 6 shows surface renderings of the averaged cortical thickness maps for the left and right hemisphere of each subject. Regions where the surface renderings show thinner cortex (darker areas) corre-spond to regions of the brain where the cortex is known to be thinner [2]. This can be seen clearly at the back of the brain (occipital lobe) in all subjects and in the top cen-tral part of the brain (central sulcus) in the first and third subjects. The standard de-viation of the thickness maps calculated for subject 1 (Fig. 6b) is less than 1mm and tends to be larger where the cortex is wider. It must be noted that the standard devia-tion also includes any small errors that arise from matching the images.

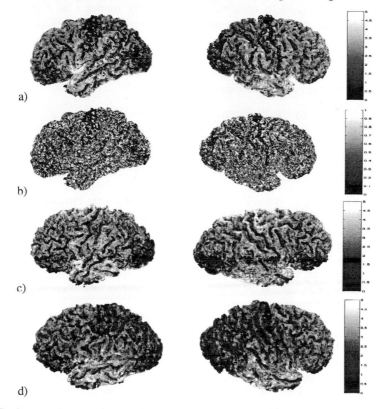

Fig. 6. Surface renderings of averaged cortical thickness maps. a) Mean of 3 coregistered aver-aged thickness maps for subject 1. b) Standard deviation of 3 coregistered averaged thickness maps for subject 1. c) and d) Averaged thickness maps for subjects 2 and 3. The shading of each surface represents the local thickness in mm corresponding to the grey scale bar. For visualization purposes, the renderings have been thresholded at a thickness of 5 mm to give an optimal intensity range

5   Summary and Conclusions

We present a method to segment deep sulci for cortical thickness measurements. The method divides the cortex into sub-layers and uses the sub-layer thicknesses to de-termine the location of sulci. Laplace's equation is solved for each sub-layer to cor-rectly determine its thickness. Our results are consistent with the literature and also show good agreement within subject.

Our approach for segmenting sulci can be considered as an automatic feature detection method that exploits the laminar structure of the cortex. In this context, our method could also provide efficient feature detection based on the underlying neuroanatomy for deformable surface models.

In this work have used the original MRI resolution of 1mm for all processing steps. However, using interpolation, our methods can be adapted to use a smaller sampling size with the disadvantage of increased processing times. The robustness of the morphological operations used to construct the final grey matter CSF border and the accuracy of the thickness measurements may be dependent on this sampling size. Therefore a full analysis of the errors related to the sampling resolution is required. This is a topic of our current work, as well as a more extensive validation using a larger number of subjects, regional analyses of cortical thickness and comparison with results using a previously published method.

This work was funded by the Wellcome Trust, London, UK.

References

1. Geyer, S., Schleicher, A., Zilles, K.: Areas 3a, 3b, and 1 of Human Primary Somatosensory Cortex 1. Neuroimage 10 (1999) 63-83.
2. Meyer, J.R., Roychowdhury, S., Russell, E.J., Callahan, C., Gitelman, D., Mesulam, M.M.: Location of the central sulcus via cortical thickness of the precentral and postcentral gyri on MR. *AJNR Am J Neuroradiol.* 17 (1996) 1699-706.
3. Rusinek, H., de Leon, M.J., George, A.E., Stylopoulos, L.A., Chandra, R., Smith, G., Rand, T., Mourino, M., Kowalski, H. Alzheimer disease: measuring loss of cerebral gray matter with MR imaging *Radiology* 178 (1991) 109-114.
4. Terry, R.D., Peck, A., DeTeresa, R., Schecter, R., Horoupian, D.S.: Some morphometric aspects of the brain senile dementia of the Alzheimer type. *An.of Neuro.*10(1981)184-192.
5. Stokking, R., Vincken, K.L., Viergever, M.A.: Automatic morphology-based brain segmentation (mbrase) from mri-T1 data. *Neuroimage* 12 (2000) 726-738.
6. Deichmann, R., Good, C.D., Josephs, O., Ashburner, J., Turner, R.: Optimization of 3-D MP-RAGE sequences for structural brain imaging. *NeuroImage* 12 (2000) 112-127.
7. Kruggel, F., Yves-von-Cramon, D.:Measuring the cortical thickness [MRI segmentation procedure] Proceedings IEEE Workshop on Mathematical Methods in Biomedical Image Analysis. IEEE Comput. Soc, Los Alamitos, CA, USA; (2000) 154-61.
8. MacDonald, D., Kabani, N., Avis, D., Evans, A.C.: Automated 3-D extraction of inner and outer surfaces of cerebral cortex from MRI. *Neuroimage* 12 (2000) 340-356.
9. Fischl, B., Dale, A..M.:Measuring the thickness of the human cerebral cortex from magnetic resonance images. *Proc Natl Acad Sci U S A.* 97 (2000) 11050-5.
10. Jones, S.E., Buchbinder, B.R., Aharon, I.: Three-Dimensional Mapping of Cortical Thickness Using Laplace's Equation. *Human Brain Mapping* 11 (2000) 12-32.
11. Ashburner, J., Friston, K.: Multimodal Image Coregistration and Partitioning-A Unified Framework. *Neuroimage* 6 (1997) 209-217.
12. Matlab 5 and Matlab 6 Copyright 1984-2000 The MathWorks, Inc. Natick, MA, USA.

Labeling the Brain Surface
Using a Deformable Multiresolution Mesh

Sylvain Jaume[1], Benoît Macq[2], and Simon K. Warfield[3]

[1] Multiresolution Modeling Group, California Institute of Technology, 256-80,
1200 E. California Blvd, Pasadena, CA 91125, USA, jaume@caltech.edu
[2] Telecommunications and Remote Sensing Lab, Université catholique de Louvain,
Place du Levant, 2, 1348 Louvain-la-Neuve, Belgium
[3] Surgical Planning Laboratory, Brigham and Women's Hospital,
Harvard Medical School, 75 Francis St, Boston, MA 02115, USA

Abstract. We propose to match a labeled mesh onto the patient brain surface in a multiresolution way for labeling the patient brain. Labeling the patient brain surface provides a map of the brain folds where the neuroradiologist and the neurosurgeon can easily track the features of interest. Due to the complexity of the cortical surface, this task usually depends on the intervention of an expert, and is time-consuming. Our multiresolution representation for the brain surface allows the automated classification of the folds based on their size. The atlas mesh is deformed from coarse to fine to robustly capture the patient brain folds from the largest to the smallest. Once the atlas mesh matches the patient mesh, the atlas labels are transferred to the patient mesh, and color coded for visualization.

Keywords: cortex labeling, cortical surface, sulci and gyri, brain segmentation, brain atlas, multiresolution mesh, progressive mesh.

1   Introduction

To diagnose a neural disorder or to preserve the main functions of the patient during a brain operation, the neuroradiologist and the neurosurgeon need to locate regions of interest relative to the folds *(sulci and gyri)* on the patient brain. Some software have been developed to ease the labeling of sulci in the patient brain scan. Since the brain geometry exhibits a high complexity and a high inter-patient variability, the labeling software usually requires the input from an expert. Unfortunately the required manual intervention makes the labeling both time-consuming and operator-dependent. Automated labeling of the sulci and gyri of the brain would be a significant aid in studying brain structure and function, with clinical applications ranging from surgical planning to the study of structural changes associated with brain disorders.

First we review some methods for automating the labeling of the cortex. At the end of this section, we briefly present our contribution and the outline of the paper.

T. Dohi and R. Kikinis (Eds.): MICCAI 2002, LNCS 2488, pp. 451–458, 2002.
© Springer-Verlag Berlin Heidelberg 2002

1.1   Related Work

Sandor et al. [1] elastically deform a reference labeled brain volume *(brain atlas)* to fit the patient brain scan. Mathematical morphology and edge detection operations convert the patient scan to a smooth representation the deformable surface can easily match. The brain atlas is parameterized with B-spline surfaces and is deformed under an energy minimization scheme. The energy attracts the atlas fold points to fold points on the patient image, and the remaining points to the patient brain surface. Finally atlas labels are transfered to the patient brain surface. However, due to the low resolution in regions of the brain scan *(partial volume effect)*, the morphological processing can accidentally disconnect or erase brain folds on the patient image. Consequently the deformable surface might be unable to capture the disconnected brain folds.

Lancaster et al. [2] use axis aligned coordinates to retrieve brain labels from the Tailarach atlas. They hierarchically subdivide the large atlas structures into substructures. For instance, the cerebrum is subdivided into lobes and sublobar structures, which are then subdivided into smaller structures. The Tailarach coordinates are addressed in a volumetric image synthesized from the Tailarach atlas. Some rules guide the segmentation and labeling of 160 contiguous regions. They compare their automated labeling with manual labeling [3] and show 70% or greater label match on 250 functional MRI scans.

Le Goualher et al. [4] extract surface ribbons that represent the median axis of the sulci for interactive sulci labeling. They build a graph where the nodes define the sulci with some geometric and anatomical attributes, and the arcs define the connections between the sulci. For every node, the expected spatial distribution of the sulci is computed and the most likely labels are returned to the operator. Then the operator needs to pick the correct label and associate it to the node. This scheme eases the task of the expert, but still requires some intervention from the user.

Lohmann et al. [5] segments the patient brain scan with a region growing method. The segmented regions, called *sulcal basins*, represent substructures of the brain folds. A point distribution model is used to match an atlas model onto the patient brain, and to label the sulcal basins. Since the geometric difference between the atlas and the patient brain can be high, the point distribution model can accidentally match an atlas sulcus to the wrong sulcus on the patient anatomy.

Hellier et al. [6] extract the sulci with an active ribbon method. Using a non-rigid registration, brain images from different subjects are matched to minimize the sum of the distances between corresponding sulci. The authors demonstrate that their scheme accurately matches six brain labels. However, it was not shown that small sulci can robustly be segmented and labeled with their non-rigid registration method.

Rivière et al. [7] use a graph representation of the brain folds similar to Le Goualher and match a graph with labels to the graph of the patient brain. For every brain fold, i.e. a node in the graph, the likelihood of assigning a particular label is computed from geometric measures and the connectivity to neighboring

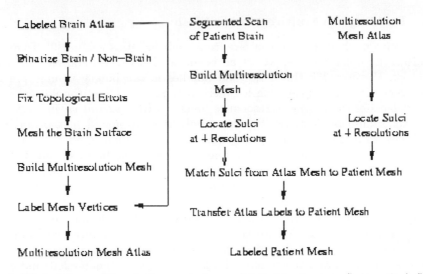

Fig. 1. We build a multiresolution mesh from a labeled brain scan *(brain atlas) (left)*. We build a similar structure for the patient mesh and detect the folds at 4 resolutions for both meshes. Then we deform the labeled mesh onto the patient mesh to match folds of similar sizes. Finally we transfer the labels to the patient mesh. *(right)*

folds. Then a matching method based on neural networks minimizes a combination of the likelihoods.

Cachier et al. [8] show that combining the previous method with feature point matching improves the registration of brain scans. They register differently the bottom line of the sulci from the upper line of the gyri, since the localization of the latter exhibits higher inter-subject variability.

1.2   Our Contribution

We propose to progressively match an atlas labeled mesh to the patient brain mesh from the largest folds to the smallest folds. Then we transfer the labels from the matched mesh to label the patient mesh without manual intervention.

2   Algorithm

First we build a multiresolution mesh of the brain surface from a reference labeled brain scan *(atlas)*. Every mesh vertex is assigned the closest label in the atlas. Then we apply some geometric operations to the multiresolution mesh to extract and classify the brain folds according to their size. Finally we match the labeled mesh onto the patient mesh and transfer the labels to the patient anatomy. To extract a surface mesh from the patient brain scan, brain tissues and non-brain tissues must be classified before the application of our algorithm. Fig 1 illustrates the steps to build a multiresolution mesh from a segmented brain scan on the left diagram. The right diagram shows the automated labeling of a patient brain mesh.

2.1 Building the Multiresolution Mesh

We create a mesh of the brain surface from a labeled atlas volume [9]. To extract a surface from the volume, we set all brain labels to white and the remaining to black. However 366 tiny holes and handles in the binary volume prevents to extract a brain surface with a spherical topology. These topological errors are artifacts of the magnetic resonance image (MRI) *(partial volume effect)* or local voxel misclassifications. We thus apply the automated method of Wood et al. [10] to remove the holes and handles with minimal modification to the binary volume. Then we generate a triangle mesh of the brain surface with the Marching Cubes [11]. Finally we associate to every mesh vertex the label of the closest structure in the atlas. The brain mesh with 35 labels is shown in Fig 2 *(left)*.

Now we build a multiresolution representation of the brain mesh to enable geometric manipulations. We use the *Progressive Mesh* structure that Hoppe [12] introduced as a sequence of vertices that progressively refines a coarse mesh. Fig 2 shows a coarse brain mesh and a refined mesh in the center left and center right images respectively. Combining the mesh hierarchy of Guskov et al. [13] and the local operator of Desbrun et al. [14], we encode for every vertex in the sequence the difference its insertion makes to the local mesh geometry. We can perform various geometric operations on the brain surface, such as smoothing and matching.

The first three images in Fig 2 shows that the multiresolution labeled mesh can be represented at various resolutions. The fine geometric information is encoded based on larger structures. This hierarchical representation will help to match the labeled mesh onto a patient brain mesh, such as the mesh shown in the fourth image.

2.2 Extracting the Sulci

We smooth the brain surface at four resolutions. The regions where the geometry significantly changes from the previous resolution define brain folds with similar sizes. We thus classify the brain folds into four size categories. Fig 3 show the brain folds classification for the reference mesh in the first row, and for a patient brain mesh in the second row. The largest folds *(light blue)* appear at the smoothest resolution, and progressively smaller folds *(green, yellow ang red respectively)*, appear on the successive representations. The regions without significant geometric difference between two representations the remaining brain surface *(dark blue)*.

2.3 Matching the Labeled Mesh onto the Patient Mesh

We take advantage of the multiresolution mesh representation and the classification of the brain folds to constrain the matching from the atlas mesh to the target mesh. A coarse to fine matching first allows large surface deformations and then more subtle deformations. We also use our fold classification as a constraint: large folds on the atlas must match large folds on the patient brain, and similarly for the small folds. We repeatedly move every vertex of the deformable mesh along its local normal to the closest intersection with the surface of the patient mesh. The last row of Fig 3 illustrates the multiresolution matching of the labeled mesh *(first row)* onto the patient mesh *(second row)*. From left to right, the matching evolves from a smooth representation to the original representation. First the smoothest representations are registered to match the center fold *(light blue)*. As smaller brain folds are introduced on the successive representations, they are matched onto the patient surface *(green, yellow, and red)*. The final match captures the brain folds on the original patient mesh.

3   Results and Discussion

We matched the labeled mesh for nine cases with a brain tumor. The tumor deforms the patient brain anatomy. The pathological deformation adds to the inter-subject variability and makes the matching of the atlas mesh to the patient mesh even more difficult. After atlas matching, we transfer and color code the atlas labels onto the patient mesh. Fig 4 shows the nine patient meshes after labeling. Visualization of the labels indicates that the multiresolution matching accurately captures the patient brain folds despite the high difference from the atlas geometry. It took less than 8 minutes on a Pentium 4 2GHz to automatically label a new patient scan. This makes the software suitable as a clinical aid. Future validations will compare our automated labeling with manually labeled data, quantify the accuracy of our method.

4   Conclusion

We match the labeled surface of a brain atlas to the patient anatomy from the largest folds to the smallest folds. A multiresolution mesh built for every brain scan allows the classification of the folds based on their size. To robustly match the atlas mesh, we first match the largest folds, and progressively match the smaller folds. Once the atlas mesh fits the smallest patient folds, the atlas labels are transfered to the patient mesh. The multiresolution matching provides the neurologist with a map of the patient brain in a short time and with no intervention. We ran our method to automatically label nine brain scans with a significant pathological deformation. Visualization of the labeled patient meshes indicates that the labels closely match the folds on the patient anatomy.

Acknowledgements: Special thanks to Zoë Wood for running her algorithm on every case, Peter Schröder and Mathieu Desbrun for insightful discussions, and Christopher Malek for making this research possible. Thanks to Ron Kikinis, Martha Shenton, Robert McCarley, and Ferenc Jolesz for sharing the atlas volume. Sylvain Jaume is working towards a Ph.D. degree with awards from FRIA and FNRS (Belgian Science Foundation). This investigation was supported by NIH grants P41 RR13218, P01 CA67165, R01 RR11747, R01 CA86879, by a research grant from the Whitaker Foundation, and by a New Concept Award from the Center for Integration of Medicine and Innovative Technology.

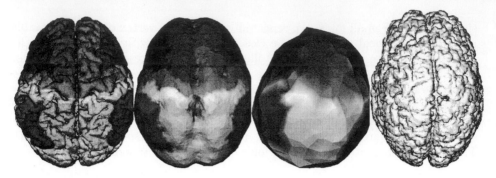

Fig. 2. We label a surface mesh from a labeled brain scan *(left)* and represent it in multiresolution *(center left and center right)*. The multiresolution representation allows the matching of the labeled mesh onto a patient brain mesh *(right)*.

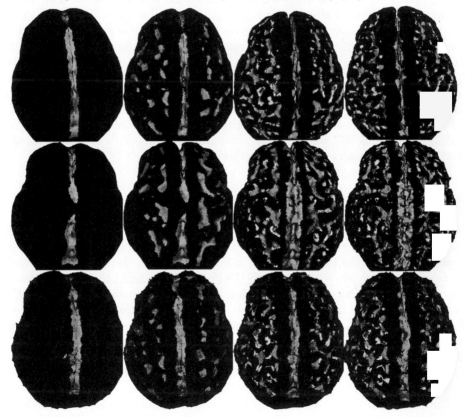

Fig. 3. The multiresolution representation of the cortex allows to distinguish the large sulci from the the small sulci. The first structure to appear is the fold between the hemispheres *(light blue)*. The remaining brain surface is colored in *dark blue*. Then the sulci appear from the largest to the smallest *(respectively green, yellow, and red)*. In the second row, we perform the sulci classification on a mesh of the patient brain. In the third row, the multiresolution mesh is progressively deformed to match the corresponding folds on the patient mesh.

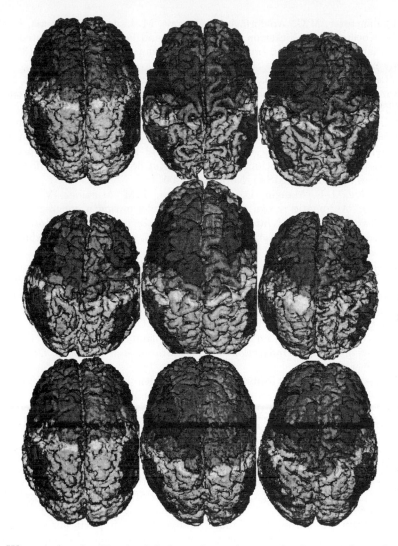

Fig. 4. We transfer the 35 atlas labels to the patient mesh after matching the atlas mesh onto nine cases. The nine cases were thus labeled without manual intervention. The visualization of the labels with color coding indicates that the labels accurately match the patient brain geometry.

References

1. S. Sandor and R. Leahy. Surface-based labeling of cortical anatomy using a deformable atlas. *IEEE Transactions on Medical Imaging*, 16(1):41–54, February 1997.
2. J.L. Lancaster, L.H. Rainey, J.L. Summerlin, C.S. Freitas, P.T. Fox, A.C. Evans, A.W. Toga, and J.C. Mazziotta. Automated labeling of the human brain: a preliminary report on the development and evaluation of a forward-transform method. *Human Brain Mapping*, 5(4):238–242, 1997.

 3. J.L. Lancaster, M.G. Woldorff, L.M. Parsons, M. Liotti, C.S. Freitas, L. Rainey, P.V. Kochunov, D. Nickerson, S.A. Mikiten, and Fox P.T. Automated tailarach atlas labels for functional brain mapping. *Human Brain Mapping*, 10(3):120–131, July 2000.
 4. G. Le Goualher, E. Procyk, D.L. Collins, R. Venugopal, G., C. Barillot, and A.C. Evans. Automated extraction and variability analysis of sulcal neuroanatomy. *IEEE Transactions on Medical Imaging*, 18(3):206–217, March 1999.
 5. G. Lohmann and D.Y. von Cramon. Automatic labelling of the human cortical surface using sulcal basins. *Medical Image Analysis*, 4(3):179–188, September 2000.
 6. P. Hellier and Barillot C. Coupling dense and landmark-based approaches for non rigid registration. Technical report, Institut de Recherche en Informatique et Systèmes Aléatoires (IRISA), November 2000.
 7. D. Rivière, J.-F. Mangin, D. Papadopoulos, J.-M. Martinez, V. Frouin, and J. Régis. Automatic recognition of cortical sulci unisng a congregation of neural networks. In *Third International Conference on Medical Robotics, Imaging and Computer Assisted Surgery - MICCAI 2000*, pages 40–49, Pittsburgh, USA, October 11-14 2000.
 8. P. Cachier, J.-F. Mangin, X. Pennec, D. Rivière, D. Papadopoulos-Orfanos, J. Régis, and N. Ayache. Multisubject non-rigid registration of brain mri using intensity and geometric features. In *Fourth International Conference on Medical Image Computing and Computer-Assisted Intervention - MICCAI 2001*, volume 2208, pages 734–742, Utrecht, The Netherlands, October 14-17 2001.
 9. Kikinis et al. A digital brain atlas for surgical planning model driven segmentation and teaching. *IEEE Transactions on Visualization and Computer Graphics*, 2(3), September 1996.
10. Z. Wood, H. Hoppe, M. Desbrun, and P. Schröder. Isosurface topology simplification. *ACM Transactions on Graphics*, 2002. submitted.
11. W.E. Lorensen and H.E. Cline. Marching cubes: a high resolution 3D surface construction algorithm. In *Proceedings of Computer Graphics SIGGRAPH*, pages 163–169, Anaheim, USA, July 1987.
12. H. Hoppe. Progressive meshes. In *Proceedings of Computer Graphics SIGGRAPH*, New Orleans, USA, August 4-9 1996.
13. I. Guskov, W. Sweldens, and P. Schröder. Multiresolution signal processing for meshes. In *Proceedings of Computer Graphics SIGGRAPH*, Los Angeles, USA, August 8-13 1999.
14. M. Desbrun, M. Meyer, P. Schröder, and A. Barr. Implicit fairing of irregular meshes using diffusion and curvature flow. In *Proceedings of Computer Graphics SIGGRAPH*, Los Angeles, USA, August 8-13 1999.

New Approaches to Estimation of White Matter Connectivity in Diffusion Tensor MRI: Elliptic PDEs and Geodesics in a Tensor-Warped Space

Lauren O'Donnell[1], Steven Haker[2], and Carl-Fredrik Westin[1,2]

[1] MIT AI Laboratory, Cambridge MA 02139, USA
odonnell@ai.mit.edu
[2] Laboratory of Mathematics in Imaging, Brigham and Women's Hospital, Harvard
Medical School, Boston MA, USA
{haker,westin}@bwh.harvard.edu

Abstract. We investigate new approaches to quantifying the white matter connectivity in the brain using Diffusion Tensor Magnetic Resonance Imaging data. Our first approach finds a steady-state concentra-
tion/heat distribution using the three-dimensional tensor field as diffu-
sion/conductivity tensors. Our second approach casts the problem in a
Riemannian framework, deriving from each tensor a local warping of
space, and finding geodesic paths in the space. Both approaches use the
information from the whole tensor, and can provide numerical measures
of connectivity.

1 Background

Diffusion Tensor Magnetic Resonance Imaging (DT-MRI) measures the self-
diffusion of water in biological tissue. The utility of this method stems from the
fact that tissue structure locally affects the Brownian motion of water molecules.
Consequently, a coherent organization of tissue (over scales comparable to that
of a voxel) will be reflected in the DT-MRI diffusion measurements.

Neural fiber tracts contain parallel axons whose membranes restrict diffusion,
so the self-diffusion of water is most probable along the tracts. Thus in DT-MRI
imagery of the brain, the local structure of the diffusion tensor can be treated
as an approximation to the local neural fiber structure. The diffusion tensor is
a low-pass, Gaussian approximation to the actual microscopic structure of the
neuroanatomy, but it provides a fast and non-invasive anatomical measurement.

In DT-MRI, the diffusion tensor field is calculated from a set of diffusion-
weighted images by solving the Stejskal-Tanner equation (eq. 1). This equation
describes how the signal intensity at each voxel decreases in the presence of
diffusion:

$$S_k = S_0 e^{-b \hat{g}_k^T D \hat{g}_k}. \tag{1}$$

Here S_0 is the non-diffusion-weighted image intensity at the voxel and S_k
is the intensity measured after the application of the kth diffusion-sensitizing

T. Dohi and R. Kikinis (Eds.): MICCAI 2002, LNCS 2488, pp. 459–466, 2002.

gradient. $\hat{g}_k$ is a unit vector representing the direction of this diffusion-sensitizing gradient, and D is the diffusion tensor, so the product $\hat{g}_k^T D \hat{g}_k$ represents the diffusivity in direction $\hat{g}_k$. In addition, b is LeBihan's factor describing the pulse sequence, gradient strength, and physical constants [1].

There is a physical interpretation of the diffusion tensor, D, which is closely tied to the standard ellipsoid tensor visualization scheme. The eigensystem of the diffusion tensor describes an ellipsoidal isoprobability surface, where the axes of the ellipsoid have lengths given by the square root of the tensor's eigenvalues. A proton which is initially located at the origin of the voxel has equal probability of diffusing to all points on the ellipsoid.

Initial work on DT-MRI connectivity focused on tractography [8, 2, 1], or the interpolation of paths through the principal eigenvector field. An extension of this method evolved a surface through the field using a discretized fast marching method, where the speed function was dependent on the principal eigenvector field [7]. Another approach iteratively simulated diffusion in a 2D tensor volume, and quantified connection strengths based on a probabilistic interpretation of the arrival time of the diffusion front [3]. The tractography approach has also been extended to much higher angular resolution diffusion data, and connectivity has been estimated using the most probable path between points [10].

Our first approach finds a steady-state concentration/heat distribution using the three-dimensional tensor field as diffusion/conductivity tensors. The steady-state flow along any path reflects connectivity. Our second approach casts the problem in a Riemannian framework, deriving from each tensor a local warping of space, and finding geodesic paths in the space. In this method, path lengths are related to connectivity. Both approaches use the information from the whole tensor, and can provide numerical measures of connectivity.

2   Diffusion Theory

Fick's first law relates a concentration difference to a flux (a flow across a unit area). It states that the flux, j, in any direction is proportional to the concentration gradient, ∇u, in the opposite direction. The proportionality constant d is the diffusivity in the direction of interest.

$$j = -d\nabla u. \tag{2}$$

For an anisotropic material, the flow field does not follow the concentration gradient directly, since the material properties also affect diffusion. Consequently, the diffusion tensor, D, is introduced to model the material locally.

$$j = -D\nabla u. \tag{3}$$

The standard model of diffusion says that over time, the concentration of the solute will change as the divergence of the flux:

$$u_t = \nabla \cdot (D\nabla u). \tag{4}$$

This is due to conservation of mass. Intuitively it means that, for example, fluid flow outward from a point (divergence) should decrease the concentration at that point while increasing the concentration at neighboring points. In the steady state, the concentration does not change; consequently the steady-state flux vector field is divergence-free.

3 PDE-Based Connectivity

Previous work has employed an iterative technique to create time-of-arrival maps of a heat diffusion front [3]. Instead, we solve directly for the steady state concentration, u, which can also be thought of as a heat distribution in the tensor field:

$$\nabla \cdot (D\nabla u) = 0. \tag{5}$$

We use this information to create the flux vector field, $j = -D\nabla u$, which describes the steady-state heat flow in the tensor volume (eq. 3). Paths in this divergence-free vector field can be compared using a connection strength metric that approximates the total flow along the path:

$$\int_P |j^T t| \, ds \tag{6}$$

where j is the flux along the path, and t is the unit tangent to the path. Normalization for the length of the path may also be included in the metric. To obtain an overall connection strength measure between two points, the value of the maximum flow path can be taken.

Of great interest in this method are the boundary conditions, or the locations of sources and sinks in the tensor field. One possibility is to set a region or regions of interest as the source, and simulate a sink at infinity. Another useful possibility is to choose one region of interest as the source, and another as the sink. In the experiments discussed in this paper, we have simulated a sink at one point of interest, and a source at another, in order to estimate the flow between the regions.

3.1 Experiments

DT-MRI Data Acquisition. DT-MRI scans of normal subjects were acquired using Line Scan Diffusion Imaging [6] on a 1.5 Tesla GE Echospeed system. The following scan parameters were used: rectangular 22 cm FOV (256x128 image matrix, 0.86 mm by 1.72 mm in-plane pixel size); slice thickness = 4 mm; interslice distance = 1 mm; receiver bandwidth = +/-6 kHz; TE = 70 ms; TR = 80 ms (effective TR = 2500 ms); scan time = 60 seconds/section. 20 axial slices were acquired, covering the entire brain. This protocol provides diffusion data in 6 gradient directions as well as the corresponding T2-weighted image. All gradients and T2-weighted images are acquired simultaneously, and thus do not need any rigid registration prior to the tensor reconstruction process. Tensors are reconstructed as described in [12] and eigenvalues are computed.

Tensor Preprocessing. We are interested in measuring connectivity in the white matter, and consequently, to de-emphasize other regions, we multiply the tensors by a soft mask. This is necessary to decrease the effect of the ventricles, where neural fiber tracts are nonexistent but water diffusion is relatively unrestricted and has large magnitude. We calculate the weights in the mask as the linear shape measure at each voxel, which lies in the range of zero to one [11, 12]

$$c_l = \frac{\lambda_1 - \lambda_2}{\lambda_1}. \tag{7}$$

In addition, we remove negative eigenvalues to ensure that each tensor is a positive definite matrix. We set a small positive lower bound for the eigenvalues to guarantee that the tensors are invertible, which is necessary when utilizing them as local metric descriptors as described below. Setting the negative eigenvalues to zero would give the closest positive semi-definite tensor in the least-squares sense, but would not ensure invertibility.

Concentration/Heat Flow between Regions. In this experiment we solve for the steady-state concentration/heat distribution in the tensor field, with boundary conditions of one source and one sink. The maximal flow is found as expected along the strong anatomical path between the source and sink, the corpus callosum. Figure 1 displays the steady-state concentration and flow.

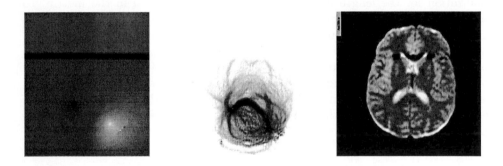

Fig. 1. Results of solving equation 5 for the steady-state heat distribution. The temperature (left) and the steady-state flow magnitude (center) demonstrate the flow from the source to the sink. In the temperature image the source is bright and the sink is dark; in the center flow image, dark means high flow magnitude. The grayscale image on the right, a non-diffusion-weighted image, shows the corresponding anatomy.

4   A Riemannian Metric Space

A natural interpretation of the "degree of connectivity" between two points is the distance between the points in some metric space. For our purposes, the distance between two anatomical locations should depend on the diffusion tensor field.

The diffusion operator (eq. 4) can naturally be associated with a Riemannian metric tensor G via the relation $G = D^{-1}$, allowing us to compute geometric quantities such as geodesic paths and distances between points in the brain. The relation between the diffusion and metric tensors is intuitive: large eigenvalues in the original DT-MRI tensor become small when the tensor is inverted to create the metric tensor. Consequently, large eigenvalues in the original tensor imply short metric distances along the direction of the corresponding eigenvector.

We will limit ourselves here to a brief discussion of the theory; see [4] for a more rigorous and thorough treatment of the connection between diffusion and Riemannian geometry. The Laplacian for a scalar function u on a manifold can in tensor notation be written as:

$$\nabla_G^2 u = (G^{kl} u_{;k})_{;l} = G^{kl} \frac{\partial^2 u}{\partial x^k \partial x^l} - \Gamma^l \frac{\partial u}{\partial x^l} \tag{8}$$

where G_{kl} is the metric tensor, and Γ is the Christoffel symbol that represents the derivatives of the basis vectors and the metric,

$$\Gamma^i = \frac{1}{2} G^{kl} G^{ij} \left(\frac{\partial G_{jk}}{\partial x^l} + \frac{\partial G_{jl}}{\partial x^k} - \frac{\partial G_{kl}}{\partial x^j} \right). \tag{9}$$

It can be noted that the Christoffel symbol is zero when the basis vectors and the metric are spatially invariant, as in the case of $\mathcal{R}^n$. Inserting the expression for the Christoffel symbol from equation 8 gives

$$\nabla_G^2 u = \frac{1}{|G|^{\frac{1}{2}}} \frac{\partial}{\partial x^k} \left(|G|^{\frac{1}{2}} G^{kl} \frac{\partial u}{\partial x^l} \right), \tag{10}$$

which is known as the Laplace-Beltrami operator, the generalization of the Laplacian to manifolds. In matrix notation the Laplace-Beltrami operator can be written as

$$\nabla_G^2 u = |G|^{-\frac{1}{2}} \nabla \cdot \left(|G|^{\frac{1}{2}} G^{-1} \nabla u \right). \tag{11}$$

It is straightforward to check from these definitions that we have the following relation between the diffusion operator in (eq. 4) and a diffusion operator in the Riemannian space characterized by G:

$$\nabla \cdot (D\nabla u) = \nabla_G^2 u - \frac{1}{2} \langle \nabla \log |G|, \nabla_G u \rangle \tag{12}$$

where the second order term on the right hand side represents simple Laplacian smoothing in the tensor-warped space, *i.e.* isotropic diffusion associated with the heat equation.

4.1   Measuring Distances in the Tensor-Warped Space

Once we have the metric tensor G, we are able to apply results from Riemannian geometry to describe geometric objects such as geodesic paths and distances between points in the brain. Unlike tractographic methods based on following the flow of principal eigenvectors of D, these geodesic paths are well-defined even in regions where the tensor diffusion is isotropic.

We have approached the measurement of distances in this space in two ways. First, we have implemented an Eikonal-type equation using level-set methods to produce a distance transform which respects the metric G. This required the derivation of a formula for the speed of an evolving front in the direction of its Euclidean normal. Second, we have implemented Dijkstra's algorithm using G to determine distances between neighboring voxels, using the formula $(w^T G w)^{\frac{1}{2}}$ where w is the vector from a voxel to its neighbor. Though it can suffer from discretization problems, Dijkstra's algorithm is fast and allows interactive display of return paths.

For our level set [9] implementation, we seek a speed function F for use in the evolution equation

$$\phi_t = F|\nabla \phi|. \tag{13}$$

This can be done using the following algorithm, which amounts to finding the length of the projection of the unit normal in the tensor-warped space onto the Euclidean normal:

1) Set $n = \frac{\nabla \phi}{|\nabla \phi|}$, the Euclidean normal to the level set.

2) Find any two linearly independent vectors t_1 and t_2 perpendicular to n. These are tangents which span the tangent space to the level set.

3) Set $w = (Gt_1) \times (Gt_2)$.

4) Set $\tilde{n} = \frac{w}{(w^T G w)^{\frac{1}{2}}}$. This is the unit normal with respect to G.

5) Set $F = |\tilde{n}^T n|$. This is the length of the projection of $\tilde{n}$ onto n.

4.2   Experiments

These experiments were performed on the same data set and with the same preprocessing as in Section 3.1.

Tensor-Warped Distances. Figure 2 shows a slice through a 3D distance transform with respect to the metric derived from the DT-MRI tensor field. The result can be viewed as a topographical map, with iso-level contours. Defining the seed point as the highest elevation, the direction of maximum connectivity will be in the direction of slowest descent.

Connectivity Measure. By comparing the geodesic path length to the Euclidean length of the same path, we produce a measure of the "degree of connectivity" between any two points. We compute the ratio of Euclidean path length to geodesic path length for all paths outward from the initial point. Figure 3 displays the connectivity measure as calculated for the distance map shown in Figure 2.

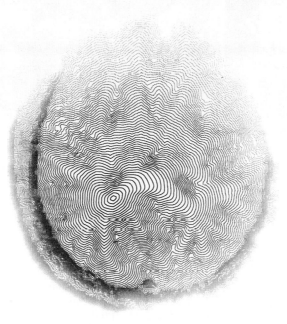

Fig. 2. Tensor-warped distance map: this contour map shows metric distance from an initial point located in the posterolateral part of the corpus callosum. The image is a slice through a 3D distance map, at the level of the initial point. The apparent "ridges" in the image indicate low metric distance, or high connectivity.

5   Discussion

The introduction of a Riemannian metric allowed us to reformulate the connectivity/diffusion simulation problem as a search for geodesic paths. In addition, we solved for a steady-state heat distribution and flow field which reflect connectivity.

The connection between the anisotropic diffusion operator and the Laplace-Beltrami operator (eq. 12) relates an anisotropic diffusion process in $\mathcal{R}^3$ to an isotropic diffusion process in a Riemannian space, where the metric is defined by the inverse of the diffusion tensor. This connection is likely responsible for the observed similarity between the results of both methods. Qualitatively, the steady-state maximal heat flow path between the source and sink appears to follow the geodesic derived from the Riemannian shortest path algorithm. The precise nature of this connection is a topic for further investigation.

Acknowledgements

This work was funded in part by a National Science Foundation Graduate Fellowship and by NIH grants P41-RR13218 and 1 R33-CA99015.

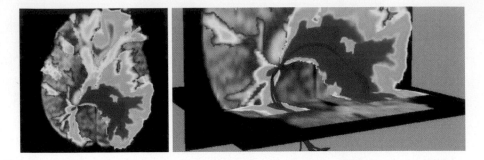

Fig. 3. Degree of connectivity, measured as Euclidean path length over geodesic path length. Very low connectivity is not shown. Purple is the highest connectivity. Traditional tractography based on following the principal eigenvector direction, with seed locations around the initial point, is displayed in red (right). Visual inspection confirms that the trace lines agree well with the region of highest connectivity.

References

1. P.J. Basser: Inferring microstructural features and the physiological state of tissues from diffusion-weighted images. *NMR in Biomedicine.* 8 (1995) 333–344.
2. P.J. Basser and S. Pajevic and C. Pierpaoli and J. Duda and A. Aldroubi: In Vivo Fiber Tractography Using DT-MRI Data. *Magn. Reson. Med..* 44 (2000) 625–632.
3. P.G. Batchelor, D.L.G. Hill, F. Calamante and D. Atkinson: Study of Connectivity in the Brain Using the Full Diffusion Tensor from MRI. *Information Processing in Medical Imaging, 17th International Conference, IPMI'01.* (2001) 121–133.
4. M.C. De Lara: Geometric and Symmetry Properties of a Nondegenerate Diffusion Process. *Annals of Probability.* 23:4 (1995) 1557–1604.
5. G. Kindlmann, D. Weinstein, D. Hart: Strategies for Direct Volume Rendering of Diffusion Tensor Fields. *IEEE Transactions on Visualization and Computer Graphics.* 6:2 (2000) 124–138.
6. H. Gudbjartsson, S. Maier, R. Mulkern, I.A. Morocz, S. Patz, F. Jolesz: Line scan diffusion imaging. *Magn. Reson. Med.* (1996) 36 509–519.
7. G.J.M. Parker, C.A.M. Wheeler-Kingshott, and G.J. Barker: Distributed Anatomical Brain Connectivity Derived from Diffusion Tensor Imaging. *Information Processing in Medical Imaging 17th International Conference, IPMI'01.* (2001) 106–120.
8. C. Poupon, C. A. Clark, F. Frouin, J. Régis, I. Bloch, D. Le Bihan, I. Bloch, and J.-F. Mangin: Regularization of Diffusion-Based Direction Maps for the Tracking Brain White Matter Fascicles. *NeuroImage.* 12 (2000) 184–195.
9. J.A. Sethian: *Level Set Methods and Fast Marching Methods.* Cambridge University Press. (1999).
10. D.S. Tuch: Diffusion MRI of Complex Tissue Structure. *Ph.D. Thesis, Division of Health Sciences and Technology, Massachusetts Institute of Technology.* (2002).
11. C.-F. Westin, S. Peled, H. Gudbjartsson, R. Kikinis and F.A. Jolesz. Geometrical Diffusion Measures for MRI from Tensor Basis Analysis. *ISMRM 97* Vancouver, Canada (1997).
12. C.-F. Westin, S.E. Maier, H. Mamata, A. Nabavi, F.A. Jolesz, and R. Kikinis.: Processing and Visualization of Diffusion Tensor MRI. *Med. Image Anal.* 6:2 (2002) 93–108.

Improved Detection Sensitivity in Functional MRI Data Using a Brain Parcelling Technique

Guillaume Flandin[1,2,3], Ferath Kherif[2,3], Xavier Pennec[1],
Grégoire Malandain[1], Nicholas Ayache[1], and Jean-Baptiste Poline[2,3]

[1] INRIA, Epidaure Project, Sophia Antipolis, France
{flandin,pennec,malandain,ayache}@sophia.inria.fr
[2] Service Hospitalier Frédéric Joliot, CEA, Orsay, France
{kherif,poline}@shfj.cea.fr
[3] IFR 49, Neuroimagerie fonctionnelle, Paris, France

Abstract. We present a comparison between a voxel based approach
and a region based technique for detecting brain activation signals in
sequences of functional Magnetic Resonance Images (fMRI). The region
based approach uses an automatic parcellation of the brain that can
incorporate anatomical constraints. A standard univariate voxel based
detection method (Statistical Parametric Mapping [5]) is used and the
results are compared to those obtained when performing detection of
signals extracted from the parcels. Results on a fMRI experimental protocol are presented and show a greater sensitivity using the parcelling
technique. This result remains true when the data are analyzed at several
resolutions.

1 Introduction

Since the discovery of fMRI [10], the analysis of these series of images has been
an extremely active field of research. One of the challenge when analyzing these
noisy data is to detect very small increase of activity in the brain. Many approaches have been proposed for this purpose. They can be classified in several overlapping categories such as multivariate versus univariate, voxel based
versus region based, parametric versus non parametric, inferential versus exploratory, etc.

Despite the number of approaches proposed, the only one that is extensively
used to detect the brain activity is to fit at each and every voxel in the brain
a linear model that represents the expected voxel time course derived from the
experimental paradigm. A test is then applied to detect voxels that have a significant part of their variance explained by the model. An obvious problem with
this technique is that the threshold controlling for the type one error (false positive rate) has to be adjusted depending on the number of tests performed, here
as many as voxels in the brain (in the order of 20000). Because voxels are spatially dependent, techniques have been developed to set this threshold such that
the correction for multiple comparison does not lead to a conservative test with
reduced sensitivity. For this purpose, the theory of random field has been extensively developed and applied in particular through the work of K. Worsley [13].

T. Dohi and R. Kikinis (Eds.): MICCAI 2002, LNCS 2488, pp. 467–474, 2002.
© Springer-Verlag Berlin Heidelberg 2002

This approach has been popularized by K. Friston and co-workers through the distribution of the SPM package[1].

Because brain regions activated by a given experimental paradigm generally spread over many contiguous voxels, spatial regularization is used through the application of spatial filters. These filters tend to increase the signal to noise ratio (SNR) and permit a partial overlapping of the signal originating from different subjects data that are not (and cannot be) perfectly aligned [7]. The correction for multiple comparison is strongly linked to the size of the spatial filter since the greater the dependence of the data, the less severe is the test correction. Clearly, activated region with size and shape similar to the one of the filter are best detected. Since activated regions can in principle have any size or shape, multi-filtering or multi-scale approaches have been investigated [11, 14]. However, the greater the filter size the less precise are the boundaries of the region.

In this work, we propose an alternative approach that consists in parcelling the analyzed brain into a user defined number of regions (or parcels). The parcelling method is able to take into account anatomical information extracted from the T_1-weighted MRI acquired together with the functional images. This should allow for the use of relatively large spatial averaging informed by the anatomy. It also should solve easily for the multiple comparison problem since functional signals extracted from parcels can in a first approximation be considered independent. In the first section, we present the parcelling technique based on a K-means algorithm with geodesic distances. The functional signal assignment to the parcels and the detection model are then presented, followed by a description of the methodology used to compare voxel and parcel based detection analyses. Comparison has been investigated with several filter sizes and corresponding numbers of parcels on an experimental protocol. We show that the method is more sensitive at several resolutions.

2   Methods

2.1   Automatic Parcellation of Brain Images

The aim is to provide a fully automatic parcellation of a certain volume of interest (the cortex in our case) at a (user supplied) adjustable resolution. Furthermore, a desired feature of such a parcellation is to obtain "homogeneous" parcels: a first intuitive guess is to use a criterion based on the cells volume but, to prevent the algorithm from finding very elongated cells, a criterion such as the sum of inertia of each cell (intra-class variance) seems more relevant, thus introducing a cell compactness concept. We propose an algorithm based on the K-means clustering [3] using geodesic distances.

Definition of the Volume of Interest. Here we restrict the functional data analysis to the cortex. A segmentation of the grey matter is performed on a T_1-weighted image [9] and a brain mask is extracted from functional images using

---

[1] http://www.fil.ion.ucl.ac.uk/spm/

an adapted threshold. The domain to parcel is then defined at an anatomical resolution as the intersection (logical and) between these two binary images.

Parcellation of the Domain. The volume of interest is described by a set of 3D coordinates $\{x_i\}$. We define parcels as connected clusters of anatomical voxels, represented by their centers of mass $\bar{x}_j$. The problem is then to find simultaneously a partition of the voxels $\{x_i\}$ into k classes C_j and the cell positions $\bar{x}_j$ minimizing the intra-class variance:

$$I_{intra} = \sum_{j=1}^{k} \sum_{i \in C_j} d^2\left(x_i, \bar{x}_j\right)$$

Such an optimization problem is efficiently solved using the well-known K-means algorithm in the classification context. After an initialization step that randomly selects k distinct voxels in the volume of interest as the initial cell positions, the criterion is solved using an alternate minimization of I_{intra} over:

1. The partition of the data (given cell positions): each voxel x_i is assigned to the class C_j that minimizes the distance to its position $\bar{x}_j$.
2. The cell positions (given a data partition): the position $\bar{x}_j$ is chosen to minimize the variance of the x_i's assigned to this class.

With spatial data, each step of the K-means algorithm can be rephrased in terms of discrete geometry.

Step 1 consists in the construction of a Voronoï diagram. Due to the non-convexity of the domain, we cannot use Euclidean distances for the computation of d. Indeed two points on opposite sides of a sulcus are close to each other in Euclidean terms but may be geodesically far apart. Thus the geodesic 3D distance (the shortest path within the volume of interest) is the most suitable. We implemented 3D discrete Voronoï diagram with geodesic distances using region growing and hierarchical queues adapted from [2].

Step 2 consists in computing the "geodesic center of mass" of each cell. Its value may be obtained by a gradient descent on the intra-class variance but in practice, most of the cells are still convex and the standard center of mass is a good approximation. In our implementation, we use the Euclidean center of mass as far as it stays within the cell, and a gradient descent otherwise.

Finally, the K-means clustering algorithm consists in repeating these two estimations until convergence, reached when voxels assignments to the cells are the same at two consecutive steps. There are proofs of the convergence even if the domain is non-convex, but in our case we use approximations with discrete distances that prevent a statement on convergence. We however observed that this algorithm always converges in a reduced number of iterations (typically a few dozens). Although implemented in 3D, we present, for display purpose, in figure 1 an example of convergence of the algorithm on a 2D cortex slice of an hemisphere with 50 parcels. The algorithm can be further improved by introducing additional anatomical constraints through the use of weighted geodesic distances.

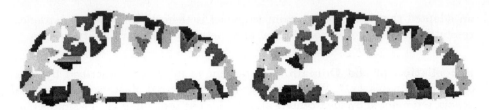

Fig. 1. 2D geodesic Voronoï diagram with 50 seeds (black dots). Left: random initialization. Right: after convergence of the K-means algorithm.

2.2 Signal Assignment

In this section, we address the method used to assign a representative time course at each parcel.

Parcellation being defined at an anatomical resolution, functional images are oversampled at this resolution using spline interpolation. Numerous strategies can then be used to provide a single temporal signal to each and every parcel using all signals belonging to the same cell: average them with mean or median, obtain the first eigenvector of their PCA or use multivariate analyses such as CCA (Canonical Correlation Analysis) to find the linear compound of signals that maximizes correlation with a model [4].

In the following, we used the sample mean in a first approximation leaving a thorough study of the best sampling technique for future work.

2.3 Statistical Detection Model

We first present the model used to detect activated signals coming from voxels or parcels. We used the General Linear Model (GLM) popularized by the SPM software. Then we present the multiple comparison problem corrections used for both voxel and parcel based analyses.

The General Linear Model. Given a column vector Y corresponding to a time course, the general linear model [5] is:

$$Y = X\beta + \epsilon$$

where X is the so-called design matrix whose columns represent the *a priori* information on expected signals, ϵ the residual error (assumed normally distributed) and β the parameters of the model.

In order to take into account the temporal autocorrelation of functional time series, the data and the model are convolved by a Toeplitz smoothing matrix K to impose a known autocorrelation $V = KK^T$ [6].

The maximum likelihood estimate of β, assuming a full rank design matrix, is:

$$\hat{\beta} = \left(X^{*T}X^*\right)^{-1} X^{*T} KY \quad \text{with} \quad X^* = KX$$

A contrast c of the parameter estimates is tested with:

$$T = \frac{c^T \hat{\beta}}{\left(Var \left[c^T \hat{\beta} \right] \right)^{1/2}} = \frac{c^T \hat{\beta}}{(c^T \hat{\sigma}^2 (X^{*T} X^*)^{-1} X^{*T} V X^* (X^{*T} X^*)^{-1} c)^{1/2}}$$

where $\hat{\sigma}^2$ is the estimated error variance. The effective degrees of freedom are given by $\nu = \frac{trace(RV)^2}{trace(RVRV)}$ with R such as $\hat{\epsilon} = RY$.

The null distribution of T may be approximated by a t-distribution with ν degrees of freedom. Thus hypotheses regarding contrasts of the parameter estimates can be tested and a threshold for a given voxel or parcel can be set to control the false detection rate.

Multiple Comparison Problem. Images contain a large number of voxels so that the risk of false positive *across voxels* will not be controlled if the statistical threshold is set as if only one test was performed: this is the so-called multiple comparison problem and is an important issue when comparing results provided by voxelwise (SPM) and parcelwise analyses. Multiple comparison correction depends on both the number of tests performed and their statistical dependence.

First, with a parcel based analysis, we may assume in a first approximation that signals are independent because, by construction, parcels signals are averaged over an important number of almost independent voxels. We can therefore apply a "Bonferroni" correction procedure that consists in adjusting the significance level α (type one error, usually 5%) for the number of tests n:

$$\alpha_{corrected} = 1 - (1 - \alpha)^{1/n} \simeq \frac{\alpha}{n}$$

Second, in a standard voxel-based analysis, the non independence of voxel intensities is obvious, due to both the initial resolution of images and to post processing smoothing. A Bonferroni correction would therefore be much too severe. A well-established correction proposed by Worsley [13] uses Random Field Theory to provide strong control over the type one error. An estimate of the field smoothness is computed, and the stringency of the correction depends on this measure and on the size of the volume analyzed. Smoothness based correction can be seen as the computation of the number of tests normalized for the global smoothness of the statistical field.

2.4   Comparing Voxel and Parcel Based Techniques

We investigated three different ways to perform such a comparison. Our goal is to provide a comparison of the detection with an equivalent spatial resolution. Given the very different natures of the two techniques, there are several ways of achieving such an equivalence. We briefly present three possible solutions:

- C_1: First, the number of parcels can be set such that it corresponds to the volume analyzed divided by a measure of the resolution of the filtered data used in the voxel based technique. The most natural measure in this instance is to consider the Full Width at Half Maximum of the point spread function (PSF) of the data. This corresponds to the applied filter combined with the intrinsic spatial dependency of the original images. When the former is large enough, the resulting number is close to the one imposed by the spatial filter. The number of parcels is set to the volume analyzed divided by the volume of the PSF at its half maximum.

- C_2: Second, the point spread function can be measured not on the original filtered volumes but on volumes corrected for the signal predicted by the model and normalized by their residual variance. This solution better reflects the statistical aspect of the problem. This corresponds to the notion of RESELS (Resolution Elements) in the work of K. Worsley [13]. The number of parcels is set as the *effective* degrees of freedom [15].
- C_3: Lastly, we can use the (corrected) p-value threshold proposed by the random field theory, compute the corresponding number of independent tests (N_B) and set the number of parcels to N_B.

We have investigated these three solutions and compared results obtained on the data described in the next section.

2.5   Application: Task and Paradigm Design

We compared detection results obtained in voxel and parcel based analyses on a cognitive paradigm that investigates the brain network involved in a motor (grasping) task [12]. The experimental protocol consisted of three activation epochs separated by three control periods (26 s. each), preceded by a 4-seconds instruction period. The subject performed this sequence twice. Repetition time (duration of one functional image acquisition) was 2 seconds for a total of 186 scans. Functional image matrix was $64 \times 64 \times 18$ with $3.75 \times 3.75 \times 3.8$ mm^3 voxel size. A T_1-weighted anatomical scan was acquired at the same time with a resolution of $0.94 \times 0.94 \times 1.5$ mm^3 ($256 \times 256 \times 124$ matrix).

Activations are investigated by setting a contrast between the control condition and the grasping one. The model X used for detection consists in one function per condition (instruction, control, and task) modeled by a box-car regressor convolved with a canonical haemodynamic response function.

3   Results and Discussion

We applied several Gaussian filters (FWHM of 8, 12 and 16 mm) on the raw functional images and computed the corresponding numbers of parcels for each comparison criterion C_1, C_2 and C_3. Results are similar for all filters and we therefore only present those corresponding to the 8 mm filtered data. Figure 2 shows results obtained with the SPM approach (top left) and the comparison with the parcel based approach with the 3 equivalent resolutions (1700 with criterion C_1, 340 with C_2 and 4900 with C_3).

We can observe a large increase in sensitivity for 340 and 1700 parcels. For instance, t-maps global maxima are respectively of 28.18 and 30.19 compared with

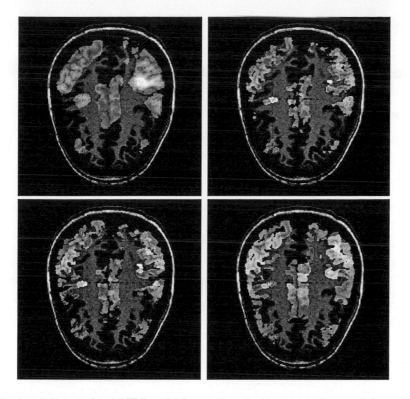

Fig. 2. Axial T_1-weighted MRI with detected activations superimposed ($p_c < 0.05$). SPM t-map with 8 mm smoothing (top left). Parcel-based t-map with 4900 parcels (top right), 1700 parcels (bottom left) and 340 parcels (bottom right).

23.25 using SPM, while the spatial localization does not seem to be degraded by the parcelling technique. With 4900 parcels, we obtain about the same sensitivity as SPM (global maxima is 22.5). However, in this case, the anatomical localization seems to be more precise with the parcel based approach. Indeed, 3D smoothing leads to the averaging of signals coming from different structures and to a poor localization of brain activity (look at the locus pointed by the cross in each image). We can maintain that the sensitivity increase is a consequence of the anatomically informed spatial smoothing performed by the parcelling technique (cortex structure taken into account), as opposed to 3D smoothing. Lastly, according to the results presented here, the criterion C_1 for the equivalent number of parcels (1700 parcels in this case) seems to be the most relevant.

4   Conclusion

This work is close in spirit with the methodology developed by Andrade [1] or Kiebel [8] performing a surface-oriented fMRI data analysis confined to the cortex since both techniques aim at incorporating anatomical information to the statistical analysis of functional time courses. The work [1] also reported increased sensitivity, but less pronounced than here. Furthermore we propose here a flexible method working at a voxel level that can be generalized to other structures than cortex, is more robust to misregistrations between functional and anatomical images and will eventually incorporate *a priori* information (anatomical and functional) in the parcellation definition.

Acknowledgments

The authors would like to thank J. Stoeckel for fruitful discussions. Many thanks also to O. Simon and S. Dehaene who provided the images.

References

1. A. Andrade, F. Kherif, J.-F. Mangin, K.J. Worsley, A.-L. Paradis, O. Simon, S. Dehaene, D. Le Bihan, and J.-B. Poline. Detection of fMRI activation using cortical surface mapping. *Human Brain Mapping*, 12:79–93, 2001.
2. O. Cuisenaire. *Distance Transformations: Fast Algorithms and Applications to Medical Image Processing*. PhD thesis, Katholieke Universiteit, Leuven, 1999.
3. R.O. Duda and P.E. Hart. *Pattern Classification and Scene Analysis*. Wiley, New York, 1973.
4. O. Friman, M. Borga, P. Lundberg, and H. Knutsson. Detection of neural activity in fMRI using maximum correlation modeling. *NeuroImage*, 15(2):386–395, 2002.
5. K.J. Friston, A.P. Holmes, J.-B. Poline, C.D. Frith, and R.S.J. Frackowiak. Statistical parametric maps in functional imaging: A general linear approach. *Human Brain Mapping*, 2:189–210, 1995.
6. K.J. Friston, O. Josephs, E. Zarahn, A.P. Holmes, S. Rouquette, and J.-B. Poline. To smooth or not to smooth? bias and efficiency in fMRI time-series analysis. *NeuroImage*, 12:196–208, 2000.
7. P. Hellier, C. Barillot, I. Corouge, B. Giraud, G. Le Goualher, L. Collins, A. Evans, G. Malandain, and N. Ayache. Retrospective evaluation of inter-subject brain registration. In *MICCAI'01*, volume 2208 of *LNCS*, pages 258–265, October 2001.
8. S.J. Kiebel, R. Goebel, and K.J. Friston. Anatomically informed basis functions. *NeuroImage*, 11(6):656–667, 2000.
9. J.-F. Mangin, V. Frouin, I. Bloch, J. Régis, and J. Lopez-Krahe. From 3D magnetic resonance images to structural representations of the cortex topography using topology preserving deformations. *J. Math. Imaging and Vision*, 5:297–318, 1995.
10. S. Ogawa, T.M. Lee, A.R. Kay, and D.W. Tank. Brain magnetic resonance imaging with contrast dependent on blood oxygenation. *Proc Natl Acad Sci USA*, 87:9868–9872, 1990.
11. J.-B. Poline and B.M. Mazoyer. Enhanced detection in brain activation maps using a multi filtering approach. *J. Cereb. Blood Flow Metab.*, 14:639–641, 1994.
12. O. Simon, J.-F. Mangin, L. Cohen, D. Le Bihan, and S. Dehaene. Topographical layout of hand, eye, calculation, and language-related areas in the human parietal lobe. *Neuron*, 31(33(3)):475–87, Jan 2002.
13. K.J. Worsley, A.C. Evans, S. Marrett, and P. Neelin. A three-dimensional statistic analysis of CBF activation studies in human brain. *J. Cereb. Blood Flow Metab.*, 12:900–918, 1992.
14. K.J. Worsley, S. Marrett, P. Neelin, and A.C. Evans. Searching scale space for activation in PET images. *Human Brain Mapping*, 4:74–90, 1996.
15. K.J. Worsley, J.-B. Poline, A.C. Vandal, and K.J. Friston. Tests for distributed, non-focal brain activations. *NeuroImage*, 2:183–194, 1995.

A Spin Glass Based Framework to Untangle Fiber Crossing in MR Diffusion Based Tracking

Y. Cointepas[1], C. Poupon[2], D. Le Bihan[1], and J.-F. Mangin[1]

[1] UNAF, Service Hospitalier Frédéric Joliot, CEA, France
cointepa@shfj.cea.fr http://www-dsv.cea.fr/
[2] General Electric Medical Systems, Clinical Software Applications, Buc, France
cyril.poupon@med.ge.com

Abstract. We propose a general approach to the reconstruction of brain white matter geometry from diffusion-weighted data. This approach is based on an inverse problem framework. The optimal geometry corresponds to the lowest energy configuration of a spin glass. These spins represent pieces of fascicles that orient themselves according to diffusion data and interact in order to create low curvature fascicles. Simulated diffusion-weighted datasets corresponding to the crossing of two fascicle bundles are used to validate the method.

1 Introduction

A number of algorithmic approaches have been recently proposed to study anatomical connectivity from MR diffusion-weighted data. For most of these approaches, the putative fascicles are revealed by the step by step reconstruction of highest diffusion 3D trajectories [11, 2]. The reconstruction is performed from a vector field made up of the local directions of highest diffusion, usually the diffusion tensor first eigenvector. Unfortunately, this approach is not robust to spurious local directions, which induce erroneous forks in the tracking process. Since partial volume averaging at the level of fiber crossing is bound to generate such spurious highest diffusion directions [12, 3], more robust tracking schemes have to be designed. A direction of research consists of simulating large scale diffusion processes throughout white matter, either at the random walk level [5], or at the macroscopic level using partial differential equation frameworks [8]. Such methods provide for each given input area a map of connectivity probability related for instance to the time required for some information to reach any brain area. Tracking information propagation streamlines may allow the mapping of the putative bundle trajectories stemming from this input area including possible forks. One new diffusion process, however, has to be simulated for each new input area. A second class of approaches relies on regularization principles leading to search for the optimal path between a pair of input points [10], or for the optimal fascicle map linking a set of points [9], combining diffusion data and a priori knowledge on fascicle curvature.

In this paper, we extend the global approach mentioned above [9], casting it into a global inverse problem framework. This framework leads to infer the fascicle map with highest likelihood from a set of observations about the water diffusion process occuring into brain white matter. Such a fascicle map is made up of a set of inter-connected fascicle pieces. The whole fascicles can be automatically reconstructed from this map

T. Dohi and R. Kikinis (Eds.): MICCAI 2002, LNCS 2488, pp. 475–482, 2002.

as paths following the links defined between these fascicle pieces. The fascicle map includes branching locations, which results in more tracking efficiency than using a path by path approach, because the chains of fascicle pieces included in several paths are investigated only one time during optimization. Once the optimal fascicle map has been inferred, an exhaustive list of pairs of points of the white matter surface linked by a putative fascicle can be provided at low cost.

The optimality of the fascicle map is defined as a trade-off between local information on voxel micro-structure provided by diffusion data and a priori information on the low curvature of plausible fascicles. This trade-off is obtained from the minimization of a global measure of the likelihood of a fascicle map knowing the diffusion data set. This likelihood is made up of two kind of terms. The first ones assess the quality of the fit between the local diffusion data and the related local pieces of fascicle. The second ones assess the contextual plausibility of the local configurations of fascicle pieces. Contextual plausibility is used to detect and regularize the spurious fascicle local directions induced by corrupted or ambiguous diffusion data. This measure is modeled using the ideas that most of the fascicles have a rather low bending in anatomical dissections and that a fascicle cannot end up inside white matter.

Our framework stems from the field of spin glasses developped in statistical physics. During our previous works, the fascicle map was including only one fascicle piece per voxel, which was unsufficient to deal correctly with bundle crossing. Moreover, only diffusion tensor models had been considered, while MR physics research should lead to much more informative high angular resolution models [3, 10]. In this paper, we show that the spin glass based approach can be extended to deal with more or less accurate diffusion data and can embed the possible existence of some crossings inside voxels. The extended model behaviour is explored using simulated data in order to get rid of the MR physics problems that have still to be overcome to understand actual MR diffusion data [1].

2   Framework

Inverse problem: The reconstruction of the white matter fascicle geometry from diffusion-weighted data may be considered as a standard inverse problem. Like many other inverse problems, fascicle map inference has to deal with acquisition artifacts and coarse data sampling. The choice of the trade-off between signal to noise, spatial and angular resolutions is important relatively to the accuracy of the fascicle map that can be reconstructed. If the fascicle map resolution is too high relatively to the relevant information included in the data, the inverse problem becomes ill-posed, which means that two different acquisitions of the same brain will yield two very different fascicle maps simply because of noise and partial volume. Any single wrong local diffusion data interpretation, indeed, may create a spurious fascicle in the map while splitting an actual one. Voxels including crossing fibers are especially difficult to deal with and may lead to different fascicle reconstructions according to the data spatial and angular sampling. It should be understood also that several different local fiber configurations may provide the same diffusion data. For instance, a flat tensor may correspond to a crossing or to a "fan shaped" fascicle. Hence, there is a need for the problem to be formulated in a way that gives the same unique solution with different acquisitions, at least for the same sampling level.

A standard approach to deal with ill-posed problems relies on the regularization principle: a priori knowledge on the regularity of the most plausible solutions allows the distinction between relevant information and noise. The family of methods proposed in the following uses the reasonable hypothesis that in case of ambiguity, the most plausible fascicle trajectory is endowed with the lowest curvature. This hypothesis and the additional knowledge that a fascicle should not end inside white matter allows the method to extrapolate the reliable fascicle segments inferred from the areas of unequivocal diffusion data to more problematic white matter areas.

Fascicle maps and spin glasses: As mentioned above, the choice of the fascicle map resolution has to be consistent with the amount of relevant information embedded in the diffusion data. Hence, the following methods aim at recovering maps including only a limited number of fascicles into each diffusion data voxel. Once the fascicle map domain has been defined, a representation has to be devised for the local pieces of fascicles. Each piece will have some degrees of freedom, which will lead to set out the inverse problem as an optimization driven issue. While a lot of different approaches may be figure out, we focus in the following on an analogy with spin glasses. Therefore, the pieces of fascicles will be called spins. Whatever the nature of the diffusion data set, it will be embedded into our framework as a non stationary external magnetic field acting on the spin orientations. The a priori knowledge on the fascicle map geometry (low fascicle curvature, no dead ends inside white matter) will be embedded as interactions between neighboring spins. The solution to the fascicle map inverse problem will be defined as the minimal energy configuration of the spin glass. The family of methods proposed in this paper includes more or less sophisticated variants related to the kind of spins that live inside the domain voxels. The simplest model, which has been used during our previous experiments [9], puts one compass needle like spin in the center of each voxel. In this paper, we introduce more sophisticated models that either relax the spin localization in order to improve the fascicle trajectory sampling, or put several spins inside each voxel in order to deal with fascicle crossing.

The external magnetic field models: For each voxel M of the fascicle domain, information on local water mobility inferred from the diffusion data can be used to build models which provide for any direction of space the likelihood of the existence of a fascicle. These models can then be converted into a virtual diffusion based local potential P_D^M acting on the orientations v_i^M of the spins i located inside M. Hence, the virtual potential field made up of these local potentials will act on the simulated spin glass as a non stationary magnetic field. Various likelihood models can be devised according to the nature of the diffusion data. As matter stands when using DTI data, these models are directly related to the hypothesis that the diffusion coefficient is higher in the fascicle direction than in neighboring directions. Recent experiments including higher angular resolution data, however, have proved that this hypothesis was not always true at the level of crossings [12, 3]. Hence, a better understanding of the crossing and compartment issues might lead to better likelihood models in the future [7, 1].

When the spin glass is embedded into such an external potential field, the spin orientations rotate in order to reach a minimum of energy, which can be simulated using a minimization algorithm. Without any spin interaction, a minimum for the whole glass is made up of minima in each voxel. With tensor data, the spin align themselves along the tensor eigenvector associated with the largest eigenvalue. Hence, the resulting spin glass configuration is equivalent to the vector field used by standard tracking algorithms [2]. In the following, spin interaction potentials are added into the glass energy in order to introduce the a priori knowledge about the low curvature of most of the fascicles. Hence, spin glass energy minima will correspond to a global trade-off between two different kinds of forces.

The interaction model: At the resolution of standard diffusion data, the geometry of the fascicle map may be related to the geometry of spaghetti plates. Therefore, the interaction potential that will embed a low curvature constraint for the fascicles is inspired by a simple model of the local bending energy accumulated by spaghetti during cooking, namely a quadratic potential based on the spaghetti local curvature [9]. Then, a spaghetti potential $P_S^M(i)$ is defined to embed the interactions between each spin i located into voxel M and the neighboring spins, namely the set $\mathcal{N}_i^M$ made up of all the other spins located into M and of the spins located in M neighboring voxels in the fascicle map domain. The neighboring spin set $\mathcal{N}_i^M$ is split first into forward and backward subsets from the spin i orientation v_i. Then one neighboring spin is selected in each half-neighborhood (respectively $f(i)$ and $b(i)$) in order to create a local fascicle trajectory $b(i) - i - f(i)$ endowed with the lowest possible curvature. Note that whatever the relative orientations of $v_{b(i)}$, v_i, and $v_{f(i)}$, a putative fascicle has to be defined because of our assumption that the fascicles can not lead to dead ends inside white matter. Each time that one half-neighborhood is empty, however, no best neighboring spin can be defined and the fascicle is supposed to leave white matter. Therefore, no bending constraint is added into $P_S^M(i)$ in that direction. Whatever the spin glass model, the lowest energy configurations induced by the spaghetti interaction potentials are made up of straight fascicles. Such configurations, indeed, have a null energy and correspond to spaghetti sets without any cooking.

Global energy and minimization: Diffusion based potentials and bending energy based spin interactions are gathered into a global energy E which is defining the solution to the inverse problem as the lowest energy configuration:

$$E = \sum_M \sum_i P_D^M(i) + \alpha \sum_M \sum_i P_S^M(i) , \qquad (1)$$

where α is a positive rigidity constant which balances the influence of the *a priori* knowledge on the fascicle low curvature. The solution is obtained using either deterministic or stochastic minimization, according to the quality of the initialization that can be provided. The fascicle map model is more flexible than the path by path method proposed by Tuch et al. [10], because chains of linked spins may split and merge during the minimization. Split and merge operations create additional paths throughout the energy landscape, which highly reduces the influence of initialisation and local minima during optimization.

3 Experiments

In the following, some experiments are proposed to show the advantage of the glass models including several spins into each voxel to deal with fiber crossing. All these experiments rely on simulated data to discard potential difficulties induced by the current weaknesses of the diffusion models used to interpret high angular resolution data [10, 3, 1]. Our goal is to provide a tracking model that will be ready to untangle fiber crossing when current MR physics problem will have been overcome. The lack of data obtained from some phantoms with known fiber geometry, indeed, prevents a reliable use of actual data to test tracking methods.

Simulation of the diffusion driven local likelihood:

In order to generate a simulated dataset including in each voxel the likelihood of the presence of a fascicle in any orientation of space, a virtual bundle crossing geometry is created (see Fig. 1). For each voxel of the mask corresponding to this geometry, the proportion of each bundle contributing to the partial volume effect is computed. Then, a direction set supposed to correspond to the direction set of the MR sequence is chosen. In order to simulate the diffusion based MR signal attenuation in one direction d, a different weighted sum of tensors [6] is used within each voxel v to represent the contribution of each fiber bundle:

$$A_v(d) = (1 - f_v^1 - f_v^2).e^{d^T.D^0.d} + f_v^1.e^{d^T.D^1.d} + f_v^2.e^{d^T.D^2.d} , \qquad (2)$$

where f_v^1 end f_v^2 denote the volume fraction of each fiber bundle ($f_v^1 + f_v^2 \leq 1$), D^0 is an isotropic tensor representing pure water, D^1 and D^2 are highly anisotropic tensors adapted to each fiber bundle direction.

For the following experiments, we have chosen to simulate the standard situation where diffusion data stem from the single tensor model, which is in our opinion unsufficient to untangle fiber crossings in a robust way. Nevertheless, this simulation is sufficient to show the superiority of multi-spin per voxel glasses and is closer to the current understanding about what can be obtained from MR diffusion. The simulated high angular resolution diffusion dataset (40 directions) is used to fit in each voxel v a single tensor, from which is computed the likelihood function proposed in [9]. For a direction d :

$$likelihood_v(d) = \frac{(e^{d^T.D_v.d} - \lambda_v^{max})^2}{\|D_v\|} , \qquad (3)$$

where D_v is the tensor estimated in voxel v and λ_v^{max} is the maximum eigen value of D_v. Figure 1 shows that anisotropic likelihoods are obtained in voxels containing homogenous fiber directions and, because of partial volume effect, flat likelihoods are obtained in voxels corresponding to fascicle crossing.

Fascicle map reconstruction:

In order to illustrate the problems that can arise in fiber tracking methods that consider only one fiber direction per voxel, we present the reconstructions obtained putting one or two spins in each voxel. These reconstructions stem from the minimisation of the global energy presented in section 2 with a stochastic method based on the Gibb's sampler [4]. Using only one spin per voxel cannot lead to a correct crossing representation.

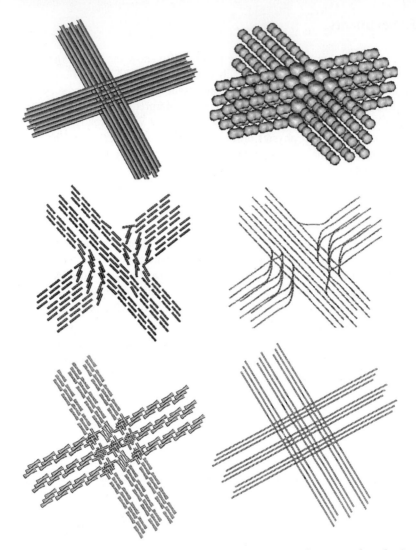

Fig. 1. Top left: *a virtual bundle crossing.* **Top right**: *the corresponding tensor based orientation likelihood functions. For the sake of understanding,* $1 - likelihood_v(d)$ *is actually shown.* **Middle** *Optimal glass configuration using one spin per voxel. One of the two bundles wins while the other is broken into two parts, which leads to spurious tracts.* **Down** *Optimal glass configuration using two spins per voxel. The crossing is correctly reconstructed.*

Therefore, during the minimization process, one bundle wins, whereas the other leads to spurious connections (cf. Fig. 1). In return, with two spins located into each voxel, the simulated geometry is correctly inferred by the minimisation. The spins located into one single bundle area are all oriented in the bundle direction, whereas in the crossing the spins are oriented along the two directions. Hence, the resulting tracts correspond to the initial geometry (cf. Fig. 1).

While the previous experiment has shown the advantage of more complex spin glasses, untangling a complex fascicle geometry will require diffusion data with higher angular resolution, which is beyond the scope of the paper. Higher angular resolution, however, will be reached at the cost of noisier data. Hence, a complex issue will be related to the choice of the optimal trade-off between this angular resolution and the number of degrees of freedom used to interpret and smooth them. With the 6 degrees of freedom single tensor model, for instance, noisy data give smooth likelihood functions. A lot of information, unfortunately, is lost about the fiber orientation into crossing areas.

Dealing with higher angular resolution models, however, requires the resolution of a local inverse problem at the level of each voxel. Indeed, converting a high angular resolution diffusion-weighted dataset into a likelihood potential is far to be straightforward. First, a model of the diffusion process has to be chosen, for instance the multi-compartment model underlying equation 3. Second the parameters of this model have to be estimated from noisy data (fractions and tensors), which is a difficult non linear estimation problem. Finally, a likelihood model has to be inferred from this MR physics model, which has to be related to the estimation variance. Without a good understanding of this process, which has to be adressed in our opinion by any tracking method, experimenting the spin glass framework with higher angular resolution models may be meaningless, which explains our current choice. This inverse problem framework, however, is sufficiently versatile to be adapted to such new physical models in a very intuitive way.

4 Conclusion

In this paper, we have formalized the reconstruction of a putative fascicle map from diffusion-weighted data as a global inverse problem. The proposed framework is flexible enough to be adapted to foreseeable evolutions of MR acquisition schemes. In our opinion, the inverse problem point of view will help to clarify what reliable information can be extracted from a diffusion-weighted dataset. More and more informative connectivity matrices will be computed from the reconstructed fascicle maps, leading to a very attractive new field of research for neurosciences, ranging from pure graph theory to brain growth or new insights into connectivity related pathologies.

References

1. P. J. Basser. Relationships between diffusion tensor and q-space MRI. *MRM*, 47(2):392–7, 2002.
2. P. J. Basser, S. Pajevic, C. Pierpaoli, J. Duda, and A. Aldroubi. In vivo fiber tractography using DT-MRI data. *MRM*, 44(4):625–632, 2000.
3. L. R. Frank. Anisotropy in high angular resolution diffusion-weighted MRI. *Magn. Reson. Med.*, 45(6):935–939, 2001.

4. S. Geman and D. Geman. Stochastic relaxation, Gibbs distributions, and the Bayesian restoration of images. *IEEE Transaction on Pattern Analysis and Machine Intelligence*, PAMI-6(6):721–741, November 1984.
5. M. Koch, D. G. Norris, and M. Hund-Georgiadis. An investigation of functional and anatomical connectivity using diffusion tensor imaging. In *ISMRM-ESMRMB, Glasgow*, page 1509, 2001.
6. D Le Bihan. *Diffusion and Perfusion Magnetic Resonance Imaging*, chapter A-2-IV, pages 50–57. Raven Press, Ltd., New-York, 1995.
7. D. Le Bihan, J.-F. Mangin, C. Poupon, C. A. Clark, S. Pappata, N. Molko, and H. Chabriat. Diffusion tensor imaging: concepts and applications. *Journal of Magnetic Reonance Imaging*, 13:534–546, 2001.
8. G. J. M. Parker, C. A. Wheeler-Kingssbott, and G. J. Barker. Distributed anatomical brain connectivity derived from diffusion tensor imaging. In *XVIIth IPMI, LNCS-2082, Springer-Verlag*, pages 372–380, 2001.
9. C. Poupon, J.-F. Mangin, C. A. Clark, V. Frouin, J. Régis, D. Le Bihan, and I. Bloch. Towards inference of human brain connectivity from MR diffusion tensor data. *Medical Image Analysis*, 5:1–15, 2001.
10. D. S. Tuch, M. R. Wiegell, T. G. Reese, J. W. Belliveau, and J. Van Wedeen. Measuring cortico-cortical connectivity matrices with diffusion spectrum imaging. In *ISMRM-ESMRMB, Glasgow*, page 502, 2001.
11. C.-F. Westin, S.E. Maier, B. Khidir, P. Everett, F. A. Jolesz, and R. Kikinis. Image processing for diffusion tensor magnetic resonance imaging. In *MICCAI'99, Cambridge, UK, LNCS-1679, Springer-Verlag*, pages 441–452, 1999.
12. M. R. Wiegell, H. B. Larsson, and V. J. Wedeen. Fiber crossing in human brain depicted with diffusion tensor MR imaging. *Radiology*, 217(3):897–903, 2000.

Automated Approximation of Lateral Ventricular Shape in Magnetic Resonance Images of Multiple Sclerosis Patients

Bernhard Sturm[1], Dominik Meier[2], and Elizabeth Fisher[1]

[1] Department of Biomedical Engineering / ND20, Lerner Research Institute,
The Cleveland Clinic Foundation, 9500 Euclid Avenue, Cleveland, Ohio 44195, U.S.A.
{sturm,fisher}@bme.ri.ccf.org
[2] Center for Neurological Imaging, Brigham & Women's Hospital, Harvard Medical School,
221 Longwood Avenue- RFB 398, Boston, Massachusetts 02115
meier@bwh.harvard.edu

Abstract. "Active surfaces" or deformable models have been proposed for the segmentation of anatomic structures in MRI data. Such algorithms are dependent on a good initial approximation of the target shape. The purpose of this work was to develop a reliable method for automatic generation of a starting point for segmentation of the lateral ventricle. The algorithm uses a parametric representation of an average lateral ventricle, which is customized for each individual by modulating the parametric coefficients based on the brain parenchymal fraction. The method was developed with a training set of 6 healthy controls and 25 patients with multiple sclerosis, and tested on an additional set of 10 patients. Compared to the average ventricle, this new approach provided a closer approximation to the manually segmented ventricular shape in 81% of the cases in the training set and 100% of the additional test set.

1   Introduction

Automated segmentation of the lateral ventricles in MRI data would be beneficial for quantification of regional atrophy, and for ongoing efforts in structure driven anatomical labeling of the brain [1]. A successful segmentation algorithm would alleviate issues of operator variability and accelerate the current method. The improved precision provided by automated segmentation is of particular value in the study of neurodegenerative diseases, where morphological changes are subtle, and a high sensitivity is required for their detection.

Approaches for segmentation of anatomic structures include algorithms such as "active surfaces" or deformable models [2]-[7]. For successful and reproducible convergence, such algorithms typically require an initialization that represents a reasonably close approximation of the target shape. Little has been reported on the selection and evaluation of such initializations. Manual identification of a starting point provides a customized initialization but can be time-consuming and introduces observer variability. Initialization from average population models is automated but potentially limited by the variability of the target population. Population based models also allow the introduction of additional prior knowledge, such as statistics to limit the extent to

T. Dohi and R. Kikinis (Eds.): MICCAI 2002, LNCS 2488, pp. 483-491, 2002.
© Springer-Verlag Berlin Heidelberg 2002

which a model can deform [4]-[7]. However, such approaches often rely solely on the average population model as their starting point. We demonstrate in this work that additional information derived automatically from the individual case can be the basis for customizing an average population model and thus lead to a better approximation of the target shape. Such an approach has direct applications to automated segmentation algorithms based on deformable models.

The purpose of this study was to test an automatically generated shape approximation of the lateral ventricle in multiple sclerosis (MS) patients and normal healthy volunteers. We propose a parametric model of ventricular shape, linked to the brain parenchymal fraction (BPF), where BPF is a size-normalized estimate of whole brain atrophy [8]-[9]. BPF calculation is fully automated and readily available. The relationship between the coefficients of a parametric description and BPF can be used to extrapolate the shape of a ventricle for any individual based on the BPF. The concept is similar to that presented in [10] where the position of anatomical structures in the brain are predicted based on the location and parameterization of the head surface.

2   Methods

2.1   Population

MR images from 25 MS patients and 6 healthy volunteers were selected to represent a sample of MS patients with varying disease type, duration and severity (13 relapsing-remitting MS, 9 secondary progressive MS, and 3 primary progressive MS). These 31 cases formed the training set for the average ventricle shape. Images from 10 additional MS patients (6 relapsing-remitting, 4 secondary progressive) were selected for testing purposes.

2.2   BPF Calculations

BPF was determined automatically on each MRI image as described in [8]-[9]. An automated 3D segmentation algorithm was applied to identify brain tissue voxels and the smoothed outer surface of the brain. The algorithm calculated the brain volume (BV) while accounting for partial volume effects. The outer brain contour volume (OCV), i.e. the volume enclosed by the smoothed outer surface of the brain, is also determined. The BPF is then defined as:

$$BPF = BV / OCV \tag{1}$$

BPF thus represents a normalized estimate of brain volume.

2.3   Spherical Harmonic Parameterization of the Lateral Ventricle

The left lateral ventricle of each case was segmented by manual tracing using customized software developed in IDL (Research Systems Incorporated, Boulder, U.S.A.). A parametric representation of each segmented left ventricle based on spherical harmonics was generated as described in [1], [11]. The Cartesian coordinates of uniformly sampled points on the surface of the ventricle can be homologically mapped onto the surface of a sphere. Spherical harmonics $Y_l^m(\theta,\phi)$ were used as the basis functions for a parametric representation of the ventricular surface, according to:

$$\mathbf{a}_{l,m} \approx \frac{4\pi}{N} \sum_{i=1}^{N} \mathbf{x}_i Y_l^m\left(\theta_i, \phi_i\right) \qquad (2)$$

$$\mathbf{x}(\theta,\phi) = \sum_{l=0}^{H} \sum_{m=-l}^{l} \mathbf{a}_{l,m} Y_l^m\left(\theta,\phi\right) \qquad (3)$$

where $\mathbf{a}_{l,m} = [a_x, a_y, a_z]^T$ is the coefficient vector for level l and order m, and $\mathbf{x}_i$ ($i=1...N$) are the Cartesian coordinates of the object surface. Spherical harmonics are defined as:

$$Y_l^m(\theta,\phi) = \sqrt{\frac{2l+1}{4\pi}\frac{(l-m)!}{(l+m)!}} P_l^m(\cos\theta)e^{im\phi} \qquad (4)$$

where P_l^m are the associated Legendre polynomials, defined by the differential equation

$$P_l^m(x) = \frac{(-1)^m}{2^k l!}(1-x^2)^{m/2}\frac{d^{l+m}}{dx^{l+m}}(x^2-1)^l \qquad (5)$$

A recursive algorithm for their computation is given in [12]. This yields a parameterization for arbitrary 3D object surfaces of genus zero. The imaginary portion of the series is ignored and only the real portion is used. Note that objects do **not** have to be star-shaped, as long as (θ,ϕ) is a homologic spherical map. To make the coefficients $\mathbf{a}_{l,m}$ view independent, each ventricle's spherical harmonic coefficients were mapped into a common reference frame by registration using a full-affine transformation.

2.4   Population Average and BPF Modulation

The average left lateral ventricle was generated by averaging the coefficients $\mathbf{a}_{l,m}$ of the first 12 harmonics across individuals included in the training set). This average model was then modulated based on the BPF to obtain an approximation of each individual ventricle. The relationship between the BPF and the magnitude of each coefficient of the first 12 harmonics (i.e. Y_l^m with l=0,...,12, and m=-l,...,0,...,l) was tested using linear regression. This process was performed in the x, y, and z directions. Coefficients where the p-values for the regression lines were less than or equal to 0.05 were identified as coefficients to modulate and were adjusted based on BPF according to:

$$\tilde{a}_{l,m} = a_{l,m} \cdot \left(\frac{\beta_{l,m} \cdot BPF + \gamma_{l,m}}{\|a_{l,m}\|} \right) \tag{6}$$

where $a_{l,m}$ is the model parameter of the average ventricle, $\tilde{a}_{l,m}$ is the modulated version approximating the individual shape, and $\beta_{l,m}$ and $\gamma_{l,m}$ are the slope and intercept of the regression line, respectively.

An initial set of customized ventricle approximations was obtained as described above for each of the 31 subjects in the training set. A "leave-one-out" approach was used to ensure that information derived from each test case was not included in the average ventricle. Thus for each case, the customized ventricle was derived from data obtained solely from the other 30 cases considered. New regression lines were determined for each test case and for each spherical harmonic coefficient.

The set of coefficients to include in the approximation model were identified as the coefficients consistently chosen for modulation during the initial "leave-one-out" tests. Thus, the coefficients modulated in at least 90% of the test cases (i.e. at least 28 of the 31 cases) were determined as being linearly related to BPF and selected as the final set of spherical harmonic coefficients to. This proposed model was also applied to the training set in a "leave-one-out" fashion and further tested on an additional test set of 10 MS patients.

2.5   Evaluation

The proposed approximation model was evaluated for each case by comparing both the average ventricle and its individualized modulation to the manual segmentation of the ventricle (gold standard) based on the kappa coefficient, κ [13]. The kappa coefficient is a measure of the overlap between two regions and is calculated according to:

$$\kappa = \frac{2(A \cap B)}{2(A \cap B) + \overline{A} \cap B + A \cap \overline{B}} \tag{7}$$

where A and B are 3D binary images of the segmented objects, A-bar and B-bar are the inverse images of A and B, and $\cap$ is the intersection operator (which, in this case, returns the volume of the intersection). Kappa $>= 0.7$ indicates excellent agreement. The two kappa coefficients were compared to determine which ventricle (customized or average) represented a closer approximation of the manually segmented ventricle.

3   Results

The BPF values measured for the training set and test cases are reported in Table 1. The BPF values ranged from 0.69 to 0.88. The mean (s.d.) BPF for the whole group was 0.806 (0.057). The BPF measures obtained for the cases involved in the study was a representative sample of the range of BPF values observed in our laboratory as shown in Figure 1.

Table 1. Population breakdown

	Type	n	BPF range	Mean BPF (s.d.)
Training	Healthy volunteer	6	0.86-0.87	0.87 (0.006)
	Relapsing-remitting MS	13	0.70-0.88	0.82 (0.046)
	Secondary-progressive MS	9	0.69-0.83	0.75 (0.043)
	Primary-progressive MS	3	0.76-0.81	0.78 (0.028)
Test	Relapsing-remitting MS	6	0.75-0.80	0.77 (0.020)
	Secondary-progressive MS	4	0.70-0.75	0.73 (0.023)

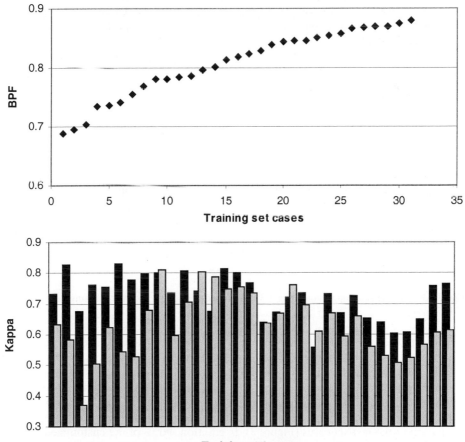

Fig. 1. Top: BPF values of the training set cases. Bottom: Kappa coefficients for the training set population. Kappa coefficient values calculated for each test case by comparing the average ventricle (gray) and customized approximation ventricle (black) to the manually segmented ventricle

The first H=12 harmonics (eq. 2) were considered for inclusion in the approxima-tion model, which was sufficient to describe the shape of the ventricles. Of the 91 spherical harmonic coefficients tested for modulation in each direction, 34 % (31 of 91) were used in the x direction, 30 % (27 of 91) in the y direction, and 37 % (34 of 91) in the z direction.

The "leave-one-out" evaluation of the proposed approximation model on the training set yielded the following results. The mean (s.d.) kappa coefficient for the average ventricles was 0.633 (0.103) versus 0.721 (0.072) for the customized ap-proximation ventricles, where a kappa coefficient greater than 0.7 indicates excellent agreement. The individual kappa coefficient values for each series are presented in Figure 1. The differences in the kappa coefficients are plotted against BPF in Figure 2. The kappa coefficients calculated from each series were compared using a paired t-test and found to be significantly different ($p < 0.0001$). Based on the kappa coeffi-cient, the custom approximation represented an improvement over the average ventri-cle in 81 % of the cases (25 of 31). Furthermore, 61 % of the custom ventricle (19 of 31) had a kappa coefficient larger than 0.7 compared to 26 % of the cases (8 of 31) for the average ventricle.

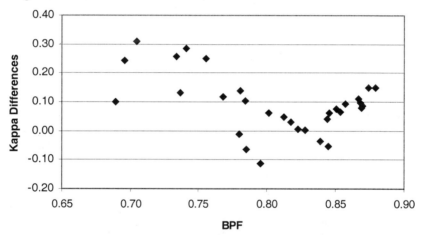

Fig. 2. Differences in Kappa coefficients (customized − average) for the training set cases vs. BPF values

The outcome was similar for the test set with 10 additional MS patients. The mean (s.d.) kappa coefficient for the average ventricles was 0.639 (0.098) versus 0.796 (0.058) for the customized approximation ventricles, which was also significantly different ($p < 0.001$). As in the leave-one-out evaluation, the customized ventricle represented a consistent improvement over the average ventricle. The kappa coeffi-cients for the customized approximation were larger than those for the average ventri-cle in each of the test set cases (Figure 3). In addition, 90 % of the customized ventri-cles had a kappa coefficient larger than 0.7, compared to 20 % for the average ventricle.

Figure 4 shows an example axial image with overlaid delineations of the average and customized ventricle boundaries. Figure 5 shows the average and customized ventricle surfaces in 3D for the same patient.

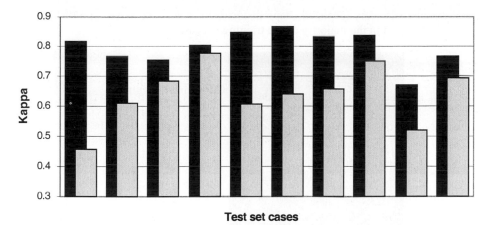

Fig. 3. Kappa coefficients for the test set. Kappa coefficient values calculated for each test case by comparing the average ventricle (gray) and customized approximation ventricle (black) to the manually segmented ventricle

4   Discussion

The proposed model reliably and automatically generated customized ventricles based on a population average and BPF. The customized ventricles represented a closer approximation of the target shape than the average ventricle in the majority of the cases (81% and 100% improvement in the training and test sets, respectively). The improvement was most pronounced for people with BPF significantly different from the mean (see Figure 2), which was expected since the customized ventricles are derived from an average ventricle model. This observation is relevant since a purely statistical model is likely to fail in producing a good instantiation from the same training set for cases with BPF far from the mean. Thus, the proposed approximation model can accommodate any individual case falling within the range of BPFs defined by the training set, regardless of whether similar cases have been observed. Outside of the defined BPF range, the proposed method will rely on extrapolation to approximate expected ventricular shape.

Sensitivity towards the initial condition is an important limitation of deformable models and the main impediment to routine use in clinical morphometry. Statistical priors derived from population averages have been shown to improve optimization efficiency [5]-[7], but an improved approximation of the target shape is likely to further increase both speed and likelihood of convergence to the global minima. The presented model proved especially effective for cases at the tails of the population distribution, where an unmodified statistical prior is likely to fail. Note also that no explicit assumption was made as to the type of deformable model to be used for the segmentation.

The proposed approximation model relies on the assumption of atrophy as a global process and thus relies on a global measure of atrophy and global shape descriptors. Under such conditions, this approach may not perform as well in cases with extreme focal atrophy (i.e. very localized shape distortions), unless the same type of focal atrophy is observed in the majority of the training set cases.

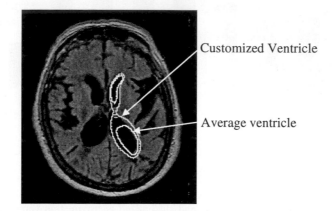

Customized Ventricle

Average ventricle

Fig. 4. Example image with ventricle outlines for the average ventricle and custom approximation of the ventricle

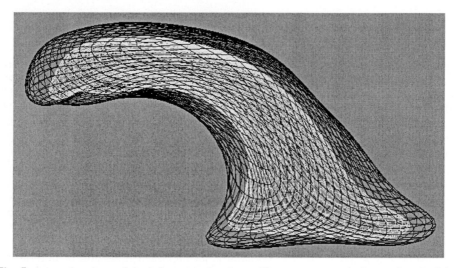

Fig. 5. Approximations of the left ventricular shape. The average ventricular surface (training set) is shown in gray while the customized ventricular surface is shown in black

The new approach was presented on the left ventricle in MS patients. There are, of course, no restrictions as to the right ventricle or other shapes, and further efforts will include additional structures in MS patients and other pathologies. Similar models for Alzheimer's disease and normal aging are of particular interest. Future work will involve applying the custom ventricle as a starting point for automated segmentation of the lateral ventricles in our clinical data.

5   Conclusion

The proposed approximation model was successful in reliably and automatically generating customized ventricles approximating the shape of individual left lateral ventricles. The approximation model relied on a training set consisting of representative MS patients and normal volunteers. The customized approximation of the ventricle was based on the spherical harmonic parameterization of the left ventricle and the associated BPF measures in the training set cases. A set of spherical harmonic coefficients was identified as being linearly related to BPF, and the customized approximation of ventricular shape was generated for a given BPF value by independently modulating the individual coefficients within that set. These customized approximations of the ventricular shape represented a reliably better approximation of the ventricular shape than the average population ventricle (especially for extreme cases), and are, therefore, appropriate for use as a good initial starting point for a variety of segmentation methods.

References

1. Meier, D.S., Fisher E.: Parameter Space Warping: Shape-Based Correspondence Between Morphologically Different Objects. IEEE Trans. Med. Imag. 21 (2002)
2. Cohen, L.D., Cohen, I.: Finite-Element Methods for Active Contour Models and Balloons for 2D and 3D Images. IEEE Trans Pattern Anal. Mach. Intell. 15 (1993) 1131-1147
3. Klingensmith, J.D., Shekhar, R., Vince, D.G.: Evaluation of three-dimensional segmentation algorithms for the identification of luminal and medial-adventitial borders in intravascular ultrasound images. IEEE Trans. Med. Imag. 19 (2000) 996-1011
4. McInerney, T., Terzopoulos, D.: Deformable Models in Medical Image Analysis: A Survey. Med Imgage Anal. 1 (1996) 91-108
5. Kelemen, A., Szekely, G., Gerig, G.: Elastic Model-Based Segmentation of 3D Neuroradiological Data Sets. IEEE Trans. Med. Imag. 18 (1999) 828-839
6. Staib, L.H., Duncan, J.S.: Model-Based Deformable Surface Finding for Medical Images. IEEE Trans. Med. Imag. 15 (1996) 720-731
7. Cootes, T.F., Taylor, C.J., Cooper, D.H., Graham, J.: Active Shape Models-Their Training and Application. Computer Vision Image Understanding, 61 (1995) 38-59
8. Fisher, E., Cothren, R.M., Tkach, J.A., Masaryck, T.J., Cornhill, J.F.: Knowledge-Based 3D Segmentation of MR Images for Quantitative MS Lesion Tracking. SPIE Med. Imag. 3034 (1997) 599-610
9. Rudick, R., Fisher, E., Lee, J.-C., et al: Use of the Brain Parenchymal Fraction to Measure Whole Brain Atrophy in Relapsing-Remitting MS. Neurology. 53 (1999) 1698-1704
10. Nikou, C. Bueno, G., Heitz, F., Armspach, J.-P.: A Joint Physics-Based Statistical Deformable Model for Multimodality Brain Image Analysis. IEEE Trans. Med. Imag. 20 (2001) 1026-1037
11. Brechbuhler, C., Gerig, G., Kubler, O.: Parametrization of Closed Surfaces dor 3-D Shape Description. Computer Vision Image Understanding, 61 (1995) 154-170
12. Press, W.H., Teutolsky, S.A. Vetterling, W.T., Flannery, B.P.: Numerical Recipes in C – the Art of Scientific Computing, 2nd edn. Cambridge University Press, Cambridge (1992)
13. Zijdenbos, A.P., Dawant, B.M., Margolin, R.A., Palmer, A.C.: Morphometric Analysis of White Matter Lesions in MR Images. IEEE Trans. Med. Imag. 13 (1994) 716-724

An Intensity Consistent Approach to the Cross Sectional Analysis of Deformation Tensor Derived Maps of Brain Shape

C. Studholme, V. Cardenas, A. Maudsley, and M. Weiner

U.C.S.F., Dept of Radiology, VAMC (114Q),
4150 Clement Street, San Francisco,
CA 94121, USA
cs1@itsa.ucsf.edu

Abstract. This paper describes a novel approach to the spatial filtering of deformation tensor derived maps of shape difference and shape change estimated in multi-subject studies of spatially normalised brain anatomy. We propose a spatial shape filter that combines tensor values locally which fall within regions of similar underlying intensity and therefore tissue. The filter additionally incorporates information derived from the spatial normalisation process to focus filtering more strongly within specific MRI intensities in regions where tissue intensities have been most consistently aligned in the spatial normalisation process. This is achieved using a statistical framework to introduce a measure of uncertainty of regional intensity correspondence. Results comparing the approach to conventional Gaussian filtering in the analysis of tensor derived measures of brain shape change in Alzheimer's disease and normal aging indicate significantly improved delineation of local atrophy patterns, particularly in cortical gray matter, without the need for explicit tissue segmentation.

1 Introduction

The use of non rigid registration transformations to capture spatial statistical measures of human anatomy is developing as a powerful tool in automated computational neuro anatomy [5, 14, 13, 6, 9, 4, 1]. These methods make use of non rigid registration of brain MRI to a common anatomy, allowing the mapping of shape difference over the entire brain. Unlike ROI based techniques, such approaches are not limited to the quantification of specific anatomically defined structures, but can capture changes in all anatomical boundaries visible in the MRI which can be brought into correspondence. Once these spatially normalizing transformations have been estimated, it is possible to use a range of approaches to quantify shape difference from measurements derived from these transformations. One such powerful approach is that of tensor based morphometry which makes use of spatial derivatives of these transformations [5, 3]. One of the challenges however in making use of this approach is how to handle the inherent spatial uncertainty in the underlying transformations, and resulting errors in the derivatives being analyzed. Spatial filtering of such fields can dramatically

T. Dohi and R. Kikinis (Eds.): MICCAI 2002, LNCS 2488, pp. 492–499, 2002.

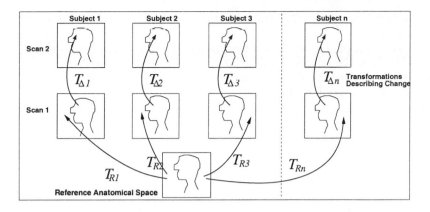

Fig. 1. Using non-rigid registration to capture local shape differences between subjects from the transformations T_{Rn}, and shape changes within subject over time from the transformations $T_{\Delta n}$. To examine common patterns across subjects, maps of shape measures derived from these transformations may be evaluated and compared in the reference anatomy.

improve the statistical power of the approach, but at the expense of losing the fine-scale localization properties of these transformations. Filtering with uniform spatial filters is inherently sub-optimal because the underlying errors in registration estimates are themselves spatially varying: some locations are consistently aligned across all subjects, while other locations are poorly aligned because of underlying differences in anatomical topology. In this paper we explore a simple and novel approach to spatial filtering of these fields which incorporates information about the inherent spatial uncertainty in the spatial normalisation, while retaining the underlying anatomical localization accuracy provided by the alignment of visible boundaries in the images.

2   Method

2.1   Tensor Morphometry: Spatial Maps of Shape from Registration

The problem addressed in this paper is that of analyzing the spatial derivative fields used to describe shape difference (in purely cross sectional studies) and shape change (in serial or longitudinal MRI studies) over a group of individual anatomies. In such approaches non-rigid registration is used to capture shape difference between an individual and a reference anatomy or between repeat scans of an individual, as illustrated in figure 1. In such a study we have either imaged or synthesized a reference anatomy, producing a map of reference intensities $i_R(\mathbf{x}_R)$ over the points $\mathbf{x}_R \in X_R$ to use as a target for spatial normalisation. We then use this reference anatomical space to study a set N of subject images with image intensities $\{i_n(\mathbf{x}_n), n \in N\}$ over points $\{\mathbf{x}_n \in X_n, n \in N\}$. In general we assume that the non-rigid registration transformation between the reference space and each subject $T_{Rn} : \mathbf{x}_R \mapsto \mathbf{x}_n$ has been estimated by a registration procedure optimising an intensity similarity criteria, $C(i_R, i_n)$ between image intensities or alternatively extrapolating transformation models from aligned corresponding features.

In cross sectional tensor based morphometry [5, 3, 6, 10], relative differences in shape between the reference and subject anatomies are described by the spatial derivatives of these transformations, evaluated at each point, to form maps of the local point-wise Jacobian,

$$\mathbf{J}_{Rn}(\mathbf{x}_R) = \frac{\partial T_{Rn}(\mathbf{x}_R)}{\partial \mathbf{x}_R}. \tag{1}$$

describing the relative local contractions or expansions of tissue from reference coordinates $\mathbf{x}_R$, to subject coordinates $T_{Rn}(\mathbf{x_R})$. To remove directional information, the determinant of this matrix is often used as a summary measure of overall contraction or expansion at each point in the reference anatomy $J_{Rn}(\mathbf{x}) = |\mathbf{J}_{Rn}(\mathbf{x})|$.

In serial MRI studies [11] a similar approach can be used to map local volumetric change between time points within a subject study using a non rigid transformation say T_n between the time point 1 to 2 scans of subject n, which has itself been spatially normalised by a transformation T_{Rn}. In the space of the common reference anatomy, these tissue contractions and expansions of an individual anatomy are described by the Jacobian mapping between time point 1 and time point 2 coordinates:

$$\mathbf{J}_n(\mathbf{x}_R) = \frac{\partial T_n(T_{Rn}(\mathbf{x}_R))}{\partial T_{Rn}(\mathbf{x}_R)}. \tag{2}$$

In this paper the approaches described to filtering local shape measures are applicable to both cross sectional and serial shape measures, and we will therefore refer to the general case of filtering shape measure J_n at location $\mathbf{x}_R$.

2.2   The Need for Spatial Filtering in Shape Analysis

When estimating spatial transformations between anatomies, there are a number of fundamental reasons why there is remains an underlying ambiguity in the transformation estimates and the shape measures derived from them, which mean that post filtering of the shape fields is desirable. These include three main factors: Firstly that registration accuracy away from anatomical boundaries in the images is inherently under-determined and dependent on both the starting estimate and estimation methodology. Secondly: Geometric constraints on the allowable transformation estimates, such as transformation invertibility [2] and resolution of transformation parameterisation prevent a complete optimisation of $C(i_R, i_n)$ and therefore residual differences between $i_R(\mathbf{x})$ and $i_n(T_{Rn}(\mathbf{x}))$ remain. Thirdly: the underlying variability of the location of disease induced effects across structures such as the cerebral cortex requires the study of their shape at both fine and coarse scales (i.e. a disease may remove local points of cortical gray matter distributed randomly within a given larger region such as the frontal lobe).

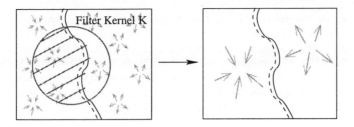

Fig. 2. An illustration of the aim of spatially filtering contractions and expansions in neighboring tissues separately so that anatomical boundaries are not lost.

2.3   Spatial Filtering of Tensor Fields

In the most direct approach to improving the signal to noise properties of the individual shape maps, we may consider applying a spatial filter to the Jacobian determinant map,

$$\tilde{J}_n(\mathbf{x}_R) = \int_{\mathbf{k} \in K} J_n(\mathbf{x}_R - \mathbf{k}).f(\mathbf{k}) \tag{3}$$

to accumulate estimates of neighboring volume change into a more stable regional estimate, where $f(\mathbf{k})$ denotes the response of the spatial filter over neighborhood $\mathbf{k} \in K$. Previous approaches have used conventional Gaussian filters [6] which also usefully force the residual field toward a Gaussian random field for the purposes of statistical analysis. However, this does not take into account the fact that different tissues are expected to exhibit different shape properties. This is a particular problem when studying patterns of opposing local shape difference in fine scale structures such as the those in contracting cortical gray matter and expanding sulcal CSF in normal aging and degenerative disease. In this work we address this limitation by modifying the filtering of shape measures using an approach derived from that of the sigma filter [7]. Specifically, we propose a general probabilistic form of shape filter:

$$\tilde{J}_n(\mathbf{x}_R) = \frac{1}{\Theta(\mathbf{x}_R)} \int_{\mathbf{k} \in K} J_n(\mathbf{x}_R - \mathbf{k}).f(\mathbf{k}).p_{xk}(\mathbf{x}_R, \mathbf{k}) \tag{4}$$

where $p_{xk}(\mathbf{x}_R, \mathbf{k})$ represents the statistical relationship between measurements at $\mathbf{x}_R$ and $\mathbf{x}_R - \mathbf{k}$ and,

$$\Theta(\mathbf{x}_R) = \int_{\mathbf{k} \in K} f(\mathbf{k}).p_{xk}(\mathbf{x}_R, \mathbf{k}) \tag{5}$$

normalizes for the volume under the local probabilistic neighborhood. The following section goes on the describe the design of a suitable formulation for $p_{xk}(\mathbf{x}_R, \mathbf{k})$.

2.4   A Measure of Association
between Neighboring Shape Measurements

One important aim is to use this filter operation to enforce the combination of shape measurements that fall in regions of similar underlying MRI intensity.

However, since we are analyzing the maps in a common averaged anatomical space, we would ideally like each filtered subject map to conform to the anatomical structure in the averaged spatially normalised MRI of the entire group under study, rather than the spatially normalised individual MRI in which the measurements are made, since this may contain local tissue misalignment errors with respect to the common averaged MRI. We therefore choose to build a measure of association derived between the averaged intensity value,

$$\mu'(\mathbf{x}_R) = \frac{1}{N} \sum_{n \in N} i_n(\mathbf{T}_{Rn}(\mathbf{x}_R)). \tag{6}$$

of all spatially normalised MRI's, at the reference anatomy location $\mathbf{x}_R$ where the filter is being applied, and the spatially normalised individual MRI value,

$$i'_n(\mathbf{x}_R) = i_n(T_{Rn}(\mathbf{x}_R)), \tag{7}$$

at neighboring point $(\mathbf{x}_R - \mathbf{k})$. In this work we examine the use of the conditional probability $p_K(i|\mu)$ as a regional filtering statistic. This is the probability of observing in region K, the spatially normalised individual MRI intensity i, given the averaged intensity of the group μ' at the same location. We derive this by first constructing a local spatially weighted estimate of the joint probability distribution $p_K(i, \mu)$ between averaged MRI intensities and individual spatially normalised MRI intensities in the filter support around location $\mathbf{x}_R$. Algorithmically this is implemented as a discrete 2D histogram such that,

$$p_K(i, \mu) = \frac{1}{\Gamma} \sum_{n \in N} \sum_{\mathbf{k} \in K} f(\mathbf{k}).\epsilon(i, i'_n(\mathbf{x}_R - \mathbf{k})).\epsilon(\mu, \mu'(\mathbf{x}_R - \mathbf{k})), \tag{8}$$

where,

$$\epsilon(\alpha, \beta) = \begin{cases} 1, \langle \frac{\alpha}{b} \rangle = \langle \frac{\beta}{b} \rangle \\ 0, otherwise \end{cases} \tag{9}$$

counts equivalent intensities falling in bins with width b, $\langle \rangle$ indicates nearest integer, and the term

$$\Gamma = \sum_{n \in N} \sum_{\mathbf{k} \in K} f(\mathbf{k}) \tag{10}$$

normalises by the weighted total number of voxels. This distribution captures the fraction of the filter neighborhood occupied by correctly aligned intensity pairs, together with the fraction of all combinations of mis-aligned intensity pairs. From this we then derive our intensity based statistical relationship between neighboring shape measurements, as the conditional probability $p_K(i|\mu)$ such that,

$$p_{xk}(\mathbf{x}_R, \mathbf{k}) = p_K(i'_n(\mathbf{x}_R - \mathbf{k})|\mu'(\mathbf{x}_R)) = \frac{p_K(i'_n(\mathbf{x}_R - \mathbf{k}), \mu'(\mathbf{x}_R))}{p_K(\mu'(\mathbf{x}_R))}, \tag{11}$$

where $p_K(\mu'(\mathbf{x}_R))$ is the marginal probability of μ'. In regions where intensities are inconsistently aligned, $p_K(i|\mu)$ contains more than one peak and thus local shape measures lying in these peaks are accepted by the filter, reflecting the uncertainty in whether shape measures in these locations have been spatially normalised to the correct tissue. Conversely, in regions where MRI intensities are consistently brought into correspondence, $p_K(i|\mu)$ has one distinct peak for μ and forces the shape filter to accept only points falling in this narrow range.

3   Results on Serial MRI Analysis in Alzheimer's Disease

To illustrate the effect of using this proposed filtering on clinically derived shape maps, we have applied the filtering approach, using Gaussian spatial kernels for the filter $f()$, to the task of mapping brain shape change over time in a serial imaging study of dementia. 10 subjects diagnosed with Alzheimer's disease and 10 aging cognitively normal volunteers were imaged twice with an interval of between 1 and 3 years. A fine lattice entropy driven B-Spline deformation registration algorithm [11] was used to deform the later scan back to match the earlier scan, and spatially differentiated to produce a map of point-wise volume change in the coordinate system of the first time point scan. The transformation mapping between each first time point subject MRI scan and a single reference MRI was then evaluated using a multi-grid and multi-resolution registration, again driven by normalised mutual information [12]. The individual maps of point-wise volume change between time points were then transformed to the coordinate system of the reference MRI. Global and local intensity inhomogeneity was removed from the intensity images and filters of three widths were then applied to each subject's atrophy map. A mean atrophy rate map was then calculated for the two groups. The results of comparing the three filter widths using conventional and intensity consistent filtering are shown in Figure 3 and enlarged for Alzheimer's in figure 4. As the filter width increases the ability of intensity consistent filter to retain fine structure in the cortex is clear. The overall level of atrophy is clearly greater in Alzheimer's over controls. The enlarged view shows the contrast detected in the atrophy rate between the white matter and gray matter ribbon over much of the cortex (note here that no explicit tissue segmentation has been applied).

4   Discussion

We have developed an approach to refining the analysis of deformation tensor fields that are derived from MRI scans of multiple subjects mapped to a common reference anatomy. It focuses filtering of local shape measures within regions of similar underlying MRI intensity and, additionally incorporates information about the local quality of the spatial normalisation of MRI intensities across the scans of subjects being studied. The filter does not require additional parameters to define its behaviour and automatically weights filtered shape measurements based on the local consistency in mapping structural image values at each point in the reference anatomy. One important factor to consider in this approach is that the filtered fields produced are fundamentally not continuous, but in fact reflect the underlying discontinuity in the anatomical structure being imaged. Statistically these fields therefore cannot be analysed using techniques based on assumptions such as those made in Gaussian random field theory. This is particularly important for correcting the statistical significance of any measurements

Alzheimer's   Cognitively Normal
4mm   8mm   12mm   4mm   8mm   12mm

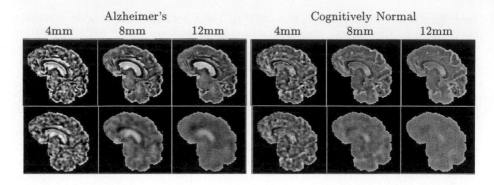

Fig. 3. Sagittal slices through reference anatomy showing the average spatially normalised maps of annualised volume change in 10 Alzheimer's patients (left) and 10 cognitively normal elderly subjects (right). Bottom row shows conventional spatially invariant Gaussian filtering, top row shows intensity consistent filtering. Averaged Jacobian determinant displayed as a gray scale thresholded at -8%(black) and +8%(white) per year.

for multiple comparisons. We are therefore developing approaches to analyzing statistical models of these fields based on permutation testing [8]. Although The approach is essentially free from spatial priors on the shape difference or change, the spatial filtering level employed is itself an implicit prior on any analysis. An interesting approach we are exploring is the multi-scale analysis possible in the non-Gaussian scale space of shape description produced by repeated application of tissue consistent spatial filters.

Acknowledgments. This work was primarily funded by the Whitaker Foundation. Image data used in this work was acquired as part of NIH grant P01 AG12435. The authors wish to thank Bruce Miller, Howard Rosen and Helena Chui for access to data and useful discussions on dementia and aging.

References

1. J. Ashburner, C. Hutton, R. Frackowiak, I. Johnsrude, C. Price, and K.J. Friston. Identifying global anatomical differences: Deformation-based morphometry. *Neuroimage*, 6:348–357, 1998.
2. G.E. Christensen and H.J. Johnson. Consistent image registration. *Transactions on Medical Imaging*, pages 568–582, 2001.
3. M. K. Chung, K. J. Worsley, T. Paus, C. Cherif, D. L. Collins, J. N. Giedd, J. L. Rapoport, and A. C. Evans. A unified statistical approach to deformation-based morphometry. *Neuroimage*, 14:596–606, 2001.
4. J.G. Csernansky, L. Wang, S. Joshi J.P. Miller M. Gado D. Kido D. McKeel, J.C. Morris, and MI. Miller. Early DAT is distinguished from aging by high-dimensional mapping of the hippocampus. *Neurology*, 55(11):1636–1643, 2000.
5. C. Davatzikos, M. Vaillant, S.M. Resnick, J.L. Prince, S. Letovsky, and R.N. Bryan. A computerised approach for morphological analysis of the corpus callosum. *Journal of Computer Assisted Tomography*, 20(1):88–97, 1996.

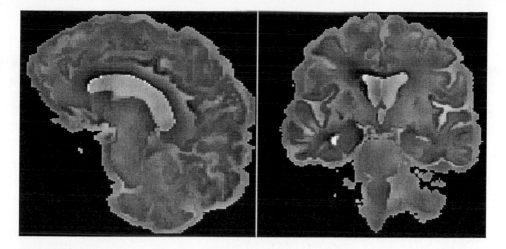

Fig. 4. Enlarged orthogonal views through the Alzheimer's average atrophy rate map, illustrating the different contraction rates visible in the cortical gray matter layer.

6. C. Gaser, H.P. Voltz, S. Kiebel, S. Riehemann, and H. Sauer. Detecting structural changes in whole brain based on nonlinear deformations- application to schizophrenia research. *Neuroimage*, 10:107–113, 1999.
7. J.S. Lee. Digital image smoothing and the sigma filter. *Computer Vision, Graphics and Image Processing*, 24(2):255–269, 1983.
8. T. E. Nichols and A. P. Holmes. Nonparametric permutation tests for functional neuroimagin: A primer with examples. *Human Brain Mapping*, 15:1–25, 2001.
9. D.J. Pettey and J.C. Gee. Using a linear diagnostic function and non-rigid registration to search for morphological differences between poluations: An example involving the male and female corpus callosum. In *Proceedings SPIE Medical Imaging*, volume 4322, page In Press, 2001.
10. C. Studholme, V. Cardenas, N. Schuff, H. Rosen, B. Miller, and M. Weiner. Detecting spatially consistent structural differences in alzheimer's and fronto temporal dementia using deformation morphometry. In *Proceedings of 4th International Conference on Medical Image Computing and Computer Assisted Interventions, 2001*, pages 41–48, 2001.
11. C. Studholme, V. Cardenas, and M. Weiner. Building whole brain maps of atrophy from multi-subject longitudinal studies using free form deformations. In *Proceedings of ISMRM 2001, Glasgow, Scotland*, 2001.
12. C. Studholme, V. Cardenas, and M. Weiner. Multi scale image and multi scale deformation of brain anatomy for building average brain atlases. In *Proceedings SPIE Medical Imaging*, volume 4322-60, pages 557–568, 2001.
13. J.P. Thirion and G. Calmon. Deformation analysis to detect and quantify active lesions in three-dimensional medical image sequences. *IEEE Transactions on Medical Imaging*, 18(5):429–441, 1999.
14. P. Thompson, R. Woods, M. Mega, and A. Toga. Mathematical/Computational challenges in creating deformable and probabilistic atlases of the human brain. *Human Brain Mapping*, 9:81–92, 2000.

Detection of Inter-hemispheric Asymmetries of Brain Perfusion in SPECT

Bérengère Aubert-Broche[1], Christophe Grova[1], Pierre Jannin[1], Irène Buvat[2], Habib Benali[2], and Bernard Gibaud[1]

[1] Laboratoire IDM, Faculté de Médecine, Université de Rennes 1, France
{berengere.broche,christophe.grova,pierre.jannin,bernard.gibaud}
@univ-rennes1.fr,
[2] INSERM U494, CHU Pitié Salpétrière, Paris
{irene.buvat,habib.benali}@imed.jussieu.fr

Abstract. This paper describes an unsupervised method to help detection of significant functional inter-hemispheric asymmetries in brain SPECT. A validation of this method was performed with realistic simulated SPECT data sets with known asymmetries (in size and amplitude) as gold standard. Detection performances were assessed through Receiver Operating Characteristic (ROC) analysis based on measures of the overlap between known and detected asymmetries.

1 Introduction

^{99m}Technetium HMPAO and ^{99m}Tc ECD Single Photon Emission Computed Tomography (SPECT) imaging is now commonly used to highlight altered regional cerebral perfusion. In partial epilepsy, SPECT imaging is considered relevant to show perfusion abnormalities, such as hyperperfusion in ictal SPECT (i.e. during epileptic seizure) and hypoperfusion in interictal SPECT (i.e. at a distance from any epileptic seizure) to help localize the epileptogenic focus [1].

Although in clinical routine the analysis of brain SPECT images is often limited to a qualitative side-by-side visual inspection of the data, recent research works have attempted to propose quantitative approaches. The relationship between blood flow and HMPAO or ECD SPECT brain uptake is non linear due to a saturation phenomenon. Absolute measurement of regional cerebral blood flow (rCBF) from HMPAO/ECD SPECT scans is thus not feasible. Only relative quantification can be used, for example using regions of interest (ROIs). ROIs may be geometric [2] or may follow the boundaries of anatomical structures [3]. They may be positioned manually or with the assistance of an anatomical atlas or template [4] or of the Magnetic Resonance images (MR) of the patient[5].

In this paper we propose a fully automatic method to detect inter-hemispheric asymmetries of brain perfusion in SPECT. The principle of this method is described as well as an assessment of its detection capabilities using realistic simulated SPECT data.

T. Dohi and R. Kikinis (Eds.): MICCAI 2002, LNCS 2488, pp. 500–507, 2002.

2   Material and Methods

The proposed method aims at detecting inter-hemispheric functional asymmetries in brain SPECT images, based on anatomical information available from MR images. For this purpose, an asymmetry map was computed at the MRI spatial resolution. For each MRI voxel, the anatomically homologous voxel in the contro-lateral hemisphere was identified. Both homologous voxel coordinates were then mapped into the SPECT volume thanks to the SPECT-MRI registration. Neighborhoods were then defined around these SPECT voxels and compared to obtain a volume of inter-hemispheric differences from which we calculated a volume reflecting the significance of this difference (called "statistical volume").

The following sections describe the major steps of the method, i.e. the SPECT-MRI registration, the identification of homologous voxels and the creation of the difference and statistical volumes. Then, we present the validation method and results based on realistic simulated SPECT data.

2.1   Detection of Inter-hemispheric Functional Asymmetries

SPECT-MRI registration: Rigid registration was performed using mutual information as described by Maes *et al.* [6]. The reliability of this registration method has already been demonstrated in SPECT-MRI registration [7].

Identification of homologous regions: For every voxel of the MRI volume, we determined the voxel which was anatomically homologous in the contro-lateral hemisphere. A first method consisted in defining manually the inter-hemispheric plane on MR images and using it as symmetry plane. A scaling factor was used to take into account the difference in size between the two hemispheres.

A second method used the spatial normalization scheme provided in the Statistical Parametric Mapping software package (SPM) [1] [8]. We used this method to compute non linear transformations between the MR scan of the patient and a symmetrical SPM T1 template. By using this transformation, we identified in the template the voxel corresponding to each point of the patient's MRI. The template being symmetric by construction, the homologous voxel in the contro-lateral hemisphere was obtained by symmetry. By using the inverse deformation fields, the coordinates of this homologous voxel in the patient's MRI were determined. These voxel coordinates were then transferred to the SPECT volume to define voxel-neighborhoods.

Creation of an inter-hemispheric difference volume: We considered two symmetrical spherical voxel-neighborhoods (diameter 1.8 centimeters) containing 33 voxels. We calculated the means ($\bar{x}_1$ and $\bar{x}_2$) and the standard deviations (σ_1 and σ_2) of the voxel intensity values in both neighborhoods. Then, we calculated the difference value : $D = \frac{\bar{x}_1 - \bar{x}_2}{\sqrt{\sigma_1{}^2 + \sigma_2{}^2}}$. This result was stored in a volume of differences at the same coordinates as the initial voxel within the MR volume. We repeated this calculation for each MRI voxel to fill the difference volume.

---

[1] http://www.fil.ion.ucl.ac.uk/spm/

Creation of a statistical volume: The statistical volume was created by testing the hypothesis H_0: $D = 0$ against H_1: $D \neq 0$ at each MRI voxel and by assigning the corresponding p-value.

Voxel values of the difference volume were strongly correlated because of the limited spatial resolution of the SPECT images and the filtering process involved in the SPECT image calculation. Correlation was also introduced by the use of overlapping adjacent voxel-neighborboods. We therefore established an empirical estimation of the probability law under the null hypothesis H_0 by selecting a set of uncorrelated voxels from the difference volume. From a study of the correlation between neighbour voxels, we estimated that samples spaced by at least 18 mm within the brain were not correlated. Since the probability law was established under the null hypothesis, outlier voxels located in asymmetric areas should be removed. These outliers should be only few since we assumed that the asymmetry size was small with respect to the total volume of the brain. We thus removed voxels below the 1% quantile and above the 99% quantile.

From these spatially decorrelated voxels, we estimated the empirical distribution which allowed us to calculate the p-value at each voxel within the difference volume. We therefore obtained a statistical volume, to which threshold values may be applied to get a map of significant voxels corresponding to those voxels for which hypothesis H_0 was rejected.

2.2   Validation Method

Our aim was to determine the ability of our method to detect functional asymmetry zones of various sizes and amplitudes, in both anatomically symmetric and asymmetric brains. Simulated realistic SPECT data sets with known functional asymmetries (in size and amplitude) were used as a gold standard. Detection performances were assessed through Receiver Operating Characteristic (ROC) analysis based on measures of the overlap between known and detected asymmetries. Area under the ROC curve (AUC) was used as quality index.

Realistic SPECT simulations: To perform realistic SPECT simulation, we need to compute at the MRI resolution photon attenuation and activity maps. We used Zubal's head phantom that consists of sixty three anatomical entities manually segmented and labeled from a normal T1-weighted MRI data set [9]. The attenuation map was derived from these entities classified into seven different classes (conjunctive tissue, water, brain, bone, muscle, fat and blood). From measures performed from the SPM SPECT template, we assigned a perfusion value to each of these entities to compute the activity map [7]. These attenuation and activity maps were input parameters of the RecLBL software package created by the Lawrence Berkeley Lab [10] to simulate SPECT projections (64 projections 128 x 128 over 360°). Physical processes including both single photon propagation (e.g. Poisson noise and tissue attenuation) and acquisition procedures (e.g. collimator and detector response) were simulated. Tomographic reconstruction used filtered back-projection with a Hann filter (cutoff frequency : 0.4 cycle per projection bin).

Functional asymmetries simulation: First, we simulated SPECT volumes without any anatomical asymmetry. We introduced functional asymmetric zones of various sizes and intensities in the grey matter of the temporal lobe. The asymmetric zones were spherical with a radius of 5, 10, 15 or 20 mm. However, to model perfusion in a realistic way, only grey matter voxels were given the increased or decreased activity value (baseline activity plus or minus 10 %, 20 %, 30 % or 40 %). Consequently, the volume of the asymmetric zone was 0.5 cm^3, 2.3 cm^3, 5.4 cm^3 or 11 cm^3, depending on the radius of the sphere. Thirty two different cases of functional asymmetries were created (combination of 4 size values and 8 amplitude values), based on an anatomically symmetric brain.

Figure 1 presents two examples of simulated SPECT volumes. The asymmetric zone extension is 11 cm^3 in both figures and amplitude values are +40% and -40%, respectively.

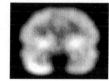
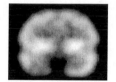

Fig. 1. Symmetric simulated SPECT with 11 cm^3 asymmetric zones with amplitude values of + 40% (left) and -40% (right) in the temporal lobe

We also assessed the ability of the method to detect asymmetric functional zones within an anatomically asymmetric brain. Therefore, we modified the spatial distribution model (based on Zubal's phantom) to introduce anatomical asymmetry. This was achieved by registering the corresponding Zubal's MRI scan to a patient's MRI scan showing obvious anatomical asymmetry of brain hemispheres. The resulting deformation fields were then applied to the spatial distribution model.

Measures of overlap: Once the asymmetry maps had been calculated (difference and statistical volumes), we calculated a degree of overlap between the actual asymmetric zone and the estimated one (at a given statistical threshold). This was achieved by counting voxels as true positives (TP), true negatives (TN), false positives (FP) and false negatives (FN). True positives are voxels belonging to both the significant zone in the statistical volume and to the actual asymmetric zone. The true negatives are voxels belonging to none of these two zones. The false positives are voxels belonging to the significant zone but not to the actual asymmetric zone. The false negatives are voxels belonging to the actual asymmetric zone but not to the significant one. Sensitivity and specificity were computed as respectively the probability to find a significant zone where there is a functional asymmetry (sensitivity = $\frac{TP}{TP+FN}$) and the probability not to detect significant zones where there is no functional asymmetry (specificity = $\frac{TN}{TN+FP}$). Receiver Operating Characteristic curves (or ROC curves) [11] were computed as plots of the true positive rate (or sensitivity) against the false pos-

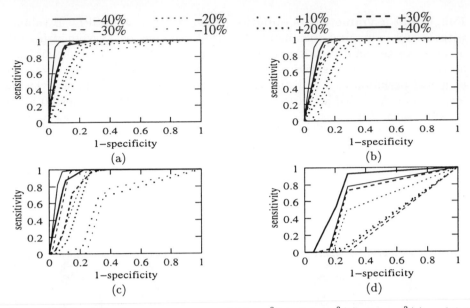

Fig. 2. ROC curves for an asymmetry of 11 cm^3(a), 5.4 cm^3(b), 2.3 cm^3(c) and 0.5 cm^3(d) simulated from a symmetric MRI

itive rate (1- specificity) for different statistical threshold values. Each point of ROC curves corresponds to a pair of sensitivity and specificity values deduced from a p-value threshold applied to the statistical volume. Detection efficiency was measured by the area under the ROC curve (AUC).

3   Results

Figure 2 shows the ROC curves obtained with the detection method applied to volumes simulated from an anatomically symmetric MRI. Symmetric voxel-neighborhoods were computed using the manually defined inter-hemispheric plane. Each figure includes eight ROC curves corresponding to the eight amplitude values of the asymmetries (plus and minus 10, 20, 30, 40 % of activity) for the considered extension. The AUC values are given in figure 3 as a function of the asymmetric zone amplitude and extension values. For the smallest asymmetric zone (0.5 cm^3), the detection efficiency expressed in terms of AUC is between 0.3 and 0.6 for amplitude values of +10, +20, -10, -20 and -30 %. It lies between 0.6 et 0.8 for the amplitude values of +40, +30 and -40 %. It is of 0.6 for an asymmetric zone of 2.3 cm^3 with a low amplitude value (+10 % and -10 %) and close to or greater than 0.8 for all higher values of the asymmetric zone extension and amplitude.

Figure 4 shows the ROC curves obtained with the method of detection applied to volumes simulated from an anatomically asymmetric MRI. Symmetric voxel-neighborhoods were calculated by means of the spatial normalization

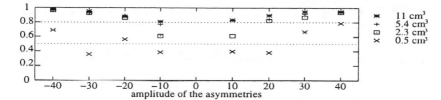
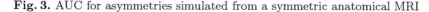

Fig. 3. AUC for asymmetries simulated from a symmetric anatomical MRI

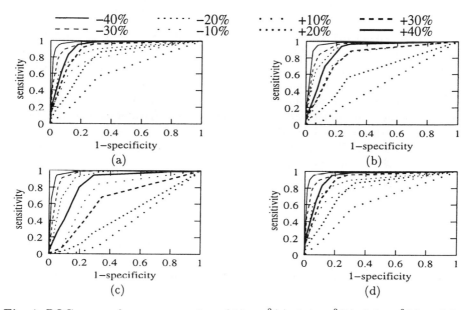

Fig. 4. ROC curves for an asymmetry of 11 cm^3(a), 5.4 cm^3(b), 2.3 cm^3(c) and 0.5 cm^3(d) simulated from an asymmetric MRI

method available in the SPM package. The AUC values are given in figure 5 as a function of the asymmetric zone amplitude and extension values. The AUC values are between 0.75 and 0.98 for asymmetric zones with decreased activity, whatever the value of the asymmetric zone's extension. In the case of increased activity in a 0.5 cm^3 asymmetric zone, the AUC value is around 0.5 whatever the asymmetry amplitude. For larger asymmetric zones, the AUC value is greater than 0.8 only for asymmetric zones with amplitude over +40 % in 2.3 cm^3 asymmetric zones, over +30 % in 5.4 cm^3 zones, and over +20 % in 11 cm^3 zones.

4   Discussion

Our results show that, as expected, the larger and the more intense the asymmetric zone, the more efficient the detection. Within a symmetric brain, all asymmetric zones with amplitude over 20% and size over 2.3 cm^3 are well detected, with AUC equal or over 0.8. These results have been obtained with the

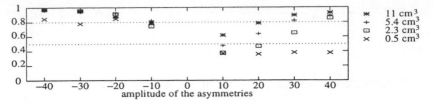

Fig. 5. AUC for asymmetries simulated from an asymmetric anatomical MRI

first way of calculating the contro-lateral homologous voxel-neighborhood (i.e. using a manual definition of the inter-hemispheric plane). The second method (based on the SPM normalization scheme) was also tested and led to slightly degraded performances (detailed results not presented here).

Within an asymmetric brain, detection performances are different depending on the sign of the asymmetry, zones with decreased uptake being better detected than zones with increased uptake. This may be related to registration errors, since a slight shift of few millimeters may change significantly the overlap degree between the actual and the detected asymmetric zone. This has to be confirmed by simulating more asymmetric zones in various locations throughout the brain.

The size of spherical voxel-neighborhood used to compute difference volumes (diameter 1.8 centimeter, 33 voxels) was a tradeoff: indeed it was large enough to take into account the spatial resolution of SPECT and to provide a sufficient number of measures, but not too large in order not to smooth and hide local differences.

An alternative to ROI or voxel-neighborhood based methods is voxel-based methods. These approaches aim at studying either inter-scan and intra-subject variability [12] or inter-scan and inter-subject variability [13],[14]. We believe that our approach studying intra-scan and intra-subject variability is different and complementary. Compared with inter-scan and inter-subject voxel-based analysis which is ¡¡fairly conservative¿¿[13], our method aims at being very sensitive and detecting most of inter-hemispheric perfusion asymmetries (with the risk to have false positive). In a second stage, our goal is to extend our detection method to determine whether this asymmetry is pathological or not, which will involve comparison with normal perfusion asymmetry measured from a control group.

5   Conclusion

We have presented an automatic and unsupervised method to detect functional asymmetry in SPECT images. A validation with computer-simulated data demonstrates the ability to detect asymmetric zones with relatively small extension and amplitude. Further validation based on simulated data will be performed to better characterize the performance, especially in asymmetric brain. A clinical validation will follow this first level of validation, with comparison to depth electrodes recordings and surgical outcome.

References

1. Devous M.D., Thisted R.A., Morgan G.F. *et al.* SPECT brain imaging in epilepsy: a meta-analysis. *J Nucl Med*, 39(2):285–293, 1998.
2. Baird A.E., Donnan G.A., Austin M.C. *et al.* Asymmetries of cerebral perfusion in a stroke-age population. *J Clin Neurosci*, 6(2):113–120, 1999.
3. Kuji I., Sumiya H., Niida Y. *et al.* Age-related changes in the cerebral distribution of 99mTc-ECD from infancy to adulthood. *J Nucl Med*, 40(11):1818–1823, 1999.
4. Migneco O., Darcourt J., Benoliel J. *et al.* Computerized localization of brain structures in single photon emmission computed tomography using a proportional anatomical stereotaxic atlas. *Comput Med Imaging Graph*, 18(6):413–422, 1994.
5. Julin P., Lindqvist J., Svensson L. *et al.* MRI-guided SPECT measurements of medial temporal lobe blood flow in alzheimer's disease. *J Nucl Med*, 38(6):914–919, 1997.
6. Maes F., Collignon A. *et al.* Multimodality image registration by maximisation of mutual information. *IEEE Trans Med Imaging*, 16(2):187–198, 1997.
7. Grova C., Biraben A., Scarabin J.M. *et al.* A methodology to validate MRI/SPECT registration methods using realistic SPECT simulated data. *LNCS(MICCAI01)*, 2208:275–282, 2001.
8. Friston K.J., Ashburner J., Poline J.B. *et al.* Spatial registration and normalization of images. *Hum Brain Mapp*, 2:165–189, 1995.
9. Zubal I.G., Harrell C.R. *et al.* Computerized three-dimensional segmented human anatomy. *Med Phys*, 21(2):299–302, 1994.
10. Huesman R.H., Gullberg G.T., Greenberg W.L. *et al.* Reclbl library users manual. Technical-report pub 214, Lawrence Berkeley Lab, Univ of California.
11. Metz C.E. Roc methodology in radiologic imaging. *Investigate Radiology*, 21(9):720–732, 1986.
12. O'Brien T.J., O'Connor M.K., Mullan B.P. *et al.* Substraction ictal SPECT co-registrated to MRI in partial epilepsy: description and technical validation of the method with phantom and patient studies. *Nucl Med Commun*, 19(1):31–45, 1998.
13. Acton P.D. and Friston K.J. Statistical parametric mapping in functional neuroimaging: beyond PET and fMRI activation studies. *Eur J Nucl Med*, 25(7):663–667, 1998.
14. Lee J.D., Kim H.J., Lee B.I. *et al.* Evaluation of ictal brain SPET using statistical parametric mapping in temporal lobe epilepsy. *Eur J Nucl Med*, 27(11):1658–1665, 2000.

Discriminative Analysis for Image-Based Studies

Polina Golland[1], Bruce Fischl[2], Mona Spiridon[3],
Nancy Kanwisher[3], Randy L. Buckner[4], Martha E. Shenton[5],
Ron Kikinis[6], Anders Dale[2], and W. Eric L. Grimson[1]

[1] Artificial Intelligence Laboratory,
Massachusetts Institute of Technology, Cambridge, MA.
[2] Athinoula A. Martinos Center for Biomedical Imaging,
Massachusetts General Hospital, Harvard Medical School, Boston, MA.
[3] Department of Brain and Cognitive Sciences,
Massachusetts Institute of Technology, Cambridge, MA.
[4] Departments of Psychology, Anatomy and Neurobiology, and Radiology,
Washington University, and Howard Hughes Medical Institute, St. Louis, MO.
[5] Laboratory of Neuroscience, Clinical Neuroscience Division, Department of
Psychiatry, VAMC-Brockton, Harvard Medical School, Brockton, MA.
[6] Surgical Planning Laboratory, Brigham and Women's Hospital,
Harvard Medical School, Boston, MA.

Abstract. In this paper, we present a methodology for performing statistical analysis for image-based studies of differences between populations and describe our experience applying the technique in several different population comparison experiments. Unlike traditional analysis tools, we consider all features simultaneously, thus accounting for potential correlations between the features. The result of the analysis is a classifier function that can be used for labeling new examples and a map over the original features indicating the degree to which each feature participates in estimating the label for any given example. Our experiments include shape analysis of subcortical structures in schizophrenia, cortical thinning in healthy aging and Alzheimer's disease and comparisons of fMRI activations in response to different visual stimuli.

1 Introduction

Statistical studies of neuroanatomy in different populations are important in understanding anatomical and neurophysiological effects of diseases when comparing patients *vs.* normal controls, or biological processes, for example, comparing different age groups. High dimensionality of the feature space and limited number of examples present a significant challenge for statistical analysis tools. Two different approaches are typically used to overcome this difficulty. The first is to simplify the feature space by using global measurements, such as volume of a structure or average thickness of an anatomical area of the cortex [6, 9, 10, 14]. However, this does not provide detailed information on the type of differences and their location. Another commonly used solution is to analyze each feature separately [2, 11, 12, 18], thus ignoring possible correlations in the feature values.

T. Dohi and R. Kikinis (Eds.): MICCAI 2002, LNCS 2488, pp. 508–515, 2002.

Using more powerful analysis techniques can potentially improve our understanding of detected differences between populations, as well as identify possible dependencies in the features. In this paper, we demonstrate experimental results of applying discriminative analysis to several different statistical studies of neuroanatomy and function. In each study, the image-based features were chosen based on the question of interest. While selecting representations for statistical analysis is an important problem, it is outside the scope of this paper. Here, we focus on the analysis techniques applicable once the features are extracted from the images.

2   Discriminative Analysis

This section provides a brief overview of discriminative modeling for population comparison (for details, see [8]). We start by training a classifier for labeling new, unseen, inputs into one of two example groups. We then extract an explicit representation for the differences between the two groups captured by the classifier function. This approach is based on the premise that in order to automatically detect statistical differences between two populations, one should try to build the best possible classifier for labeling new examples. In the optimal case, the classifier function will exactly represent the important differences between the two classes, while ignoring the intra-class variability.

Training. We use the Support Vector Machines (SVMs) learning algorithm [17] to arrive at a classification function. In additional to the sound theoretical foundations of SVMs, they have been demonstrated empirically to be quite robust and seemingly free of the over-fitting problems to which other learning algorithms, such as neural networks, are subject.

Given a training set of l pairs $\{(\mathbf{x}_k, y_k)\}_1^l$, where $\mathbf{x}_k \in \mathbb{R}^n$ are observations and $y_k \in \{-1, 1\}$ are corresponding labels, and a kernel function $K : \mathbb{R}^n \times \mathbb{R}^n \mapsto \mathbb{R}$, the SVM learning algorithm produces a classification function

$$f_K(\mathbf{x}) = \sum_{k=1}^{l} \alpha_k y_k K(\mathbf{x}, \mathbf{x}_k) + b,$$

where the coefficients α_k's and b are chosen to maximize the margin between the two example classes. Training vectors with non-zero α's are called support vectors, as they define, or "support", the separating boundary. In the simplest case of the linear kernel, $K(\mathbf{u}, \mathbf{v}) = \langle \mathbf{u} \cdot \mathbf{v} \rangle$, the separating boundary is a hyperplane whose normal is $\mathbf{w} = \sum_k \alpha_k y_k \mathbf{x}_k$. For non-linear classification, we employ the commonly used Gaussian Radial Basis Function (RBF) kernel family $K(\mathbf{u}, \mathbf{v}) = e^{-\|\mathbf{u}-\mathbf{v}\|^2/\gamma}$ (parameter γ determines the width of the kernel). One of the important properties of this family of classifiers is its locality: moving a support vector slightly affects the separation boundary close to the vector, but does not change it in regions distant from the vector.

We use leave-one-out cross-validation to estimate the expected accuracy of the resulting classifier and, in the non-linear case, to select the optimal set of parameters (e.g., the width γ for the Gaussian RBF kernels).

Classifier Interpretation. We use the previously introduced *discriminative direction* [7, 8] to explicitly represent the spatial pattern of differences between populations implicitly captured by the classifier function. Intuitively, the discriminative direction defines the optimal direction of change that makes an input vector look to the classifier more like the examples from the other class while introducing as little irrelevant change as possible. It is easy to see that for the linear classifier, the discriminative direction corresponds to the normal to the separating hyperplane $\mathbf{w}$, which is also the gradient of the classifier function. It can be shown that moving along the gradient of the classifier function minimizes irrelevant changes for the RBF kernels as well. More precisely, the classifier gradient $\nabla f_K(\mathbf{x})$ defines the discriminative direction for the class with label -1, while the discriminative direction for the class with label 1 is $-\nabla f_K(\mathbf{x})$. The gradient of the linear classifier function is the same at every point in the input space, but it varies spatially for non-linear classifiers. This suggests that the most appropriate points for evaluation of the discriminative direction for the non-linear case are the points close to the separating boundary, i.e., the support vectors.

To summarize the steps of the analysis, given a training set of feature vectors and their class labels, we train a classifier (linear and/or RBF), estimate its cross-validation accuracy and compute its gradient, which can be directly visualized in the original input space.

3   Experimental Studies

In this section, we present the results of the analysis for several statistical studies. For each experiment, we describe the original data and the feature extraction procedure, report statistical analysis results and show the discriminative direction identified by the technique. The cross-validation accuracy is reported with the corresponding 95% confidence interval. The online version of the paper (in www.ai.mit.edu/people/polina) contains color images.

Hippocampus-Amygdala Complex in Schizophrenia. This study contains MRI scans of 15 schizophrenia patients and 15 matched controls [14]. The hippocampus-amygdala complex was manually segmented. We used volumetric signed distance transforms as feature vectors defining the shape of the structure, aligning the shapes by bringing them into a "canonical" pose defined by the first and the second order moments. Since the volumetric discriminative direction is difficult to interpret, we project it onto the space of possible deformations of the shape boundary and visualize the resulting surface deformation instead [8].

The linear classifier performance was very close to the 50% baseline, while the best RBF classifier achieved 76.7%($\pm$15.1%) and 70.0%($\pm$16.3%) accuracy for the right and the left hippocampus respectively. Thus, we expect the non-linear classifier to capture relevant structure in the data that allows it to achieve above the baseline performance. In order to visualize the differences represented by the classifier, we compute the discriminative direction for the support vectors.

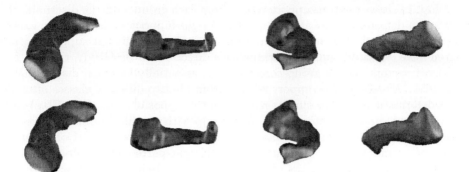

(a) Right hippocampus, the first two support vectors.

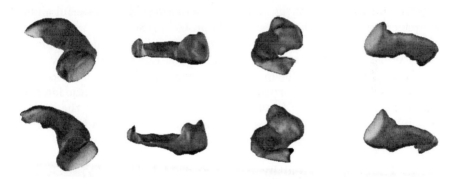

(b) Left hippocampus, the first two support vectors.

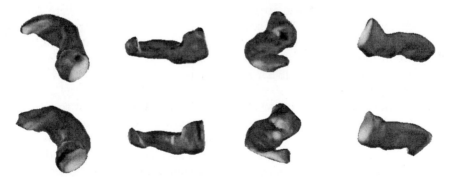

(c) Left hippocampus, the next two support vectors.

Fig. 1. Example support vectors for the hippocampus-amygdala study, shown in pairs of a normal control (top) and a schizophrenia patient (bottom). Four views of each shape are shown (one row per shape). The color indicates the amount of deformation, from blue (moving inwards) to red (moving outwards).

Fig. 1a shows the top support vector from each group with the discriminative direction detected by the algorithm for the right hippocampus. In many experiments, we find that even for the non-linear classifiers, different support vectors often have (visually) similar discriminative direction. In this study, the first four support vectors in each group correspond to essentially identical discriminative direction. Moreover, the support vectors from the two different classes often define deformations of very similar nature, but of opposite signs. Fig. 1(b,c) show the top two support vectors from each group with the discriminative direction for the left hippocampus. Note the deformation in the anterior part of the structure, of a similar nature but localized in different parts of the bulbous head of the amygdala in the two pairs of examples shown. Besides the obvious explanation that the location of this deformation is not fixed in the population, it could also be caused by our method's sensitivity to alignment. Misalignments of the structures in the feature extraction step can cause such size differences to be detected in different areas of the anatomical structure. More powerful alignment technique can potentially help resolve this problem [16].

This example demonstrates the amount of detail in the description of the shape differences between the two populations that can be detected by our technique. This information can help guide the exploration of the relationship between the changes in the subcortical structures and the symptomatic information on the disease (e.g., memory functions and their degradation in the hippocampus study). If a better shape representation is suggested, it can be directly used in conjunction with the presented statistical analysis framework.

Cortical Thinning in Healthy Aging and Alzheimer Type Dementia. In this study, we compared the thickness of the cortex in 31 young controls, 38 old controls and 37 patients diagnosed with dementia of the Alzheimer type (DAT) [13]. The gray/white matter interface and the pial surface were automatically segmented from each MRI scan [1, 5], followed by a registration step that brought the surfaces into correspondence by mapping them onto a unit sphere while minimizing distortions and then non-rigidly aligning the cortical folding patterns [3, 4]. The cortical thickness was densely sampled at the corresponding locations for all subjects.

The performance of the linear classifier was virtually identical to that of the RBF classifier in both comparisons. Consequently, we only show the gradient of the linear classifier (i.e., the discriminative direction for the second class). The cross-validation accuracy was 98.4%(±3.1%) for the aging study (young vs. old controls) and 77.3%(±9.5%) for the dementia study (old controls vs. DAT patients). Fig. 2 shows the discriminative direction for the two studies. The images show both hemispheres inflated so that the entire cortical surface is visible in the rendering. Grayscale is used to display the sulcal pattern, while color is used to show the differences in the cortical thickness. We can see that the two patterns are significantly different, suggesting that the effects of the Alzheimer's disease on the brain are distinct from those of healthy aging. While the aging pattern is aligned with major sulci, the differences in dementia patients are more localized and confined to a few areas on the cortex. Such analysis could

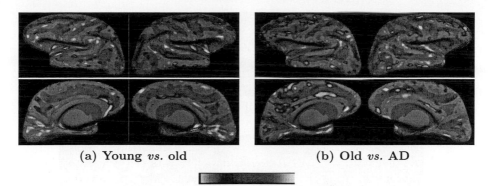

(a) Young *vs.* old   (b) Old *vs.* AD

Fig. 2. Discriminative direction maps for cortical thickness studies. Two views are shown for each hemisphere: lateral (top) and medial (bottom). The color is used to indicate the weight of each voxel, from light blue (negative) to yellow (positive).

potentially be useful for investigating various hypotheses on the development of the disease and its affects on brain structure.

Categorical Differences in fMRI Activation Patterns. This experiment is significantly different from the others in this paper, as it compares the patterns of fMRI activations in response to different visual stimuli in a *single* subject. We present the results of comparing activations in response to face images to those induced by house images, as these categories are believed to have special representation in the cortex [2, 11]. The comparison used 15 example activations for each category (for details on data acquisition, see [15]). The fMRI scans were aligned to the structural MRI of the same subject using rigid registration. For each scan, the cortical surface was extracted using the same techniques as in the study of cortical thickness, and the average activation values were sampled along the cortical surface. A surface-based representation models the connectivity of the cortex and is therefore well suited for fMRI activation studies.

Linear classification achieves 96.3%(±6.8%) cross-validation accuracy for this experiment. Fig. 3a shows the discriminative direction for the linear classifier for the face class. The fMRI images did not cover the entire cortical surface, leaving out the frontal area. We can see several localized areas that were detected as highly predictive of the stimulus category, in general confirming previous findings based on a point-wise t-test. Investigating the differences between the pattern in Fig. 3a and the t-test map will help us understand the spatial correlations between different regions of the cortex.

An additional advantage of using the discriminative approach is that it becomes possible to evaluate how predictive of the category certain sub-regions of the brain are without sacrificing the detailed representation. Fig. 3b shows the resulting discriminative direction if only the "visually active" region of the cortex is considered. The mask for the visually active voxels was obtained using a separate visual task. Note that in general, the method produces a map that is very similar to the corresponding subset of the one in Fig. 3a, indicating robust-

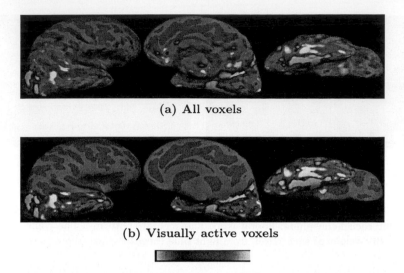

(a) All voxels

(b) Visually active voxels

Fig. 3. Discriminative direction map for the face class in comparison with the house class. Three views of the right hemisphere are shown: lateral (left), medial (center) and inferior (right). The color is used to indicate the weight of each voxel, from light blue (negative) to yellow (positive).

ness of the estimation. Interestingly, the cross-validation accuracy increased to 100% (i.e. the classes are completely separable) in this case, suggesting that the rest of the surface had a lot of noisy voxels making the learning task harder.

4   Conclusions

We presented experimental results for several substantially different image-based studies using the same statistical analysis framework based on discriminative modeling, i.e., training a classifier to label new examples based on the structure in the training data set. The analysis considers all features simultaneously, thus accounting for possible dependencies among the features. By estimating the expected error of the classifier we can effectively assess how separable the populations are with respect to the chosen set of features. Furthermore, visualizing the gradient of the classifier function provides us with detailed information on how predictive individual features and groups of features are of the class label.

Our experience with the technique has suggested several interesting questions to be explored next. Understanding the effects of variability within each population on the detected differences will allow us to provide a better interpretation of the estimated classifier function in terms of the true differences between the populations. Another important problem is assessing significance of the obtained results, especially in light of high dimensionality of the data and small number of samples. Answering these questions will lead towards improving the accuracy and the reliability of the resulting hypotheses of differences between populations.

Acknowledgements. This research was supported in part by NSF IIS 9610249 grant and Athinoula A. Martinos Center for Biomedical Imaging collaborative research grant. The Human Brain Project/Neuroinformatics research is funded jointly by the NINDS, the NIMH and the NCI (R01-NS39581). Further support was provided by the NCRR (P41-RR14075 and R01-RR13609). The authors would like to acknowledge Dr. Kanwisher's grants EY 13455 and MH 59150, Dr. Shenton's grants NIMH K02, MH 01110 and R01 MH 50747 grants, Dr. Kikinis's grants NIH PO1 CA67165, R01RR11747, P41RR13218 and NSF ERC 9731748. Dr. Buckner would like to acknoledge the assistance of the Washington University ADRC, James S McDonnell Foundation, the ALzheimer's Association, and NIA grants AG05682 and AG03991.

References

1. A. M. Dale, *et al.* Cortical Surface-Based Analysis I: Segmentation and Surface Reconstruction. *NeuroImage*, 9:179-194, 1999.
2. R. Epstein and N. Kanwisher. A cortical representation of the local visual environment, *Nature* 392:598-601, 1998.
3. B. Fischl, *et al.* Cortical Surface-Based Analysis II: Inflation, Flattening, a Surface-Based Coordinate System. *NeuroImage*, 9:195-207, 1999.
4. B. Fischl, *et al.* High-resolution intersubject averaging and a coordinate system for the cortical surface. *Human Brain Mapping*, 8:272-84, 1999.
5. B. Fischl, *et al.* Measuring the thickness of the human cerebral cortex from magnetic resonance images. *In PNAS*, 26:11050-5, 2000.
6. G. Gerig, *et al.* Shape versus Size: Improved Understanding of the Morphology of Brain Structures. *In Proc. MICCAI'01*, LNCS 2208, 24-32, 2001.
7. P. Golland, *et al.* Deformation Analysis for Shaped Based Classification. *In Proc. IPMI'01*, LNCS 2082, 517-530, 2001.
8. P. Golland. Statistical Shape Analysis of Anatomical Structures. PhD Thesis, MIT, August 2001.
9. C. Good, *et al.* A voxel-based morphometric study of aging in 465 normal adult human brains. *Neuroimage*, 14:21-36, 2001.
10. T. L. Jernigan, *et al.* Effects of age on tissues and regions of the cerebrum and cerebellum. *Neurobiol. Aging*, 22:581-94, 2001.
11. N. Kanwisher, *et al.* The Fusiform Face Area: a module in human extrastriate cortex specialized for face perception. *J. Neurosciences* 17:4302-4311, 1997.
12. D. J. Pettey and J. C. Gee. Using a Linear Diagnostic Function and Non-rigid Registration to Search for Morphological Differences Between Populations: An Example Involving the Male and Female Corpus Callosum. *In Proc. IPMI'01*, LNCS 2082, 372-379, 2001.
13. D. H. Salat, *et al.* Early and widespread thinning of the cerebral cortex with normal aging. *Submitted*, 2002.
14. M. E. Shenton, *et al.* Abnormalities in the left temporal lobe and thought disorder in schizophrenia: A quantitative magnetic resonance imaging study. *New England J. Medicine*, 327:604-612, 1992.
15. M. Spiridon and N. Kanwisher. How distributed is visual category information in human occipito-temporal cortex? An fMRI study. *Submitted*, 2002.
16. S. J. Timoner, *et al.* Performance Issues in Shape Classification, *To Appear in Proc. MICCAI 2002.*, September 2002.
17. V. N. Vapnik. Statistical Learning Theory. *John Wiley & Sons*, 1998.
18. P. Yushkevich, *et al.* Intuitive, Localized Analysis of Shape Variability. *In Proc. IPMI'01*, LNCS 2082, 402-408, 2001.

Automatic Generation of Training Data for Brain Tissue Classification from MRI

Chris A. Cocosco, Alex P. Zijdenbos, and Alan C. Evans

McConnell Brain Imaging Centre, Montreal Neurological Institute,
McGill University, Montreal, Canada
crisco@bic.mni.mcgill.ca

Abstract. A novel fully automatic procedure for brain tissue classification from 3D magnetic resonance head images (MRI) is described. The procedure uses feature space proximity measures, and does not make any assumptions about the tissue intensity distributions. As opposed to existing methods, which are often sensitive to anatomical variability and pathology (such as atrophy), the proposed procedure is robust against morphological deviations from the model. Starting from a set of samples generated from prior tissue probability maps (the "model") in a standard, brain-based coordinate system ("stereotaxic space"), the method reduces the fraction of incorrectly labeled samples in this set from 25% down to 5%. The corrected set of samples is then used by a supervised classifier for classifying the entire 3D image. Validation experiments were performed on both real and simulated MRI data; the Kappa similarity measure increased from 0.83 to 0.94.

1 Introduction

Fully automatic, accurate, and robust brain tissue classification[1] from anatomical magnetic resonance images (aMRI) is of great importance for research and clinical studies of the normal and diseased human brain. Operator-assisted segmentation methods are impractical for large amounts of data, and also are highly subjective and non-reproducible [1].

Existing methods for fully automatic brain tissue classification typically rely on an existing anatomical model. This makes them sensitive to any deviations from the model due to pathology, due to aging, or simply due to normal anatomical variability between individuals. Also, there may be situations when the only model available was constructed from a different human population than the image to be classified. Moreover, many of the published feature-space classification methods assume multi-variate Normal (Gaussian) tissue intensity distributions. It has been shown that this is a poor assumption for multi-spectral anatomical brain MRI [2, 3].

---

[1] In the context of this paper, "classification" means the labeling of individual image voxels as one of the main tissue classes in the brain: cerebro-spinal fluid (CSF), grey matter, and white matter; a fourth class ("background") denotes everything else.

T. Dohi and R. Kikinis (Eds.): MICCAI 2002, LNCS 2488, pp. 516–523, 2002.
© Springer-Verlag Berlin Heidelberg 2002

sample MRI: CSF TPM: Grey-matter TPM: White-matter TPM:

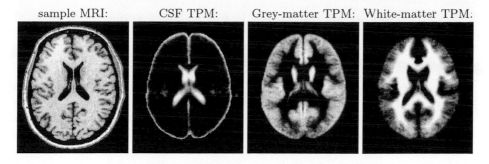

Fig. 1. All 3D image volumes are spatially registered to the same stereotaxic space. The tissue probability map (TPM) values range from 0 (black) to 1 (white).

The MRI intensity scale has no absolute meaning, and is dependent on the pulse sequence and other variable scanner parameters. An aspect that is ignored by most brain MRI intensity-based classification schemes is the *fully automatic* generation of a *correct* set of training samples for the classifier, when given a never-seen-before MRI brain dataset. Existing approaches to fully automatic classification include:

- EM-style schemes were proposed by Van Leemput [4] and by Ashburner [5]. Both use a probabilistic brain atlas to initialize and constrain the tissue classification. However, both authors report failures on atypical (significantly different than the atlas) brain scans, such as child or pathological brains.
- The use of stereotaxic space tissue probability maps for automating supervised classification algorithms was originally proposed by Kamber [6], and subsequently used by other researchers [1, 7]. The maps are used to select training samples from spatial locations that are very likely to contain a given tissue type. This approach's limitations are described in the next section.

The main contribution of this paper is a novel method for fully automatic generation of correct training samples for tissue classification. The method is non-parametric, hence does not make any assumptions about the feature space distributions. It is based on a prior tissue probability map in stereotaxic space (the "model"), and is designed to accommodate subject anatomies that are significantly different than the model.

2   Problem Statement

A stereotaxic space tissue probability map (TPM) of a given tissue is a spatial probability distribution representing a certain subject population. For each spatial location in a standard, brain-based, coordinate system (stereotaxic space), the TPM value at that location is the probability of the given tissue being observed there, for that particular population.

Once imaging data is spatially registered (normalized) to the stereotaxic space, TPM-s provide an a-priori spatial probability distribution for each tissue

(Fig. 1). This distribution can be used to automatically produce a training set for the supervised classifier [6]: for example, choose spatial locations that have a TPM value $\geq \tau = 0.99$ (99%). The lower the τ, the more qualifying spatial locations there will be. However, this simplistic approach has two limitations:

1. Mis-labeled samples ("false positives"): Since the morphology of the human brain is so variable, even among the locations with very high a-priori probability of being a given tissue, some of them will be wrongly labeled as one tissue class when in fact they are from another class. The fraction of false positives in the training set will increase when τ is decreased. Also, for a given τ, this fraction will be larger when the subject is from a different population than the population represented by the TPM.

2. Intensity distribution estimation: For highest τ (where the false positive rate is lowest) the qualifying sample points give a very limited coverage of the brain area, especially for CSF (Fig. 1). Intuitively, this will not give a good estimate of the true tissue intensity distributions (which is needed by a supervised classifier), for two reasons:

- Brain tissue, as seen in aMRI, is not homogeneous throughout the brain [8].
- MRI artifacts, such as intensity non-uniformity (INU), introduce additional spatial variations in the measured tissue signal.

Thus, sampling at a lower τ would be beneficial for the intensity distribution estimation; however, a lower τ also means more false positives.

Our novel contribution is a way to address these two limitations. Specifically, a "pruning" of the raw set of points obtained from the TPM is performed, with the goals of eliminating the false positives caused by anatomical difference, and of allowing for a lower TPM τ. The only requirement for the TPM is that the majority of training points it provides, for a given τ, are correctly labeled.

3   Method

The following presents a fully automatic, non-parametric, brain tissue classification procedure based on feature space proximity measures. Non-parametric classifiers are attractive because they do not make any assumptions about the underlying feature space data density functions. The procedure consists of two stages:

1. A semi-supervised classifier, using a minimum spanning tree graph-theoretic method, and stereotaxic space prior information. It produces a set of training samples customized for the particular individual anatomy subjected to classification. This stage will be referred to as the "pruning" stage.
2. A supervised classifier, using the classic k-nearest-neighbor (kNN) algorithm [9]. It is trained on the set of samples produced by the first stage. In this work: $k = 45$, and the classifier had > 3000 training points per class.

The image features used are only signal intensities of one or more MRI modalities (contrasts). The feature space proximity measure used is the common Euclidean distance in d-dimensional space. However, for $d > 1$ the Euclidean distance is not invariant to independent scaling of the different axes, and the MRI scanner raw output has no absolute nor guaranteed scale. This problem is addressed by a pre-processing step that normalizes the intensities of the input multi-spectral MRI-s. A simple intensity histogram range-matching procedure is used: points located at a small percentile away from the absolute minimum/maximum of the histograms are matched between MRI modalities.

3.1   Pruning Stage

The pruning works on a set of input sample points that are selected through random sampling from the qualifying locations in the respective tissue probability map (TPM); an equal number of samples is selected for each tissue class (background, CSF, grey matter, white matter). The qualifying locations are locations where the TPM value (i.e. the prior probability) is $\geq \tau$, where τ is the threshold parameter.

The pruning technique makes use of a minimum spanning tree (MST) in feature space. This method is referred to as "semi-supervised" because, unlike in traditional unsupervised classification ("clustering" techniques), some prior information exists in this application: the number of main clusters, and their relative position in feature space is known. Furthermore, each sample point has an initial labeling suggested by the TPM-based point selection process (section 2). The purpose of the pruning is to reject the points with incorrect labeling.

Here are the three main steps of the pruning method:

1. The minimum spanning tree of the input set of points is constructed in feature space (Fig. 2).
2. Iteratively, the graph is broken into smaller trees (connected components, or clusters) by removing "long", or "inconsistent", edges from the initial MST. At each step, the *main clusters* are identified and labeled by using prior knowledge, and a stop condition is tested on them. If the condition is not satisfied, the graph breaking is continued.
3. At the end, the points that are in the right cluster (i.e. have the same initial labeling as their cluster) are deemed to be true positives and kept; all the other points are deemed to be incorrectly labeled and discarded.

MST breaking: A heuristic method (inspired by [9]) was implemented and experimentally evaluated (section 4). It uses a threshold value T, which is decreased at each iteration of the algorithm and tested on all edges of the graph in parallel:

– an edge (i, j) is removed if $length(i, j) > T \times A(i)$ or if $length(i, j) > T \times A(j)$, where $A(i)$ is the average length of all the other edges incident on node i.

Main clusters identification: The main clusters are the best guesses for the true background, CSF, grey matter, and white matter clusters in feature space. Under the assumption that the majority of points have correct initial labels, the best guess for each class is the cluster which contains the largest number of points labeled as that class.

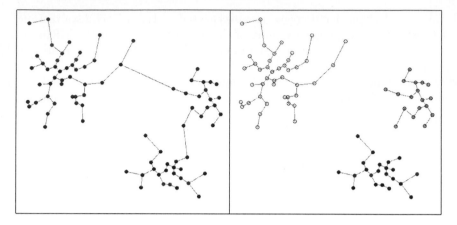

Fig. 2. *Left*: minimum spanning tree (MST) of a set of points in the plane. *Right*: the result of removing the "inconsistent" edges (section 3.1), for a $T = 1.45$.

Stop condition: If the above determined main clusters are found to be four distinct clusters, and the relative cluster locations in feature space correspond to prior knowledge, the iterative graph breaking stops.

4   Experiments and Results

Experiments were performed in order to validate the training set pruning method, and also the entire brain tissue classification scheme proposed here. All experiments were performed with repetitions, for assessing the statistical significance of each resulting data point. The performance on both subject brains similar to the TPM used and, more importantly, on brains with significant morphological differences from the TPM, was explored using the following MRI datasets:

1. Realistic simulations [10] driven by a new custom set of "phantoms" (digital anatomical models) resembling elderly brains. These phantoms were produced using a non-linear spatial registration procedure between real MRI-s of elderly subjects (aged 60-70) and a standard anatomical model [10]; the resulting deformation field was inverted and used for deforming the standard phantom. Multi-spectral MRI-s (T1, T2, PD) were simulated as $1\,mm^3$ isotropic voxel acquisitions, with 3% noise and 20% INU (intensity non-uniformity).

2. Real T1-T2-PD scans of a young normal individual (aged 36), $1\,mm^3$ resolution. INU correction was performed using MNI-N3 [11]; the different acquisitions were spatially normalized to each other using a linear (affine) registration procedure. The head T1 scan was completely manually segmented (except the cerebellum) by a human expert – a trained neuroanatomist.

3. Real multi-spectral scans of 31 ischemia patients, who exhibit brain atrophy. T1: $1\,mm^3$ resolution; T2/PD: 1x1x3.5 mm resolution; same processing as for 2 above. Only a qualitative evaluation was performed on these data.

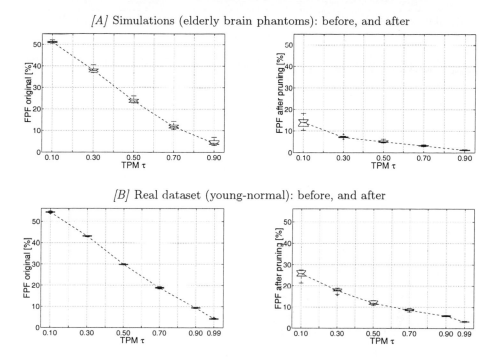

Fig. 3. Multi-spectral aMRI (T1-T2-PD) operation: false positives fraction (FPF) in the point set. *[A]:* 10 repetitions, each with a different phantom (anatomical model). *[B]:* 10 repetitions, each with a different initial point set. It can observed that for all experiments the pruning significantly reduces the FPF. The results for T1-only (single-feature) operation are similar.

For the quantitative measurements (on 1 and 2 above), the "gold standard" was the anatomical model used for the simulations, and the manual classification for the real dataset. For each pruning experiment, 7500 candidate points per class were selected based on the TPM-s (section 3.1); the TPM-s used were produced [7] from a group of 53 young normal subjects (aged 18-35).

An intuitive figure of merit for the pruning method is the rate of false positives (mis-labeled samples) left in the point set. A low such rate is desired in the pruned point set, as it corresponds to a "mostly correct" training set for the final supervised tissue classification stage (Fig. 3).

However, it is more important to study how the pruning influences the final tissue classification result. For a quantitative measure of performance, the *Kappa* measure (a chance-corrected similarity measure between two labelings [12]) was computed against the gold standard, over the intra-cranial area. For comparison, Figs. 4-5 also show the result for an experiment with $\tau = 0.99$ and no pruning ("raw") [7]: the final kNN classifier was simply trained with the raw samples extracted from the TPM at $\tau = 0.99$.

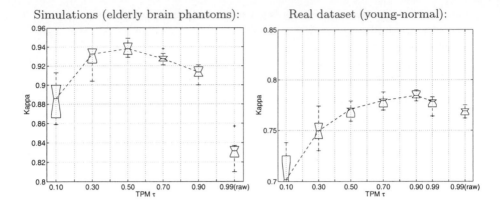

Fig. 4. Multi-spectral aMRI (T1-T2-PD) operation: final classification Kappa (repetitions same as Fig. 3). *Left:* the pruning gives a clear improvement over the "raw" (no pruning) operation. *Right:* for $\tau \geq 0.7$, the pruning produces a small, but statistically significant, improvement over "raw" (box notches do not overlap: $p < 0.05$).

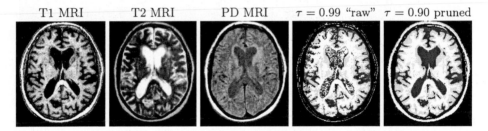

Fig. 5. Real dataset (ischemia patient): multi-spectral aMRI, and classified images (the different gray levels correspond to the different tissues). This subject exhibits severe brain atrophy (i.e. significant morphological difference from the "young normal" model), which is the likely cause for the poor performance of the "raw" method (no pruning). The pruning method, for $\tau = 0.90$, gives significantly better classification.

5   Discussion and Conclusion

Based on the experimental results presented above, it can be concluded that the MST-based pruning method achieves its goal of reducing the rate of mis-labeled samples in the point set selected using the TPM-s. Moreover, the pruning improves the final tissue classification compared to the "raw" method. This improvement is substantial for some ischemia patients (Fig. 5).

Limitations: Not all of the false positives are "pruned", and part of the true positives in the original training set are discarded as well. The cause of this is the partial overlap of the tissue class distributions in feature space – an inherent limitation of anatomical brain MRI.

This paper describes a fully automatic procedure for brain tissue classification from MR anatomical images. As opposed to existing methods, it does not make any assumptions about the image intensity distributions, or about the close morphological similarity between the subject's brain and the anatomical model. This procedure (which can operate on both single-spectral and multi-spectral aMRI) will provide improved tissue segmentation for research and clinical studies of the development, functioning, and pathology of the human brain.

Acknowledgements

John Sled, Steve Robbins, Peter Neelin, Jean-François Mangin, Noor Kabani, Louis Collins.

References

1. Zijdenbos, A., et al.: Automatic quantification of MS lesions in 3D MRI brain data sets: Validation of INSECT. In: Proc. of MICCAI, Cambridge (1998) 439–448
2. Clarke, L. P., et al.: MRI: stability of three supervised segmentation techniques. Magnetic Resonance Imaging **11** (1993) 95–106
3. DeCarli, C., et al.: Method for quantification of brain, ventricular and subarachnoid CSF volumes from MR images. Journal of Computer Assisted Tomography **16** (1992) 274–284
4. Van Leemput, K., et al.: Automated model-based tissue classification of MR images of the brain. IEEE Trans. on Medical Imaging **18** (1999) 897–908
5. Ashburner, J., Friston, K.J.: Voxel-based morphometry — the methods. NeuroImage **11** (2000) 805–821
6. Kamber, M., et al.: Model-based 3-D segmentation of multiple sclerosis lesions in magnetic resonance brain images. IEEE Trans. on Medical Imaging **14** (1995) 442–53
7. Kollokian, V.: Performance analysis of automatic techniques for tissue classification in magnetic resonance images of the human brain. Master's thesis, Concordia University, Montreal, Canada (1996)
8. Kandel, E.R., et al.: Principles of Neural Science. fourth edn. McGraw Hill (2000)
9. Duda, R.O., Hart, P.E., Stork, D.G.: Pattern classification. 2nd edn. Wiley (2001)
10. Brainweb – simulated brain database. (http://www.bic.mni.mcgill.ca/brainweb/)
11. Sled, J.G., et al.: A non-parametric method for automatic correction of intensity non-uniformity in MRI data. IEEE Trans. on Medical Imaging **17** (1998) 87–97
12. Cohen, J.: A coefficient of agreement for nominal scales. Educational and Psychological Measurements **20** (1960) 37–46

The Putamen Intensity Gradient in CJD Diagnosis

A. Hojjat[1], D. Collie[2], and A.C.F. Colchester[1]

[1] Medical Image Computing, Kent Institute of Medicine and Health Sciences,
University of Kent at Canterbury, UK
[2] National CJD Surveillance Unit, Western General Hospital, Edinburgh, UK
a.colchester@ukc.ac.uk

Abstract. The deep grey matter structures of the brain have been reported to show MR hyperintensity in the sporadic form of Creutzfeldt-Jakob disease (sCJD), but the criteria for visual judgment of this are not well defined. We carried out a quantitative study of T2 weighted and proton density scans comparing 10 sCJD patients with 10 non-CJD dementia controls (NCD) and also with 11 patients suffering from the new variant form of CJD (vCJD). Scans were acquired in a clinical context and came from many hospitals. Absolute intensities varied widely and did not allow any useful discrimination. In all groups the putamen had a gradient of reducing intensity from anterior to posterior on T2 scans. In both s- and v- CJD patients this gradient was increased. Sensitivity and specificity (S&S) for sCJD against NCD were 89%. The T2 and PD intensities of the putamen relative to the other grey matter structures studied were not useful for distinguishing between any of the patient groups. The ratio of putamen to frontal white matter T2 intensity was significantly increased in vCJD compared to NCD and also to sCJD, while sCJD and NCD were indistinguishable by this test. We conclude that: (1) in our preliminary study, the putamen gradient appears to be important diagnostically for sCJD; (2) intensities of deep grey matter structures vary systematically and intensity-based segmentation methods used in patients and normals should take account of this.

Introduction

The deep grey matter structures of the cerebral hemispheres include the basal ganglia, which are mainly involved in motor control, and the thalamus, which is mainly involved in sensory processing. The basal ganglia include the caudate nucleus, the putamen and the globus pallidus. All these structures are anatomically distinct and are easily recognised in axial and coronal MR images of the brain. They are subject to a wide variety of acute and chronic pathological processes, which may selectively affect sub-parts of the deep grey structures, for example in Creutzfeldt Jakob disease (CJD) in which intensity abnormalities have been reported [9,11]. There is strong evidence from visual analysis that increased signal in the posterior part of the thalamus may be diagnostic for the new variant form of CJD (vCJD) [1,3,4,8]. There is less clear evidence that increased signal in the caudate nucleus and/ or the putamen may be diagnostic for the classical sporadic form of CJD (sCJD) [2,5].

We have been using quantitative analyses to validate and extend these observations [1]. For a particular structure, absolute MR intensities obtained using a particular sequence vary widely according to several poorly controlled parameters, even for

T. Dohi and R. Kikinis (Eds.): MICCAI 2002, LNCS 2488, pp. 524–531, 2002.

"standard" sequences (e.g. "T2 weighted"), so it is difficult to compare data from different scanners. Thus, for a rare disease like CJD, when data are often acquired at different hospitals using different scanner manufacturers and different settings, it is notable that visual analyses indicate that significant intensity differences are still identifiable. A central issue in quantitative analysis is how to define a normalisation method to *reduce* the variability of intensity estimates *within* diagnostic patient groups, while *preserving* or *increasing* the variability *between* diagnostic groups. The most obvious approach is to identify in the same scan specific reference structures against which the abnormal structures can be compared. For variant CJD we have recently evaluated different reference structures and shown that very high sensitivity and specificity for vCJD diagnosis can be achieved when MR examinations from a wide variety of scanners are analysed [1].

In the present work we examined putamen intensity changes using different normalisation approaches. It has been noted that intensity appears to reduce gradually from front to back on T2 axial slices [2]. Systematic study of putamen T2 intensities thus requires either (1) averaging the whole putamen cross-section, or (2) division of the putamen into reproducible sub-parts within which the intensities are recorded, or (3) quantifying the spatial rate of intensity change within the putamen. We evaluated these approaches in the context of CJD diagnosis. The results have relevance not only to this clinical condition but also to a range of other MR applications including intensity-based tissue class segmentation.

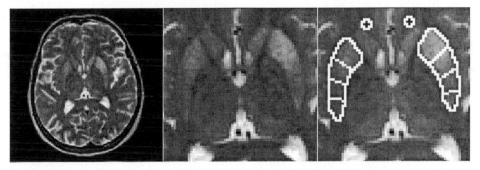

Fig. 1. (Left) T2-weighted axial MR slice through level of the putamen. **(Middle)** Magnified view of region containing the putamen. **(Right)** Outline shows putamen (segmented into 4 segments) and frontal white matter region

Methods

Dual echo (simultaneously acquired PD and T2-weighted) scans from three groups of patients with (1) sporadic CJD, (2) variant CJD and (3) non-CJD dementia (NCD) were studied. Prior to any intensity analyses, all available scans were graded for quality by visual inspection on two predefined 5-point subjective scales (5 being top quality), one scale for the level of contrast/noise and the other one for freedom-from-movement-artefact. Of a total of 73 scans, 32 scans were rejected as being very poor quality (graded 1 or 2 on either scale). This rejection rate reflects the fact that scans were obtained in clinical circumstances from a variety of hospitals, in patients who were often confused and uncooperative. Two additional scans were rejected because there was a focal lesion such as a lacunar infarct visible in one putamen. The remaining 39 scans (all scoring at 3 or greater on both scales) were included in the quantitative analyses.

There were 12 scans from 10 patients aged 50-76 with sporadic CJD, 11 scans from 11 patients aged 17-36 with variant CJD, and 16 scans from 10 patients aged 14-76 with dementia in whom CJD had been excluded. All patients had dual echo, fast spin-echo MR scans with repetition time values ranging from 2862 to 4200msec, and echo time values from 12-22msec for PD and from 80-120msec for T2 scans. Slice thickness ranged from 3 to 5mm. Data were all manipulated digitally; no hard copies were used.

Partial volume error (PVE) is an important potential confounding factor in any intensity analysis. The height of the putamen, in the cranio-caudal direction, is about 20mm for much of its antero-posterior extent. We decided to restrict the present work to analysis of the axial (i.e. approximately parallel to the anterior commissure-posterior commissure line) which passed through the putamen at mid-height (c.f. Fig 1, left). This meant that most or all of the observed antero-posterior gradation of T2 intensity could not be a result of PVE.

In each scan the putamen and a region of interest in the frontal white matter were segmented interactively by a trained observer who viewed both the T2 and corresponding PD slice on the same display. The PD and T2 images were linked so that each anatomical structure could be outlined using either or both of the two images. In order to study the gradation of intensity, the putamen was subdivided into four parts of similar antero-posterior length, Fig 1 (middle). For each segment the average intensity was calculated and normalised by expressing intensities as ratios of different possible reference structures. Considering the putamen segments starting at the front, the ratio of the first and second part was similar to the ratio of the second and third part. We therefore fitted a straight line to the log transformed intensity ratios and examined the gradient of this line.

For each of the four putamen segments, the T2 and PD indices (raw values, normalised values etc) obtained from different patients were plotted. There was a strong linear correlation between T2 and PD values. To evaluate the simultaneous use of T2 and PD values in discriminating between patient groups, a straight line was fitted to the data on the scatter plot, and a line perpendicular to this was used as a threshold. Sensitivities and specificities using different thresholds were then calculated. These results were plotted as receiver operator characteristic (ROC) curves which showed the performance of the index in discriminating between sCJD and NCD, vCJD and NCD, and between sCJD and vCJD. One ROC curve plotted the true positive fraction (number of correctly categorised patients divided by the total number of patients with this diagnosis) versus the false positive fraction (number of incorrectly categorised control patients divided by the total number of these controls) [6]. The true positive fraction (TPF) is sensitivity and false positive fraction (FPF) is (1- specificity). Each ROC curve showed how sensitivity and specificity varied according to different thresholds. It is important to note that the optimum threshold selected for a diagnostic test depends on the clinical circumstances in which the test is being used, which may require high sensitivity at the expense of some loss of specificity, or high specificity at the expense of some loss of sensitivity. The ROC curve shows this pay-off graphically. One important point on the ROC curve is where the sensitivity and specificity are equal, and the value at this point was noted as a simple way to compare different indices.

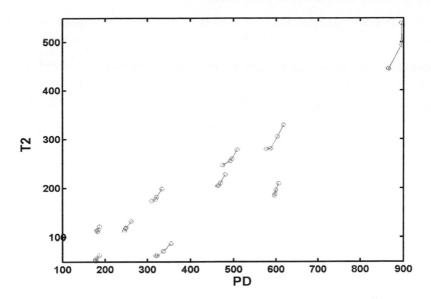

Fig. 2. Scatter plot of absolute T2 and PD values in four segments of the putamen in the vCJD group. Values of consecutive segments from one patient (corresponding right and left segments having been averaged) are connected by a line

Results

As expected, the absolute values of T2 and PD intensities for the putamen varied very widely between patients (T2 range 50-600; PD range 180-950). The range of variation within one putamen was very small compared to this (T2 range 15-150; PD range 20-120). Fig 2 shows the putamen values for the vCJD clinical group. The anterior three segments of the putamen showed progressive reduction of T2 intensity from front to back in nearly all patients (c.f. Fig 2). The posterior segment was more variable and subsequent analyses mainly focused on the front three parts.

Indices based on the ratio of putamen intensity divided by the frontal white matter intensity were examined. Results were similar whether the whole putamen or specific segments were used. Fig 3 (left) shows the scatter plot of the log of this index calculated for the whole putamen, averaged left and right, for T2 and for PD, with different clinical groups identified by different symbols. Fig 3 (left) shows that PD values did not help to discriminate between groups. However, for T2 there was hyperintensity of the putamen relative to frontal white matter in vCJD patients allowing good discrimination from both NCD controls and from sCJD patients, but sCJD patients were indistinguishable from NCD. For a particular discrimination - e.g. sCJD versus non-CJD dementia, the effect of using a chosen threshold for this index on the T2 axis can readily be visualised, and quantified by calculating the TPF (the proportion of sCJD patients correctly categorised) and FPF, (the proportion of non-CJD dementia patients incorrectly categorised as sCJD). The line k1= 1.25 in Fig 3 (left) is the threshold value for the T2 index which generates approximately equal sensitivity and specificity for sCJD against control group. For a full range of possible thresholds, the TPF and FPF values can be plotted as an ROC curve (Fig 3 (right)).

ROC curves derived from a limited number of data points are jagged (curve 1 in Fig 4 (left)). We chose to smooth the raw ROC curve using five iterations of a simple 3-point filter rather than fit a parametric function [6]. The resulting curves (both curves in Fig 3 (right) and curve 2 in Fig 4 (left)) follow the trend of the data closely and allow simple interpolation.

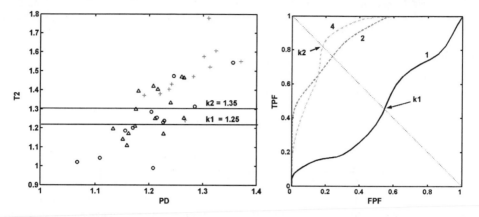

Fig. 3. (Left) Scatter plot of log intensity ratios (averaged left and right) for whole putamen divided by frontal white matter (FWM) in T2 versus PD. Circles = sCJD; pluses = vCJD; triangles = non-CJD dementia (NCD) controls. Horizontal lines: examples of T2 thresholds which generate approximately equal sensitivity and specificity: k1 for sCJD vs NCD and k2 for sCJD vs vCJD. **(Right)** ROC curve for T2 log intensity ratios (averaged left and right), for whole putamen divided by frontal white matter (FWM). TPF = true positive fraction (or sensitivity); FPF = false positive fraction (or 1 - specificity). Curve 1 = sCJD vs NCD; curve 2 = vCJD vs NCD; curve 4 = vCJD vs sCJD

Various methods of estimating rate of reduction of intensity along the putamen (anterior to posterior segments) were examined and gave good discriminatory results. Fig 4 (left) shows the ROC curve for the following method. For each patient the intensity of the second most anterior putamen segment was divided by the anterior putamen segment, for the right side and the left side separately. The smaller of the log ratios (corresponding to the steeper gradient) was noted for this patient. Very good discrimination of sCJD from NCD was achieved using this method, with the sensitivity and specificity balanced at approximately 89%.

The ROC curves show how the TPF and FPF vary with respect to each other as the threshold is changed, but they do not show what specific thresholds generated which points on the ROC curve. We therefore show this mapping explicitly in Fig 4 (right) for the same data that are shown in Fig 4 (left). The log threshold ratio is plotted on the horizontal axis, against the sensitivity and specificity.

Discussion

Following published reports that putamen MRI signal intensities are high in sCJD, we expected normalisation using white matter (which has not been observed to show MR abnormalities in CJD) to provide reasonable discrimination between sCJD and non-CJD dementia (NCD) controls. We could not verify this quantitatively. However, we were able to demonstrate a clear difference in intensity in vCJD patients and this meant that putamen intensities normalised in this way could be used to discriminate with high confidence between vCJD and sCJD in our patients.

Within the putamen, the T2 intensity is varies systematically. We observed that the rate of reduction of log T2 intensity of the putamen from front to back was approximately linear in all patient groups. The within-structure changes allowed us to normalise one part of the putamen with respect to another, with impressive results for discriminating sCJD patients from NCD. Our results were achieved without the use of bias field correction techniques; normalisation using nearby structures will reduce the effect of intensity inhomogeneity artifacts on the normalised indices.

Our approach allows us to select a different balance of sensitivity and specificity by varying the threshold. For diagnosis of sCJD from the T2 ratio mid-anterior / anterior putamen (Figs 4), we balance sensitivity and specificity at a ratio threshold of 0.93. However, in a clinical context such as screening a large group of patients with the goal of picking up almost all sCJD cases, Fig 4 (right) shows that the ratio threshold can be increased to 0.95 (e.g. an intensity change over 5% is labeled as abnormal) in order to increase sensitivity to 99%, at the cost of reducing of specificity to about 75%. In contrast, at times one may require a very high specificity, for example in a context where a risky but potentially curative treatment is under consideration. While the specificity of our test could be increased to 99% by reducing the threshold to 0.89 (e.g. 11% intensity change), this would be at a cost of a substantial fall in sensitivity to about 39%, which would probably be unacceptable.

An important group of methods for MR brain segmentation depend on the differences in MR signal intensity between grey matter, white matter and cerebrospinal fluid. These methods usually attempt to classify the deep grey matter structures into a single class of voxels. The present paper has drawn attention to the systematic and wide variation of intensity which may occur within a single grey matter structure. This variation increases errors when using current intensity-based segmentation methods. Future work should consider how modeling such variation could be used to improve accuracy.

Conclusions

1. Nearly all discriminatory diagnostic information came from T2 weighted images. However, if co-registered PD scans are available (usually this implies dual echo acquisition), some increased confidence in diagnosis can be achieved.
2. Quantitative processing allowed intensities to be measured reproducibly. While visual inspection is good for judging which of the two structures is the brighter, computer processing can provide additional information, for example allowing non-unity ratios to be quantified. Another benefit was that the threshold used for discrimination can be varied, to prioritise sensitivity or specificity for different applications. Plotting the sensitivity and specificity against the threshold contained all the information in a traditional ROC curve and had some advantages.
3. Putamen intensities normalised to a frontal white matter region do not discriminate between sCJD and non-CJD dementia (NCD) controls. However, a putamen/ frontal white matter intensity ratio of 1.35 or greater was a useful test for distinguishing between sCJD and vCJD (82% sensitivity and specificity) and a ratio of 1.4 or greater had 78% sensitivity and specificity for vCJD against NCD.

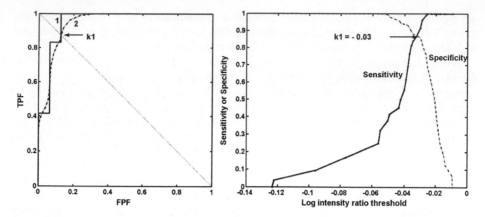

Fig. 4. (Left) ROC curve for diagnosis of sCJD versus non-CJD dementia using log T2 intensity ratios of mid-anterior putamen divided by anterior putamen (minimum of right ratio or or left ratio). TPF = true positive fraction (sensitivity); FPF = false positive fraction (1 - specificity). Curve 1 = raw data; curve 2 = smoothed ROC curve. The smoothed ROC curve data and point k are also used to generate the right figure. **(Right)** Graph showing log intensity ratio threshold (horizontal axis) versus sensitivity and specificity. The threshold k= -0.03 is a putamen gradient of 0.93 (i.e. 7% reduction in intensity from the anterior segment to the second segment along the putamen)

4. The rate of change of intensity along the putamen (the putamen gradient) on T2 scans was higher in sCJD and in vCJD than in non-CJD dementia controls. A gradient of 0.93 (i.e. a fall of 7%) or greater between one segment and another along the putamen has high sensitivity and specificity for diagnosis (89%).
5. Differences between hemispheres were slight and the ratio of indices for one hemisphere divided by those for the other were of no value in differential diagnosis.

Acknowledgements

This work was supported by the EU-funded project "Quantitative Analysis of MR scans in CJD (QAMRIC)" BMH 4-98-6048. The authors are grateful to Emily Colchester who carried out the interactive segmentation of anatomical structures.

References

1. Colchester, A. C. F., Hojjat, S. A., Will, R. G., and Collie, D. A. Quantitative validation of MR intensity abnormalities in variant CJD. Journal of Neurology, Neurosurgery of Psychiatry, in Press, 2002.
2. Collie, D. A., Sellar, R. J., Zeidler, M., Colchester, A. C. F., Knight, R., and Will, R. G. MRI of Creutzfeldt-Jakob disease: imaging features and recommended MRI protocol. Clinical Radiology 56, 726-739. 2001.
3. Collie, D. A., Sellar, R. J., Ironside, J., and et al. New variant Creutzfeldt-Jakob disease: diagnostic features on MR imaging with histopathologic correlation. Proceedings 36th Meeting of American Society of Neuroradiology , 139. 1998.

4. Coulthard, A., Hall, K., English, P. T., and et al. Quantitative analysis of MRI signal intensity in new variant Creutzfeldt-Jakob disease. British Journal of Radiology 72, 742-748. 1999.
5. Finkenstaedt, M., Szudra, A., Zerr, I., Poser, S., Hise, J. H., Stoenbner, J. M., and Weber, T. MR Imaging of Creutzfeldt-Jakob disease. Radiology 199, 793-798. 1996.
6. Metz, C. E., ROC methology in radiologic imaging, 1986, Invest. Radiol. 21, 720-733.
7. Uchino, A., Yoshinaga, M., Shiokawa, O., Hata, H., and Ohno, M. Serial MR imaging in Creutzfeldt-Jakob disease. Neuroradiology 33, 364-367. 1991.
8. Zeidler, M., Sellar, R., Collie, D. A., Knight, R., Stewart, G. E., Macleod, M-A., Ironside, J., Cousens, S. N., Colchester, A. C. F., Hadley, D. M., and Will, R. G. The pulvinar sign on magnetic resonance imaging in variant Creutzfeldt-Jakob disease. *Lancet*, 355(9213):1412-1418, April 2000.

A Dynamic Brain Atlas

D.L.G. Hill[1], J.V. Hajnal[2], D. Rueckert[3], S.M. Smith[4], T. Hartkens[1], and K. McLeish[1]

[1] Computational Imaging Science, King's College London
Derek.Hill@kcl.ac.uk
[2] Imaging Sciences Department, Clinical Sciences Centre, Imperial College London
[3] Computer Science Dept. Imperial College London
[4] FMRIB, University of Oxford

Abstract. We describe a dynamic atlas that can be customized to an individual study subject in near-real-time. The atlas comprises 180 brain volumes each of which has been automatically segmented into grey matter, white matter and CSF, and also non-rigidly registered to the Montreal BrainWeb reference dataset providing automatic delineation of brain structures of interest. To create a dynamic atlas, the user loads a study dataset (eg: a patient) and queries the atlas database to identify similar subjects. All selected database subjects are then aligned with the study subject using affine registration, and average tissue probability maps and structure delineations produced. The system can run on distributed data and distributed CPUs illustrating the potential of computational grids in medical image analysis.

Introduction

Neuro-imaging research is a successful example of web-enabled science. The web enables exchange of standardized datasets (atlases) [1,2,3,4,5] and research software tools[1] and facilitates collaboration between individual research sites. But you cannot analyze data on the web. The "web-science" paradigm involves downloading software and / or data, and running algorithms for data analysis locally. This limits collaboration, and is one of the main reasons why neuroimaging research papers typically involve small cohorts of research subjects collected by one site.

This pattern of research is fairly typical of web-enabled science. The web has facilitated certain types of collaboration, but large scale group working is difficult to achieve. Computational grids [6] have the potential to extend the functionality of the internet in ways that will make collaborative science involving large amounts of data and sophisticated algorithms much more straightforward. Scientific collaboration built on computational grids can go beyond web-science by transparently integrating data repositories, sophisticated algorithms and distributed computing.

Similar issues are also important in healthcare. Digital image archive systems are becoming more widespread in hospitals, and image data is being incorporated into multimedia patient records. This will make widespread computational analysis of *clinical* (as opposed to *research*) images possible for the first time. The capabilities

---

[1] See, for example: www.cma.mgh.harvard.edu/tools

T. Dohi and R. Kikinis (Eds.): MICCAI 2002, LNCS 2488, pp. 532–539, 2002.

provided by computational grids could make it possible to use the huge quantity of distributed on-line patient images for decision support in diagnosis.

In this paper we describe a proof of concept demonstrator that illustrates this potential through a network application that constructs brain atlases on the fly from selected subsets of a cohort of subjects 180 subjects.

Method

Our approach involved the following stages: assembling the data, and loading it onto an internet accessible database'; implementation of a network interface to launch data processing that creates new data rather than just retrieving stored data.; pre-processing the images to label tissue types and structures of interest; interactive use of the system to synthesize brain atlases specific to any individual on the fly.

Assembling the Data

The data comprised 180 whole brain magnetic resonance (MR) images of normal controls and patients with a variety of non-space-occupying brain lesions. All images were rf spoiled T1 weighted gradient echo volume acquisitions acquired on a 1T MR scanner (Philips Medical Systems, Cleveland Ohio), interpolated to approximately 1mm cubic voxels. All data was anonymised prior to transfer to the database.

The database, constructed using the open source MySQL (www.mysql.com), recorded subject age at scan date, gender, study group, and the URL of the image file. The database was automatically populated with the study data by parsing the filenames and image headers. Although we used a single server, different parts of the dataset could have been stored on servers at separate sites.

Network Interface

A TCL/TK interface incorporated into an interactive image viewer provides a user-friendly environment to query the database, transfer images using the secure grid protocol globus-url-copy (www.globus.org) and securely launch processing on a distributed computing cluster using globus and condor-g (www.cs.wisc.edu/condor).

Data Preparation

Database images were segmented into tissue types, and anatomical structures of interest delineated. The very substantial computation required for these automated analysis stages was carried out on computing hardware distributed across three sites (University of Oxford, King's College London and Imperial College London). The database was automatically populated with the analysis results.

Tissue Type Segmentation

Each brain volume was segmented into grey matter, white matter, and CSF using a statistical classifier implemented as part of the publicly available FSL package (www.fmrib.ox.ac.uk/fsl), running on a 16 CPU alpha server with 16Gbytes of RAM.

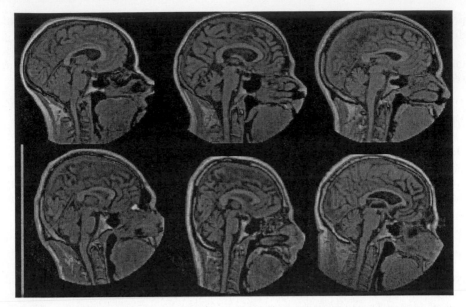

Fig. 1. Mid-sagittal sections through six of the 180 database subjects

Anatomical Structure Delineation

Anatomical structures were automatically delineated from the brain scans by registering the Montreal Brainweb reference image [9] to each scan in turn using a non-rigid registration algorithm based on manipulating a uniform array of B-spline control points (separation 2.4mm) while optimizing normalized mutual information [7]. The Brainweb reference image is implicitly segmented into grey matter, white matter and CSF (plus some other tissue types), and we had additionally delineated some anatomical structures including the caudate nucleus and lateral ventricles. After registration, the deformation field calculated was used to warp the segmented tissue labels and delineated structure boundaries to each of the 180 images, automatically segmenting and labeling each dataset to the accuracy of the registration algorithm. The non-rigid registration took 2 hours per dataset, and on a condor cluster of sixteen 1.4GHz Athlon PCs running linux, could process all 180 datasets in 24 hours.

Interactive Use to Calculate Atlases

The dynamic aspect of the system is the ability to generate an atlas specific to a particular subject in near real-time, rather than making use of a pre-computed atlas that may not be appropriate. The user loads a dataset of interest onto their local computer (we refer to this patient or research subject as the *study subject*). The user then queries the network database to identify *database subjects* that are close to the study subject in age, gender and/or other attributes stored in the database). The user then specifies the number of computers from the remote condor cluster they wish to make use of. Finally, the user launches the analysis. The study subject and instructions are then securely transferred to the computer cluster using globus protocols. Each of the

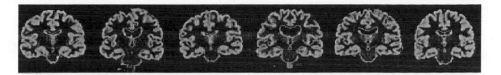

Fig. 2. Coronal sections through 6 example grey matter tissue probability maps selected from the 180 database subjects. Note intersubject variability

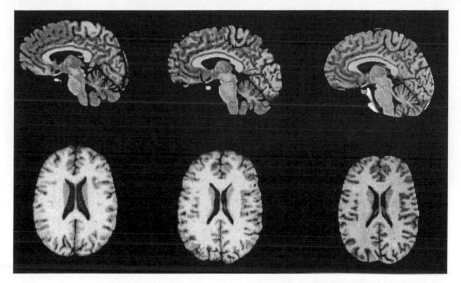

Fig. 3. Sagittal (top) and axial (bottom) slices through the Brainweb reference dataset (left), an example subject (right), and the reference dataset after warping to the subject (center). The reference dataset was warped to all 180 database subjects as part of pre-processing, effectively delineating all structures segmented in the reference dataset

selected database subjects is then registered to the study subject using an affine registration algorithm running on the condor cluster, and the resulting transformation is used to transform all the segmented tissue maps and delineated structures into the coordinate frame of the study subject and generate an atlas that comprises an average image of the tissue types and structure boundaries that can be used to assist in interpretation or subsequent analysis of the study subject. The results are securely transferred back to the local computer. On our cluster of 16 linux PCs, an atlas of up to 16 subjects could be generated in about 3 minutes.

Results

Pre-processing

Figure 1 shows some example sagittal sections through some of the 180 subjects in the database. Figure 2 shows example tissue probably maps for grey matter, for six

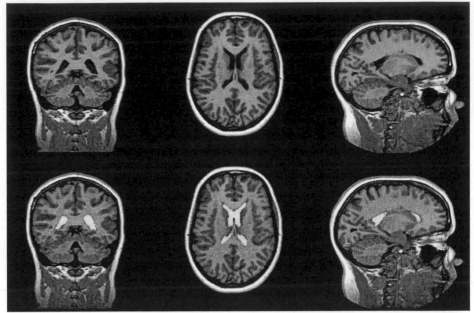

Fig. 4. Example coronal, axial and sagittal slices through a subject before and after delineation of the lateral ventricles using warping of the reference dataset

different subjects, reformatted in the coronal plane. Figure 3 shows an axial slice through the Brainweb reference dataset before, and after non-rigid registration to one of the subjects in the database. Figure 4 shows the subject image with the delineated structure warped from the reference dataset. These example results are shown as two-dimensional slices, but the analysis was done in 3D on all 180 database subjects.

Example Dynamically Generated Atlases

Figures 5 shows CSF maps from example atlases generated for study subjects of three different ages: For a 25 year old subject, the atlas was generated from images in the database from 30 subjects between 16 and 35 years of age, each registered to the study subject, then with the pre-computed segmentations and delineations trans-formed into the study subject's coordinates and averaged. For a 45 year old subject, the process was repeated using database subjects between 35 and 65 years of age, and for a 75 year old subject, the atlas was generated from database subject over 70 years old. Although we show example images, the user can generate a new atlas by loading in a study subject of choice, querying the network database as they choose, and launching the data-analysis on the remote computer facility.

Figure 6 shows a study subject with the 50 percentile boundary of the lateral ventricles from a similar-aged group of database subjects overlaid. Similar overlays could be produced for any delineated structure in the reference image.

Dicussion

We have implemented a network application using computational grid protocols that allows the user to dynamically generate brain atlases customized to a selected study

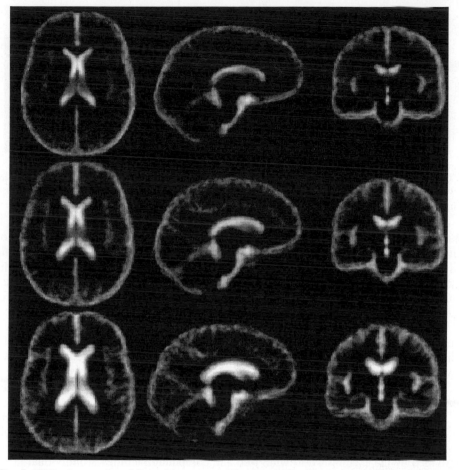

Fig. 5. CSF atlas produced for subjects aged 25 years (top), 45 years (middle) and 75 years (bottom). Note increasing size of CSF spaces with age. The dynamic atlas enables an atlas for any subject (selected by age or gender) to be calculated within a few minutes

subject. It provides a network interface that can be used to launch processing that creates new data, rather than just retrieving stored data. One of the characteristics of our network application and of grid applications in general is that they are scaleable, and it should be straightforward to extend them to much larger distributed collections of images and massive distributed computing facilities within multicentre collaborations. As the grid protocols evolve, it should make it increasingly easy to build and use large scale network applications of this type.

Dynamically configurable atlases have considerable value in neuroimaging research and in healthcare. In neuroimaging research, "static" web brain atlases are widely used to assist in data analysis and in cohort studies. A dynamic atlas could easily be configured to the research question of interest, which may provide added sensitivity to the analysis. In healthcare, MR imaging is being used more and more often in the management of patients with subtle or diffuse brain disease. Diagnosis of

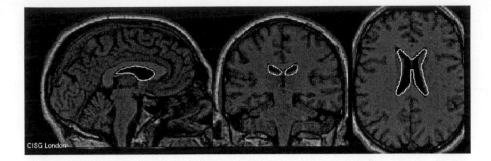

Fig. 6. Study subject with 50% boundary of lateral ventricles from age-mathed dynamic atlas overlaid as white boundary. This sort of functionality could provide decision support by assisting a radiologist in quantifying the degree of abnormality in a patient

such cases by conventional visual inspection of the images may be hard because of difficulties in precisely identifying what is abnormal about a subject's images. This process could be made more straightforward by providing an atlas made up of individuals of the same age, gender and possibly even co-morbidity as the study subject. Such an atlas could assist a radiologist by providing decision support that could in future be implemented on large healthcare image archives.

A natural extension of the dynamic atlas would be to add a knowledge discovery component. Rather than registering the images to a study subject, the network application could register the images to one-another in order to discover relationships between the data. The value of such a facility would increase with increasing numbers of subjects, and larger amounts of non-image information about the subjects, potentially including genetic information.

Future neuro-imaging research is going to require analysis of much larger cohorts of data in order to add to our understanding of brain development, aging and pathology. Such large scale projects will require better data analysis infrastructure than is provided by the existing world wide web and computing facilities at individual laboratories. We believe that this dynamic brain atlas project indicates the sort of capability that will be needed in such research programmes in the future.

Acknowledgements

This work was funded by the UK Department of Trade and Industry / Engineering and Physical Sciences Research Council e-science core programme as a technology demonstrator. We are grateful for the use of the MRI data, which was collected under the supervision of Professor Graeme Bydder, Dr Basant Puri and Dr Angela Oatridge. We thank Philips Medical Systems for supporting the MRI aspects of this work.

References

1. Sandor S. Leahy R. Surface-based labeling of cortical anatomy using a deformable atlas. *IEEE Transactions on Medical Imaging. 16(1):41-54, 1997*
2. Woods RP. Dapretto M. Sicotte NL. Toga AW. Mazziotta JC. Creation and use of a Talairach-compatible atlas for accurate, automated, nonlinear intersubject registration, and analysis of functional imaging data. *Human Brain Mapping. 8(2-3):73-9, 1999*

3. van Leemput K. Maes F. Vandermeulen D. Suetens P. Automated model-based bias field correction of MR images of the brain. *IEEE Transactions on Medical Imaging. 18(10):885-96, 1999*

4. Thompson PM. Mega MS. Woods RP. Zoumalan CI. Lindshield CJ. Blanton RE. Moussai J. Holmes CJ. Cummings JL. Toga AW. Cortical change in Alzhcimer's disease detected with a disease-specific population-based brain atlas. *Cerebral Cortex. 11(1):1-16, 2001*

5. Chung MK. Worsley KJ. Paus T. Cherif C. Collins DL. Giedd JN. Rapoport JL. Evans AC. A unified statistical approach to deformation-based morphometry. *Neuroimage. 14(3):595-606, 2001*

6. Foster, C. Kesselman, S. Tuecke The Anatomy of the Grid: Enabling Scalable Virtual Organizations.. *International J. Supercomputer Applications*, 15(3), 2001.

7. Rueckert D, Sonoda LI, Hayes C, Hill DLG, Leach MO, Hawkes DJ. Non-rigid Registration using Free-Form Deformations: Application to Breast MR Images *IEEE Trans. Medical Imaging* 18(8): 712-721 1999

8. D. L. Collins, A. P. Zijdenbos, V. Kollokian, J. Sled, N. J. Kabani, C. J. Holmes, and A. C. Evans. Design and construction of a realistic digital brain phantom. *IEEE Transactions on Medical Imaging.* 17,(3),463-468, 1998.

Model Library for Deformable Model-Based Segmentation of 3-D Brain MR-Images

Juha Koikkalainen[1] and Jyrki Lötjönen[2]

[1] Laboratory of Biomedical Engineering, Helsinki University of Technology, P.O.B. 2200, FIN-02015 HUT, Finland
jkoikkal@cc.hut.fi
[2] VTT Information Technology, P.O.B. 1206, FIN-33101 Tampere, Finland
Jyrki.Lotjonen@vtt.fi

Abstract. A novel method to use model libraries in segmentation is introduced. Using similarity measures one model from a model library is selected. This model is then used in model-based segmentation. The proposed method is simple, straightforward and fast. Various similarity measures, both voxel and edge measures, were examined. Two different segmentation methods were used for validating the functionality of the proposed procedure. Results show that a statistically significant improvement in segmentation accuracy was achieved in each study case.

1   Introduction

In some applications the slow manual segmentation of complicated pathological organs may be acceptable. However, the manual segmentation is usually too slow for the segmentation of normal healthy organs, especially in studies where a large number of cases is necessary. Many kinds of automatic segmentation methods have been developed. One group of methods is segmentation using deformable models [1]. A commonly known problem with deformable models is the need for a good initialization. If the initialization is not good, a model may attract to wrong features or it may have problems in converging to complicated boundaries.

One way to make segmentation results more accurate and robust is to use a bigger set of models, i.e. a model library or a training set. Cootes and Taylor proposed an approach based on statistical models [2]. The idea is to allow all legal transformations of shape and spatial relations of structures, but at the same time prohibit all deformations that are not typical to the organ. Information on shapes, their spatial relations and gray-level appearance in the training set are used in establishing the statistical model. The normal procedure is to use principal component analysis (PCA) to calculate from the training set the modes of shape variation, which reflects variations in the training set. Usually a small number of modes, those with the highest eigenvalues, can explain most of the variation. Maximum variations in the eigenmode space can be also limited [3]. Wang and Staib used this kind of statistical shape information from the

T. Dohi and R. Kikinis (Eds.): MICCAI 2002, LNCS 2488, pp. 540–547, 2002.

training set in non-rigid registration [4]. The fundamental problem with statistical models is the need for a point correspondence. The manual definition of landmarks is slow and subjective, especially in three dimensions (3-D). One possibility to automate this is to use the parameterization of shapes, like spherical harmonics [3]. Davies *et al.* found the point correspondence via an optimization problem [5]. Rueckert *et al.* applied PCA to the deformation fields that were got by registering the volumes in a training set to a reference volume [6].

We propose a new way to utilize training set to improve segmentation accuracy. This method partly overcomes initialization problems. Our method has similarities with object recognition, like face recognition (e.g. [7]) and shape recognition (e.g. [8]), i.e. the model, which was the most similar to a target volume, i.e. the volume to be segmented, in terms of some similarity measure was searched. Instead of transforming the training set into a statistical form, a normal unconstrained segmentation was performed. The model used in segmentation was selected from the model library. The target volume was first rigidly transformed to the coordinate system of the model library. Thereafter, the model that was the most similar to the target volume was selected from the library based on a similarity measure, and used in segmentation. The proposed method is simple and straightforward. There is no need for defining the point correspondence. Selecting one model gives more freedom to the shape of the segmentation target. The topology of the model is not anymore bound, assuming that the model library is a representative sample of the target shape. The method can be used in segmentation as well as in registration.

2   Methods

2.1   Model Library

In this study, eight T1-weighted brain MR-volumes were used to build a model library. The size of the volumes was $128 \times 128 \times 90$ and the voxel size was about 2 mm $\times$ 2 mm $\times$ 2 mm. In each volume five organs were manually segmented using triangulated surfaces: skin, brain envelope, cerebellum, corpus callosum (CC) and midbrain. The intensity of the volumes was normalized by scaling histograms between values 0 and 255.

For establishing the model library, one volume was selected to be a reference volume. All other volumes were aligned with this volume using a registration method that optimizes seven parameters: 3 for translation, 3 for rotation and 1 for isotropic scaling. The optimization was based on mutual information. One slice from each model in the library is shown in Fig. 1.

An alternative possibility for initialization would be to use a coordinate system based on anatomical landmarks. The most popular approach is the Talairach-coordinate system which was used by Keleman *et al.* [3] for global alignment of head volumes. In this system 12 affine transformations are done based on anterior and posterior commissures (AC and PC) and the extreme limits of the brain.

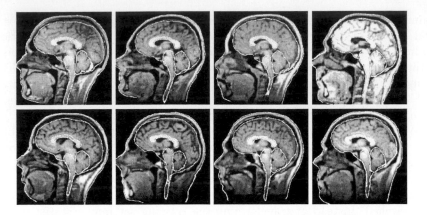

Fig. 1. An example of the model library. Eight volumes are manually segmented and registered in to a common coordinate system

2.2 Model Selection

A new target volume was first rigidly aligned with the reference volume. The model that was used in segmentation was selected based on similarity measures. Similarity measures are commonly used in image registration in cost and energy functions. These measures can be divided into two classes: voxel similarity measures which use gray-level information and edge measures which use edge information.

Voxel similarity measures are very popular in different registration applications. There exists a large selection of different measures [9, 10]. Measures based on correlation, like mean-square-distance (MSD), Pearson's cross correlation (NCC) and correlation ratio (CR) [11], are mainly for monomodal registration, except CR. Another class is voxel similarity measures based on entropy: e.g. entropy of the difference image (EDI), mutual information (MI) and normalized versions of MI, like normalized mutual information (NMI) [12]

$$\text{NMI}(F, G) = \frac{H(F) + H(G)}{H(F, G)} \tag{1}$$

and entropy correlation coefficient (ECC) [13]

$$\text{ECC}(F, G) = \frac{2MI(F, G)}{H(F) + H(G)} . \tag{2}$$

In these equations $H(F)$ and $H(G)$ are the entropies of the target volume F and the model volume G, respectively. $H(F, G)$ is the joint entropy of these volumes. These measures are applicable also in multimodal registration, because they make no assumptions about the form of the relationship between gray-levels in two images.

The idea of edge measures is to measure how near the model surface is to a strong edge. After all, the optimal segmentation is usually close to strong edges.

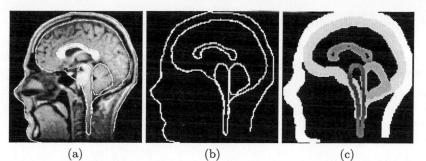

(a)   (b)   (c)

Fig. 2. a) A manually segmented volume. b) A binary volume of surfaces. c) Dilated volumes that were used as masks in computing similarity measures

Information on edge directions can be also incorporated in these measures, so that surfaces must be both near strong edges and edges in the model and the target volumes must be parallel. In this work we tested 24 edge measures such as

$$\text{edge1}\,(F, G) = \frac{1}{N} \sum_{i=1}^{N} \frac{\nabla f_i \cdot \nabla g_i}{|\nabla f_i||\nabla g_i|} |\nabla f_i| \tag{3}$$

and [14]

$$\text{edge2}\,(F, G) = \frac{1}{N} \sum_{i=1}^{N} \frac{\nabla f_i \cdot \nabla g_i}{|\nabla f_i||\nabla g_i|} \min\left(|\nabla f_i|, |\nabla g_i|\right) . \tag{4}$$

N is the number of nodes in the model surface and f_i and g_i are voxels in the target volume and the model volume, respectively. Edge volumes were made using Canny-Deriche operator, which gives also edge directions.

The values of these similarity measures are usually computed from the whole overlapping image volume in registration. Since the segmentations of separate organs are searched for in this study, similarity measures should take into account only the organ of interest. In this work a binary volume was made from the model's boundary (Fig. 2 (b)). Then a dilation operation was executed 1-3 times, depending on the size and the surroundings of the organ (Fig. 2 (c)). This volume was used as a mask when the similarity between the model volume and the target volume was computed. In this way only the alignment and the shape of that organ affected on the similarity measure. Edge-based similarity measures were computed mainly on the model surface.

The complementary information produced by voxel- and edge-based measures was merged to improve the accuracy and robustness in [14, 15]. The approach was adopted also in this work. The optimal combination of different measures was determined using regression analysis. The dependent variable was the final segmentation error and the independent variables were the values of similarity measures. A group of regression equations was achieved using the stepwise regression. The regression equation predicts the final segmentation error based on similarity measures. Therefore, the model that produced the lowest predicted value was chosen in the model selection phase.

2.3   Final Segmentation

The model selection procedure was validated by two segmentation algorithms, i.e. the chosen model was used as a prior model in the algorithms [16, 15].

In [16], a surface template consisting of triangulated surfaces was non-rigidly matched to edges in MR volumes using a free-form deformation (FFD) grid in the multiresolution framework. The energy measure to be minimized consisted of two components: 1) the distance of the model surfaces from the edges in MR volumes using oriented distance maps, and 2) the change of the model shape during the deformation.

A volumetric template consisting of a gray-scale volume and triangulated surfaces of objects of interest was used in [15]. Instead of applying FFD, the deformation was accomplished by deformation spheres. The energy term had three components. The first one was a voxel similarity measure; MSD was used in this monomodal study. The second term was a gradient term, which took into account edge intensities and directions in target and model volumes. The third term regulated the change of the model shape.

3   Results

Our image database was composed of nine volumes. Since the database was reasonably small, the jack-knife procedure was used to validate the model selection procedure, i.e. each volume was once regarded as a target volume and the rest eight volumes composed the model library (Fig. 1). The target volume was initialized to the common coordinate system and all similarity measures (in total 31) were calculated for all model volumes. Then the final segmentation was done and the segmentation error was determined as an average distance from the nodes of the model surface to the manually segmented target surface.

The following procedure was used to validate the model selection. For each target volume i, where $i \in 1, 2, ..9$, each library model ($N = 8$) was used separately as a prior model in the segmentation algorithm. The minimum m_i and the average a_i errors were defined. The minimum error is achieved if the best model was chosen in the model selection. The average gives an idea of the error if the model is chosen arbitrarily from the library. As the model selection was used, the error was s_i. The quality of the model selection is defined by the improvement percent, $p_i = 100 \frac{a_i - s_i}{a_i - m_i}$. If the best model is chosen, $p_i = 100\%$. To get an idea of the real error values, $a = 0.986$, $m = 0.686$ and $s = 0.724$ voxels (for the similarity measure NMI) for the skin as the values were averaged over all target volumes.

Tables 1 and 2 present results averaged over nine target volumes for both segmentation methods and for all organs. The results are reported only for similarity measures that produced the best improvement percents. The second row is the percentage of cases, where the best model was selected, and the last row the percentage of cases, where a model better than the average was selected. In the two last columns, the same similarity measure was used for all organs. In the column "many models", each organ was chosen independently from the

Table 1. Results using surface-based segmentation

	skin	brain env	cerebellum	CC	midbrain	many models	one model
improvement (%)	65	90	61	47	78	53	26
best model (%)	22	33	33	22	44	36	18
better than average (%)	89	100	89	78	100	84	71

Table 2. Results using intensity-based segmentation

	skin	brain env	cerebellum	CC	midbrain	many models	one model
improvement (%)	87	94	57	60	92	63	35
best model (%)	44	67	11	44	67	44	29
better than average (%)	100	100	89	78	100	84	71

model library. In the column "one model", one model was selected from the model library and it was used to segment all organs. The improvements in the accuracy were statistically significant ($p < 0.05$), as tested with Wilcoxon signed rank test.

In overall, the best similarity measures were voxel measures. The best results using one similarity measure for all organs were achieved by using NMI. ECC was also good, as were NCC and EDI in some cases. The edge similarity measures presented in Eqs. 3 and 4 were almost as good as voxel measures. One and the same similarity measure was not the best one for each organ. However, using the same measure for all organs gave a reasonable good improvement, as can be seen from the two last columns.

The best model was not found every time. In some cases the selected model was even worse than the average. However, in these cases the model was almost as good as the average. These results indicate, that the selected model was generally good but not necessarily the best. Models, which gave a very poor segmentation, were never selected. So when a surface is attracted severely to a wrong edge, this model is discarded, as in the example in Fig. 3.

Tables 3 and 4 correspond to Tables 1 and 2, except that regression equations were utilized in the model selection. In these equations, two to five similarity

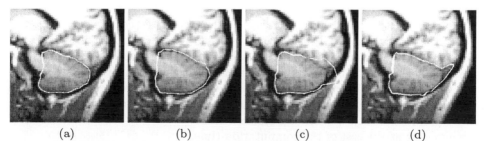

| (a) | (b) | (c) | (d) |

Fig. 3. An example of the segmentation of cerebellum: a) and b) the best two models, and c) and d) the worst two models after the final segmentation

Table 3. Results using regression analysis and surface-based segmentation

	skin	brain env	cerebellum	CC	midbrain	many models	one model
improvement (%)	74	91	72	54	84	55	33
best model (%)	33	44	56	33	56	33	29
better than average (%)	100	100	89	89	100	84	73

Table 4. Results using regression analysis and intensity-based segmentation

	skin	brain env	cerebellum	CC	midbrain	many models	one model
improvement (%)	86	94	58	60	95	64	43
best model (%)	44	67	33	44	56	40	27
better than average (%)	100	100	100	89	100	87	71

measures were used. Despite of the complementary information in the selection, the results are only slightly better than using only one similarity measure.

The time needed for computing the values of similarity measures is short compared to the computation time of the segmentation methods. The initial alignment is necessary in these segmentation methods even if the model selection is not done. So the method proposed for model selection does not increase the computational burden of the segmentation practically at all. Obviously, if the library contained hundreds of models, the computation time of similarity measures might become significant.

4   Discussion

Deformable model-based segmentation is a powerful tool but suffers from problems related to the model initialization and complicated shapes. The results show convincingly that the presented method improves the segmentation accuracy by selecting one model from the model library. These improvements were statistically significant.

The proposed method is very simple and easy to realize. Any parameterization or definition of point correspondence is not necessary. The topology of segmented subject can vary, if this variation is presented in the model library as well. Also, this method can be combined with methods that use training set to make a statistical model of the shape. The model library could consist of statistical models from which the best one would be selected.

Initialization was done using rigid registration. Another possibility is to use the Talairach-coordinate system. According to our studies with a smaller database, this method may be better than the rigid registration. However, it can be used only for brain images whereas the method used in this paper can be generalized to other applications. Also elastic registration methods could be used in initial registration instead of linear transformations. This would improve results, but at the cost of the computation time.

In the future the library must be enlarged, manual segmentation improved and new, more complex organs studied. New segmentation methods, parameters and especially different initialization methods should be also studied. The method will be tested also in other applications.

Acknowledgements

Research was supported by Tekes, the National Technology Agency, Finland. The authors express thanks to The Department of Radiology, Helsinki University Central Hospital, Finland, for providing volume images.

References

1. T. McInerney, D. Terzopoulos. Deformable Models in Medical Image Analysis: a Survey. *Medical Image analysis*, 1(2): 91–108, 1996.
2. T.F. Cootes, C.J. Taylor. Statistical models of appearance for medical image analysis and computer vision. *Proc. SPIE*, 2001.
3. A. Kelemen, G. Székely, G. Gerig. Elastic Model-Based Segmentation of 3-D Neuroradiological Data Sets. *IEEE Trans. Medical Imaging*, vol 18(10):828–839, 1999.
4. Y. Wang, L.H. Staib. Elastic Model Based Non-Rigid Registration Incorporating Statistical Shape Information. *Proc. MICCAI 1998*, 1162–1173, 1998.
5. R.D. Davies, T.F. Cootes, J.C.Waterton, C.J. Taylor. An Efficient Method for Constructing Optimal Statistical Shape Models. *Proc. MICCAI 2001*, 57–65, 2001.
6. D. Rueckert, A.F. Frangi, J.A. Schnabel. Automatic Construction of 3D Statistical Deformation Models Using Non-rigid Registration. *Proc. MICCAI 2001*, 77–84, 2001.
7. B. Moghaddam, A. Pentland. Face Recognition using View-Based and Modular Eigenspaces. *Automatic Systems for the Identification and Inspection of Humans, SPIE*, vol 2277, July 1994.
8. S. Sclaroff, A.P. Pentland. Modal Matching for Correspondence and Recognition. *IEEE Trans. Pattern Analysis and Machine Intelligence*, vol 17(6): 545–561, 1995.
9. D.L.G. Hill, D.J. Hawkes. Across-Modality Registration Using Intensity-Based Cost Functions. Handbook of Medical Imaging Processing and Analysis, I.N. Bankman ed., Academic Press, 2000.
10. M. Holden, D.L.G. Hill, E.R.E. Denton, J.M. Jarosz, T.C.S. Cox, T. Rohlfing, J. Goodey, D.J. Hawkes. Voxel Similarity Measures for 3-D Serial MR Brain Image Registration. *IEEE Trans. Medical Imaging*, vol 19(2): 94–102, 2000.
11. A. Roche, G. Malandain, X. Pennec, N. Ayache. Multimodal Image Registration by Maximation of the Correlation Ratio. Rapport de recherche, INRIA, 1998.
12. C. Studholme, D.L.G. Hill, D.J. Hawkes. An overlap invariant entropy measure of 3D medical image alignment. *Pattern Recognition*, 32(1): 71–86, 1999.
13. J. Astola, I. Virtanen. Entropy correlation coefficient. A measure of statistical dependence for categorized data. *Proc. Univ. Vaasa, Discussion Papers*, 44, 1982.
14. J.P. Pluim, J.B.A. Maintz, M.A. Viergever. Image Registration by Maximation of Combined Mutual Information and Gradient Information. *IEEE Trans. Medical Imaging*, vol 19(8): 809–814, 2000.
15. J. Lötjönen, T. Mäkelä. Elastic matching using a deformation sphere. *Proc. MICCAI 2001*, 541–548, 2001.
16. J. Lötjönen, P-J. Reissman, I.E. Magnin, T. Katila. Model extraction from magnetic resonance voluma data using the deformable pyramid. *Medical Image Analysis*, vol. 3(4): 387–406, 1999.

Co-registration of Histological, Optical and MR Data of the Human Brain

É. Bardinet[1], S. Ourselin[2], D. Dormont[4], G. Malandain[1], D. Tandé[3],
K. Parain[3], N. Ayache[1], and J. Yelnik[3]

[1] INRIA, Epidaure Project, Sophia Antipolis, France
[2] CSIRO Telecom. and Industrial Physics, PO Box 76, Epping NSW 1710 Australia
[3] INSERM U289, Salpêtrière Hospital, France
[4] Neuroradiology Dept and LENA UPR 640-CNRS, Salpêtrière Hospital, France
ebard@sophia.inria.fr

Abstract. In order to allow accurate pre-operative localisation of functional targets in functional neurosurgery, we aim at constructing a three dimensional registrable cartography of the basal ganglia, based on histology. For doing this, a *post mortem* MR study was conducted on a cadaver's head, and the brain was then extracted and processed for histology. The *post mortem* MR image will allow to report the cartography on the patient's anatomy, by its registration with the patient's MR image. In this paper, we focus on the problem of co-registering the histological and *post mortem* MR data of the same subject. First, realignment of the histological sections into a reliable three dimensional volume is performed. Then the reconstructed volume is registered with the *post mortem* MR image. To insure three dimensional integrity of the histological reconstructed volume, a reference volume is first constructed from photographs of the unstained surface of the frozen brain. This reference is then used as an intermediate volume for, on the one hand, independant alignment of each histological section with its corresponding optical section and on the other hand, three dimensional registration with the *post mortem* MR image.

1 Introduction

Advances in image guided stereotactic neurosurgery and stimulation technology have given rise to a reappearence of the use of functional neurosurgery for the treatment of movement disorders, e.g. Parkinson's disease or dystonia. The intervention is based on the stereotactic introduction of electrodes in disease-specific nuclei of the basal ganglia, e.g. for Parkinson's disease a small, deeply located, nucleus called the subthalamic nucleus (STN) [6]. The nucleus is targeted on pre-operative stereotactic MR acquisitions [1]. In these procedures, the surgical success depends primarily on the accurate localisation of the target.

MR imaging of the basal ganglia, despite technological and clinical progress over the last decade, appears to be intrinsically limited by two factors. First, the resolution of clinical routine MR images is nowadays around 1mm^3, thus limiting the level of detail of the images to the gross features of the basal ganglia;

T. Dohi and R. Kikinis (Eds.): MICCAI 2002, LNCS 2488, pp. 548–555, 2002.

second, and more fundamentally, the MR signal, being a measure of tissue physical properties, provides us with a representation of the underlying anatomical reality of the organ being imaged. The relationship between the measured signal and the real anatomy is not always completely understood. For example, for Parkinson's disease, the STN is targeted on pre-operative MR acquisitions (T1 and T2-weighted) [1]. On the T1 image (acquired in stereotactic conditions), this nucleus is undistinguishable, and on the T2 image (not in stereotactic conditions, due to geometric distortions), an hyposignal at the STN level is observed, but a clearly defined relationship between this signal and the STN is still debated. This introduces uncertainty on the nucleus localisation. Consequently, electrophysiological study and clinical testing are performed during the intervention to refine the pre-operatively determined target position. This causes the intervention to last on average 10 hours. Therefore, allowing more accurate pre-operative locatisation of the functional targets appears to be a key issue.

Detailed and accurate cartography of the basal ganglia can be performed on histological serial sections. Indeed, histology, consisting in the study of postmortem autopsy tissues, overcomes the limitations of MR imaging, allowing higher level of detail and direct observation of anatomical reality [11, 7]. Moreover, staining of histological sections can provide functional information, e.g. Nissl stain which can reveal cytoarchitectonic details of cerebral regions, or Calbindin immunoreactivity which can distinguish the associative and sensori-motor territories of the striatum [2]. Therefore, anatomical and functional cartography of the complete basal ganglia can be performed on histology, and the corresponding features accurately outlined. Nevertheless, before to use such a cartography for target localisation in functional neurosurgery, reliable three dimensional reconstruction from the histological sections must be done, as histology being by nature two-dimensional, i.e. histological data consist of a series of discontinuous serial sections. Also, this cartography has to be registrable with the MR acquisitions of the patient, in order to report the outlined features on the patient's anatomy.

Resuming, we aim at constructing a three dimensional, anatomical and functional, as well as registrable, cartography of the basal ganglia, based on histology. For doing this, a *post mortem* MR study was conducted on a cadaver's head, 36 hours after death, insuring the MR signal to be very similar to an *in vivo* MR image, and the brain was then extracted and processed for histology. The *post mortem* MR image will allow to report the cartography on the patient's anatomy, by its registration with the patient's MR image.

In this paper, we focus on the problem of co-registering histological and *post mortem* MR data of the same subject. First, realignment of the histological sections into a reliable three dimensional volume has to be performed. Then this reconstructed volume has to be registered with the MR image. Because histological sections suffered independant two dimensional geometric distortions, direct alignment of these sections would not allow to get a reliable three dimensional volume, lacking a three dimensional reference. In order to build such a reference, photographs were taken during brain sectionning. Their alignment provides us with a reference volume, which is then used as an intermediate volume for, on the one hand, alignment of the histological sections with their corresponding optical sections, and on the other hand, three dimensional registration with the *post mortem* MR image.

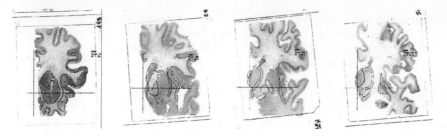

Fig. 1. Nissl stained histological sections with outlines of basal ganglia structures and territories superimposed.

2   Material and Methods

2.1   Material

A human brain was obtained 36 hours after death. First an MR study (T1 and T2-weighted acquisitions) was conducted, before extraction of the brain. Then the brain was stored in 4% paraformaldehyde for 8 days and in phosphate buffer with sucrose for 7 days. One hemisphere was sectioned into 3 blocks (1.5 cm thick) in order to favour a better fixation, and stored frozen at $-40°$C. The blocks were cut into $70\,\mu$m thin sections which were collected serially. Sectioning was done on a Tetrander Jung freezing microtome. During cutting, some sections at the bottom and top of the blocks were lost as the cryomicrotome could not reach them. Sections were treated according to different immunohistochemical procedures. One out of ten sections (thus every $700\,\mu$m) was stained for Nissl to reveal cytoarchitectonic details of cerebral regions. After staining, histological sections were scanned, and structures and territories of the basal ganglia were outlined (Figure 1). During sectioning, photographs of the unstained surface of the frozen brain, together with part of the cryomicrotome including 6 screws, were taken for one out of ten sections (Figure 2). There was therefore a corresponding optical section for each histological stained section.

2.2   Fusion of Histological and *Post Mortem* MR Data

As explained in section 1, realignment of the histological sections has to be performed first, followed by the registration of the reconstructed volume with the *post mortem* MR image.

Alignment of histological serial sections into a three dimensional volume can be done following a straightforward method. It consists in the registration of consecutive sections two by two and further three dimensional reconstruction by composition of the resulting transformations [4, 3, 5, 9]. Nevertheless, this method is not adequate when the sections have suffered independant two dimensional geometric distortions. Indeed, rigid registration of contiguous sections would not compensate for the distortions, and non rigid registration, which could partially cope with distortions, followed by transformation composition, would not allow to get a reliable three dimensional histological volume in the absence of a three dimensional reference.

In order to build such a reference, following [12, 8], photographs of the unstained surface of the frozen brain were taken. Feature-based alignment of these

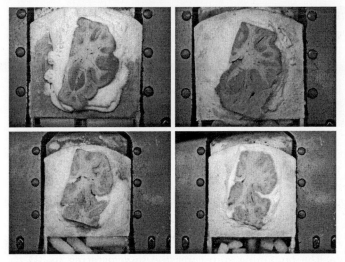

Fig. 2. Photographs of the unstained surface of the frozen brain taken during brain sectioning, together with part of the cryomicrotome including 6 screws.

photographs, the screws of the cryomicrotome acting as fiducial markers, yields a reference volume. This reference is then used as an intermediate volume for, on the one hand, independant alignment of each histological section with its corresponding optical section (this guarantees the three dimensional integrity of the reconstructed histological volume) and on the other hand, three dimensional registration with the *post mortem* MR image.

Feature-based alignment of the optical sections. In order to reconstruct a reference three dimensional volume from the optical sections, we used a feature-based registration method (rigid ICP - Iterative Closest Point algorithm), where the 6 screws of the cryomicrotome served as fiducial markers. These screws were detected automatically by combination of thresholding and connected component analysis. Alignment of the optical sections using these markers guaranteed the integrity of the resulting three dimensional reconstruction. The resulting volume presented intensity variations from slice to slice, due to the photographs acquisition and scanning process. In order to get an homogeneous volume, these variations were corrected by histogram equalisation.

Reconstruction of the histological volume. Using the optical reconstructed volume as a geometrical reference, each histological section was registered with its corresponding optical section. The 2D registrations were performed with the block matching algorithm [10], an intensity-based two-steps method consisting in selective local-based correspondance computation, followed by robust transformation estimation, these two steps being embedded in an iterative multi-scale scheme (typically 6 levels). Correlation coefficient was used as the similarity measure for computation of the correspondances, and 2D affine transformations, one for each section, were estimated.

Selective local-based correspondance computation and robust estimation of the transformation made this algorithm particularly adapted to the problem, capable to cope with distortions due to the processing of the histological sections. Indeed, most of the correspondances were found in highly contrasted regions,

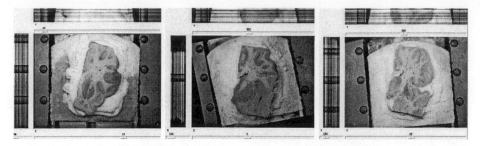

Fig. 3. Rigid alignment of the optical sections. Three orthogonal views of each of the three brain blocks (see text for details)

i.e. around the basal ganglia, and irrelevant correspondances were considered as outliers during robust estimation.

Registration with the _post mortem_ MR data. To achieve the fusion of histology and MR data, the remaining step consisted in registering in 3D the intermediate reference optical volume with the T1-weighted _post mortem_ MR image. Again, this registration was performed with the block matching algorithm [10], and a unique three dimensional affine transformation was estimated.

3   Results and Discussion

First, feature-based alignment of the optical sections was performed. As explained in section 2.1, the brain (one hemisphere) was first sectioned into 3 blocks (1.5 cm thick) in order to favour a better fixation, before histological sectioning in thin sections. Consequently, photographs taken during sectioning consisted in three series, for which feature-based registration, using cryomicrotome screws as fiducial markers, lead to reliable three dimensional alignments (three orthogonal views of the alignments are shown Figure 3 - note the alignment of the cryomicrotome on lateral views, as well as intensity variations from slice to slice). To get the complete optical volume, alignment of the last section of the first (resp. second) block with the first section of the second (resp. third) block was then performed manually by an expert, to insure perfect structural continuity between the blocks around the basal ganglia. Alignment of the complete optical sections followed by correction of intensity variations can be seen in Figure 5 (left).

Then, each histological section was independantly registered with its corresponding optical sections. On Figure 4, some results are presented: optical sections (first row), registered corresponding histological sections (second row), and both sections fused (third row), in order to visually assert the quality of the registrations. Stacking-up the registered histological sections lead to a reliable three dimensional histological volume (Figure 5, right). As said in section 2.1, some histological sections at the top and bottom of the blocks were lost during brain cutting. The two gaps in the sagittal and axial views of the reconstructed histological volume on Figure 5 correspond to these missing sections.

Registration of the reference optical volume with the T1-weighted _post mortem_ MR image was finally performed, as well as registration of the T1 and T2-weighted MR images.

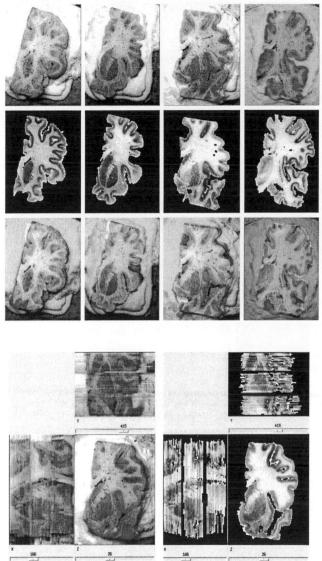

Fig. 4. Two dimensional registration of histological and optical sections. First row: four optical sections along the anteroposterior axis; second row: corresponding histological sections after registration; third row: both sections fused with an opacity factor, allowing to visually assert the good correspondence for the basal ganglia.

Fig. 5. Three orthogonal slices through the optical (left) and histological (right) reconstructed volumes (see text for details).

For registration of the histological sections as well as fusion of the optical volume with the T1-weighted MR image, our interest being the basal ganglia, the block matching algorithm was particularly adapted, as correspondances were found in highly contrasted regions, i.e. around the basal ganglia, and irrelevant correspondances were considered as outliers during robust estimation of the transformations.

Once co-registration of the histological, optical and MR data was achieved, we reported structures and territories of the basal ganglia outlined on the histological Nissl-stained sections onto the histological, optical and *post mortem* MR

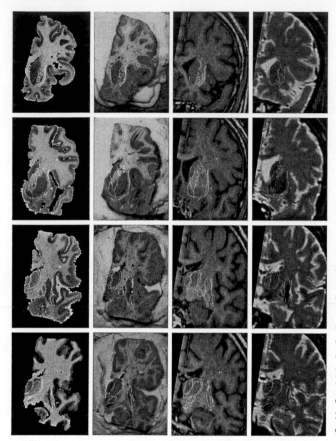

Fig. 6. Histological, optical and *post mortem* (T1 and T2-weighted) MR volumes co-registered. Four sections along the antero-posterior axis. Structures of the basal ganlia outlined on the histological sections are reported on the four volumes (including caudate nucleus, putamen, pallidum, claustrum, accumbens, nuclei of the thalamus, subthalamic nucleus and substancia nigra).

volumes using the corresponding transformations. On Figure 6, four sections of these volumes, along the antero-posterior axis, are shown, with contours of the basal ganlia superimposed (including caudate nucleus, putamen, pallidum, claustrum, accumbens, nuclei of the thalamus, subthalamic nucleus and substancia nigra).

4   Conclusion

In this study, we have carried out co-registration of histological and *post mortem* MR data of the same subject. This work is part of a project which aims at constructing a three dimensional, anatomical and functional, as well as registrable, cartography of the human basal ganglia, based on histology, in order to improve accuracy of the pre-operative localisation of targets in functional neurosurgery.

Realignment of the Nissl-stained histological sections into a reliable three dimensional volume was first performed. Then the reconstructed volume was registered with the *post mortem* MR image. To insure three dimensional integrity of the histological reconstructed volume, an intermediate reference volume was first constructed from photographs of the unstained surface of the frozen brain.

Co-registration of the histological, optical and MR data allowed us to report structures and territories of the basal ganglia outlined on the histological sections onto the *post mortem* MR volumes.

In order to use this three-dimensional cartography of the basal ganglia for pre-operative planning in functional neurosurgery, the remaining step consists in an accurate registration of the *post mortem* MR data with the patient's MR data, that will allow to report this cartography on patient's anatomy.

References

1. B.P. Bejjani, D. Dormont, B. Pidoux, J. Yelnik, P. Damier, and I. Arnulf. Bilateral subthalamic stimulation for parkinson's disease by using three-dimensional stereo-tactic magnetic resonance imaging and electrophysiological guidance. *Journal of Neurosurgery*, 92:615–625, 2000.

2. C. François, J. Yelnik, G. Percheron, and D. Tandé. Calbindin d-28k as a marker for the associative cortical territory of the striatum in macaque. *Brain Research*, 633:331–336, 1994.

3. E. Guest and R. Baldock. Automatic reconstruction of serial sections using the finite element method. *Bioimaging*, 3:154–167, 1995.

4. L.S. Hibbard and R.A. Hawkings. Objective image alignment for three-dimensional reconstruction of digital autoradiograms. *Journal of Neuroscience Method*, 26:55–74, 1988.

5. B. Kim, J.L. Boes, K.A. Frey, and C.R. Meyer. Mutual Information for Automated Unwarping of Rat Brain Autoradiographs. *Neuroimage*, 5:31–40, 1997.

6. P. Limousin, P. Pollak, D. Benazzouz, D. Hoffmann, J.F. Le Bas, E. Broussolle, J.E. Perret, and A.L Benabid. Effect of parkinsonian signs and symptoms of bilateral subthalamic nucleus stimulatiom. *Lancet,* 345, 1995.

7. J. Mai, J. Asscheuer, and G. Paxinos. *Atlas of the Human Brain. Academic Press,* 1997.

8. M.S. Mega, S.S. Chen, P.M. Thompson, R.P. Woods, T.J. Karaca, A. Tiwari, H.V. Vinters, G.W. Small, and A.W. Toga. Mapping Histology to Metabolism: Coregistration of Stained Whole-Brain Sections to Premortem PET in Alzheimer's Disease. *Neuroimage*, 5:147–153, 1997.

9. S. Ourselin, E. Bardinet, D. Dormont, G. Malandain, A. Roche, N. Ayache, D. Tande, K. Parain, and J. Yelnik. Fusion of histological sections and MR images: towards the construction of an atlas of the human basal ganglia. In W.J. Niessen and M.A. Viergever, editors, *4th Int. Conf. on Medical Image Computing and Computer-Assisted Intervention (MICCAI'01)*, volume 2208 of *LNCS*, pages 743–751, Utrecht, The Netherlands, October 2001.

10. S. Ourselin, A. Roche, S. Prima, and N. Ayache. Block Matching: A General Gramework to Improve Robustness of Rigid Registration of Medical Images. In A.M. DiGioia and S. Delp, editors, *International Conference on Medical Image Computing And Computer-Assisted Intervention*, pages 557–566, Pittsburgh, Pennsylvania USA, October 11-14 2000.

11. G. Schaltenbrand and W. Wharen. *Atlas for Stereotaxy of the Human Brain.* Stuttgart: Georg Thieme Verlag, 1977.

12. T. Schormann, M. Von Matthey, A. Dabringhaus, and K. Zilles. Alignment of 3-D Brain Data Sets Originating From MR and Histology. *Bioimaging*, 1:119–128, 1993.

An Automated Segmentation Method of Kidney Using Statistical Information

Baigalmaa Tsagaan[1], Akinobu Shimizu[1],
Hidefumi Kobatake[1], and Kunihisa Miyakawa[2]

[1] Graduate School of Bio-Applications and Systems Engineering,
Tokyo University of Agriculture and Technology,
2-24-16 Naka-cho, Koganei-shi, Tokyo 184-8588, Japan
{tsagaan,simiz,kobatake}@cc.tuat.ac.jp
[2] Department of Radiology, National Cancer Center Hospital,
5-1-1 Tsukiji, Chuo-ku, Tokyo 104-0045, Japan
kmiyagaw@ncc.go.jp

Abstract. This paper presents a deformable model based approach for auto-mated segmentation of kidneys from tree dimensional (3D) abdominal CT im-ages. Since the quality of an input image is very poor and noisy due to the large slice thickness, we use a deformable model represented by NURBS surface, which uses not only the gray level appearance of the target but also statistical information of the shape. A shape feature vector is defined to evaluate geomet-ric character of the surface and its statistical information is incorporated into the deformable model through an energy formulation for deformation. Principal curvature on the model surface, which is invariant to rotation and translation, is adopted as a component of the vector. Furthermore, automated positioning pro-cedure of an initial model is presented in this paper. We applied the proposed method to the 33 abdominal CT images whose slice thickness is 10mm and evaluated the effectiveness of the proposing method.

1 Introduction

The segmentation in medical images remains difficult task due to variation in image quality and requires a laborious work especially in three dimensional (3D) images. The medical images are often corrupted by noise which can cause difficulties when applying the conventional methods, such as thresholding and region growing approaches[1]. To address these problems, deformable models have been offering accurate and robust approach, which ensures smoothly connected extracted regions for noisy edges of an image[2]. In more sophisticated deformable models, the prior information about geometrical shape or the location of organs is used to constrain shape and appearance, as well as the statistical variation of these quantities[2,3]. For example, Cootes et al.[4-6] have proposed the active shape model (ASM), which uses PCA to analyze model's shape variation. ASM represents the object shapes by a set of boundary points. Thus some preprocessing, such as adjustment of the point coordinates for the affine transformation of an input images, is necessary. Recently, hierarchically organized models with affine-invariant statistical information, in conjunction with point correspondences are presented, and the results seem to be excellent [7].

The most common example of parameterized deformable model is Fourier model, which can represent the smooth shapes compactly and whose a prior information can

T. Dohi and R. Kikinis (Eds.): MICCAI 2002, LNCS 2488, pp. 556–563, 2002.
© Springer-Verlag Berlin Heidelberg 2002

be derived from probability distributions of the Fourier coefficients [9]. However, it is not easy to deform the model instinctively, especially in the case of 3D segmentation [10].

In this paper, we present an automated segmentation procedure of kidneys in abdominal CT images. The image quality in our research is very poor and noisy, due to low spatial resolution between slices (Fig.1). In addition, the surrounding organs such as the liver and spleen whose CT values are similar to those of kidney, are very close to or in contact with a part of kidney. Therefore we adopt a deformable model, which uses not only the gray value of the target but also statistical information of the shapes [11]. Our model is defined by NURBS surface in order to achieve easy manipulation and representation of the smooth shapes [12].

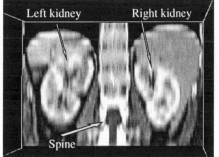

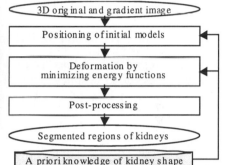

Fig. 1. An example of 3D abdominal CT image (coronal and axial plane)

Fig. 2. Flowchart of kidney segmentation process

2   Method for Segmenting the Kidney

The flowchart is shown in Fig.2. First, initial models of left and right kidneys are located in an image automatically. Next, we deform the models so that the energy functions can be minimized. Here, statistical information about the shape variation is considered via the energy function. Finally, the post-processing extracts hilum of kidneys.

In the following sub-sections, we first describe the model representation of the kidney. Then the shape feature vector and its statistical information are defined. Next, we present automated positioning procedure of initial models. Finally, definition of the energy function and post-processing are described.

2.1   Model Description

A kidney model is defined by a Non-Uniform Rational B-Spline (NURBS) surface,

$$S(u,v) = \frac{\sum_{i=0}^{N_u-1}\sum_{j=0}^{N_v-1} w_{i,j} B_i^{\,n}(u) B_j^{\,n}(v) P_{i,j}}{\sum_{i=0}^{N_u-1}\sum_{j=0}^{N_v-1} w_{i,j} B_i^{\,n}(u) B_j^{\,n}(v)} \tag{1}$$

where $u, v (\in R)$ are parameters of surface $S(u,v)$, $P_{i,j}$ and $w_{i,j}$ are coordinate vector and weight of control point, respectively. N_x is number of control points in the direction x $(= u, v)$, and B_x^n denotes B-Spline basis function of order n in the direction x. The reason of using the NURBS surface is that it has high flexibility for designing a large variety of objects and can be easily modified by moving the control points[12]. The details how we represent kidney's shape by this NURBS surface are given in [13]. An example of kidney models with control points ($N_u = 9, N_v = 12$) is shown in Fig.3(a). Here, with white boxes are control points, where as black ones are sampling points at regular intervals on the surface model to reduce computational cost of deformation. Shape feature vectors and energy functions are defined with respect to the sampling points, as described in the following subsections.

2.2   Shape Feature Vector and Its Statistical Information

Shape feature vector x is defined at each sampling point and its components are principal curvatures of 13 sampling points of interest, as it is shown in Fig.3(b),

$$x_{UV} = (x_1, \ldots, x_{26}) = \{ k_1 (S_{U'V'}), k_2 (S_{U'V'}) \} \qquad (U', V' \in \eta_{UV}) \qquad (2)$$

where $U (\text{or } V)$ represents a sampling point number in the direction u (or v). k_1, k_2 are minimum and the maximum of curvatures on the surface point (U', V'), and η_{UV} is a set of numbers of neighboring points of the (U,V)th sampling point. Here, it should be noticed that our shape feature vector defined by curvatures remains unchanged under rotation and translation of an input image.

Statistical information about the shape variation is computed as mentioned below. We extracted true surfaces of kidney directly manipulating control points of NURBS model. Shape feature vectors were computed at each sampling point on the extracted surfaces. Then their average vector $\bar{x}_{UV}$ and covariance matrix Σ_{UV} of the feature vectors were calculated after deciding the correspondence between control points of different surfaces manually. These statistical information about the geometric feature of the kidney are incorporated into the deformable model via an internal energy function in subsection 2.4.

2.3   Positioning of Initial Model

An initial guess for shape, scale and position of the model can influence the segmentation accuracy significantly. In our early work, we have placed the initial model in an image manually [11]. Here we describe a procedure for estimation of size (scale) of the initial model and the position at which the initial model should be located. Fig.4(a) shows a flowchart of the procedure.

Step1: Extract skin line and spine position by using thresholding.

Step2: Set two ROIs for left and right kidney using spine position and circumscribed rectangular of the skin line, as it is shown in Fig.4(b). The following steps are applied to each of ROIs.

Step3: Estimate the position, where correlation coefficient between CT image and 3D gray template of kidney is maximum. Here, the templates (see Fig.4(c)) are generated from the training data set. During the matching process, size of the template is rescaled in order to estimate the scale of the target. To reduce the computational cost, this matching process is applied to the image whose slice interval is 10mm.

Step4: Estimate more precise initial position by using fine-scale image, which is reconstructed by cubic interpolation (slice interval=1mm). In this process, we use a mean surface model, which is calculated from the manually segmented regions. First, the mean surface model is rescaled by using the target's scale parameters and place it at the position derived from Step3. Then we move the model to its neighborhood and find the position, where the standard deviation of CT values of all sampling points is minimum.

Step5: Locate the initial models at the searched positions in Step4.

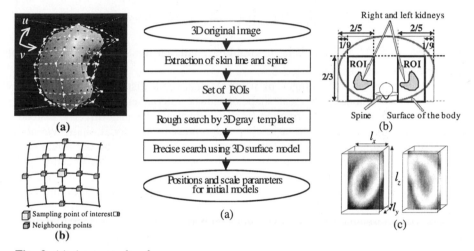

Fig. 3. (a) An example of kidney model. (b) Neighboring points for shape feature vector

Fig. 4. (a) An automated positioning process for the initial models, (b) Definition of ROIs, (c) Coronal planes of 3D gray templates for left and right kidneys

2.4 Deformation by Minimizing Energy Function and Post-processing

The total energy function to be minimized is defined as follows,

$$E^i = E^i_{ext} + w_{int} E^i_{int} \qquad (w_{int}: \text{weight}, \ i = \text{left, right kidney}) \qquad (3)$$

where E^i_{ext} is an external energy and E^i_{int} is an internal energy. A greedy deformation algorithm was used for minimization of energy function [13].

External energy function is defined as follows,

$$E^i_{ext} = -\sum_{U=0}^{M_U-1} \sum_{V=0}^{M_V-1} \left| Dir(S_{UV}) G_\sigma * \nabla_d f(S_{UV}) \right| \qquad (4)$$

where ∇_d means a gradient operator with difference distance d, G_σ is a Gaussian function with standard deviation σ and f denotes an original image. Here, function *Dir* defines the similarity between direction of image gradient vector and that of normal vector of the surface. The value ranges from 0(dissimilar) to 1(similar). Since the external energy is based on the gradient, it deforms the model to be close to boundary of the object. However, quality of the image is very poor, especially in the direction of body axis. Therefore we prepare two pairs of σ and d , and deform the model hierarchically to avoid local minima and to reduce computational cost. First, we use large values of σ and d to generate a gradient image with broad valley around the boundary and fit the model to the boundary roughly. Then, we use gradient image with small σ and d , and deform the model to be closer to the boundary.

The sum of Mahalanobis distances of the shape feature vectors is used as E_{int}^{i} ,

$$E_{int}^{i} = \sum_{U=0}^{M_U -1} \sum_{V=0}^{M_V -1} (x_{UV} - \bar{x}_{UV})^t \Sigma_{UV}^{-1} (x_{UV} - \bar{x}_{UV}) \tag{5}$$

where M_U and M_V are numbers of sampling points on the surface. Other symbols are explained in subsections 2.1, 2.2.

We expect several advantages of using Mahalanobis distance. If the deformed model becomes similar to the mean shape of kidney, internal energy becomes smaller. Our model uses statistical information from the covariance matrix directly, instead of using PCA. Covariance matrix at each point represents the local shape variability around that point. A part of surface with small variation can not be deformed easily, while a part with large variation can be deformed greatly. In addition, our model considers curvature correlation between the neighboring points.

In the post-processing, a region growing method[13], is applied to the region extracted by deformable models and extract the hilum of kidney, where the ureter and vessels connect to kidney in a very complicated way.

3   Experiments

The 33 abdominal CT images were used to evaluate the performance of the procedure. The size of image is 512x512x18(~24) voxels, the resolution in slice (=size of pixel) is 0.625 (or 0.63)mm and slice thickness are 10mm. We interpolated gray values to make the isotropic voxel (1mm³/voxel). To compute statistical information of left and right kidneys, all images are used.

Segmentation accuracy of extracted region is evaluated by two criterions [11]. First criterion is the degree of correspondence between the segmented region and the true (manually segmented) one, which ranges from 0 and 1. The high value means that the two regions are overlapped each other. Second criterion is an average distance between the extracted surface and the true one. It ranges from 0 to ∞ . The small value means that the two surfaces are close to each other.

3.1   Experimental Results and Discussion

To evaluate the accuracy of initial positioning process, we measured the distance between a gravity point of an automatically located initial model and that of a manually segmented region. The average displacement was 4mm for right kidneys (maximum: 10mm) and 4mm for left kidneys (maximum: 9mm). The major direction of displacements was the direction parallel to body axis where the image resolution is low. Table1 gives quantitative comparison between extracted regions based on an automatic positioning of initial models and that based on manual positioning. Difference between the evaluation values of two regions are not significant. However it is confirmed that the difference for right kidney is slightly larger than that of left kidney. Main cause of failure is that CT value of the surrounding organs such as liver and spleen are similar to those of kidney.

Fig.5(a),(c) are the segmentation results without the internal energy and Fig.5(b), (d) show the results with the internal energy. Here, left and center figures are axial and coronal slice images, respectively. The black line denotes border of the segmented region, and the white line means border of true one. The deformation with the internal energy avoides local minima and yields a result far better than the deformation without it. Moreover, it is confirmed that the segmentation with the internal energy is robust even in the cases of poor initialization. When we use the internal energy, the average degree of correspondence is approximately 86.5% and the aforementioned average distance is 1.13 voxels. Both of the values are superior to those of the segmentation without the internal energy and the differences are 2.8% (maximum: 15.4%) and 0.26 voxels (maximum: 1.51 voxel), respectively. In these circumstances, we conclude that the statistical information about the shape works effectively and gives the relatively reliable results. However, the segmentation has failed in some cases where the true contour was affected by the surrounding organs.

Examples of final extracted regions (after post-processing) of left and right kidneys are shown in Fig.6. All results were evaluated by a physician. He observed boundary curves of extracted regions slice by slice and rated them on a 3-point scale: 1=good, 2=fair, 3=failure. Here "fair" means that the segmentation result is almost good but failure in parts. The 30 of left kidneys were rated to be satisfactorily good or fair, while the remaining three were failure. The 28 of right kidneys were rated good or fair and five were failure. The segmentation accuracy of right kidneys was slightly lower than the left one. The main reason of failure is poor initialization, in conjunction with a notable variation of shape and pose of right kidneys, which is occurred due to stress by liver. The increasing number of training samples will definitely improve the results, in the future.

Table 1. Quantitative evaluation of segmentation results between automatic positioning of initial models and manual positioning. [Average±SD.]

	a. Degree of Correspondence (%)		b. Average Distance(voxel)	
Initial Positioning Method	manual	automatic	manual	automatic
Left Kidney	87.3±2.5	87.1±2.3	1.08±0.17	1.09±0.17
Right Kidney	86.5±2.2	85.7±3.4	1.14±0.18	1.18±0.26
Both Kidneys	86.9±2.3	86.5±2.8	1.12±0.18	1.13±0.22

4   Conclusion

In this paper, we have presented a deformable model for automatically segmenting of kidney. In this model, the shape feature vector is defined at each sampling point on the surface and its statistical information is calculated from a manually segmented

562   B. Tsagaan et al.

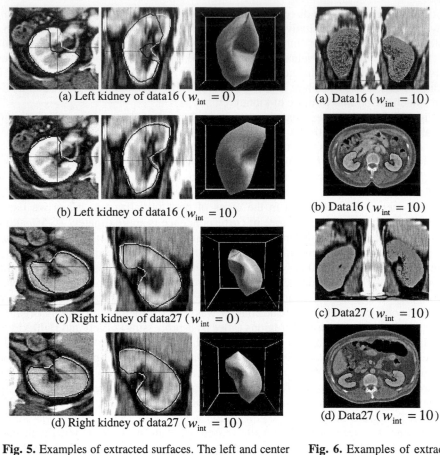

(a) Left kidney of data16 ($w_{int} = 0$)

(a) Data16 ($w_{int} = 10$)

(b) Left kidney of data16 ($w_{int} = 10$)

(b) Data16 ($w_{int} = 10$)

(c) Right kidney of data27 ($w_{int} = 0$)

(c) Data27 ($w_{int} = 10$)

(d) Right kidney of data27 ($w_{int} = 10$)

(d) Data27 ($w_{int} = 10$)

Fig. 5. Examples of extracted surfaces. The left and center figures are axial and coronal slice images. Here, the black contour denotes cross curve of segmented region, while the white one denotes the manually segmented one. The right is 3D resultant surface rendered in perspective

Fig. 6. Examples of extracted regions. (a),(c) Volume region with coronal slice image, (b),(d) Axial slice with extracted curves.

training data. The shape variability is incorporated into the model through formulation of an internal energy. The experimental results in the 3D abdominal CT images were promising. Our current work focuses on extending the proposed model to include statistical information about the global feature of the target, such as pose or orientation [8].

Acknowledgements

The authors would like to thank colleagues of Kobatake & Shimizu laboratory for their help and advice. This work is supported by Grant-in-Aid for Scientific Research from Ministry of Education, Culture, Sports, Science and Technology, Japan and Grant-in-Aid for Cancer Research from Ministry of Health, Labour and Welfare in Japan.

Reference

1. Duncan,J., Ayache,N.: Medical Image Analysis: Progress Over Two Decades and Challenges Ahead, IEEE Trans. Patt. Anal. Mach. Intell., vol.22 (2000) 85-106
2. McInerney,T., Terzopoulos,D.: Deformable Models in Medical Image Analysis: A Survey, Med. Imag. Anal. vol. 1(2) (1996) 91-108
3. Shimizu,A.: Segmentation of Medical Images Using Deformable Models : A Survey, Med. Imag. Tech. in Japan. vol.20(1) (2002) 3-12
4. Cootes,F., Taylor,L., Cooper,H.: Active Shape Models;Their Training and Application, CVIU vol.61(1) (1995) 38-59
5. Jacob,G., Noble,A., Blake,A.: Evaluating a Robust Contour Tracker on Echocardiographic Sequences, Med. Imag. Anal. vol.3(3) (1998) 63-75
6. Fleute,M., Lavallee, M., Julliard,S.: Incorporating a Statistically Based Shape Model Into a System for Computer-Assisted Anterior Cruciate Ligament Surgery, Med. Imag. Anal. vol.3(3) (1999) 209-222
7. Shen,D., Herskovits,E.H., Davatzikos,C.: An Adaptive- Focus Statistical Shape Model for Segmentation and Shape Modeling of 3-D Brain Structure, IEEE Trans. Med. Imag., vol.20(4) (2001) 257-270
8. Hamarneh,G., McInerney,T., Terzopoulos,D.: Deformable Organisms For Automatic Medical Image Analysis, MICCAI (2001) 66-76
9. Staib,L.H., Duncan,J.S.: Boundary Finding with Parametrically Deformable Models, IEEE Trans. Patt. Anal. Mach. Intell., vol.14(11) (1992) 1061-1075
10. Szekely,G., Kelemen,A. : Segmentation of 2-D and 3-D Objects From MRI Volume Data Using Constrained Elastic Deformations of Flexible Fourier Contour and Surface Models, Med. Imag.Anal., vol.1(1) (1996) 19-34
11. Tsagaan,B., Shimizu,A., Kobatake,H., Miyakawa,K., Hanzawa,Y.: Segmentation of Kidney by Using Deformable Model, ICIP, vol.3 (2001) 1059-1062
12. Terzopoulos,D., Qin,H.,: Dynamic NURBS with Geometric Constraints for Interactive Sculpting", ACM Trans. Graphics, vol.13(2) (1994) 103-136
13. Tsagaan,B., Shimizu,A., Kobatake,H., Miyakawa,K.: Development of Extraction Method of Kidneys From Abdominal CT Images Using 3-D Deformable Model, Trans. of IEICE in Japan, vol.J85(D-II) (2002) 140-148
14. Williams,D., Shan,D., Shan,M.,: A Fast Algorithm for Active Contours, CVGIP:Imag. Under. , vol.55(1) (1992) 14-26

Incorporating Non-rigid Registration into Expectation Maximization Algorithm to Segment MR Images

Kilian M. Pohl[1], William M. Wells[2], Alexandre Guimond[3],
Kiyoto Kasai[4], Martha E. Shenton[2,4], Ron Kikinis[2],
W. Eric L. Grimson[1], and Simon K. Warfield[2]

[1] Artificial Intelligence Laboratory, Massachusetts Institute of Technology,
Cambridge MA, USA   {kpohl,welg}@ai.mit.edu, http://www.ai.mit.edu
[2] Surgical Planning Laboratory, Harvard Medical School and Brigham and Women's
Hospital, 75 Francis St., Boston, MA 02115 USA
{sw,kikinis,warfield}@bwh.harvard.edu, http://www.spl.harvard.edu
[3] Center for Neurological Imaging, Harvard Medical School and Brigham and
Women's Hospital, 221 Longwood Av., Boston, MA 02115 USA
guimond@bwh.harvard.edu
[4] Clinical Neuroscience Division, Laboratory of Neurosciene, Department of
Psychiatry, Harvard Medical School, VA Boston Healthcare System, Brockton
Division, and Harvard Medical School, 940 Belmont St., Brockton, MA 02301 USA
kasaik@bwh.harvard.edu, martha_shenton@hms.harvard.edu

Abstract. The paper introduces an algorithm which allows the automatic segmentation of multi channel magnetic resonance images. We extended the Expectation Maximization-Mean Field Approximation Segmenter, to include Local Prior Probability Maps. Thereby our algorithm estimates the bias field in the image while simultaneously assigning voxels to different tissue classes under prior probability maps. The probability maps were aligned to the subject using non-rigid registration. This allowed the parcellation of cortical sub-structures including the superior temporal gyrus. To our knowledge this is the first description of an algorithm capable of automatic cortical parcellation incorporating strong noise reduction and image intensity correction.

1   Introduction

Quantitative medical image analysis often involves segmentation to assess the shape and volume of anatomical structures. Progress has been made for major tissue classes, however, segmentation of other structures is still difficult. Manually segmenting hundreds of cases is not only time consuming but also has large variations. Given these factors, the need for automatic and validated segmentation methods is clear.

There are several approaches to achieve this goal. The Level Set Method introduced by Osher and Sethian [1] segments images by evolving predefined shapes to fit the image. Leventon [2], Tsai [3] and Baillard [4] introduced this method to the clinical field by using complex anatomical information. These methods ignore the intra-scan inhomogeneities, often caused by the radiofrequency (RF) coils, or acquisition sequences. Comprehensive validation studies are still needed regarding these methods.

T. Dohi and R. Kikinis (Eds.): MICCAI 2002, LNCS 2488, pp. 564–571, 2002.

Using registration for segmentation is another approach. These methods use a previously segmented brain and align it with the subject. The result of this alignment is the segmentation. Fischl et el. [5] uses a detailed atlas with over 30 different labels to segment the brain. The ANIMAL+INSECT algorithm [6] on the other hand uses two algorithms at the same time. The ANIMAL is responsible for the non-rigid alignment of an atlas with the subject. The INSECT corrects the intensity inhomogeneity in the image. Nevertheless, segmentation by registration approaches cannot segment structures, which are not projected from the atlas onto the subject. For example, white matter lesions, which are common in several neurological diseases, cannot be identified with such an approach. As an alternative, some algorithms have been proposed which combine intensity based classification with segmentation by registration (Warfield [7]).

A very different approach introduced to the medical field by Wells [8], is the Adaptive Segmentation, which uses an Expectation Maximization (EM) Algorithm. It simultaneously labels and estimates the intensity inhomogeneities artifacts in the image. To add more robustness through noise rejection, Kapur [9] incorporated the Mean-Field Approximation (MF) for the labeling mechanism. However, the algorithm lacked any shape information. Van Leemput [10] improved this handicap by including prior probability maps (PPM) of tissue class spatial distribution into the initial formulation of Wells togther with a MF. He used affine registration to align PPMs with the subject. He iteratively updated the tissue class distributions and the labeling of the image simultaneously. To date, the published results indicate that 'the method may occasionally fail, due to poor initialization ... This problem may be overcome by using non rigid rather than affine registration for matching.' [10] Additionally Van Leemput did not consider parcellation of the cortex.

Like Van Leemput, we used the Expectation Maximization-Mean Field Approximation (EM-MF) Algorithm for the segmentation itself, however, we align the PPM through non-rigid registration. Compared to registration alone, this approach has the advantage of segmenting tissue classes relative to each other. Therefore, it can better cope with large artifacts in the image, such as significant intensity differences between the subject and the atlas. It allows us to parcellate substructures of the cortex, e.g. amygdala or parrahippocampal gyrus. We demonstrate the clinical usefulness of our new algorithm by carrying out validation experiments on the task of superior temporal gyrus (STG) segmentations.

2   Method

As mentioned, the Expectation Maximization - Mean Field Approximation - Local Prior Algorithm (EM-MF-LP) first registers PPMs to the subject. The method then uses the EM-MF algorithm, defined through Expectation-Step (E-Step) and Maximization-Step (M-Step), to segment the subject. The E-Step is responsible for calculating the weights, representing the likelihood of tissue classes, using the aligned PPMs. The M-Step calculates the bias field, which models the intensity inhomogeneity artifact. These two steps are repeated until the algorithm converges.

The PPMs used in this paper were derived from 82 different subjects using a statistical atlas construction method described by Warfield [11]. This method projects anatomy from a source to a target, such as white matter from subject a to subject b. The result is a minimum entropy anatomical model and a statistical volume or probability map for each tissue class.

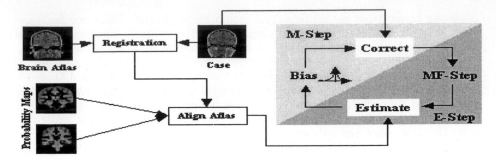

Fig. 1. The structure of the EM-MF-LP Algorithm

2.1 Non-rigid Registration

In order to use these PPMs, we must register them to our subject. We register the SPGR corresponding to the target of the statistical atlases to the subjects SPGR, and project the PPMs using the same transformation. To do so, we use a deformable registration procedure [12, 13]. It finds the displacement $v(x)$ for each voxel x of a target image T to match the corresponding anatomical location in a source image S. The solution is found using the following iterative scheme:

$$v_{n+1}(x) = G_\sigma \otimes (v_n + \frac{S_n^\star \circ h_n(x) - T(x)}{||\nabla S_n^\star \circ h_n(x)||^2 + [S_n^\star \circ h_n(x) - T(x)]^2} \nabla S_n^\star \circ h_n(x)) \quad (1)$$

where G_σ is a Gaussian filter with a variance of σ^2, $\otimes$ denotes convolution, $\circ$ denotes the composition, ∇ is the gradient operator and the transformation $h(x)$ is related to the displacement $v(x)$ by $h(x) = x + v(x)$. $S_n^\star$ is an intensity corrected version of S computed at the nth iteration to help capture intensity variations present between the images to register.

Equation (1) finds voxel displacements in the gradient direction $\nabla S_n^\star \circ h_n(x)$. Convolution with a Gaussian kernel G_σ is performed to model a smoothly varying displacement field. As is common with registration methods, multi-resolution techniques are used to accelerate convergence.

2.2 EM-MF

When segmenting magnetic resonance images (MRI) it is hard to determine the inhomogeneities without knowing the tissue type of every voxel. On the other hand, one cannot find out the tissue type without knowledge of the inhomogeneities. Therefore, the adaptive segmentation approach [8] will try to solve for these two unknowns simultaneously.

In the Expectation Step (E-Step), the algorithm calculates the expected value of the weight (also see Kapur [9])

$$\overline{W}_T(x,y,z) \leftarrow \frac{1}{N} P(Y(x,y,z)|D_T, \beta(x,y,z)) P(T) e^{E_T(x,y,z)} \quad (2)$$

where Y(x,y,z) is the log intensity and $\beta(x,y,z)$ is the bias of the image at voxel (x,y,z), T is the tissue class, D_T is the tissue class distribution, and N is the normalizing factor of weight W_T. The energy function $E_T(x, y, z)$, representing the mean field approximation, is defined as

$$E_T(x, y, z) = E(\overline{W}_T(x, y, z)|W_T(s), s \in U) = \sum_{s \in U} \sum_{i=1}^{M} J_{Ti} \overline{W}_i(s) \qquad (3)$$

where M is the number of classes, $U = U(x,y,z)$ is the neighborhood of (x,y,z) and

$$J_{Ti} = \frac{\#\ \text{tissue T appears next to class i in the training set}}{\#\ \text{tissue class T appears in the training data}} \qquad (4)$$

is the 'Tissue Class Interaction Matrix' (CIM).

The Maximization Step (M-Step) calculates the maximum a-posteriori (MAP) estimate of the bias field assuming the weight calculation in the previous step is correct for every voxel.

$$\hat{\beta}(x, y, z) = \arg \max_{\beta} p(\beta|Y) = H\overline{R} \qquad (5)$$

where $\overline{R}$ is the mean residual, defined by D_T, $\overline{W_T}$ and Y, and H is determined by the mean tissue class covariances and the bias covariance (see Wells [8]).

2.3   The EM-MF-LP

The EM-MF Algorithm, described in Section 2.2, assumed that the probability for a given tissue class $P(T)$ does not change throughout the image. For the EM-MF-LP algorithm this assumption will be dropped. $P(T)$, in equation (2), will be substituted with $P(T|x, y, z)$. Thus the weight in the E-Step will be updated as follows:

$$\overline{W}_T(x, y, z) \leftarrow \frac{1}{N} P(Y(x, y, z)|D_T, \beta(x, y, z)) P(T|x, y, z) e^{E_T(x,y,z)} \qquad (6)$$

The EM-MF-LP Algorithm works in two phases (see Figure 1). First, it registers the brain atlas with the subject. The resulting deformation field is used to align the PPMs to the subject. The aligned PPMs define the local prior probability $P(T|x, y, z)$. In the second phase, it segments the image using EM-MF Algorithm with the updated E-Step (see Equation 6).

3   Implementation and Experiments

The algorithm is fully integrated in the 3D Slicer [14], which is a software package for medical image analysis. A basic version of the described method is publicly available at http://www.slicer.org. The user interface guides the user through the segmentation process. Tissue definitions for the actual image can be done manually or automatically. Graphs and other tools help to verify the results.

To show the improvements of the EM-MF-LP method over other approaches, the different strategies will be compared on one MRI Scan with 256x256 pixels. Both Spoiled Gradient Recalled Acquisitions in the Steady State(SPGR) and T2 weighted intensity features were. The resulting segmentations are displayed

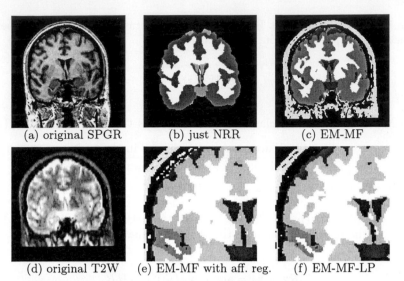

(a) original SPGR   (b) just NRR   (c) EM-MF

(d) original T2W   (e) EM-MF with aff. reg.   (f) EM-MF-LP

Fig. 2. Segmenting up to 7 tissue classes with different methods. Methods used in (b) and (c) do not allow the parcelation of cortical substructures. In (e) the misclassifcation of the scalp is visible as described in [10]. These errors are eliminated in our result shown in(f).

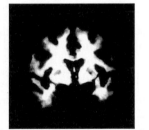
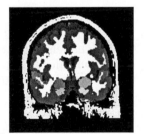

Fig. 3. Segmenting brain with 11 tissue classes including left and right amygdala, superior temporal gyrus and parrahippocampal gyrus

(a) White Matter Tissue Atlas (b) EM-MF-LP with 11 classes

in Figure 2. The first method is simply using brain mapping with non-rigid Registration (NRR). After the atlas brain is registered with the subject, the PPMs are then aligned. Each voxel is assigned to the tissue class with the highest a posteriori probability. This approach is very similar to Fischl[5], Pachai[15], and Collins[6]. The segmentation is only a rough estimate, which is too 'stiff' for the subject. Especially the CSF at the outside of the brain is underestimated.

The EM-MF Algorithm is more flexible than NRR (see Figure 2(c)). In addition, the algorithm better incorporates the image inhomogeneities. However, voxels are still seen independently, which causes additional noise. Segmenting cortical substructures is not possible, as opposed to NRR. Again, the need for increased usage of spatial information is very apparent. In Figure 2(f), we use the method described in Section 2. Figure 2(e) is the same method, but the non-rigid registration is substituted with an affine one, similar to Van Leemputs' approach. Comparing 2(e) to 2(f) the dangers of including local priors into the EM-MF Algorithm are readily apparent. The STG in Figure 2(e) is expanding into neighboring structures like the middle temporal gyrus. Also as in Van Leem-

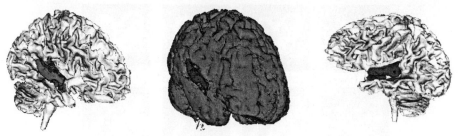

(a) WM and Left STG   (b) GM and Left STG   (c) WM and Right STG

Fig. 4. These figures show high quality, volumetric brain segmentations higlighting left and right STG

Table 1. Comparing the average DSC for one case and Warfield/Zou/Wells Measure between Rater A, B, C and the EM-MF-LP algorithm. The fraction in Table (b) is defined as $\frac{sensitivity}{specificity}$. - means value was not available.

(a) DSC Measure for one case

Rater	A	B	C	EM
A	1.0	0.828	0.742	0.778
B	0.828	1.0	0.744	0.825
C	0.742	0.744	1.0	0.715
EM	0.778	0.825	0.715	1.0

(b) Warfield/Zou/Wells Measure

Rater\Case	1	2	3	4
A	$\frac{0.99945}{0.836294}$	$\frac{0.99969}{0.753}$	$\frac{1.0}{0.520}$	$\frac{0.99996}{0.760}$
B	$\frac{0.99994}{0.73514}$	$\frac{-}{-}$	$\frac{0.99963}{0.908}$	$\frac{0.9998}{0.853}$
C	$\frac{0.99952}{0.817932}$	$\frac{0.99990}{0.670}$	$\frac{0.99972}{0.856}$	$\frac{0.99939}{0.747}$
EM	$\frac{0.99954}{0.814183}$	$\frac{0.99910}{0.840}$	$\frac{0.99771}{0.885}$	$\frac{0.99933}{0.909}$

put's paper [10] additional misclassification at the outside of the brain can be observed in Figure 2(e). This is primarily due to poor alignment of the atlases. It can readily be seen that these effects are eliminated in Figure 2(f), where the more accurate non-rigid registration method is used.

Figure 3(b) shows a segmentation with 11 different tissue classes. Increasing the number of tissue classes does not cause a problem for the algorithm in terms of convergence. The algorithm will only take more time for every iteration step because it has to consider more classes. However, as mentioned, more classes restricts the system further and therefore lets the algorithm converge faster.

4   Validation

To validate this new approach, the left and right STG of four subjects were manually segmented by three raters. We used the Dice Similarity Measure (DSC) described by Zijdenbos et al. [16] to compare manual and EM-MF-LP segmentations. The DSC $= 2 * \frac{|A_1 \cap A_2|}{|A_1| + |A_2|}$ is derived from the kappa statistic, where A_1 and A_2 are the two segmented areas. DSC $> 70\%$ is regarded as an excellent agreement between the two. In our approach, in all cases the similarity measure for the automatic segmentation was within the variance of the manual ones or above 70% (see Table 1(a)), which can also be observed in Figure 5.

The results were also compared with the performance measure introduced by Warfield et al. [17] (see Table 1(b)). This measure combines a maximum likelihood estimate of the 'ground truth' segmentation from all the segmentations,

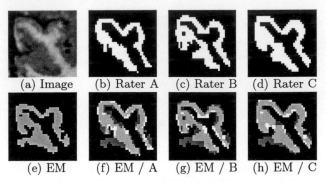

(a) Image   (b) Rater A   (c) Rater B   (d) Rater C

(e) EM   (f) EM / A   (g) EM / B   (h) EM / C

Fig. 5. Comparing manual and automatic (EM-MF-LP) segmentation of the right STG where dark gray is EM-MF-LP only, light gray overlapping of manual and automatic, and white manual only segmentation.

and a simultaneous measure of the quality of each expert. The quality measure is composed of a sensitivity and specificity measures. A value of 1.0 for both is seen as perfect. Again, in all cases the automatic segmentation does as well as the manual ones. However, unlike manual segmentations, the algorithm can occasionally spread out over the ends of the STG into the middle temporal gyrus. In this segmentation the STG's local priors do not compete with other neighbouring cortical substructures. Adding additional local tissue classes, like the middle temporal gyrus, would eliminate this effect and therefore further increase the accuracy of the automatic segmentation. Overall, the validation shows that the algorithm produces reliable results when compared with manual segmentations.

5   Discussion and Conclusion

In this paper we showed the benefits of integrating local tissue priors through non-rigid registration into the EM-MF. We validated the method by comparing it to manual segmentations of the STG. The results showed that the segmentation is comparable to manual ones. Through examples we showed that the algorithm performs better than some previous methods and is capable of more detailed segmentation including parcellation of the cortical structures. It also runs rapidly and robustly enough for further use in the real medical environment.

We believe the accuracy of the algorithm could be further increased by re-aligning the PPMs with the subject, by using the results of the segmentation and then re-segmenting the images again. When segmenting smaller structures, small errors can have large effects on the topology of the object,e.g. a voxel is assigned to a wrong class causing a structure to be separated. This effect could be limited by using higher order spatial information.

We believe that this approach is a step towards fully automated medical image processing, enabling the automatic segmentation of cortical sub-structures.

Acknowledgements: This investigation was supported by NIH grants P41 RR13218, P01 CA67165,R01 RR11747, R01 CA86879, by a research grant from the Whitaker Foundation, and by a New Concept Award from the Center for Integration of Medicine and Innovative Technology. We would especially like to thank for the helpful discussions with Dave Gering, Lauren O'Donnell and Samson Timoner.

References

1. S. Osher, J. A. Sethian, "Fonts propagating wiht curvature-dependent speed: Algorithms based on hamilton-jacobi formulations," *J. Comp. Physics*, vol. 79, pp. 12–49, 1988.
2. M. E. Leventon, *Statistical Models in Medical Image Analysis*. PhD thesis, Massachusetts Institute of Technology, 2000.
3. A. Tsai, A. Yezzi, W. Wells III, C. Tempany, D. Tucker, A. Fan, W. Grimson, A. Willsky, "Model-based curve evolution technique for image segmentation," *IEEE Conference on Computer Vision and Pattern Recognition*, 2001.
4. C. Baillard, P. Hellier, C. Barillot, "Segmentation of 3d brain structures using level sets," *Rapport interne IRISA*, vol. 1291, 2000.
5. B. Fischl, D. H. Salat, E. Busa, M. Albert, M. Dieterich, C. Haselgrove, A. van der Kouwe, R. Killiany, D. Kennedy, S. Klaveness, A. Montillo, N. Makris, B. Rosen, A. M. Dale, "Whole brain segmentation: Automated labeling of neuroanatomical structures in the human brain," *Neuron*, vol. 33, 2002.
6. D. L. Collins, A. P. Zijdenbos, W. F. C. Barre, and A. C. Evans, "Animal+insect: Inproved cortical structure segmentation," *Proc. of the Annual Symposium on Information Processing in Medical Imaging*, vol. 1613, 1999.
7. S. K. Warfield, J. Rexilius, M. Kaus, F. A. Jolesz, R. Kikinis, "Adaptive, template moderated, spatial varying statistical classification," *Med. Image Analysis*, vol. 4, no. 1, pp. 43–55, 2000.
8. W.M. Wells III, W.E.L Grimson, R. Kikinis, F.A Jolesz, "Adaptive segmentation of MRI data," *IEEE Transactions on Medical Imaging*, vol. 15, pp. 429–442, 1996.
9. T. Kapur, *Model based three dimensional Medical Imaging Segmentation*. PhD thesis, Massachusetts Institute of Technology, 1999.
10. K. Van Leemput, F. Maes, D. Vanermeulen, P. Suetens, "Automated model-based bias field correction of MR images of the brain," *IEEE Transactions on Medical Imaging*, vol. 18, no. 10, pp. 885–895, 1999.
11. S. K. Warfield, J. Rexilius, P. S. Huppi, T. E. Inder, E. C. Miller, W. M. Wells, G. P. Zientara, F. A. Jolesz, R. Kikinis, "A binary entropy measure to assess nonrigid registration algorithm," in *MICCAI*, pp. 266–274, Oct. 2001.
12. J.-P. Thirion, "Image matching as a diffusion process: an analogy with Maxwell's demons," *Medical Image Analysis*, vol. 2, no. 3, pp. 243–260, 1998.
13. A. Guimond, A. Roche, N. Ayache, J. Meunier, "Three-dimensional multimodal brain warping using the demons algorithm and adaptive intensity corrections," *IEEE Transactions in Medical Imaging*, vol. 20, pp. 58–69, Jan. 2001.
14. D. Gering, A. Nabavi, R. Kikinis, N. Hata, L. O'Donnell, E. Grimson, F. Jolesz, P. Black, W. Wells, "An integrated visualization system for surgical planning and guidance using image fusion and an open MR," *J. Magn. Reson. Imaging*, vol. 13, pp. 967–975, 2001.
15. C. Pachai, Y. M. Zhu, C. R. G. Guttmann, R. Kikinis, F. A. Jolesz, G. Gimenez, J.-C. Froment, C. Confavreux, and S. K. Warfield, "Unsupervised and adaptive segmentation of multispectral 3d magnetic resonance images of human brain: a generic approach," pp. 1067–1074, 2001.
16. A. P. Zijdenbos, B. M. Dawant, R. A. Margolin, A. C. Palmer, "Morphometric analysis of white matter lesions in MR images: Method and validation," *IEEE Transactions on Medical Imaging*, vol. 13, no. 4, pp. 716–724, 1994.
17. S. K. Warfield, K. H. Zou, W. M. Wells, "Validation of image segmentation and expert quality with an expectation-maximazation algorithm," in *MICCAI*, 2002.

Segmentation of 3D Medical Structures Using Robust Ray Propagation

Hüseyin Tek, Martin Bergtholdt, Dorin Comaniciu, and James Williams

Imaging and Visualization, Siemens Corporate Research, Inc.
755 College Road East, Princeton NJ 08540, USA

Abstract. A robust and efficient method for the segmentation of 3D structures in CT and MR images is presented. The proposed method is based on 3D ray propagation by mean shift analysis with a smoothness constraint. Specifically, ray propagation is used to guide an evolving surface due to its computational efficiency. In addition, non-parametric analysis and shape priors are incorporated to the proposed technique for robust convergence. Several examples are depicted to illustrate its effectiveness.

1 Introduction

The segmentation of 3D structures in CT and MR images is an inherently difficult and time consuming problem. The accurate localization of object surfaces is influenced by the presence of significant noise levels, generated through partial-volume effects and by image acquisition devices. In addition, the processing in 3D space implies an increased computational complexity, which makes impractical the 3D extension of most two-dimensional segmentation algorithms.

Deformable models have been popular for the segmentation of 3D medical images [18, 5, 10, 17, 23, 22, 13, 24, 15]. These approaches can produce good segmentation results if the initialization is done properly. However, choosing proper initialization of deformable models is typically a difficult task. In addition, the current deformable model approaches are computationally expensive. This is due to the additional dimension in the case of level set methods [12, 4, 9], or expensive reinitialization of parameters in the case of explicit surface evolution techniques [18, 5].

In this paper, we present an efficient, robust, and user-friendly method for the interactive segmentation of 3D medical structures, e.g., aneurysm from contrast enhanced CT or MR data. The primary innovation of the method is the boundary propagation by mean shift analysis combined with a smoothness constraint. As a result, our technique is robust to both outliers in the data and missing data structures. The first property is guaranteed by the mean shift procedure, while the second is obtained through the use of a priori information on boundary smoothness. Furthermore, due to our computationally efficient framework based on ray propagation, the entire processing is fast, allowing real-time user interaction (under 10 seconds on a Pentium III 1Ghz). A two-dimensional version of this approach was first presented in [16] for detecting 2D vessel boundaries in cross-sectional views in contrast enhanced CT and MR images. In this paper, we extend the technique to the segmentation of 3D medical structures and demonstrate it on aneurysms in 3D CTA data.

T. Dohi and R. Kikinis (Eds.): MICCAI 2002, LNCS 2488, pp. 572–579, 2002.
© Springer-Verlag Berlin Heidelberg 2002

Within the proposed segmentation method, the user specifies the structure to be segmented by placing a single seed inside it. A boundary surface is then automatically generated via the propagation of rays from the seed point. The propagation is guided by the image forces defined through mean shift analysis and smoothness constraints. The gradient-ascent mean shift localizes edges accurately in the presence of noise and provides good computational performance, being based on local operators. Currently, we employ the mean curvature for the smoothness constraint, however, other geometric smoothing techniques, such as the Mean-Gaussian curvature [11] can be applied. Figure 1 summarizes the goal of this paper and the method described here. Currently, we are working on validating our technique with phantoms of known ground-truth and data from clinical practice.

2   Deformable Surfaces for 3D Volume Segmentation

Deformable model-based segmentation algorithms can be divided into explicit methods and implicit methods based on how the deformable surface is represented. In explicit methods, deformable surfaces are represented by triangular mashes [23], superquadrics [18], and others [5, 10, 8]. In implicit methods, the popular choice for deformable surface representation is the level set methods. Level set methods [12, 4, 9, 21, 17, 15] have been popular because they are topologically flexible and can represent complex shapes without any computationally expensive reparametrization step. One of the main shortcomings of level set methods is the computational complexity due to the additional embedded surface requirement for simulations. To overcome the complexity, narrow band level set evolutions have been proposed [9, 1, 21] [1]. However, these methods are still not fast enough for real-time volume segmentation. Thus, in this paper, we rely on ray propagation for fast image segmentation.

2.1   Ray Propagation

Let the front be represented by a 3D surface $\psi(\xi, \eta, t) = (x(\xi, \eta, t), y(\xi, \eta, t), z(\xi, \eta, t))$ where x, y and z are the Cartesian coordinates, ξ, η parameterize the surface, and t is time. The front evolution is governed by

$$\begin{cases} \frac{\partial \psi}{\partial t} = S(x, y, z) \boldsymbol{N} \\ \psi(\xi, \eta, 0) = \psi_0(\xi, \eta) \end{cases} \tag{1}$$

where $\psi_0(\xi, \eta) = (x(\xi, \eta, 0), y(\xi, \eta, 0), z(\xi, \eta, 0))$ is the initial surface, and $\boldsymbol{N}$ is the unit normal vector and $S(x, y, z)$ is the speed of the surface at point (x, y, z).

The approach that we consider is based on explicit front propagation via normal vectors. The surface is sampled and the evolution of each sample is followed in time by rewriting the Eikonal equation [14] in vector form, namely,

---

[1] Similarly, Sethian [14] proposed fast marching methods for simulating the monotonically advancing front. This method does not require any additional surface, but it is limited to simulate one directional flows, i.e., no curvature smoothing, thus its use in segmentation is rather limited.

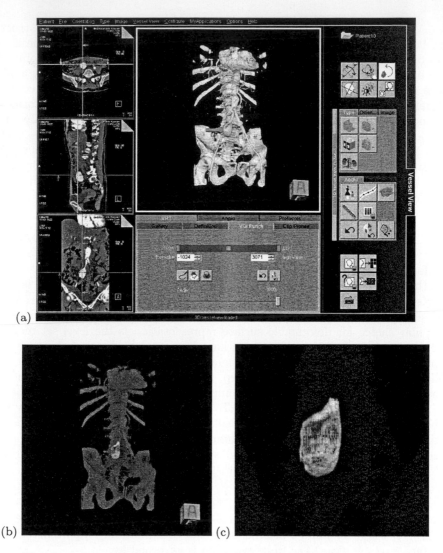

Fig. 1. This figure summarizes the method described in this paper. (a) illustrates the original (CE-CTA) data in multi-planar reformats (MPRs) and volume rendering. This data set contains an aneurysm which is indicated by the arrow. In addition, MPRs (orthogonal views) are centered on this pathology. The system allows the radiologist quickly detect pathologies from different visualizations. The next step is the quantification of these pathologies. The goal of this work is to provide a mechanism such that an user can quickly measure the volume of blob-like structures by simply clicking on them. In this example, the user clicks on a structure of interest and the 3D ray propagation algorithm detects the boundary of the structure and computes its volume. (b) The detected aneurysm (lumen boundary) is blended with the original data. (c) Segmented aneurysm (lumen boundary).

$$\begin{cases} x_t = S(x,y,z)\frac{N_x}{||N||} \\ y_t = S(x,y,z)\frac{N_y}{||N||} \\ z_t = S(x,y,z)\frac{N_z}{||N||} \end{cases} \quad (2)$$

This evolution is the "Lagrangian" solution since the physical coordinate system moves with the propagating wavefront. In general, the applications of ray propagation for surface evolution have been limited. Since the normals to the wavefront may collide (formation of shocks), this approach exhibits numerical instabilities due to an accumulated density of sample points, thus requiring special care, such as reparametrization of the wavefront. Also, topological changes are not handled naturally, an external procedure being required.

Previously, we have successfully used the 2D ray propagation method for segmentation of vessel boundary cross-sections in contrast enhanced CT and MR images [16]. In this paper, we advocate ray propagation from a single point source for the segmentation of blob-like structures found in medical images, such as aneurysm and brain tumors. In fact, ray propagation is well suited for these problems because it is very fast, no topological changes are necessary and no shocks form during the propagation, since rays from a single source point do not collide with each other.

Observe that the speed function $S(x,y,z)$ plays an important role in the quality of the segmentation results. In this paper, the speed of rays, $S(x,y,z)$ depends on image information and shape priors. Specifically, we propose to use $S(x,y,z) = S_0(x,y,z) + \beta S_1(x,y,z)$ where $S_0(x,y,z)$ measures image discontinuities, $S_1(x,y,z)$ represents shape priors, and β balances these two terms.

2.2   Robust Measure of Discontinuities: Mean-Shift Analysis

Traditionally, image gradients are used to guide deformable models to object boundaries [4, 9]. However, they are not robust to noise, and outliers in the data can significantly influence the result. A solution to this problem is to use robust measures of discontinuities.

Our approach is based on a new representation of image data which uses kernel density estimation [6, 7]. Let us consider a 1-dimensional intensity profile (ray) obtained from a gray level image. Each pixel along the ray is characterized by a location x and an intensity value I. As a result, an input ray of N pixels is represented as a collection of 2-dimensional points $\{x_i, I_i\}_{i=1,...,N}$. The 2-dimensional space constructed as before is called the joint spatial-intensity domain. Note that this construction generalizes for standard gray-level image data (3-dimensional space with 2 dimensions for coordinates and one for intensity), color data (5-dimensional space with 2 dimensions for coordinates and three for color), multi-modal data, or image sequences.

The task of identifying image discontinuities reduces to the partitioning of the joint space according to the probability density estimated in this space. The number of segments is determined by the number of peaks (modes) of the underlying density. The iterative mean shift procedure [7] is used to find the modes in the joint space and assign each data point to a mode in its neighborhood. Denote by $\{x^*_i, I^*_i\}$ the mode associated to $\{x_i, I_i\}$ where $i = 1, ..., N$. Since the modes delineate regions with high concentration of similar data, the robustness to outliers is guaranteed. The overall analysis is related to robust anisotropic diffusion [3] and bilateral filtering [19].

Let $\{d_i = x^*{}_i - x_i\}_{i=1,\ldots,N}$ be the oriented spatial distance from a point to its assigned mode. We will further refer to this quantity as the displacement vector. The displacement vectors always point away from discontinuities and they play a dominant role in our propagation technique. The iterative, mean shift-based algorithm for finding the displacement vectors is

For each $i = 1, \ldots, N$
1. Initialize $k = 1$ and $(x_i^k, I_i^k, d_i) = (x_i, I_i, 0)$
2. Compute

$$x_i^{k+1} = \frac{\sum_{j=1}^{M} x_j e^{\frac{-(x_i^k - x_j)^2}{2\sigma_x^2}} e^{\frac{-(I_i^k - I_j)^2}{2\sigma_I^2}}}{\sum_{j=1}^{M} e^{\frac{-(x_i^k - x_j)^2}{2\sigma_x^2}} e^{\frac{-(I_i^k - I_j)^2}{2\sigma_I^2}}}$$

$$I_i^{k+1} = \frac{\sum_{j=1}^{M} I_j e^{\frac{-(x_i^k - x_j)^2}{2\sigma_x^2}} e^{\frac{-(I_i^k - I_j)^2}{2\sigma_I^2}}}{\sum_{j=1}^{M} e^{\frac{-(x_i^k - x_j)^2}{2\sigma_x^2}} e^{\frac{-(I_i^k - I_j)^2}{2\sigma_I^2}}}$$

(3)

until convergence.
3. Assign $(x^*{}_i, I^*{}_i) = (x_i^{k+1}, I_i^{k+1})$
4. Assign $d_i = (x^*{}_i - x_i)$

where σ_x and σ_I are the bandwidths of Gaussian kernels in the spatial and intensity domain, respectively. For details and explanatory figures on displacement vector computation we refer the reader to [16].

The first part of the speed term can be now defined by

$$S_0(x, y, z) = \frac{f(x, y, z)}{1.0 + |\nabla d(x, y, z)|^2}$$

(4)

The function $d(x, y, z)$ is obtained by summarizing the information provided by the displacement vectors. For a given location along a ray, $d(x, y, z)$ is positive when the corresponding displacement vector is pointing outbound and negative when the vector points towards the seed point. The term $f(x, y, z)$ is given by

$$f(x, y, z) = \begin{cases} -sign(d(x, y, z)) & if |\nabla d(x, y, z)| < threshold \\ 1 & else \end{cases}$$

(5)

where the gradient of $d(x, y, z)$, namely $\nabla d(x, y, z)$ is computed along the ray. In this formulation, rays propagate freely towards the object boundaries when they are away from them and slow down in the vicinity of boundaries. If a ray crosses over a boundary, it returns to the boundary. The parameter *threshold* is determined from the statistical measures computed from the density function of displacement vectors. It is assumed that locations of small gradients (less than *threshold*) in the displacement function are not part of any object boundary.

2.3 Smoothness Constraints

Problems related to missing data are common in the segmentation of medical structures. A solution to missing data is to exploit apriori knowledge by imposing smoothness constraints on the evolving surface. We use two types of smoothness constrains in this work, one on the speed of neighboring rays, the other on the local curvature of the front.

Thus, the speed function $S_0(x, y, z)$ of a ray is filtered by employing the speed information in a neighborhood. In addition, the speed term, $S_1(x, y, z)$ imposes the smoothness of the front. Currently, we employ the mean curvature given by $S_1(x, y, z) = \frac{\kappa_1 + \kappa_2}{2}$ where κ_1 and κ_2 are the principal curvatures. However, other geometric smoothing techniques, such as the Mean-Gaussian curvature [11] can be used.

2.4   Implementation

For the initialization of rays we use an algorithm that provides an approximation to equidistant placement of points on a sphere by employing several subdivisions of an octahedron. The octahedron is initialized with the six points $(1, 0, 0)$, $(-1, 0, 0)$, $(0, 1, 0)$, $(0, -1, 0)$, $(0, 0, 1)$ and $(0, 0, -1)$ and connections between neighboring points give the first primitive triangulization of the unit sphere. In the subdivision process each triangle is subdivided into four new ones by placing one new point on the middle of every edge, projecting it onto the unit sphere and connecting the neighboring points. Rays are then shot from the seed point along the direction given by this approximation of the unit sphere.

To estimate the surface curvature at the current position of a ray we use the following algorithm [20, 2]: Compute the first matrix S

$$S = \left(\frac{1}{2N} \sum_{i=1}^{N} \mathbf{n}_i \mathbf{n}_i^t \right) + \frac{1}{2} \mathbf{p} \mathbf{p}^t$$

where N is the number of neighbors, $\mathbf{n}_i$ denotes the vector to the current position of the i-th neighbor and $\mathbf{p}$ is the vector to the current position of the ray in question. The positive definite matrix S is called *structure tensor* or *scatter matrix*. A principle component analysis provides the eigenvalues $\sigma_1 \geq \sigma_2 \geq \sigma_3$ and eigenvectors $\mathbf{v}_1, \mathbf{v}_2, \mathbf{v}_3$ of S. The eigenvector $\mathbf{v}_1$ corresponding to the largest eigenvalue σ_1 is in normal tangential direction. The other two eigenvectors point into the directions of the principal curvatures. Though the corresponding eigenvalues σ_2 and σ_3 already give an estimate of the degree of curvature in these directions they do not give information of their orientation, forcing us to include another step. Therefore, for every neighbor we also calculate the dot product of the neighbor vector and the principal curvature vector. This coefficient is then multiplied with the difference of $\frac{\pi}{2}$ and the angle between the normal tangential vector $\mathbf{v}_1$ and the vector connecting $\mathbf{p}$ and the neighbor. The sum over this weighted angle differences is positive for convex areas and negative for concave areas. Hence, the final formulas for principal curvatures are: $\kappa_1 = \sum_{i=1}^{N} \frac{|\mathbf{v}_2 \cdot \mathbf{n}_i|}{|\mathbf{v}_2||\mathbf{n}_i|} \left(\arccos \left(\frac{\mathbf{v}_1 \cdot (\mathbf{n}_i - \mathbf{p})}{|\mathbf{v}_1||\mathbf{n}_i - \mathbf{p}|} \right) - \frac{\pi}{2} \right)$ and $\kappa_2 = \sum_{i=1}^{N} \frac{|\mathbf{v}_3 \cdot \mathbf{n}_i|}{|\mathbf{v}_3||\mathbf{n}_i|} \left(\arccos \left(\frac{\mathbf{v}_1 \cdot (\mathbf{n}_i - \mathbf{p})}{|\mathbf{v}_1||\mathbf{n}_i - \mathbf{p}|} \right) - \frac{\pi}{2} \right)$.

3   Results and Conclusions

In this paper, we have presented a user-friendly 3D volume segmentation algorithm. Figures 1 and 2 show the segmentation of the inner boundary of an

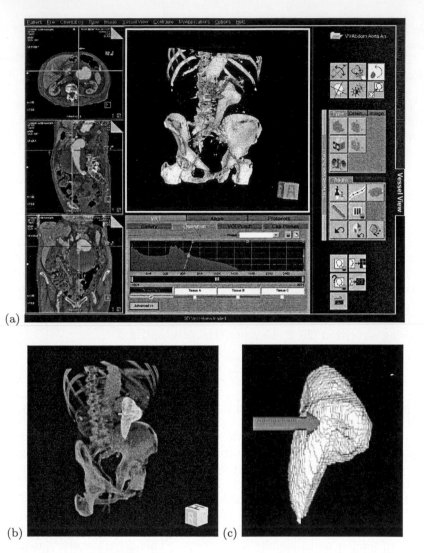

Fig. 2. This figure illustrates one-click segmentation algorithm. (a) illustrates the original image (CE-CTA) image in multi-planar reformats (MPRs) and volume rendering. This data set contains an aneurysm which is indicated by the (green) arrow. (b) The detected aneurysm (lumen boundary) is blended with the original data. (c) The segmented aneurysm (lumen boundary).

aneurysm on CE-CTA data. This proposed algorithm is very fast due to ray propagation. Second, the analysis based on mean shift makes our algorithm robust to outliers inherent in CT and MR images. Third, the use of shape priors such as smoothness constraints implies a reduced sensitivity of the algorithm to missing data, i.e., surfaces that are not well defined or missing. Fourth, our algorithm is user-friendly since one-click inside the 3D medical structure is often sufficient.

References

1. D. Adalsteinsson and J. Sethian. A fast level set method for propagating interfaces. *J. Comput. Phys*, 118:269–277, 1995.
2. J. Berkmann and T. Caelli. On the relationship between surface covariance and differential geometry.
3. M. Black, G. Sapiro, D. Marimont, and D. Heeger. Robust anisotropic diffusion. 7:421–432, 1998.
4. V. Caselles, F. Catte, T. Coll, and F. Dibos. A geometric model for active contours in image processing. TR No 9210, CEREMADE, 1992.
5. L. Cohen and I. Cohen. Finite element methods for active contour models and balloons for 2-d and 3-d images, 1993.
6. D. Comaniciu and P. Meer. Mean shift analysis and applications. In *ICCV*, pages 1197–1203, 1999.
7. D. Comaniciu and P. Meer. Mean shift: A robust approach toward feature space analysis. *IEEE Trans. on PAMI*, 24(5):To appear, 2002.
8. D. DeCarlo and D. N. Metaxas. Blended deformable models. *IEEE Transactions on Pattern Analysis and Machine Intelligence*, 18(4):443–448, 1996.
9. R. Malladi, J. A. Sethian, and B. C. Vemuri. Shape modelling with front propagation: A level set approach. *IEEE Trans. on PAMI*, 17, 1995.
10. T. McInerney and D. Terzopoulos. A dynamic finite element surface model for segmentation and tracking in multidimensional medical images with application to cardiac 4D image analysis. *Comp. Med. Imaging and Graphics*, 19:69–83, 1995.
11. P. Neskovic and B. B. Kimia. Three-dimensional shape representation from curvature-dependent deformations. TR-128, LEMS, Brown University, 1993.
12. S. Osher and J. A. Sethian. Fronts propagating with curvature dependent speed: Algorithms based on Hamilton-Jacobi formulations. *J. of Comp. Phy*, 79, 1988.
13. T. B. Sebastian, H. Tek, J. J. Crisco, S. W. Wolfe, and B. B. Kimia. Segmentation of carpal bones from 3d CT images using skeletally coupled deformable models. In *MICCAI*, pages 1184–1194, 1998.
14. J. A. Sethian. *Level Set Methods and Fast Marching Methods*. Cambridge University Press, Second Ed., New York, 1999.
15. K. Siddiqi, A. Tannenbaum, and S. Zucker. Area and length minimizing flows for image segmentation. *IEEE Trans. Image Processing*, 7:433–444, 1998.
16. H. Tek, D. Comaniciu, and J. Williams. Vessel detection by mean shift based ray propagation. In *Work. on Math. Models in Biomedical Image Analysis*, 2001.
17. H. Tek and B. B. Kimia. Volumetric segmentation of medical images by three-dimensional bubbles. *CVIU*, 64(2):246–258, February 1997.
18. D. Terzopoulos and D. Metaxas. models with local and global deformations : Deformable superquadrics. *IEEE PAMI, vol. 13, no. 7, pp. 703-714, 1991.*, 1991.
19. C. Tomasi and R. Manduchi. Bilateral filtering for gray and color images. In *ICCV*, Bombay, India, pages 839–846, January 1998.
20. B. Vemuri, A. Mitiche, and J. Aggarwal. Curvature-based representation of objects from range data. *Image and Vision Computing*, 4:107–114, 1986.
21. R. Whitaker. Algorithms for implicit deformable models. In *ICCV95*, pages 822–827, 1995.
22. R. Whitaker, D. Breen, K. Museth, and N. Soni. Segmentation of biological volume datasets using a level set framework. *Volume Graphics*, pages 249–263, 2001.
23. C. Xu and J. Prince. Snakes, shapes, and gradient vector flow. *IEEE Trans. Image Proc*, pages 359–369, 1998.
24. A. Yezzi and S. Kichenassamy and A. Kumar and P. Oliver and A. Tannenbaum" A Geometric Snake Model for Segmentation of Medical Imagery IEEE Transactions on Medical Imaging, 16(2), 1997.

MAP MRF Joint Segmentation and Registration

Paul P. Wyatt* and J. Alison Noble

Medical Vision Laboratory, Oxford University Dept. Eng. Science
{wyatt,noble}@robots.ox.ac.uk

Abstract. The problems of segmentation and registration are traditionally approached individually, yet the accuracy of one is of great importance in influencing the success of the other. We aim to show that more
accurate and robust results may be obtained through seeking a joint solution to these linked processes. The outlined approach applies Markov
random fields in the solution of a *Maximum a Posteriori* model of segmentation and registration. The approach is applied to synthetic and
real MRI data.

1 Introduction

Two of the most fundamental problems in medical image analysis, and indeed
within computer vision as a whole, are those of segmentation: processing raw
data to obtain meaningful labels, and registration: putting information from
multiple datasets into alignment. In most previous work the decision has been
taken to separate these problems. This separation means the benefits inherent
in the fusion of the data and communication between processes are lost.

Recently, interest has been growing in the potential of integrating segmentation and registration, driven by a clinical demand for more accurate and robust
diagnostic tools. One instance is the min-max entropy approach of [2] for registration of $2D$ X-Ray portal and $3D$ CT images. An active contour approach is
proposed in [12] where registration is based on contour propagation. We favour
a Markov random field approach, within which we seek to obtain a *maximum a
posteriori* estimate of the segmentation and registration.

Combined segmentation and registration should produce two principal advantages over their separate application. First, combination of registered datasets
provides multiple measurements at a pixel/voxel. In a number of imaging modalities noise decorrelates with movement, which should allow more accurate classification from the combined statistics. Second, registration succeeds or fails based
on the discriminatory ability of a similarity measure. This measure may be designed to use class information, so benefitting the registration. By improving the
accuracy and stability of both processes, this method may benefit areas where
each process fails separately. Additionally, the proof in appendix A shows that
segmentation accuracy should increase for any distribution model, upon combination, so is not limited to special cases or functions.

* PW gratefully acknowledges the financial support of the UK EPSRC for funding
this research.

T. Dohi and R. Kikinis (Eds.): MICCAI 2002, LNCS 2488, pp. 580–587, 2002.

2 Integrating Segmentation and Registration

Our goal is to *obtain the best possible estimate, in some predefined sense, for the segmentations of multiple data sets degraded by non-stationary noise, which are related through some geometric transformation, and to recover the geometric transformation.* We cast this as a *maximum a posteriori* (MAP) estimation of the segmentation labels $\mathcal{S}$, transformation(s) $\mathcal{T}$ given n datasets $\mathbf{X}_1, \mathbf{X}_2, ... \mathbf{X}_n$ and pose the solution using Markov Random Fields (MRFs).

Using MRFs and Bayesian MAP estimation requires a model to be defined for the segmentation and registration processes, conditioned upon the data. This is important, as no matter how detailed the prior information available for a given class of problems, the data determines a specific instance of that problem. The choice of a prior model, for joint segmentation and registration, is also critical as it determines the expected relationship between images and, critically, image classes.

The Bayesian problem may be stated for two datasets A and B as:

$$P(\mathcal{S}, \mathcal{T}/\mathbf{X}_A, \mathbf{X}_B) = \frac{P(\mathbf{X}_A, \mathbf{X}_B/\mathcal{S}, \mathcal{T})P(\mathcal{S}, \mathcal{T})}{P(\mathbf{X}_A, \mathbf{X}_B)} \tag{1}$$

If we assume dataset independence, equation 1 would simplify to:

$$P(\mathcal{S}, \mathcal{T}/\mathbf{X}_A, \mathbf{X}_B) = \frac{P(\mathbf{X}_A/\mathcal{S})P(\mathbf{X}_B/\mathcal{S})P(\mathcal{S})}{P(\mathbf{X}_A)P(\mathbf{X}_B)} \tag{2}$$

Our algorithm switches between equation 1 and 2 as their validity changes. Details of how this is done are provided later.

In the proposed method equation 1 and 2 are not implemented directly. Instead we expand $P(\mathcal{S}, \mathcal{T})$ using Bayes' rule and take the logarithms of both sides. The denominator is dropped as it is constant for any data, giving:

$$\ln P(\mathcal{S}, \mathcal{T}/\mathbf{X}_A, \mathbf{X}_B) \propto \ln P(\mathbf{X}_A, \mathbf{X}_B/\mathcal{S}, \mathcal{T}) + \ln P(\mathcal{S}/\mathcal{T}) + \ln P(\mathcal{T}) \tag{3}$$

Throughout this paper, we refer primarily to joint estimation of segmentation and registration; it is therefore necessary to distinguish it from simultaneous estimation. We define **simultaneous** estimation as *updating the estimation of both the classes and transforms relating any (two) datasets in a single step optimisation.* **Joint** estimation may, or may not, use the same model of segmentation and registration, but alternates between *updating the classes of any (two) datasets and updating the transforms between them in a two, or more, step optimisation.*

To illustrate this, with respect to equation 3, the joint scheme would be[1];

$$\ln P(\mathcal{S}_{n+1}, \mathcal{T}_n/\mathbf{X}_A, \mathbf{X}_B) \propto P(\mathbf{X}_A, \mathbf{X}_B/\mathcal{S}_n, \mathcal{T}_n) + \ln P(\mathcal{S}_n/\mathcal{T}_n) + \ln P(\mathcal{T}_n) \tag{4}$$
$$\ln P(\mathcal{S}_{n+1}, \mathcal{T}_{n+1}/\mathbf{X}_A, \mathbf{X}_B) \propto \ln P(\mathbf{X}_A, \mathbf{X}_B/\mathcal{S}_{n+1}, \mathcal{T}_n) + \ln P(\mathcal{S}_{n+1}/\mathcal{T}_n) + \ln P(\mathcal{T}_n)$$

and the simultaneous estimation;

$$\ln P(\mathcal{S}_{n+1}, \mathcal{T}_{n+1}/\mathbf{X}_A, \mathbf{X}_B) \propto \ln P(\mathbf{X}_A, \mathbf{X}_B/\mathcal{S}_n, \mathcal{T}_n) + \ln P(\mathcal{S}_n/\mathcal{T}_n) + \ln P(\mathcal{T}_n) \tag{5}$$

---

[1] Segmentation is performed first as the class labels are then used in registration.

The difference between these schemes depends significantly upon the models for segmentation and registration and their interdependance. As they become more independent the differences recede. As the models become more reliant, so the gains in simultaneous estimation appear. However, joint estimation is significantly quicker than simultaneous estimation [2]. More importantly, in this paper we principally consider *rigid* registration and consequently the registration criteria is evaluated over the image as a whole. This leads to small changes in segmentation having negligible effect.

3   Registration of Images

We use a class-based information theoretic criteria similar to Mutual Information[9, 10] (MI). At each step of the Joint Segmentation and Registration (JS&R) estimation a sub-optimal set of segmentation labels exist. Consider the following measure;

$$\mathcal{I}_{\mathcal{S}_A, \mathcal{S}_B} = \sum_{k \in \mathcal{K}} \mathcal{P}_k(\mathcal{S}_A, \mathcal{S}_B) \ln \mathcal{P}_k(\mathcal{S}_A, \mathcal{S}_B) \tag{6}$$

calculated from the joint **class** histogram of the two images, instead of the joint **intensity** histogram. This similarity measure is based upon image class and is conceptually similar to the MI entropy measure. This class based information measure is fast to calculate, as we have typically 2-5 class labels versus (approximately) 256 intensity levels. The smaller matrix size means fewer calculations are required for equation 6 compared to MI.

Equation 6 can be combined with the class pixel MAP probabilities if desired, to increase specificity, and is implementable for elastic registration. The MAP probabilities result from the MRF MAP ICM (Iterated Conditional Modes[3]) segmentation as calculated from the image data and prior image models.

Using the segmentation labels in the registration criteria allows estimation of the convergence of the registration. The K-means algorithm allows the estimation of the weightings of each distribution present in the $1\mathcal{D}$ datasets. These weights appear, under Maximum Likelihood classification, as the row (column) sums of the match matrix of equation 6 and are similar under MAP. The coefficient of convergence can be evaluated as the ratio of the entropy of the class match matrix, at the nth iteration, to the match matrix where maximal correlation, i.e. a 1:1 correspondence, exists.

$$\text{Coeff}_{convergence} = \frac{\sum_{k \in \mathcal{K}} \mathcal{P}_k(\mathcal{S}_{A,cur}, \mathcal{S}_{B,cur}) \ln \mathcal{P}_k(\mathcal{S}_{A,cur}, \mathcal{S}_{B,cur})}{\sum_{k \in \mathcal{K}} \mathcal{P}_k(\mathcal{S}_{A,max} \mathcal{S}_{B,max}) \ln \mathcal{P}_k(\mathcal{S}_{A,max}, \mathcal{S}_{B,max})} \tag{7}$$

Equation 7 thereby allows switching between equations 1 and 2, at some user set threshold of convergence. This avoids obtaining a poor registration which will lead to decreased accuracy in the joint segmentation.

---

[2] This results simply from the number of classes to be considered. If there are $\mathcal{K}$ distributions and we allow the registration classes to be $\pm \delta \mathcal{T}$ in each dimension $\mathcal{D}$ then for joint estimation we consider $\mathcal{K} + (2\mathcal{D} + 1)$ classes and for simultaneous estimation $\mathcal{K}(2\mathcal{D} + 1)$, i.e. additive versus multiplicative.

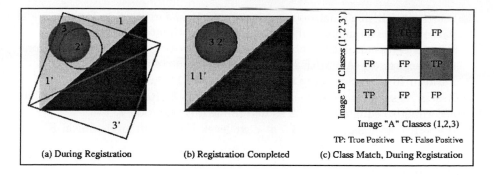

(a) During Registration   (b) Registration Completed   (c) Class Match, During Registration

Fig. 1. Diagram of the Joint Class Histogram obtained during Registration.

4   The Match Matrix and Segmentation

We propose the Gaussian mixture model (GMM) to model the image data. The GMM is ideal for simply illustrating the benefit of our approach compared to sequential segmentation and registration, though other models could easily be substituted. From the individual datasets, by applying a K-Means algorithm, we obtain a $1\mathcal{D}$ GMM for the data. As registration proceeds, classes become better correlated allowing the switch from $1\mathcal{D}$ Gaussian intensity classes to $2\mathcal{D}$ Gaussian intensity classes. This substantially improves the separation of the data. Figure 1 shows a diagram of the class match matrix; which forms the prior $\mathcal{P}(\mathcal{S}/\mathcal{T})$, in equation 1. As registration proceeds, the false positives tend towards a residual dependent upon classification errors. The relative weights reflect belief in different class combinations, which can be fixed if known *a priori*. The underlying principle is similar to Mutual Information[10], using entropy of classes rather than intensities.

The GMM required for the data model of equation 1 is formed when the registration convergence is satisfactory (equation 7). Depending whether we believe a 1:1 correspondence exists between classes in the different datasets, we can allow either a greater or smaller number of classes to be included in the GMM. This allows flexibility in modelling registration as either pure motion (1:1 correspondence) or as change between the classes in different images; for example in chemotherapy treatment of tumours.

4.1   JS&R Algorithms

We assume a familiarity with Markov fields and Bayesian estimation in this section[4, 6, 7], particularly the Iterated Conditional Modes (ICM) algorithm[3]. Let $\hat{s}$ represent class labels and $\mathbf{x}$ data. We seek, at each step;

$$\hat{s} = \arg \max_{s \in \mathcal{S}} \{ \mathcal{P}(\mathbf{x}|s)\mathcal{P}(s) \} \tag{8}$$

The JS&R algorithm may then be summarised as follows:

1. Starting with single datasets, perform a *K-Means* estimation for the model parameters. The number of classes $\mathcal{K}$ can be estimated[3] or given.
2. Form a Gaussian multiresolution hierarchy. Starting at the coarsest resolution perform a MAP MRF ICM[3] segmentation using equation 2.
3. Perform Registration using the Powell method[11] and equation 6.
4. Assess registration convergence, using equation 7. Reprocess segmentation, according to equation 1, or 2 as determined by equation 7.
5. If JS&R converged; repeat 3-5 at next level. If done all levels finish. Else 3.

5   Results

Figure 2 (a,d) show two synthetic images. These have been simulated using Gaussian classes with means $[25, 50, 100, 150, 200, 225]$ (gray levels). In (a) classes have variance ~ 20 and in (d) ~ 12 (gray levels). Image (d) is obtained from (a) through a rotation of $0.15^c, (8.59°)$ and translation of $[12, 13]^t$ pixels. Figure 2 (b,e) show the segmentation of (a,d) using a GMM based MRF on each image separately. Images (c,f) show the segmentation of (a,d) using the JS&R algorithm. The segmentation accuracies[4] are: (b) 0.908 (c) 0.956 (e) 0.977 (f) 0.986. The transformation was correctly recovered by both registration using MI of intensities and the JS&R algorithm to within the user specified tolerance (± 0.1 pixels translation and $\pm 0.1°$ rotation). However, using equation 6, as opposed to MI, speeded evaluation of the registration criteria by a factor of ~ 10. This results from the smaller matrix size required for the class based criterion versus intensity based.

Figure 3 shows five frames, approximately $\frac{1}{2}$ a cycle, of an MRI mouse heart sequence. The first column shows the MRI images, the second the single dataset segmentations. The third and fourth columns show the paired segmentations obtained using JS&R on pairs of adjacent images. The combined segmentation appears better than the separate; maintaining separation of left and right ventricles. The registrations obtained from conventional MI and the combined JS&R algorithms were the same within the specified tolerance.

6   Conclusion

We have demonstrated that a combined approach to segmentation and registration can improve the accuracy of segmentation and speed up registration, using Markov Random Fields and Bayesian estimation. The JS&R algorithm uses simple data and prior models suggesting an improved model should improve performance further. Although more testing is required, particularly on low quality medical data where the method should be of particular use, the benefits have been demonstrated; theoretically and practically.

---

[3] Using Minimum Description Length[8] (MDL) or otherwise.

[4] As the images were simulated, the actual segmentations were known. The accuracy measure used was the fraction of correctly classified pixels.

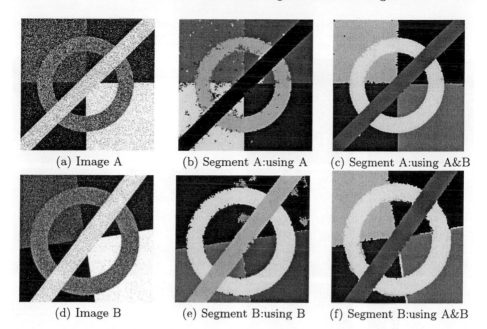

(a) Image A   (b) Segment A:using A   (c) Segment A:using A&B

(d) Image B   (e) Segment B:using B   (f) Segment B:using A&B

Fig. 2. 2 Images with 6 Classes, Gaussian Noise. (size A:250×250, B:212×221 pixels.)

A Improved Separability of Functions in Higher Dimensions

If we can prove, for any N-dimensional function $\mathcal{F}$, that the error of Maximum Likelihood (ML) classification is upper-bounded by the $1\mathcal{D}$ case then this proves that ML classification from the fusion of registered datasets yields equal or more accurate results than those possible for any single dataset.

Consider 1D functions $\mathcal{F}_1(x_1), \mathcal{F}_2(x_1)$, with ML error $\delta\mathcal{E}_1$ (about point a);

$$\delta\mathcal{E}_1 = \int_{a-\delta a}^{a+\delta a} \min\left[\mathcal{F}_1(x_1), \mathcal{F}_2(x_1)\right] dx_1 \tag{9}$$

In 2D these form, after fusion with other data, functions $\mathcal{G}_{2,1}(x_1, x_2), \mathcal{G}_{2,2}(x_1, x_2)$. The fractional error for the same data becomes;

$$\delta\mathcal{E}_2 = \int_{a-\delta a}^{a+\delta a} \int_{-\infty}^{\infty} \min\left[\mathcal{G}_{2,1}(x_1, x_2), \mathcal{G}_{2,2}(x_1, x_2)\right] dx_2 dx_1 \tag{10}$$

Iff the data is independent then $\mathcal{G}_{2,(1\cup 2)}(x_1, x_2) = \mathcal{F}_{(1\cup 2)}(x_1)\mathcal{G}(x_2)$ and equation 10 becomes;

$$\delta\mathcal{E}_2 = \int_{a-\delta a}^{a+\delta a} \int_{-\infty}^{\infty} \min\left[\mathcal{G}(x_2)\mathcal{F}_1(x_1), \mathcal{G}(x_2)\mathcal{F}_2(x_1)\right] dx_2 dx_1$$

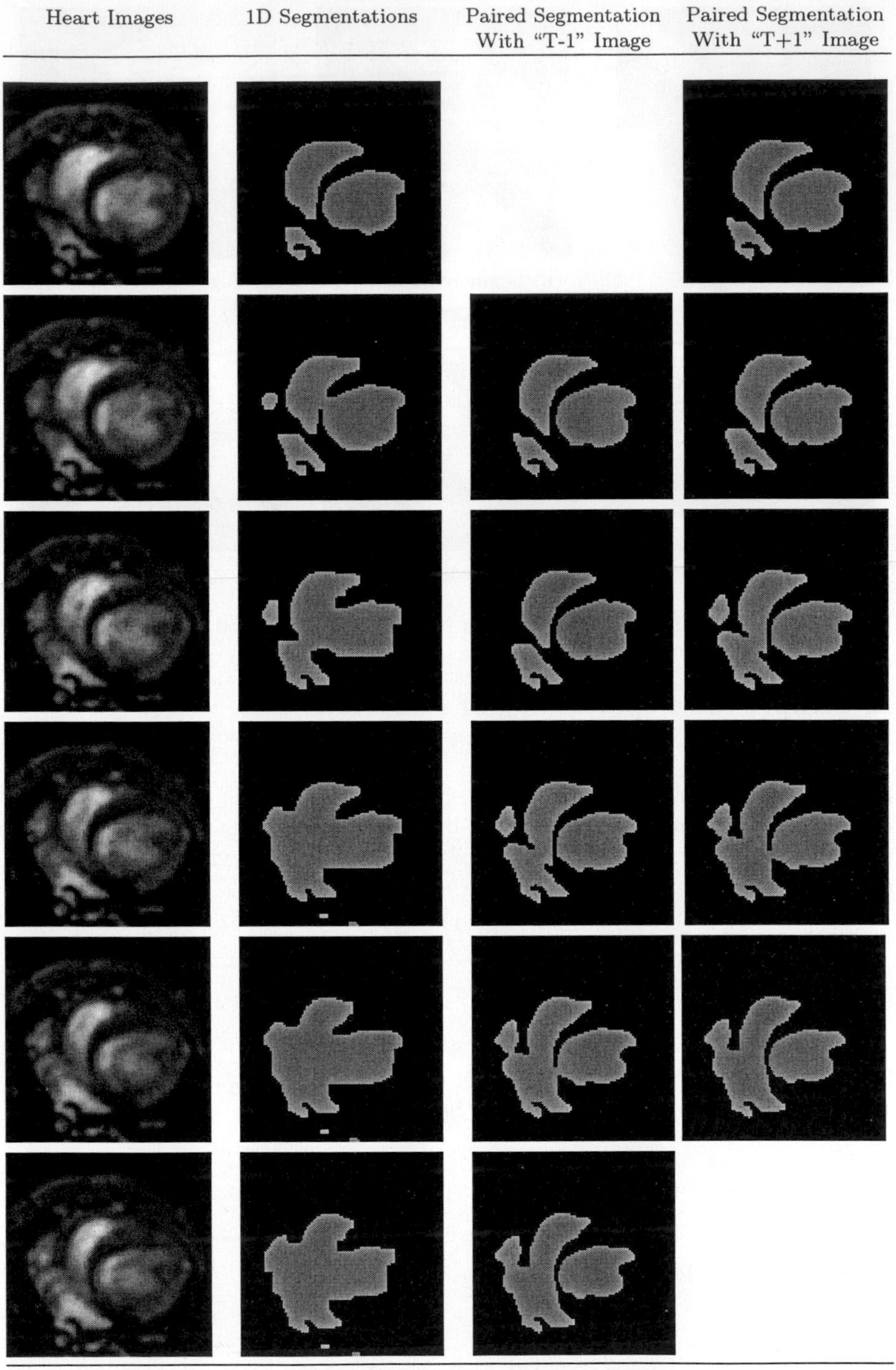

Heart Images	1D Segmentations	Paired Segmentation With "T-1" Image	Paired Segmentation With "T+1" Image

Fig. 3. Segmentations, of $\sim \frac{1}{2}$ cycle, of an MRI Mice Heart Sequence

$$= \int_{-\infty}^{\infty} \mathcal{G}(x_2) \mathrm{d}x_2 \int_{a-\delta a}^{a+\delta a} \min \left[\mathcal{F}_1(x_1), \mathcal{F}_2(x_1) \right] dx_1$$

$$= \int_{a-\delta a}^{a+\delta a} \min \left[\mathcal{F}_1(x_1), \mathcal{F}_2(x_1) \right] dx_1 \tag{11}$$

Hence, the error for $2\mathcal{D}$ is equal to that for $1\mathcal{D}$. This also implies that the ratio $\frac{\mathcal{F}_1(x_1)}{\mathcal{F}_2(x_1)} = \mathcal{K}$, a constant. However, if $\mathcal{G}_{2,(1\cup2)}(x_1, x_2) \neq \mathcal{F}_{(1\cup2)}(x_1)\mathcal{G}(x_2)$ then the ratio $\frac{\mathcal{G}_{2,1}(x_1, x_2)}{\mathcal{G}_{2,2}(x_1, x_2)} \neq \mathcal{K}$. The maximum ML misclassification must be $\delta \mathcal{E}_1$, as the maximum union of $\mathcal{F}_1(x_1), \mathcal{F}_2(x_1)$ is $\min \left[\mathcal{F}_1(x_1), \mathcal{F}_2(x_1) \right]$. Consequently, extending this logic to the whole domain;

$$\text{Iff } \frac{\mathcal{G}_{N,1}(x_1, x_2, \cdots, x_{N-1}, x_N)}{\mathcal{G}_{N,2}(x_1, x_2, \cdots, x_{N-1}, x_N)} \geq \cdots \geq \frac{\mathcal{G}_{2,1}(x_1, x_2)}{\mathcal{G}_{2,2}(x_1, x_2)} \geq \frac{\mathcal{F}_1(x_1)}{\mathcal{F}_2(x_1)} \text{ then } \delta \mathcal{E}_2 \leq \delta \mathcal{E}_1 \tag{12}$$

References

1. R Bansal and LH Staib et al., *A Novel Approach for the Registration of 2D Portal and 3D CT Images for Treatment Setup Verification in Radiotherapy*, MICCAI 1998, p1075-1086
2. R Bansal and LH Staib et al., *Entropy-Based Multiple Portal to 3D CT Registration for Prostate Radiotherapy Using Iteratively Estimated Segmentation*, MICCAI 1999, p567-578
3. J Besag, *On the Statistical Analysis of Dirty Pictures*, Journal of the Royal Statistical Society - Series B 48(3), p259-302, 1986
4. J Besag, *Spatial Interaction and the Statistical Analysis of Lattice Systems*, Journal of the Royal Statistical Society - Series B(36), p192-236, 1974
5. C Bishop, *Neural Networks for Pattern Recognition*, Oxford University Press, 1995
6. S Geman and D Geman, *Stochastic Relaxation, Gibbs Distributions, and the Bayesian Restoration of Images*, IEEE PAMI 1984, 6(6), p721-741.
7. DM Greig and BT Porteos and AH Seheult, *Exact Maximum A Posteriori Estimation for Binary Images*, Journal of the Royal Statistical Society - Series B 51(2), p271-279, 1989
8. YG Leclerc, *Constructing Simple Stable Descriptions for Image Partitioning*, IJCV, (3) p73-102 , 1989
9. JBA Maintz and MA Viergever, *A Survey of Medical Image Registration Methods*, Medical Image Analysis, 2(1), p1-36,1998
10. A Roche and G Malandain and N Ayache, *Unifying Maximum Likelihood Approaches in Medical Image Registration*, INRIA France, Tech Report RR-3741, 1999
11. WH Press and SA Teukolsky et al, *Numerical Recipes in C*, Cambridge University Press, 1992
12. A Yezzi and L Zollei and T Kapur *A Variational Framework for Joint Segmentation and Registration* IEEE Proc. MMBIA, p44-52, 2001

Statistical Neighbor Distance Influence in Active Contours

Jing Yang[1], Lawrence H. Staib[1], and James S. Duncan[1]

Yale University, P.O. Box208042, New Haven CT 06520-8042, USA
{j.yang,lawrence.staib,james.duncan}@yale.edu

Abstract. In this paper, we propose a new model for segmentation of images containing multiple objects. In order to take advantage of the constraining information provided by neighboring objects, we incorporate information about the relative position and shape of neighbors into the segmentation process by defining a new "distance" term into the energy functional. We introduce a representation for relative neighbor distances, and define a probability distribution over the variances of the relative neighbor distances of a set of training images. By minimizing the energy functional, we formulate the model in terms of level set functions, and compute the associated Euler-Lagrange equations. The contours evolve both according to the relative distance information and the image grey level information. Several objects in an image can be automatically detected simultaneously.

1   Introduction

Medical image segmentation is an important and challenging problem and a necessary first step in many image analysis and quantitation methods. Sophisticated automated and semi-automated techniques are required.

Since the original work by Kass et al. (1987) [1], extensive research has been done on active contour models or "snakes", where an initial contour is deformed towards the boundary of the object to be detected by minimizing an energy functional.

In the problem of curve evolution, level set methods [2] have been used extensively, because they allow for automatic changes in the topology. Novel geometric models of active contours have been proposed based on curve evolution and geometric flows [4] [5] [6]. By using the level-sets based numerical algorithm, several objects can be segmented simultaneously.

Recently, Chan and Vese [3] have proposed an active contour model, based on techniques of curve evolution, using a Mumford-Shah functional for segmentation with a level sets. In the level set formulation, the problem becomes a "mean-curvature flow". This model can detect objects whose boundaries are not necessarily defined by gradient.

The idea of incorporating prior information into image segmentation has received a large amount of attention in recent years and has been approached

T. Dohi and R. Kikinis (Eds.): MICCAI 2002, LNCS 2488, pp. 588–595, 2002.
© Springer-Verlag Berlin Heidelberg 2002

using point distribution models (Cootes,et al.)[7], Fourier parameters (Staib and Duncan)[8], and statistical shape inforamtion (Leventon et al.)[9].

In many cases, objects to be detected have one or more neighboring structures which have a consistent location and shape that provides a configuration and context that aids in the delineation. The relative positions or distances among these neighbors can also be modeled based on statistical information from a training set. Though applicable in many domains these models are particularly useful for medical applications. For example, the anatomical structures that appear in magnetic resonance (MR) or computed tomography (CT) scans are often segmented for use in surgical planning, navigation, simulation, diagnosis and therapy evaluation. Without a prior model to constrain the segmentation, the algorithms often fail due to difficult challenges such as poor image contrast, noise, and missing or diffuse boundaries. It can be made easier if suitable models of the relative distances among neighboring structures are available.

We incorporate relative position and shape information of neighbors by defining a new "distance" term into the energy functional. We introduce the representation for relative neighbor distances, and define a probability distribution over a training set. By minimizing the energy functional, we formulate the model in terms of level set functions, and compute the associated Euler-Lagrange equations. The contours evolve both according to the relative distance information and the image grey level information.

2 Probability Distribution of Neighbor Distances

2.1 Binary Shape Alignment

Consider a training set of N images, with M objects or structures in each image. Let the training set consist of a set of MN binary images $\{I_i^n | i = 1, 2, ...M; n = 1, 2, ..., N\}$, each with values one inside and zero outside object i. To compute the relative distances in the training set, we first transform each binary image, I_i^n, into another binary image $I_j^n, j \neq i$ to jointly align them with a similarity transformation. The idea is to calculate the set of transformation matrices $\{T_{ij}^n | i, j = 1, 2, ...M \cap j \neq i\}$, where T_{ij}^n transforms the coordinates of I_i^n into the coordinates of $I_j^n, j \neq i$. T_{ij}^n consists of translation, scale and axis rotations. In 2D, the transformed binary image $\tilde{I}_{ij}^n$ is defined as: $\tilde{I}_{ij}^n = I_i^n(T_{ij}^n \cdot [x, y, 1]^T)$

An effective way to calculate T_{ij}^n is to descend along the energy functional:

$$E_{ij\,align}^n = \frac{\int_\Omega (\tilde{I}_{ij}^n - I_j^n)^2 dA}{\int_\Omega (\tilde{I}_{ij}^n + I_j^n)^2 dA} \qquad (1)$$

Where Ω denotes the image domain. By minimizing (1), we minimize the difference between $\tilde{I}_{ij}^n$ and I_j^n [10]. To illustrate, Figure 1 shows two neighboring objects where the dotted curves are the aligned versions of the two boundaries.

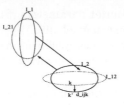

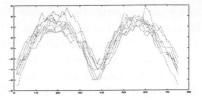

Fig. 1. Shape alignments of 2 objects and neighbor distance definition.

Fig. 2. Relative distance distribution of the two shapes in Figure 3a.

2.2 Neighbor Distances Definition

We define d_{ijk}^n as the nearest distance of the k th point on the boundary of object i in $\tilde{I}_{ij}^n$ to object j in I_j^n along $\pm n$, where n is the normal direction at the k th point of object i, as shown in Figure 1. The training set, D, consists of a set distance matrices $D = \{D^1, D^2, ..., D^N\}$, where $D^n = \{d_{ijk}^n | i, j = 1, 2, ..., M; k = 1, 2, ..., K\}$ is the distance matrix of the n th image in the training set. Note that d_{ijk}^n is not necessarily equal to $d_{jik'}^n$ because the optimal transformation may differ. Our goal is to build a statistical model over this distribution of distance matrices, under a Gaussian assumption $N(\bar{d}_{ijk}, \sigma_{ijk})$. $\bar{d}_{ijk}$ and σ_{ijk}^2 are the mean and variance of d_{ijk}^n. Figure 3 shows the outlines of two objects in a training set with 9 images. The computed relative distance matrices D of the training set in Figure 3 are shown in Figure 2. The yellow '*' curve is the mean relative distance between the two shapes.

3 Description of the Model

3.1 Energy Functional

Our method defines the segmentation problem in terms of minimizing an energy functional. Given the distribution of the relative neighbor distances, the prior information about the relative positions of all the objects of interest in an image can be modeled as an energy term. The corresponding term in the level set evolution equation of the model pulls the surface in the direction such that d_{ijk} approaches its maximum likelihood estimation $\hat{d}_{ijk}$ in the final segmentation.

Assume C_i is the evolving curve corresponding to object i in Ω, C_{i0} is the boundary of object i. Now, let us consider the following energy terms:

$$E_{ineighbor} = \sum_{j=1, j\neq i}^{M} \int_{C_i} [d_{ij}(x, y) - \hat{d}_{i,j}(x, y)]^2 dx dy , \quad E_{neighbor} = \sum_{i=1}^{M} E_{ineighbor}$$

(2)

It is obvious that C_{i0}, the boundary of object i, is the minimizer of $E_{ineighbor}$. Boundary $C_0 = \{C_{i0} | i = 1, 2, ..., M\}$ of the M objects of interest is the minimizer of $E_{neighbor}$. In our active contour model, we will minimize the energy term

$E_{neighbor}$ and we will add image gray level information based energy terms and regularizing terms, like the length of the curve C_i and (or) the area of the region inside C_i. Here, we use the energy terms defined by Chan [3] as the gray level information based energy terms. Therefore, we introduce the energy functional of each object of interest i as $E_i(c_{1i}, c_{2i}, C_i)$, defined by:

$$
\begin{aligned}
E_i(c_{1i}, c_{2i}, C_i) &= E_{ineighbor} + E_{ilength} + E_{iarea} + E_{iimage} \\
&= \sum_{j=1, j \neq i}^{M} w_{ij} \int_{C_i} [d_{ij}(x, y) - \hat{d}_{i,j}(x, y)]^2 dx dy \\
&\quad + \mu_i \cdot Length(C_i) + \nu_i \cdot Area(inside(C_i)) \\
&\quad + \lambda_{1i} \int_{inside(C_i)} |I(x, y) - c_{1i}|^2 dx dy \\
&\quad + \lambda_{2i} \int_{outside(C_i)} |I(x, y) - c_{2i}|^2 dx dy
\end{aligned}
\tag{3}
$$

Where w_{ij}, μ_i, ν_i, λ_{1i}, and λ_{2i} are non-negative fixed parameters. I is the image. C_i is the evolving curve of object i, and the constants c_{1i}, c_{2i}, depending on C_i, are the averages of I inside C_i and respectively outside C_i. We wish to minimize the total energy of all the objects of interest in the image $E_{total}(c_1, c_2, C)$:

$$
\min_{c_1, c_2, C} E_{total}(c_1, c_2, C) = \min_{c_1, c_2, C} \sum_{i=1}^{M} E_i(c_{1i}, c_{2i}, C_i)
\tag{4}
$$

Where $C = \{C_i | i = 1, 2, ...M\}$, $c_1 = \{c_{1i} | i = 1, 2, ...M\}$, $c_2 = \{c_{2i} | i = 1, 2, ...M\}$. This minimization problem can be formulated and solved using the level set method. In this way, we can realize the segmentation of multiple objects simultaneously.

3.2   Estimation of Relative Neighbor Distances

In the functional $E_{total}(c_1, c_2, C)$, we include terms that incorporate information of the relative neighbor distances of the objects being segmented. For each given evolving curve C_i, we seek the maximum likelihood estimate of the relative neighbor distances d_{ijk} of the final curve:

$$
\hat{d}_{ijk} = \arg \max_{\hat{d}_{ijk}} p(\tilde{d}_{ijk}/d_{ijk}) = \arg \max_{\hat{d}_{ijk}} \frac{p(d_{ijk}/\tilde{d}_{ijk}) p(\tilde{d}_{ijk})}{p(d_{ijk})}
\tag{5}
$$

The first term in the numerator computes the probability of the relative neighbor distance among certain evolving curves given the relative neighbor distances among the final curves. It is reasonable to model this term as a Gaussian function: $N(\tilde{d}_{ijk}, \sigma_{ijk})$. The second term in the numerator of (5) is based on our prior models, as described in section 2.2. Finally, we discard the normalization term in the denominator of (5) as it does not depend on $\tilde{d}_{ijk}$.

3.3   Level Set Formulation of the Model

In the level set method, C_i is the zero level set of a higher dimensional surface Ψ_i corresponding to the i th object being segmented, i.e., $C_i = \{(x, y) | \Psi_i(x, y) = 0\}$.

The evolution of the curve C_i is given by the zero-level curve at time t of the function $\Psi_i(t,x,y)$. We define that Ψ_i is positive outside C_i and negative inside C_i. Each of the M objects being segmented in the image has its own C_i and Ψ_i. Thus, we have M level set functions.

For the level set formulation of our model, we replace C with Ψ in the energy functional in (3) using regularized versions of the Heaviside function H and the Dirac function δ [3], denoted by H_ε and δ_ε:

$$E_i(c_{1i},c_{2i},C_i) = \sum_{j=1,j\neq i}^{M} w_{ij} \int_\Omega [d_{ij}(x,y) - \hat{d}_{i,j}(x,y)]^2 \delta_\varepsilon(\Psi_i(x,y))|\nabla\Psi_i(x,y)|dxdy$$

$$+ \mu_i \int_\Omega \delta_\varepsilon(\Psi_i(x,y))|\nabla\Psi_i(x,y)|dxdy + \nu_i \int_\Omega (1-H_\varepsilon(\Psi_i(x,y)))dxdy$$

$$+ \lambda_{1i} \int_\Omega |I(x,y)-c_{1i}|^2 (1-H_\varepsilon(\Psi_i(x,y)))dxdy$$

$$+ \lambda_{2i} \int_\Omega |I(x,y)-c_{2i}|^2 H_\varepsilon(\Psi_i(x,y))dxdy \tag{6}$$

To compute the associate Euler-Lagrange equation for each unknown level set function Ψ_i, we keep c_{1i} and c_{2i} fixed, and minimize E_{total} with respect to $\Psi_i(i=1,2,...M)$ respectively. Parameterizing the descent direction by artificial time $t \geq 0$, the equation in $\Psi_i(t,x,y)$ is:

$$\frac{\partial \Psi_i}{\partial t} = \delta_\varepsilon(\Psi_i) \cdot div[\frac{\nabla\Psi_i}{|\nabla\Psi_i|}] \sum_{j=1,j\neq i}^{M} w_{ij}[d_{ij}(x,y)-\hat{d}_{ij}(x,y)]^2 \tag{7}$$

$$+ \sum_{j=1,j\neq i}^{M} 2w_{ji}\delta_\varepsilon(\Psi_j) \cdot |\nabla\Psi_j|[d_{ji}(x,y)-\hat{d}_{ji}(x,y)]$$

$$+ \delta_\varepsilon(\Psi_i)[\mu_i \cdot div[\frac{\nabla\Psi_i}{|\nabla\Psi_i|}] + \nu_i + \lambda_{1i}|I(x,y)-c_{1i}|^2 - \lambda_{2i}|I(x,y)-c_{2i}|^2]$$

3.4 Evolving the Surface

We approximate H_ε and δ_ε as follows [3]: $H_\varepsilon(z) = \frac{1}{2}[1+\frac{2}{\pi}\arctan(\frac{z}{\varepsilon})]$, $\delta_\varepsilon(z) = \frac{\varepsilon}{\pi(\varepsilon^2+z^2)}$. c_{1i} and c_{2i} are defined by: $c_{1i}(\Psi_i) = \frac{\int_\Omega I(x,y)\cdot(1-H(\Psi_i(x,y)))dxdy}{\int_\Omega (1-H(\Psi_i(x,y)))dxdy}$, $c_{2i}(\Psi_i)$ $= \frac{\int_\Omega I(x,y)\cdot H(\Psi_i(x,y))dxdy}{\int_\Omega H(\Psi_i(x,y))dxdy}$.

Given the surfaces $\Psi_i(i=1,2,...M)$ at time t, we seek to compute evolution steps that bring all the zero level set curves to the correct final segmentation based on the prior relative distance information and image information. At each stage of the algorithm, we recompute the relative distances d_{ij} and estimation $\hat{d}_{ij}$ as well as the constants c_{1i} and c_{2i}. We then update the Ψ_i. This is repeated until convergence.

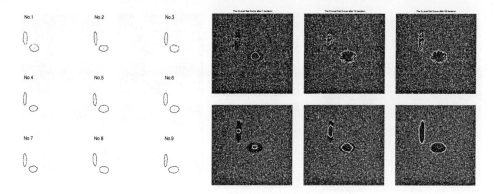

Fig. 3. Training set: Outlines of 2 shapes in 9 images.

Fig. 4. Initial, middle, and final steps in the segmentation of two shapes in a synthetic image.

The parameters w_{ij}, μ_i, ν_i, λ_{1i}, and λ_{2i} are used to balance the influence of the relative distance information model and the image information model. The tradeoff between relative distance and image information depends on how much faith one has in the distance model and the imagery for a given application. We set these parameters empirically for particular segmentation tasks, given the general image quality and the prior relative distance information.

4 Experimental Results

We have used our model on various synthetic and real images, with at least two different types of contours and shapes. We have generated a training set of synthetic images of two elliptic objects with the addition of Gaussian noise, as shown in Figure3. Figure 2 shows the distance distribution. Figure 4 illustrates several steps in the segmentation of two synthetic objects in a noisy image. The result of using neighbor information (lower row) is much better than only use the image grey level information (upper row).

Figure 5 shows the construction of a two object model (left ventricle and right ventricle) from 2D MRI heart images. In Figure 6, we show an example delineation of the ventricles with the initial, middle, and final steps in the curve evolution process. The experiment was first performed without using neighbor distance information, as shown in Figure 6 top. The evolving curves stopped at a place where there is a bigger change of the grey level. They cannot lock onto the shape of the objects. We then use the relative distance information to segment the same image again, as shown in Figure 6 bottom. By taking the statistical relative distance information of the two shapes from the training set shown in Figure 5, the curves are able to converge on the desired boundaries even though some parts of the boundaries are too blurred to be detected using only grey level information. Both of the segmentations converged in several minutes on an SGI Octane with a 255MHz R10000 processor.

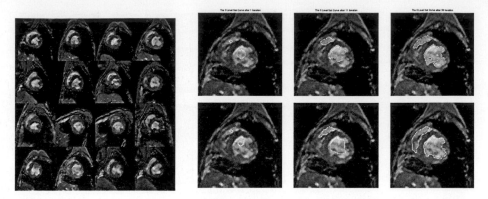

Fig. 5. Training set: 16 MR heart images.

Fig. 6. Initial, middle, and final steps in the segmentation of two shapes in a heart image.

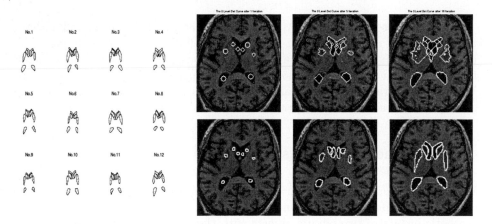

Fig. 7. Training set: outlines of 8 shapes in 12 MR brain images.

Fig. 8. Initial, middle, and final steps in the segmentation of 8 shapes in a brain image.

In Figure 8, we show that our model can detect multiple objects of different intensities, and with blurred boundaries in a 2D MR brain image. Figure 8 top shows the result of using the model based only on grey level information. The lower (posterior) portions of the lateral ventricles can be segmented perfectly since they have clearer boundaries. But for the other six structures, their boundaries are so blurred that they cannot be detected using grey level information alone. To incorporate neighbor information, we used a training set as shown in Figure 7. We also ran our algorithm to segment eight different objects: the lateral ventricles, heads of the caudate nucleus, and putamen. Segmenting all eight subcortical structures took approximately twenty minutes.

To assess the segmentation results, we computed the undirected distance between the computed boundary $A(N_A$ points) and the manual boundary B:
$$H(A, B) = \max(h(A, B), h(B, A)), \quad h(A, B) = \frac{1}{N_A} \sum_{a \in A} \min_{b \in B} \|a - b\|.$$

For our experiments, we showed improvement in all the three cases comparing with/without neighbor influence: synthetic 2.1/5.3, heart 2.6/4.2, brain 2.8/9.6.

5   Conclusions

A new model for automated segmentation of images containing multiple objects by incorporating the information about the relative position and shape of neighbors in the segmentation process has been presented. Our model is based on defining a new "distance" term into the energy functional. We introduce the representation for relative neighbor distances, and define a probability distribution over the variances of the relative neighbor distances of a set of training images. By minimizing the energy functional, we formulate the model in terms of level set functions, and compute the associated Euler-Lagrange equations. The contours evolve both according to the relative distance information and the image grey level information. Multiple objects in an image can be automatically detected simultaneously. We believe that our model can also be extended to 3D image segmentation.

References

1. M. Kass, A. Witkin, D. Terzopoulos.: Snakes: Active contour models. Int'l Journal on Computer Vision, 1 (1987) 321–331
2. S. Osher and J. A. Sethian.: Fronts propagating with curvature-dependent speed: Algorithms based on Hamilton-Jacobi Formulation. J. Comp. Phy. 79 (1988) 12–49
3. T. Chan, L. Vese.: Active Contours Without Edges. IEEE Transactions on Image Processing, vol.10 No. 2 (2001) 266–277
4. V. Caselles, F. Catte, T. Coll, and F. Dibos.: A geometric model for active contours in image processing. Numer. Math. 66 (1993) 1–31
5. V. Caselles, R. Kimmel, and G. Sapiro.: Geodesic active contours. Int. J. Comput. Vis. vol.22 No. 1 (1997) 61–79
6. R. Malladi, J. A. Sethian, and B. C. Vemuri.: A topology independent shape modeling scheme. Proc. SPIE Conf. Geometric Methods Computer Vision II, vol.2031 (1993) 246–258
7. T. Cootes, C. Beeston, G. Edwards, and T. Taylor.: Unified framework for atlas matching using active appearance models. Information Processing in Medical Imaging, (1999)
8. L.Staib, J. Duncan.: Boundary finding with parametrically deformable models. PAMI, 14(11) (1992) 1061–1075
9. M. Leventon, E. Grimson, and O. Faugeras.: Statistical shape influence in geodesic active contours. IEEE Conf. on Comp. Vision and Patt. Recog. 1 (2000) 316–323
10. A. Tsai, A. Yezzi, et al.: Model-based curve evolution technique for image segmentation. IEEE Conf. on Comp. Vision and Patt. Recog. vol.1 (2001) 463–468

Active Watersheds: Combining 3D Watershed Segmentation and Active Contours to Extract Abdominal Organs from MR Images

R.J. Lapeer[1], A.C. Tan[2], and R. Aldridge[1]

[1] School of Information Systems, University of East Anglia, Norwich NR4 7TJ, UK
[2] Department of Medical Physics and Bioengineering, University College London (UCL), London WC1E 6JA, UK

Abstract. The three-dimensional segmentation of regions of interest in medical images, be it a 2D slice by slice based approach or directly across the 3D dataset, has numerous applications for the medical professional. These applications may involve something as simple as visualisation up to more critical tasks such as volume estimation, tissue quantification and classification, the detection of abnormalities and more. In this paper we describe a method which aims to combine two of the more popular segmentation techniques: the watershed segmentation and the active contour segmentation. Watershed segmentation provides unique boundaries for a particular image or series of images but does not easily allow for the discrete nature of the image and the image noise. Active contours or snakes do possess this generalisation or smoothing property but are difficult to initialise and usually require to be close to the boundary of interest to converge. We present a hybrid approach by segmenting a region of interest (ROI) using a 3D marker-based watershed algorithm. The resulting ROI's boundaries are then converted into a contour, using a contour following algorithm which is explained during the course of the paper. Once the contours are determined, different parameter settings of internal/external forces allow the expert user to adapt the initial segmentation. The approach thus yields a fast initial segmentation from the watershed algorithm and allows fine-tuning using active contours. Results of the technique are illustrated on 3D colon, kidney and liver segmentations from MRI datasets.

1 Introduction

Segmentation of images, and more specifically medical images, is a field which has sparked exciting research throughout the last few years. However it has also caused as much controversy due to divided opinions on the benefits and drawbacks of particular segmentation techniques for particular tasks. Three standard groups of segmentation are distinguished typically as: region-based, edge-based and classification-based [3]. Most segmentation techniques in medical imaging focus on a well-defined task, for example a certain structure or tissue of a particular image modality; often this is even further specialised for a certain objective,

T. Dohi and R. Kikinis (Eds.): MICCAI 2002, LNCS 2488, pp. 596–603, 2002.

for example volume estimation and quantification or diagnosis of abnormal tissues. The aim of the research, as presented in this paper, is to create a more general, hierarchical segmentation methodology which allows a trade-off between speed and accuracy. At this stage, the initial segmentation uses a 3D marker-based watershed algorithm which gives fast results but not necessarily with the expected accuracy as little consideration is given to image noise and discretisation. To overcome this difficulty, the resulting watersheds are converted into active contours using a contour following algorithm. Active contours possess the smoothing properties which watershed lack, however the latter solves the initialisation and connectivity problems of the former.

In the next sections we discuss the established watershed and active contour models that we have used and elaborate on the contour following algorithm. The final section shows, and discusses, results on colon, liver and kidney segmentations. Also, in the final section, we discuss the technique as it currently stands together with possible extensions to create a more versatile and 'intelligent' system which automatically selects appropriate techniques for different medical image segmentation tasks.

2   Methodology

2.1   3D Marker-Based Watershed Segmentation

Watershed segmentation is a morphological region-based segmentation technique. Although first applied to grey-scale images as early as 1979 by Buecher and Lantuéjoul [1] the technique only became popular in the early 90's in a variety of fields in need of automatic image segmentation. This was as a result of the publication of a watershed algorithm by Vincent and Soille [10] and the rapid growth of the computational power of workstations. This algorithm uses a 2D grey-scale image as an input (which can be extended to a full 3D dataset), typically pre-processed to produce a smoothed gradient image. For ease of understanding the watershed principle, let us momentarily forget the 3D extension and assume a 2D image and its different grey-levels represented as a relief. Imagine this relief (looking like a landscape with hills and troughs) to be flooded by water. Water will settle first in a basin - typically called a catchment basin - and raise until it meets one or more neighbouring catchment basins. To avoid water spilling from one basin to the other we construct a dam of single-pixel width, which is higher than the highest peak(s) in the image relief. When the water has reached the highest peak(s) in the image, the resulting dams form the watershed lines which separate the basins. As the catchment basins represent different regions in the image, we arrive at a mosaic-like segmentation of that image. The problem with the standard approach is that depending on the noise in the image, too many regions (possibly belonging together) are separated, which means the image is over-segmented (see Fig.1(b)). Techniques to counteract over-segmentation are mainly based on morphological pre-processing using automatically generated internal and external markers - an overview of

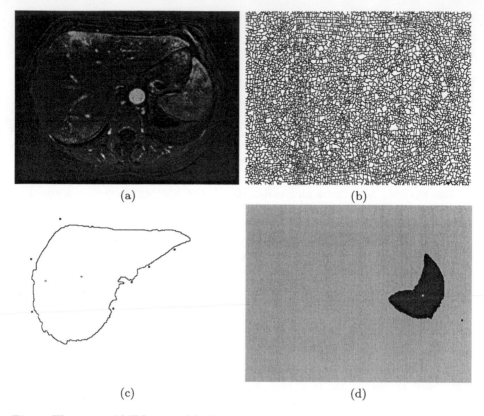

Fig. 1. The original MRI image (a), the over-segmented image using the standard Vincent and Soille algorithm (b), and avoiding this problem using manually placed internal (light) and external (dark) markers for liver segmentation showing the watershed boundary (c) and spleen segmentation showing the internal and external catchment basins (d).

such techniques can be found in [4]. Although the techniques have proved successful for certain images (e.g histological images), they often require several trials using different pre-processing combinations and, even then, are not always capable of producing unambiguous segmentation results. Therefore, we opted for a semi-interactive approach, using manually placed internal and external markers. The method requires the user, typically a medical expert, to place one or more internal markers in the ROI and one or more external markers in the rest of the image (see Fig.1(c) and (d)). If the final segmentation is unsuccessful more markers can be added or removed to yield a satisfactory result. This approach also guarantees a segmentation into two distinct regions, i.e. the region of interest (ROI) and the background.

The algorithm can be extended easily from 2D to 3D as the principle of the image 'flooding' is based on the ordering of pixels in each slot of a cumulative distribution of grey-values of the image (typically 0-255 for 8 bit); each grey-level containing an array of all pixels having that grey-value. Thus, any grey-scale image or dataset of finite dimension can be processed using the same algorithm provided the gradient calculations are adapted.

2.2 A Contour Following Algorithm to Convert the Watershed into an Active Contour

The watershed boundaries are unfortunately not perfect; they may consist of a boundary of several pixels wide, rather than one, and may contain gaps and glyphs (e.g. pixels 10N-10Q in Fig.2). We have implemented a tree-based contour following algorithm using 8-connectednes to create a closed contour with edges of neighbouring pixels:

step 1 Search from the top downwards, the first leftmost pixel in the binary bitmap - e.g. pixel D8 in Fig.2.
Make this pixel the *initial* and *current* pixel.

step 2 From the *current* pixel which is at level 0 in the tree, process in clockwise direction (just a convention ...).
Find the next boundary pixel(s) in the 8-connected neighbourhood whilst ignoring pixels in the invalid direction.
IF only one valid boundary pixel exist make this pixel the *common* pixel. Go to **step 4**.
IF no valid boundary pixels exist (which means there is a gap) expand non-boundary pixels in the right direction. Keep expanding the tree breadth-first until a level is reached containing a *common* single pixel - e.g. in Fig.2 pixel G12, will expand in valid non-boundary pixels G11,G13,H11-13, which will eventually all end in I14.
IF multiple candidate boundary pixels exist, expand until the tree reaches a level with a *common* single pixel - e.g. pixel P11 will yield three valid boundary pixels: O10,P10 and Q10. They will eventually all yield pixel P9 at the next level. Pixel N10, spawned by O10 would eventually 'die' as it has no valid successors (as only at level 0, non-boundary pixels are spawned).

step 3 From the *common* pixel at the bottom of the tree, find the 'least-effort' path. The latter implies a path with average curvature.

step 4 Connect the *current* pixel to the *common* pixel using this path and make the *common* pixel the *current* pixel.

step 5 Go back to **step 2** until the *current* pixel is the *initial* pixel.

Notes:

- A queue structure is required to expand the tree in breadth-first fashion.
- A previous current pixel (that is a pixel which is now part of the contour) becomes an invalid pixel when expanding its successors.
- Previously visited pixels which did not become part of the contour because they failed the 'least-effort' path test, become invalid too.
- When expanding the tree, valid pixels already in a higher level in the tree are not considered (which avoids a 'shortest path' test).

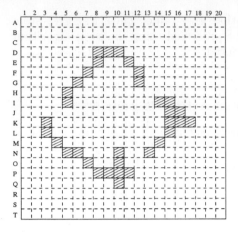

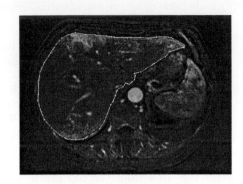

Fig. 2. A model boundary of a watershed containing gaps, multi-pixel width and glyphs.

Fig. 3. The segmented liver with active contour turned watershed.

- The final contour can be post-processed to turn edges with the same slope into a single edge.

2.3   Active Contours

Active contours have become popular as a model for image segmentation mainly by Kass, Witkin and Terzopoulos [5]. They have since then been subjected to several optimisation models and 3D extensions of which a fairly recent update is given in [11]. In this paper, we used the standard simplified active contour model (without inertial term):

$$\gamma \frac{\partial \mathbf{X}}{\partial t} = F_{int}(\mathbf{X}) + F_{ext}(\mathbf{X}) \tag{1}$$

with $\mathbf{X}(s)$, the position vector of a contour element (s being the curve parameter), internal (smoothing) forces, $F_{int}(\mathbf{X})$, and external forces (Gaussian potential force derived from the image), $F_{ext}(\mathbf{X})$. The factor γ is a damping coefficient. A finite difference scheme can be used for numerical implementation.

3   Preliminary Segmentation Results

Fig.3 shows a processed active contour, initially derived from the watershed, as shown in **Fig.1(c)**, using the contour following algorithm. **Fig.4(a)** shows the result of a 3D watershed segmentation. **Fig.4(b)** shows the result after application of active contours on the watershed contours in each slice of the MR dataset. The dataset is of size $512 \times 512 \times 56 \times 16$ bit. Four internal markers

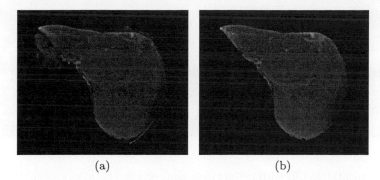

(a)   (b)

Fig. 4. 3D segmentation of liver with original texture-map in the segmented region: initial segmentation using a 3D watershed algorithm (a); smoothed segmentation after active contour fitting (b). MRI data of $512 \times 512 \times 56 \times 16$ bit was used.

and twenty external markers were needed for the watershed segmentation. The processing time was about 3 minutes on an SGI Onyx InfiniteReality. **Fig.5(a)** shows two kidneys segmented from a $256 \times 256 \times 128 \times 8$ bit MR dataset. Only two internal and three external markers in just one slice (out of 128) was needed. No active contour smoothing was applied. **Fig.5(b)** and **(c)** show segmentation of the colon from the same dataset. Only one internal and three external markers were needed, no smoothing. Note that the original texture was mapped into the segmented regions to visualise the internal structures.

4   Discussion

The example in Fig.4(a) and (b) typically shows the shortcomings of the watershed algorithm. Even with the application of a sufficient number of markers, the 3D segmentation of the liver remains prone to 'noisy' regions, caused by the internal ROI's catchment basin 'leaking' into inherently external regions. Adding external markers to the boundaries where these regions merge avoids this problem but usually results in under-segmentation. This means that parts of the (internal) ROI have now become part of the (external) background. The case of liver segmentation is a difficult task because of its inhomogeneous and lobe-like structure. Here, the watershed method by itself fails to produce a noise-free segmentation. The subsequent use of active contours smoothens out the noisy (background) regions. The results from segmenting the colon and kidneys can be further smoothed using active contours, however the watershed segmentation appears to cope very well. A good indicator to its success is the number of internal and external markers needed to produce a relatively noise-free segmentation. For the colon segmentation, which can be used typically for virtual colonoscopy, we also tested a seed-growing approach. We concluded that the watershed algorithm outperforms this method as it copes better with connectivity problems due to its more rigorous boundary criteria.

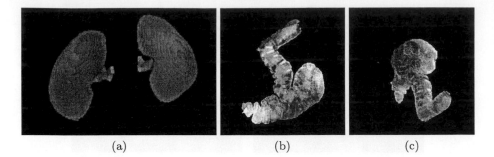

Fig. 5. Segmentation (3D with texture map using original data) of kidneys (a) and two views, (b) and (c), of a segmented colon from a $256 \times 256 \times 128 \times 8$ bit MRI dataset.

Although we know that each individual method is capable of successful segmentation of particular organs for particular modalities, the sum of the two should not normally be worse than each individual method. Care has to be taken however to avoid that one method renders the results of the other method void. For example, the watershed may settle around an undesirable boundary, which subsequently used by the active contour as its initial state, may render the latter's segmentation incorrect or more cumbersome as compared to using the active contour without the watershed. Also the active contour segmentation may destroy the original watershed segmentation for the same reason.

Currently the watershed uses 3D gradient information and the active contours use a 2D (within-slice) gradient. To allow for this discrepancy, the watershed could be used in a 2D slice-by-slice mode (which still produces a 3D segmentation) so both methods use 2D gradient information. A better alternative is to use active surfaces instead of active contours. The 3D watershed regions are iso-surfaces which can be used as an initial model to an adaptive deformable triangulated surface [8] after triangulation (e.g. using a marching-cubes technique [7]). This could be a better alternative to the use of multi-resolution volume pyramids in [8]. As this extension would require more processing resources, the current immersion-based water shed algorithm can be speeded up using a rainfall algorithm [9].

Using automatically generated markers as an alternative to manually placed markers can be further investigated using morphological filters [2], pixel statistics based methods or boundary extraction using transparency functions [6].

To further test the method, different image modalities and structures have to be investigated. For example, deformable models have been widely used for brain segmentation because of the complex geometry of brain structures. However, in [2] it is shown that marker-based watershed segmentation is also capable of successfully segmenting the ventricles, hippocampus, corpus callosum and cerebellum. It would be interesting to evaluate the combined watershed/active contour approach to the segmentatio n of these structures.

Finally, the tool could be extended to incorporate some form of artificial intelligence (AI) by selecting the appropriate methods for certain tasks. It was already pointed out that the number of markers needed for the watershed segmentation proves to be a good indicator of its potential success. Quantitative information like this together with prior (expert) information could then be used to make automatic decisions for optimal segmentation.

5 Conclusion

The combination of watershed segmentation and active contours proves to be a potentially promising tool for medical image segmentation. We currently have successfully tested the method on a limited number of MR datasets for the segmentation of abdominal organs. More tests are anticipated to further test its potential on different structures using different imaging modalities.

References

1. S. Buecher and C. Lantuéjoul. Use of watershed in contour detection. In *Proc. Int. Workshop Image Processing, Real-Time Edge and Motion Detection/Estimation, Rennes, France*, pages 17–21, September 1979.
2. G. Bueno, O. Musse, F. Heitz, and J.P Armspach. Three-dimensional segmentation of anatomical structures in MR images on large databases. *Magnetic Resonance Imaging*, 19:73–78, 2001.
3. B.M. Dawant and A.P. Zijdenbos. Chapter 2: Image segmentation. In J.M Fitzpatrick and M. Sonka, editors, *Handbook of Medical Imaging. Vol.2 Medical Image Processing and Analysis*, pages 71–127. SPIE, London, June 2000.
4. J. Goutsias and S. Batman. Chapter 4: Morphological methods for biomedical image analysis. In J.M Fitzpatrick and M. Sonka, editors, *Handbook of Medical Imaging. Vol.2 Medical Image Processing and Analysis*, pages 175–272. SPIE, London, June 2000.
5. M. Kass, A. Witkin, and D. Terzopoulos. Snakes: active contour models. *Int.J.Comp.Vis.*, 1(4):321–331, 1987.
6. G. Kindlmann and J. Durkin. Semi-automatic generation of transfer functions for direct volume rendering. In *Proc. IEEE Symposium on Volume Rendering*, October 1998.
7. W.E. Lorensen and H.E. Cline. Marching cubes: a high resolution 3d surface construction algorithm. *Computer Graphics*, 21(4):163–169, 1987.
8. J-Y. Park, T. McInerney, D. Terzopoulos, and M-H. Kim. A non-self-intersecting adaptive deformable surface for complex boundary extraction from volumetric images. *Computers & Graphics*, 25:421–440, 2001.
9. P. De Smet and D. De Vleeschauwer. Performance and scalability of a highly optimized rainfalling watershed algorithm. In *Proc. of the 1998 Int.Conf. on Imaging Science, Systems and Technology, CCIST'98 - Las Vegas*, pages 266–273, July 1998.
10. L. Vincent and P. Soille. Watersheds in digital spaces: An efficient algorithm based on immersion simulations. *IEEE Trans. Patt.Anal.Mach.Int.*, 13(6):583–598, June 1991.
11. C. Xu, D.L. Pham, and J.L. Prince. Chapter 3: Image segmentation using deformable models. In J.M Fitzpatrick and M. Sonka, editors, *Handbook of Medical Imaging. Vol.2 Medical Image Processing and Analysis*, pages 175–272. SPIE, London, June 2000.

Coronary Intervention Planning
Using Hybrid 3D Reconstruction

O. Wink[12], R. Kemkers[1], S.J. Chen[2], and J.D. Carroll[2]

[1] Cardiovascular X-ray, Philips Medical Systems North America,
Bothell, Washington, 98041 USA
{onno.wink,richard.kemkers}@philips.com
[2] Division of Cardiology, Department of Medicine,
University of Colorado Health Sciences Center, Denver, Colorado, 80262 USA
{james.chen,john.carroll}@uchsc.edu

Abstract. A new method is presented to assist the clinician in planning a interventional procedure while the patient is already on the catheterization table. Based on several ECG-selected projections from a rotational X-ray acquisition, both a volumetric cone-beam reconstruction of the coronary tree as well as a three-dimensional surface model of the vessel segment of interest are generated. The proposed method provides the clinician with the length and diameters of the vessel segment of interest as well as with an 'optimal working view'. In this view, the gantry is positioned such that the vessel segment of interest is the least foreshortened and vessel overlap is minimized during the entire heart cycle. Examples on a phantom object and on patient data demonstrate the accuracy and feasibility of the approach.

1 Introduction

Coronary artery disease remains the major cause of morbidity and mortality in the United States. Over the past years, there has been a marked increase in the number of catheterizations procedures performed. The number of catheterizations is expected to furher increase due to recent advances in stent technology (*e.g.* eluting stent), imaging capabilities and an aging of the polulation. Coronary catheterizations are performed using X-ray angiography. Choosing the correct stent dimensions is often difficult using the traditional 2D projection images due to vessel foreshortening and overlap. Based on the specific anatomy of the coronary branch and skill of the clinician, several angiographic images from different viewing angles are acquired in order to derive the length and diameter of the stent to be used for subsequent intervention. Once the clinician decides upon the stent dimensions, a 'working view' is chosen for the actual interventional procedure. In this view, it is expected that the vessel segment of interest is the least foreshortened and not blocked from sight. This 'trial-and-error' method of selection of appropriate viewing angles potentially exposes the patient to large amounts of contrast medium (dye) and radiation, even before the actual treatment of the patient begins.

T. Dohi and R. Kikinis (Eds.): MICCAI 2002, LNCS 2488, pp. 604–611, 2002.
© Springer-Verlag Berlin Heidelberg 2002

In order to avoid the 'trial-and-error' approach, several researchers have proposed various methods to construct a three-dimensional surface model of the coronaries using two or three acquisitions from different viewing angles (*e.g.* [1–5]), generally needing considerable user interaction. As a result, the clinician has the ability to view the entire three-dimensional coronary tree from any angle and to choose the 'optimal working view' without the use of extra radiation or dye.

In the last few years, rotational angiography (RA) has proven to be a very accurate and effective diagnostic tool in the treatment of cerebral vessel malformations. In this approach, the C-arm rotates rapidly around the patient while several X-ray projections are acquired. The reconstructed vessels can be viewed from different viewing angles, while only one contrast injection is given. It has been demonstrated that the use of rotational angiography for coronary vessel acquisitions yields better stenosis severity estimations and reveals lesions that were missed by only applying the traditional acquisitions [6]. Due to the high reproducibility of the rotational acquisitions, the fast rotation speed, and the nature of the cerebral vessels, the projections can be used for volumetric reconstruction providing very high detail and accuracy [7], and is completely automated.

However, straightforward volumetric reconstruction of coronary arteries has several difficulties due to the beating of the heart and respiratory motion, yielding a rough representation of the coronaries (see also left frame of Fig. 2). Although recent developments with alternative reconstruction schemes are very promising [8], an accurate reconstruction that can directly be used for lesion sizing in human subjects is not yet available. Even if a suitable volumetric reconstruction could be performed, additional user interaction is needed to arrive at the correct stent dimensions.

In this paper, a method is proposed that combines the complementary features of volume -and surface based reconstruction techniques. The rotational acquisition is used to minimize contrast medium and X-ray exposure. The projections that correspond to the same phase of the cardiac cycle are used to create an accurate surface-based model of the coronary segment of interest and to create an overview of the main coronary vessels. The presented method is unique in several ways. First, the creation of a surface model of the coronaries based on projections from a rotational acquisition has not been demonstrated before. Second, the method allows a model to be built based on every projection that captured the heart at the same phase. Third, the combination with the automatic volumetric reconstruction can be used for visualization of the main vessels of the coronary tree and to determine the 'optimal working view' without vessel overlap and without the need to manually create a surface model of the entire coronary tree. Fourth, to our knowledge, a unique study is presented about the volumetric reconstruction of the main coronary arteries of actual patients with the use of a C-arm system.

In Section 2 the method is described in more detail and the concept of the 'Optimal View Map' is explained. In Section 3 the method is applied to a static

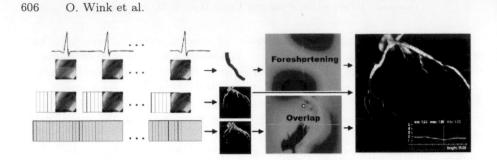

Fig. 1. Flow of the method resulting in the dimensions of a coronary segment and an optimal viewing angle to perform the actual intervention.

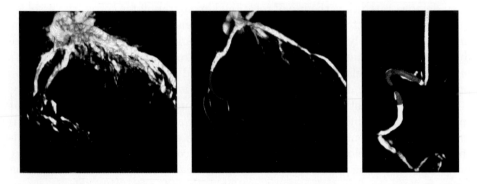

Fig. 2. Reconstruction using all projections (left). Hybrid visualization of a surface model and volumetric reconstruction based on ECG based selection of projections (middle and right).

phantom and a catheter with radiopaque markers in a patient to asses its accuracy. The discussion and conclusions are given in Section 4.

2   Description of the Method

In Fig. 1 the different phases of the method are shown. After the X-ray projections are acquired using a rotational C-arm system (Philips Integris Allura 12 inch monoplane), the images are sent to a workstation (Silicon Graphics Octane). Based on the ECG signal, two projections are chosen that correspond to the same phase of the cardiac cycle to create the central vessel axis followed by the computation of the foreshortening map. Other projections captured at the same phase can be used to refine the surface model of the segment of interest. The projections that are approximately of the same phase are used to visualize the coronary tree, while all the acquired projections are used to compute the overlap map.

2.1   Acquisition

The C-arm is placed near the head-position of the table in order to perform a calibrated propeller acquisition from 120 RAO (right side of patient) to 120 LAO (left side of patient). The C-arm rotates at 55 degrees per second and acquires images at 30 frames per second during 4 seconds while the patient is asked to hold his/her breath. A total of 8 to 12 cc's of contrast medium (Omnipaque 350) is injected during the acquisition and started 1 second before the gantry starts rotating. Since this acquisition has been calibrated in an earlier stage (see [7]), the individual projections can be corrected for the earth magnetic field and pincushion distortion and transformed to a common world coordinate system.

2.2   Surface-Based Modeling

Based on the ECG signal, the projections that correspond to the same phase of the cardiac cycle are chosen to model the segment of the artery of interest. To construct the central axis, those projections are chosen where the segment of interest is clearly visible and the angle between the two projections is around 90 degrees. Since on average five to six heartbeats are captured during the run, the user generally can choose the corresponding projections with a clear view of the lesion. The central axis of the arterial segment is manually identified by adding point pairs. A point in projection A yields an epipolar line in projection B, which is the ray coming from projection A towards the X-ray source. Once a point is set in one projection, the user has to define the corresponding point along the epipolar line in the other projection to construct the central axis of the model. By using this 'epipolar constraint', it is guaranteed that the corresponding epipolar lines do intersect and define a 3D axis point. Once the axis of the lesion is created, the user has the opportunity to delineate the borders of the lumen in every projection that corresponds to the same phase of the heart in order to create and refine a surface model of the lumen. The average time to create a model for a segment of interest once two corresponding projections are found is less than a minute on a SGI Octane.

2.3   Volumetric Reconstruction

An adapted version of the Feldkamp backprojection [9] algorithm is applied for the volumetric reconstruction. The projections are weighted according to the speed of the C-arm, where the projections acquired at a constant rotation speed have a higher weight than those acquired during startup and slowing down of the C-arm. If all available projections are used, the reconstruction contains information about several phases of the heart simultaneously, and is often difficult to interpret (left frame of Fig. 2). If only those projections are used that correspond to the same time point in the cardiac cycle used to build the surface model, the reconstructed volume is better suited for simultaneous visualization and inspection of the artery (middle and right frame of Fig. 2).

2.4   Optimal View Determination

The view that is chosen to perform the intervention is based on a combination of the amount of foreshortening of the segment of interest and the overlap of other structures [2]. The idea behind using a map is that only those gantry angles are computed that can actually be achieved. In general, the cranial (toward the head of the patient) and caudal (toward the feet of the patient) angulation should not exceed 45 degrees from the anterior-posterior (AP) plane since the image intensifier is very likely to hit the patient otherwise. The RAO and LAO thresholds can be set according to the capabilities of the imaging system and are currently set to a maximum of 60 degrees from the AP plane to avoid collision of the image intensifier with the operating table or the patient. The different values within the predefined range of angles are visualized using an interactive color coded map. In the examples used in this paper, a green color in the maps corresponds to the best viewing angle while the red color corresponds to the worst viewing angle. The left of the map corresponds to a RAO position (right with LAO) while the top of the map corresponds to a cranial position (bottom with caudal). The user has the opportunity to inspect the different viewing angles in the map by clicking at a position in the map and to toggle between the different maps. The amount of foreshortening and overlap are given in the lower right hand side of the viewport.

Foreshortening Map. The foreshortening map is computed by comparing the length of the modeled segment to the projected length of this segment as if it were viewed from a typical viewpoint as defined by the range of angles in the map [2].

Overlap Map. Although the volumetric reconstruction of all the acquired projections yields a rough representation of the coronaries, it does provide information where the vessels and other objects (*e.g.* the spine, ribs and pacemaker or ECG-leads) are located during **all** the phases of the heart. The overlap map is computed by taking the integral of all the grey values from the reconstructed volume along the rays that intersect the modeled segment. This is very efficiently implemented in OpenGL using space-leaping techniques and the Stencil Buffer [10] in combination with the special purpose graphics hardware of the SGI Octane.

Optimal View Map. The optimal view map can be constructed by taking a weighted sum of normalized values of the foreshortening map and overlap map (see Fig. 3). For a practical implementation and efficient computation, the vessel overlap is generally only estimated for those gantry angles where the vessel foreshortening has been minimized in order to obtain the resultant optimal working view.

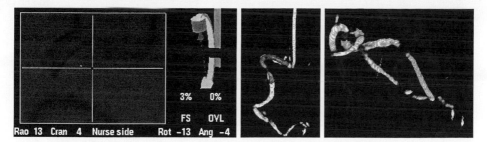

Fig. 3. Example of the optimal view map and the corresponding gantry configuration. The middle and right frame correspond to the best and worst viewing angle as determined by the the optimal view map.

3   Evaluation

Although the method has been applied to over 40 patients, the evaluation focuses on the accuracy and the feasibility of the proposed approach. A phantom with known dimensions is employed for accuracy assessment on length and diameter and the overlap map. Furthermore, the accuracy of the modeling approach is investigated using a marked catheter placed in the left ventricle of the heart.

3.1   Phantom

The employed phantom is a perspex cube of 3 x 3 x 3 cm, containing three aluminum rods with a diameter of 2 mm, oriented in the three main directions and 3 spheres with a diameter of 3 mm as shown in figure 4. The 13-th and 63-th projection are chosen from the rotational acquisition to model the rod that is vertically positioned. To quantify the accuracy, four borders are carefully drawn to define the associated diameter of the rods. All the projections are used to reconstruct the volume for both visualization and computation of the overlap map. The projection corresponding to the worst viewing angle is shown in the right frame of figure 4. From the hybrid visualization in the right frame of figure 4, it can be derived that the generated model is very similar to the reconstructed volume. Four different propeller acquisitions are performed with the image-intensifier set to 12, 9, 7 and 5 inch, respectively. The average diameter of the modeled rod is 1.84 mm, while the average length of the rod is 30.02 mm. The underestimation of the diameter of the rod can be explained by the reduced contrast between the material of the rod and its surrounding perspex. This is not the case in the determination of the rod's length which is therefore much more accurate.

3.2   Marked Catheter

A marked catheter (Cook Royal Flush II pigtail) is placed in the left ventricle of the heart of two patients. The catheter has two radio-opaque markers at the tip that are 22 mm apart (see left and middle frame of Fig. 5). Based on

Fig. 4. The perspex phantom (left frame). The overlap map (middle frame), clearly displaying the 'orbits' of the spheres where they are overlapping with the rod of interest. Hybrid visualization of the modeled (vertical) rod and reconstructed phantom having the most overlap (right frame).

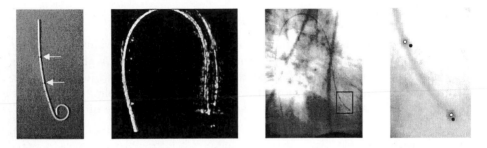

Fig. 5. The catheter with the radio-opaque markers (leftmost frame). The volumetric reconstruction displaying the movement of the catheter tip (middle left frame). A projection displaying the markers while positioned in the left ventricle of a patient (middle right frame). The determination of the accuracy of the projected 3D position of the markers (black dots) compared to the manually determined position of the markers (white dots in rightmost frame).

two projections A and B from the rotational acquisitions using an II-size of 12 inch, the 3D location of the markers is determined. The resulting 3D position is projected on the third projection (C) that corresponds to the same phase of the heart as projections A and B. The average difference between the projected 3D points and the position of the corresponding markers in projection C for both patients is 3.52 pixels.

4   Discussion and Conclusions

A hybrid reconstruction scheme is proposed that provides the clinician with the three-dimensional quantitative measurement of an arterial segment and an optimal working view throughout the cardiac cycle. This information can be provided in less than a minute and used to plan the intervention while the patient is still on the catheterization table. The accuracy of the method is validated using a static phantom and a marked catheter placed in a beating heart during a rotational acquisition. The study found the modeling approach to be accurate if the segment of interest is clearly visible in the different projections that correspond to the same time point in the heart cycle.

Acknowledgments

We would like to acknowledge Rolf Suurmond, Paul Desmedt and Wiet Lie from Philips X-ray pre-development in Best, The Netherlands, for their active support in creating the prototype environment. Babak Movassaghi and Reiner Koppe from Philips Research Laboratories in Hamburg are acknowledged for their help on calibration issues. The many anonymous patients are respectfully acknowledged for consenting in the use of their image data. Franklin Schuling is acknowledged for establishing the cooperation between Philips Research and the Cardiac Cath Lab of the University of Colorado Health Sciences Center.

References

1. S. J. Chen and J. D. Carroll, "3-D reconstruction of coronary arterial tree to optimize angiographic visualization," *IEEE Transactions on Medical Imaging*, vol. 9, no. 4, pp. 318–336, April 2000.
2. S. -Y. J. Chen and J. D. Carroll, "Computer assisted coronary intervention by use of on-line 3D reconstruction and optimal view strategy," in *Proc. Medical Image Computing and Computer-Assisted Intervention*, 1998, pp. 377–385.
3. A. Wahle, E. Wellnhofer, I. Mugaragu, H. U. Sauer, H. Oswald, and E. Fleck, "Assesment of diffuse coronary artery disease by quantitative analysis of coronary morphology based upon 3 D reconstruction from biplane angiograms," *IEEE Transactions on Medical Imaging*, vol. 14, no. 2, pp. 230–241, June 1995.
4. A. C. M. Dumay, J. H. C. Reiber, and J. J. Gerbrands, "Determination of optimal angiographic viewing angles: Basic principles and evaluation study," *IEEE Transactions on Medical Imaging*, vol. 12, no. 1, pp. 13–24, 1994.
5. U. Solzbach, U. Oser, M. Romback, H. Wollschläger, and H. Just, "Optimum angiographic visualization of coronary segments using computer-aided 3D reconstruction from biplane views," *Computers and Biomedical Research*, vol. 27, pp. 178–198, 1994.
6. G. Tommasini, A. Camerini, A. Gatti, G. Derchi, A. Bruzzone, and C. Vecchio, "Panoramic coronary angiography," *JACC*, vol. 31, no. 4, pp. 871–877, March 1998.
7. R. Koppe, E. Klotz, J. op de Beek, and H. Aerts, "Digital stereotaxy/stereotactic procedures with C-arm based rotational-angiography (RA)," in *Computer Assisted Radiology*, H. U. Lemke et al., Ed. 1996, pp. 17–22, Elsevier Publishers, Amsterdam.
8. V. Rasche, A. Buecker, M. Grass, R. Koppe, J. op de Beek, R. Bertrams, R. Suurmond, H. Kuehl, and R.W. Guenther, "ECG-gated 3D-rotational coronary angiography," in *Proc. Computer Assisted Radiology and Surgery*, H. U. Lemke, Ed., 2002, accepted for publication.
9. L. A. Feldkamp, L. C. Davis, and J. W. Kress, "Practical cone-beam algorithms," *Journal of the Opt. Society of America*, vol. A, no. 6, pp. 612–619, 1984.
10. M. Woo, J. Neider, T. David, and D. Shreiner, *OpenGL Programming Guide, Version 1.2*, Addison Wesley, Reading, Mass, 1999.

Deformation Modelling Based on PLSR
for Cardiac Magnetic Resonance Perfusion Imaging

Jianxin Gao[1], Nick Ablitt[1], Andrew Elkington[2], and Guang-Zhong Yang[1,2]

[1] Royal Society/Wolfson Foundation MIC Laboratory, Imperial College, London, UK
[2] Royal Brompton Hospital, London, UK
{jxg,naa99,gzy@doc.ic.ac.uk}

Abstract. This paper introduces a novel approach to deformation modelling based on partial-least-squares-regression and its application to the registration of first-pass magnetic resonance perfusion image sequences. The method relies on the extraction of intrinsic correlations between the latent factors of both the input and output signals for deriving a simple yet accurate deformation model. The strength of the technique has been demonstrated with both numerically simulated data sets and a myocardial perfusion study which involves nine patients with known coronary artery disease. The method represents a step forward for the commonly used principal component analysis for salient motion feature extraction. The proposed technique should be applicable to studies that involve deformation prediction such as motion adaptive radiotherapy and imaging, where the deformation of the target organ can be predicted from externally measurable signals.

1   Introduction

Magnetic Resonance (MR) myocardial perfusion imaging is a relatively new technique for distinguishing ischemic myocardium from healthy tissue [1,2]. It offers the possibility of non-invasively determining the location and extent of ischemia or infarction at transmural resolutions. First-pass techniques using fast gradient echo (turboFLASH) or echo-planar (EPI) sequences are now common practice in clinical research and quantitative results have been achieved in animal studies with intravascular agents (polylysine-Gd-DTPA) as a macromolecular blood pool marker [3-5]. At the same time, semi-quantitative results have also been established in humans with conventional extracellular agents (Gd-DTPA). Either approach has an impact on the detailed characterisation of the relationship between functional and perfusion abnormalities.

For first-pass perfusion imaging, a complete 2D or volumetric data set has to be acquired for each cardiac cycle [6-8]. Cardiac and respiratory induced motion is a major problem during both imaging and subsequent perfusion analysis. With standard perfusion sequences, a typical single slice short axis image of the myocardium may take about 100 *ms* to acquire. Even with limited coverage of three to four slices of the left ventricle, the acquisition window within each cardiac cycle can still become excessive. During this period, cardiac motion can cause the myocardium imaged through different image planes to be mis-registered, *i.e.*, some parts of the myocar-

T. Dohi and R. Kikinis (Eds.): MICCAI 2002, LNCS 2488, pp. 612–619, 2002.
© Springer-Verlag Berlin Heidelberg 2002

dium may be imaged multiple times whereas other parts may be missed out completely. This type of mis-registration is difficult to correct for by using post-processing techniques. In a previous study, we have proposed a novel 4D motion-decoupling technique based on the use of motion tagging and slice tracking [9]. This has simplified the problem to multiple 2D temporal free-form image registration tasks. In this case, the deformation within the imaging plane is normally caused by respiration during the acquisition period, typically lasting for about 50 cardiac cycles. Breath-holding has been suggested, but for most patients, particularly those with coronary artery disease, this has proven to be impractical. This renders accurate image registration of cardiac deformation a crucial step in the quantification of perfusion indices. Thus far, several image registration approaches have been proposed for in-plane motion correction [10,11]. The purpose of this paper is to introduce the concept of partial-least-squares-regression (PLSR) [12] to derive intrinsic characteristics of the deformation model both for improving the internal consistency of the registration process and for predicting myocardial deformation due to respiration.

2   Material and Methods

2.1   Myocardial Motion Prediction

Existing research in cardiac imaging has shown that there is significant correlation between myocardial deformation and respiratory motion patterns. In MR coronary imaging, for example, respiratory navigators have been extensively used to sample the movement of the diaphragm in order to predict the distortion of the epicardial surface, thus allowing real-time adaptive tracking of the coronary arteries to be used to avoid breath-holding for patient studies. Research has also shown that the internal correlation between respiration and cardiac deformation is subject specific, but intra-patient characteristics remain relatively consistent throughout the imaging period. Inspired by these findings, we propose to use the varying intensity distribution of the chest and diaphragm as predictors of myocardial deformation.

Historically, models for respiratory induced cardiac motion have been based on cardiac landmarks. This has the advantage of simplifying the derivation of motion models but has the major drawbacks in accuracy. Respiratory motion and its induced cardiac deformation are highly complex. In our proposed motion prediction model, principal modes of intensity variation related to the diaphragm and chest are extracted to correlate with deformation vectors of the myocardium, leading to a reliable motion prediction approach. Figure 1 illustrates the basic concepts involved in the motion prediction model. The use of free-form image registration allows the extraction of intra-frame tissue deformation, resulting in a dense displacement vector field within the image plane. To relate motion fields reflecting respiration to those of cardiac deformation, non-linear correlation techniques need to be employed. This, however, is not trivial especially when the model parameters are unknown and patient specific. By observing the fact that there is a large amount of redundancies and internal correlations in intensity distribution of the chest wall and the motion vectors of the myocardium, deformation modelling based on PLSR can be applied.

In PLSR, principal component analysis (PCA) is first applied to extract the intrinsic patterns, *i.e.* latent factors, of the original data sets. Then the focus is put on these latent factors rather than the original data that carries redundancies. A relationship can subsequently be established between these latent factors through linear regression. In practice, this is implemented as a learning process, *i.e.*, by feeding the model with both input (intensity distributions around the chest wall and diaphragm) and observed output (motion vectors of myocardial deformation). Since intra-patient motion characteristics are relatively consistent throughout the imaging period, a short segment of the image sequence can be used for extracting the deformation model such that cardiac deformation can be automatically predicted from the intensity variations at the chest wall or the diaphragm. This removes the need of using image registration for the remaining images within the sequence. Of course, the same process can also be used for processing the entire sequence during learning so as to derive an internally consistent motion model to regulate the deformation vectors calculated from the registration algorithm.

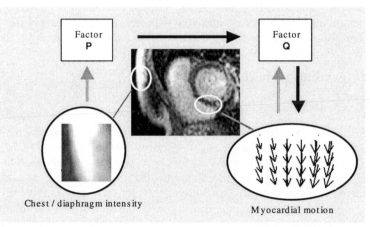

Fig.1. A schematic illustration of using PLSR for deformation modelling. In this example, multiple measurements of the intensity distribution near the chest wall, reordered as long vectors, are used as the input, from which input latent factors are extracted. A similar process is also applied to the observed output data, in this case the deformation vectors of the heart derived from normal free-form image registration. A model that reflects the intrinsic correlation between input/output can then be derived from these factors. At the prediction stage, the path along the dark arrows is followed, *i.e.*, myocardial deformation can be directly predicted from the intensity pattern measured at the chest wall

2.2 PLSR Implementation

Let $\mathbf{X}$ denote the intensity pattern of the chest wall and/or the diaphragm, $\mathbf{Y}$ the free-form deformation vectors of the myocardium, each with a dimensionality of p and m. When n image frames are used for learning, their intrinsic relationship can be expressed as

$$\mathbf{Y} = \mathbf{XC} + \mathbf{E} \tag{1}$$

where $\mathbf{C}$ is a p by m coefficient matrix, $\mathbf{E}$ represents noise and higher order terms that are not accounted for in the above relationship, with the same rank of $\mathbf{Y}$. In PLSR, both the input $\mathbf{X}$ and output $\mathbf{Y}$ are used for extracting the factors, also called scores, in forming the coefficient matrix $\mathbf{C}$. The regression is implemented based on these factors rather than the original input and output matrix themselves. That is, PCA is applied to decompose **X** and **Y** as

$$X = TP + E_1 \tag{2}$$
$$Y = TQ + E_2 \tag{3}$$

In Equation (2) and (3), **T** is the factor score matrix of n by c, **P** the factor loading matrix of c by p, **Q** the coefficient loading matrix of c by m, here c is the number of predominant latent vectors kept in the PCA computation; and E_1 and E_2 represent, respectively, parts of **X** and **Y** that are unaccounted for, with the same ranks as of **X** and **Y**.

The latent vectors are the eigenvectors of the covariance matrix $(X'Y)'(X'Y)$, through which a weighting matrix **W** can be computed iteratively such that $T=XW$. This means that the factor score matrix **T** is the weighting result of input matrix **X**. The weighting matrix **W** is generated in such a way, that each of its columns will maximize the covariance between the response matrix and the corresponding factor scores. By applying a normal regression procedure, matrix **Q** can be derived which describes the relationship between **Y** and **T**. For a predefined number of principal components c, usually much less than the number of predictors, the iteration procedure, known as the NIPALS algorithm [13,14], is as follows:

1. *Initialise $A=X'Y$, $M=X'X$, $B=I$;*
2. *For $k=1$ to c, begin iteration:*
3. *Compute coefficient loading vector q_k, being the first eigenvector of $A'A$;*
4. *Compute weighting (column) vector $w_k=BAq_k$, normalize $w_k=w_k/\|w_k\|$;*
5. *Compute factor loading vector (column) $p_k=Mw_k/f$, where $f=w_k'Mw_k$;*
6. *Renew the coefficient loading vector q_k as $q_k=A'w_k/f$;*
7. *Renewal for A and M: $A=A-fp_kq_k'$, $M=M-fp_kp_k'$;*
8. *Renewal for B: $B=B-w_kp_k'$;*
9. *If $k>c$ or M vanishes, stop iteration; otherwise return to step 3.*

where p_k, q_k, w_k are the vectors of the corresponding matrix **P**, **Q** and **W**. Once **P**, **Q** and **W** are computed, the regression matrix in equation (1) can be determined by $C=WQ$.

The above computation corresponds to a learning process. For new image frames, the myocardial motion can then be predicted according to the intensity distribution at the chest and/or diaphragm by using the established regression matrix **C**. In the current study, we used 40% of the image frames located at the end of the perfusion sequence for learning. Only the first five principal components of the covariance matrix are kept in extracting the regression matrix **C**, since they cover around 90% or more of total covariance.

2.3 Validation and *in vivo* Data Acquisition

To validate the effectiveness of the proposed model extraction scheme for motion prediction, a simulated MR myocardial perfusion image sequence has been created. This data set is used to validate the registration process in a situation where the correct deformation is known. This also allows us to test the method in a variety of different conditions. The structure of the image was based on an example short axis slice of the heart. The images consisted of 6 anatomical features: myocardium of the left ventricle, myocardium of the right ventricle, blood pool of the left ventricle, blood pool of the right ventricle, the diaphragm, the chest wall. In addition, we introduced two distinct defects in the myocardium of the left ventricle these being a sub-endocardial defect and a transmural defect. This gave nine distinct regions that were spatially defined by a static bitmap image. The temporal intensity of these regions was defined by time series curves based on real values from example data sets. Subsequently, the image sequence was warped so as to simulate respiratory motion. This motion vector was based on a real motion vector from the inverse of the motion vector produced from the registration of a real sequence. This dataset was used to evaluate the proposed 2D free form registration, self-adaptive learning and prediction with PLSR. After numerical verification, nine *in vivo* data sets acquired from patients with known coronary artery disease were used to further validate the proposed technique. These images were obtained using a 1.5T Siemens Sonata scanner (200 *T/m/s*; 40 *mT/m*) with a four-element phased-array receiver coil. The first-pass perfusion data was acquired with a FLASH sequence (Tr=3.7 *ms*) that consists of three saturation-recovery short-axis slices per cardiac cycle, for 50 cycles during the first-pass of Gd-DTPA (cubital vein, 0.1 *mmol/kg*, 3 *ml/s*) with a field of view of 400 *mm* (128 pixels) by 300 *mm* (64 pixels).

The accuracy of the deformation correction technique for the patient data sets was assessed by two independent observers by using an image analysis package (CMRtools, Imperial College). The scoring was done through the measurement of displacements in millimeters of predefined landmarks on the septal, anterior and posterior segments. The derived values were then averaged over the entire sequence, and between the three chosen locations.

3   Results

Figure 2 illustrates the internal correlation between respiration and myocardial deformation. For simplicity, a single input trace is given and patterns of respiration at 18, 26, 31, 35, 40, and 46 cardiac cycles from the beginning of the acquisition are provided. Figure 3(a) demonstrates the accuracy of the free-form image registration technique and the modeling approach based on PLSR. The temporal trace of the input bolus is also provided as a reference. It is evident that the overall accuracy of the PLSR approach is significantly better than that of using the normal registration method. The reason for the registration technique to perform poorly at the beginning the sequence was due to the application of an inversion pulse to nullify signals from the myocardium before the arrival of the contrast bolus. Figure 3(b) shows the corresponding assessment results for the patient data sets, illustrating the overall improvement of the motion correction results where only 40% of the image frames are used for motion prediction.

4   Discussion and Conclusions

Image registration is a crucial step in quantifying myocardial perfusion images. The use of conventional image registration is useful in aligning inter frame object deformations. For first-pass MR myocardial perfusion imaging, a direct application of the method can be problematic, especially before/during the arrival of the contrast bolus. During this period, the signal from the myocardium is minimum, and thus leads to large registration errors. This effect has clearly been demonstrated in our simulation data as shown in Figure 3. PLSR is a method for motion prediction where both the input and the output response data contain significant redundancies. In our study, we have used the latter 40% of the total image sequence for learning, since these images have a relatively clear structure for almost all of the anatomy. The predicted deformation distribution has shown to be reliable. This not only reduces the number of frames requiring traditional registration down to 40%, but also significantly improves the consistency of the derived deformation vectors. The study represents the first attempt of using PLSR for deformation modelling, which should have important value for other deformation prediction applications including motion adaptive radiotherapy and imaging, where the deformation of the target organ can be predicted from externally measurable signals.

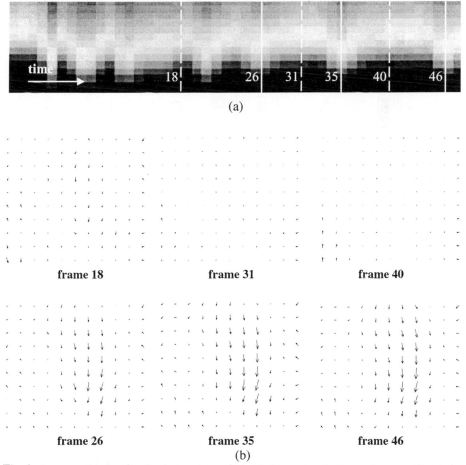

Fig. 2. An example showing the internal correlation between respiration and myocardial deformation. (a) A typical intensity distribution over time obtained from the chest wall and (b) the associated displacement vectors of the myocardium at six different time instants of the perfusion sequence

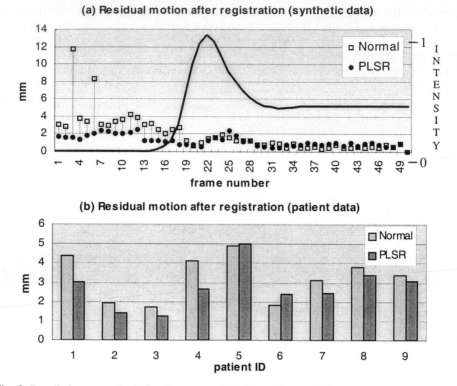

Fig. 3. Detailed error analysis for the proposed PLSR motion modeling approach with (a) synthetically generated perfusion data and (b) first-pass perfusion images from 9 patients with known coronary artery disease

References

1. Wilke N, Simm C, Zhang J, Ellermann J, Ya X, Merkle H, Path G, Ludemann H, Bache RJ, Ugurbil K. Contrast-enhanced first pass myocardial perfusion imaging: correlation between myocardial blood flow in dogs at rest and during hyperemia. *Magn Reson Med.* 1993; 29(4): 485-97.
2. Wilke N, Jerosch-Herold M, Stillman AE, Kroll K, Tsekos N, Merkle H, Parrish T, Hu X, Wang Y, Bassingthwaighte J, et al. Concepts of myocardial perfusion imaging in magnetic resonance imaging. *Magn Reson Q.* 1994; 10(4): 249-86.
3. Keijer JT, van Rossum AC, van Eenige MJ, Karreman AJ, Hofman MB, Valk J, Visser CA. Semiquantitation of regional myocardial blood flow in normal human subjects by first-pass magnetic resonance imaging. *Am Heart J.* 1995; 130:893-901.
4. Schwitter J, Debatin JF, von Schulthess GK, McKinnon GC. Normal myocardial perfusion assessed with multishot echo-planar imaging. *Magn Reson Med.* 1997; 37(1): 140-7.
5. Beache GM, Kulke SF, Kantor HL, Niemi P, Campbell TA, Chesler DA, Gewirtz H, Rosen BR, Brady TJ, Weisskoff RM. Imaging perfusion deficits in ischemic heart disease with susceptibility-enhanced T2-weighted MRI: preliminary human studies. *Magn Reson Imaging.* 1998; 16(1): 19-27.

6. Wilke N, Kroll K, Merkle H, Wang Y, Ishibashi Y, Xu Y, Zhang J, Jerosch-Herold M, Muhler A, Stillman AE, et al. Regional myocardial blood volume and flow: first-pass MR imaging with polylysine-Gd-DTPA. *J Magn Reson Imaging*. 1995; 5(2): 227-37.

7. Larsson HBW, Stubgaard M, Søndergaard L, Henriksen O. In vivo quantification of the unidirectional influx constant for Gd-DTPA diffusion across the myocardial capillaries with MR imaging. *J Magn Reson Imaging*. 1994; 4: 433-40.

8. Cullen JH, Horsfield MA, Reek CR, Cherryman GR, Barnett DB, Samani NJ. A myocardial perfusion reserve index in humans using first-pass contrast-enhanced magnetic resonance imaging. J *Am Coll Cardiol*. 1999; 33: 1386-94.

9. Ablitt N, Gao JX, Gatehouse P, Yang GZ. Motion Decoupling and Registration for 3D Magnetic Resonance Myocardial Perfusion Imaging. International Conference on Computational Science. Amsterdam, The Netherlands, 2002.

10. Delzescaux T, Frouin F, De Cesare A, Philipp-Foliguet S, *et al.* Adaptive and self-evaluating registration method for myocardial perfusion assessment. *Magn Reson Mater Phys Med*. 2001; 13: 28-39.

11. Veeser S, Dunn MJ, Yang GZ. Multiresolution image registration for two-dimensional gel electrophoresis. *Proteomics*. 2001; 1: 856-870.

12. Wold, H. Soft modelling with latent variables: the nonlinear iterative partial least squares approach. Perspectives in probability and Statistics: Papers in honour of M.S. Barlett, (J. Gani, ed). London: Academic Press. 1975: 114-142.

13. Bhupinder S. Dayal, Jhon F. MacGregor. Recursive exponentially weighted PLS and its applications to adaptive control and prediction. *J Proc Cont*. 1997; 7: 169-179.

14. Blanco M, Coello J, Elaamrani M, Iturriaga H, Maspoch S. Partial least-squares regression for the quantitation of pharmaceutical dosages in control analyses. *J Pharm. Biomed Anal*. 1996; 15: 329-338.

Automated Segmentation of the Left and Right Ventricles in 4D Cardiac SPAMM Images

Albert Montillo[1], Dimitris Metaxas[2], and Leon Axel[3]

[1] University Of Pennsylvania, Philadelphia, PA 19104, USA
montillo@seas.upenn.edu
[2] Biomedical Engineering Department, Rutgers University, New Brunswick, NJ 08854 USA
dnm@cs.rutgers.edu
[3] New York University, NY, NY 10016 USA
leon.axel@med.nyu.edu

Abstract. In this paper we describe a completely automated volume-based method for the segmentation of the left and right ventricles in 4D tagged MR (SPAMM) images for quantitative cardiac analysis. We correct the background intensity variation in each volume caused by surface coils using a new scale-based fuzzy connectedness procedure. We apply 3D grayscale opening to the corrected data to create volumes containing only the blood filled regions. We threshold the volumes by minimizing region variance or by an adaptive statistical thresholding method. We isolate the ventricular blood filled regions using a novel approach based on spatial and temporal shape similarity. We use these regions to define the endocardium contours and use them to initialize an active contour that locates the epicardium through the gradient vector flow of an edgemap of a grayscale-closed image. Both quantitative and qualitative results on normal and diseased patients are presented.

1   Introduction

Cardiovascular disease is the leading cause of death in many developed countries. To reduce morbidity, quantifying the motion of the heart is valuable for understanding normal and abnormal physiology and for patient diagnosis. SPAMM [1,2], is a promising non-invasive technique for measuring the shape and motion of the heart. Parallel sheets of tissue are magnetically tagged at end-diastole and they appear as dark lines when imaged in the direction normal to the sheets. This paper presents a completely automated method to find the epicardium and endocardium contours in tagged MR images. The endocardium segmentation is challenging because the tag lines obscure these contours and the images tend to have low contrast between the blood and the myocardium and because the intensities of the tissue change as the tags fade and new blood enters the heart. Epicardium segmentation is challenging because the boundary is occluded by adjacent structures such as the liver or a layer of fat.

Tracking the motion of the tag sheets provides 3D information about the motion of the myocardium and there has been significant research [3-8] into methods for automating tag sheet tracking. These methods are more accurate [3,4] when the epicardium and endocardium contours are provided because the contours restrict the search

T. Dohi and R. Kikinis (Eds.): MICCAI 2002, LNCS 2488, pp. 620–633, 2002.
© Springer-Verlag Berlin Heidelberg 2002

space for tag sheets to the myocardium. Methods that do not use the epicardium and endocardium contours have limited applicability in the thin walled structures such as the RV (right ventricle) where there is a sparsity of tags to track. It has been shown [9] that if the epicardium and endocardium contours could be segmented then measuring the 3D shape deformation in thin walled structures such as the RV becomes possible through finite element analysis. It has also been shown [10-12] that endocardium and epicardium contours can be used in conjunction with tag sheet tracking to determine a low dimensional, clinically relevant description of the motion of the LV (left ventricle). Moreover, the contours help identify and track key anatomical features useful for the inter-subject comparison of strain fields recovered from these tag tracking. The contours can also be used directly to measure ejection fraction, and wall thickening. Several researchers have developed methods for locating the contours of the heart in tagged MR images. The system proposed by Guttman *et al.* [13] was able to delineate the contours of the LV on radially tagged SA (short axis) slices using a dynamic programming method based on a minimum cost algorithm after the user indicated the center of the LV cavity and the region of interest. Goutsias [14] proposed a watershed segmentation method to locate the contours of the LV in SA images. While we have not directly used these techniques due to their inapplicability to our problem, these papers have influenced our work. Our method does not require any user interaction to segment the left and right ventricles. Some of these systems appear to require dark blood. Procedures such as "black blood" imaging add complexity and some time to the image acquisition procedure. Our method does not require this extra step. Another advantage of our method is that it requires only raw SPAMM data acquisition, not CSPAMM data acquisition which can substantially increase acquisition time which is problematic for the patient with cardiac disease, not accustomed to long periods of continual breath holding.

We have found that 80% or 4 of the 5 hours required to analyze tagged SPAMM data sets involves the outlining the contours of the ventricles. We present a method that directly addresses this most significant portion of the analysis time by segmenting the endocardium and epicardium contours without requiring user input. In section 2, we describe how we remove background intensity variation in each volume to prepare the volumes for segmentation. In section 3 and 4 we describe how we locate the heart and segment the endocardium and epicardium in the corrected volumes. We provide qualitative and quantitative results in section 5 and our conclusions in section 6.

2   Volumetric Intensity Correction

Tagged images are acquired mostly with one and sometimes with two surface coils. While the coils increase image contrast, they can also cause the same tissue to have different intensities depending on its location in the image. We use a new scale-based correction procedure to correct the background intensity variation throughout each volume. A variety of techniques have been employed to correct background intensity variation in MRI, few meet the following requirements that make them clinically useful: (1) no user input is needed on a per volume basis (2) the method is pulse sequence and surface coil independent (3) intensity distributions for tissue classes need not be known. Details on this method, including its performance on non-cardiac images can be found in [15]. We present an overview of the method and a modification that works well for all of the subjects that we have processed. We have found empirically that iterating the steps below 10 times works well for all subjects. Fig. 1 shows a sample slice from a corrected volume.

1. Given a volume $f(\bar{x})$, define the foreground volume as:

$$f_{foreground}(\bar{x}) = \begin{cases} 1 & f(\bar{x}) > mean\ (f(\bar{x})) \\ 0 & otherwise \end{cases}$$

2. Compute the scale volume $f_{scale}(\bar{x})$ for the pixels where $f_{foreground}(\bar{x})=1$. Scale at a pixel is defined as the radius of the largest ball centered at the pixel for which a pixel intensity homogeneity measure [15] is preserved.

3. Let S_{max} be the maximum value in $f_{scale}(\bar{x})$ and let the set *PixelsOfSmax* be the set of all pixels in the scale image that have a scale of S_{max}. Compute the mean μ and standard deviation σ of the intensities in $f(\bar{x})$ for the pixels of *PixelsOfSmax*. Let the set *objectPixels* be the set of pixels in the volume that have intensities in the interval $[\mu - \alpha\sigma, \mu + \beta\sigma]$. For tagged MR, the objects we are most interested in correcting are the bright objects (the myocardium and blood regions) and we find empirically that setting $\alpha = 1.0$ and $\beta = 5.0$ works well for all subjects.

4. To estimate the background intensity variation, a 2nd order polynomial $\beta(\bar{x})$ is fitted to the normalized intensities in *objectPixels* by minimizing
$$\sum_{v \in objectPixels}[\beta(v) - f(v)/\mu_{objectPixels}]^2$$

5. In MRI, background intensity variation is typically modeled as multiplicative noise, therefore image is corrected by replacing $f(\bar{x})$ with $f(\bar{x})\big/\beta(\bar{x})$.

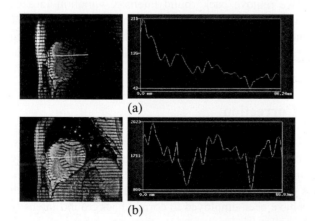

(a)

(b)

Fig. 1. 1D intensity profiles are plotted for the white lines shown in the images: (a) before correction (b) after correction. Intensity through the heart is much more uniform after correction; the two prominent intensity valleys are caused from the sampling line skimming two tags which remain dark after correction

3   Endocardium Segmentation

The endocardium contours are the boundaries between the blood filled ventricular cavities and the myocardium. To locate these boundaries reliably we look for strong image features that are present for every subject. Since we are not using "black blood" imaging, the blood appears bright and we leverage this fact to accurately locate the salient blood filled cavities of the LV and RV and the inflow and outflow tracts of the RV. In all our images from the second time (second volume) the motion of the blood has washed out the tags. We begin our endocardium segmentation in this volume by applying a 3D grayscale morphological opening operation. Let the given volume be $f(\overline{x})$ where $\overline{x}$ is an element of the domain of $f : \overline{x} \in D_f$ and let the structuring element be $b(\overline{x})$ where $\overline{x} \in D_b$. Then the gray-scale opening of f by b is written as $f \circ b = (f - b) \oplus b$ where $f - b$ is the gray-scale erosion of f by b defined in eqn (1a) and $f \oplus b$ is the gray-scale dilation of f by b defined in eqn (1b)

(a) $(f - b)(\overline{s}) = \min \left\{ f(\overline{s} + \overline{x}) - b(\overline{x}) \mid \overline{s} + \overline{x} \in D_f ; \overline{x} \in D_b \right\}$ (1)

(b) $(f \oplus b)(\overline{s}) = \max \left\{ f(\overline{s} - \overline{x}) + b(\overline{x}) \mid \overline{s} - \overline{x} \in D_f ; \overline{x} \in D_b \right\}$

The intensity value at a pixel $\overline{x}$ in the opened volume is the maximum of the minimum values in the pixels covered by the structuring element when centered at $\overline{x}$. We use a binary 3D cylinder shaped structuring element whose radius, R1, is 1.5 times the tag separation width and whose length L1 spans 4 image planes. We have found that this structuring element gives the best initial segmentation of the blood filled regions of the images. The radius is sufficient to cover at least 2 tags; therefore even if noise has corrupted one tag, the other tag covered by the structuring element will enable the opening result to reflect the presence of tags. Fig. 2b shows sample slices from the opening of a volume at time 2.

An important advantage in this cavity-locating method is that it can be applied without change in all the slices through the heart. For example the bifurcation of the right ventricle into inflow and outflow tracts can be located (see first column in Fig. 4d). In slices through the tip of the apex (not shown), a blood filled region is detected only if present. This property is important since in some subjects the apex of the LV cavity is inferior to the apex of the RV cavity, while for other subjects the reverse is true. We note that this gray-scale opening based method can detect whether there are blood filled regions are present –down to the size of the structuring element used in the opening operation. For our images this is rarely a significant limitation since the tags are closely spaced (6 pixel spacing), yielding a small-diameter structuring element.

Next, we threshold the images and fill the holes with a binary morphological closing operation. To select the threshold in this initial time, we use the threshold that minimizes the variance of the pixels grouped into the foreground object. The results of thresholding these images are shown in Fig. 2c.

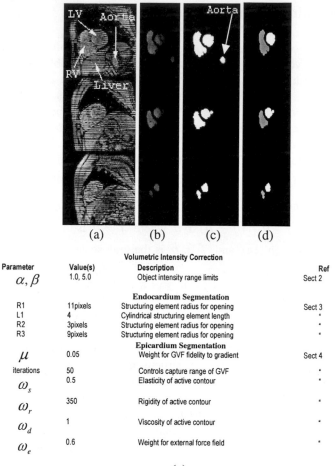

(a)   (b)   (c)   (d)

Parameter	Value(s)	Description	Ref
		Volumetric Intensity Correction	
α, β	1.0, 5.0	Object intensity range limits	Sect 2
		Endocardium Segmentation	
R1	11pixels	Structuring element radius for opening	Sect 3
L1	4	Cylindrical structuring element length	"
R2	3pixels	Structuring element radius for opening	"
R3	9pixels	Structuring element radius for opening	"
		Epicardium Segmentation	
μ	0.05	Weight for GVF fidelity to gradient	Sect 4
iterations	50	Controls capture range of GVF	"
ω_s	0.5	Elasticity of active contour	"
ω_r	350	Rigidity of active contour	"
ω_d	1	Viscosity of active contour	"
ω_e	0.6	Weight for external force field	"

(e)

Fig. 2. Steps to find the endocardium (a) 3 slices from original volume (b) grayscale opened volume (c) thresholded volume (d) pruned volume using shape similarity. Note the aorta has been pruned away. (e) Algorithm parameters

To identify which of these binary regions are from the ventricles, we first find the binary regions corresponding to the LV and RV on a *mid-ventricular* slice. To identify a mid ventricular slice, as well as the pair of regions forming the LV and RV cavities on that slice, *we find the most spatially consistent pair of regions*. We describe this measure formally with the following definitions and the accompanying drawing (Fig 3a).

We are given a short axis dataset consisting of a set V of N volumes: $V = \{v_k\}$ where $k \in [1..N]$ Each volume consists of a set S of M slices: $S = \{s_j\}$ where $j \in [1..M]$. After thresholding a morphologically opened volume, the jth slice on the kth frame consists of a set R of B(j,k) regions $R = \{r_i\}$ where $i \in [1..B(j,k)]$.

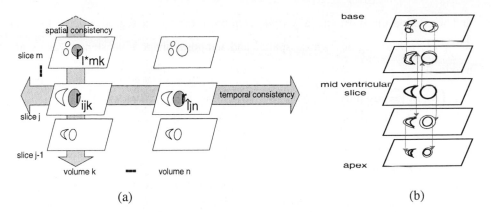

(a)   (b)

Fig. 3. (a) For a given region r_{ijk} , the regions on slice m in volume k are searched to find the most spatially similar region r_{l^*mk} . The regions on slice j in volume n are searched to find the most temporally similar region, $r_{\tilde{l}jn}$ (b) Orthographic projection to form the LV and RV cavities

We define the similarity in eqn 2., as in [16]. The similarity between region r_{ijk} (the ith region on the jth slice of the kth volume) and the region r_{ljm} (the lth region on the mth slice of the nth volume) is

$$Sim\left(r_{ijk}, r_{lmn}\right) = \frac{area\left(\cap\left\{r_{ijk}, r_{lmn}\right\}\right)}{area\left(\cup\left\{r_{ijk}, r_{lmn}\right\}\right)} \qquad (2)$$

the area of their intersection divided by the area of their union. For a given region r_{ijk} the most similar region r_{l^*mk} spatially and the most similar region $r_{\tilde{l}jn}$ temporally are defined as:

$$r_{l^*mk} = \operatorname*{arg\,max}_{l\in B(m,k),\, m\neq j} Sim\left(r_{ijk}, r_{lmk}\right) \qquad r_{\tilde{l}jn} = \operatorname*{arg\,max}_{l\in B(j,n),\, n\neq k} Sim\left(r_{ijk}, r_{ljn}\right) \qquad (3)$$

To find the LV or the RV on the mid ventricular slice we define the *spatial shape consistency* and *temporal shape consistency* of a region r_{ijk} as:

$$ssc\left(r_{ijk}\right) = \sum_{m=1,\, m\neq j}^{M} Sim\left(r_{ijk}, r_{l^*mk}\right) \qquad tsc\left(r_{ijk}\right) = \sum_{n=1,\, n\neq k}^{N} Sim\left(r_{ijk}, r_{\tilde{l}jn}\right) \qquad (4)$$

To find the **pair** of LV and RV regions on the mid ventricular slice we define the spatially *consistent* region pair $\left(r_{\tilde{i}jk}, r_{\tilde{l}jk}\right)$ as:

$$\left(r_{\tilde{i}jk}, r_{\tilde{l}jk}\right) = \operatorname*{arg\,max}_{\substack{j\in[1..M]\\ i,l\in B(j,k),\, i\neq l}} \left\{ssc\left(r_{ijk}\right) + ssc\left(r_{ljk}\right)\right\} \qquad (5)$$

and we define the most spatially *and* temporally consistent region *pair* as the pair $\left(r_{\widetilde{ijk}}, r_{\widetilde{ljk}}\right)$ of regions whose spatial and temporal shape consistency values are maximal:

$$\left(r_{\widetilde{ijk}}, r_{\widetilde{ljk}}\right) = \arg \max_{\substack{j \in [1..M] \\ k \in [1..N] \\ i,l \in B(j,k),\ i \neq l}} \left\{ ssc\left(r_{ijk}\right) + tsc\left(r_{ijk}\right) \ + \ ssc\left(r_{ljk}\right) + tsc\left(r_{ljk}\right)\right\} \tag{6}$$

The RV bifurcates at the base of the heart into inflow and outflow tracts and has a tapered lobe below the base, while the cavity of the LV resembles a prolate spheroid cropped at the top. Consequently, in the thresholded images, three regions appear in the base (RV inflow and outflow tracts and the LV cavity), two relatively large regions appear in the mid-ventricular images and two small regions appear near the apex. Because of these characteristics, the most spatially consistent region pair in the thresholded images is the pair of regions from the mid ventricular slice from the LV and RV. The LV and RV regions near the apex are too small to be the most spatially consistent pair and the inflow and outflow tracks at the base prevent the base slices from being the slice containing the most consistent pair. In addition the regions from the aorta are not part of the most spatially consistent pair because they receive low spatial shape consistency scores because the aorta does not run throughout the whole short axis volume and because the aorta is typically not oriented perpendicular to the short axis image planes. Regions from the blurring of tags due to motion artifacts, which can appear on an individual slice, are also not in the most spatially consistent pair because they do not extend throughout the short axis volume.

The mid-ventricular slice is the slice with the pair of most spatially consistent regions. We attach the regions in the superior and inferior slices that have sufficient intersection with these pairs. We determine which regions overlap through orthographic projection. To form the **base** volume of the cavities, we project the regions on the current slice (initially the mid ventricular slice) up to the next slice orthographically (see Fig 3b). *The regions that overlap are connected to the regions from the previous slice*. To form the **apical** volume of the cavities, we project the regions on the current slice (initially the mid ventricular slice) down to the next slice orthographically and the regions that overlap are connected to the regions from the previous slice. The boundaries of the cavities define the boundary between the blood and the myocardium and thereby yield the endocardium.

For subsequent times we begin the processing by opening the volumes with the 3D structuring element described above. To choose a threshold for the opened images, we use the segmentation map from the prior time. As shown in Fig. 4 (a)-(c), the endocardium regions found in the previous time are propagated onto the grayscale-opened image of the current time.

The ventricular cavity regions on the mid-ventricular slice (Fig 4a) from the previous volume are eroded by a disk of radius 3 pixels and their boundaries are propagated to the same slice on the next volume. We estimate the mean intensity of the pixels in the *blood region* on the opened image by computing the mean of the intensities of the pixels in this region (Fig. 4b). To compute the mean of the intensity of the *myocardium* portion of the opened volume we form a ring shaped sampling region by *dilating* the LV endocardium region from the previous volume's mid ventricular slice by a disk of radius, R4 of 3 pixels and a disk of radius, R3 of 9 pixels. This band is propagated to the same slice on the next volume and is located roughly in the center of the myocardium of the LV (Fig. 4c).

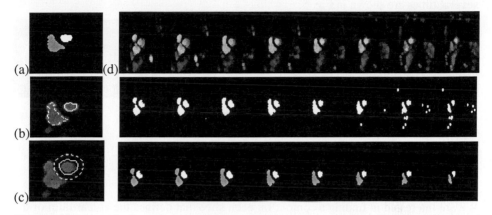

Fig. 4. (a) Mid ventricular regions from the previous time. Contours from these two regions are used to delineate regions on the same slice for the current time to sample blood tissue, [the regions inside the contours in (b)] and to sample the myocardium [using the region in between the contours in (c)]. In (d) the endocardium processing steps are shown for all slices for one time. First row: opened images. Second row: results from adaptive thresholding. Third row: results from shape similarity pruning

We identified which region was the LV from the pair of regions on the mid ventricular slice in the previous volume by noting which orthographically connected region bifurcated in the base (the RV bifurcates) or if neither has then the LV is identified as the region which has a smaller volume above the mid ventricular slice. In our datasets this provides an accurate determination of the RV and LV because the RV is typically larger than the LV and the RV volume includes the inflow and outflow tracks. Also it is important to use our knowledge of the mid ventricular slice: propagating contours from the mid ventricular slice to the same slice on the next volume works well, however if we propagated contours from a base slice to the same slice on the next volume, topological changes in the RV (see Fig. 5) can render the blood intensity sampling less accurate.

The opened images from the current time are then thresholded with the mean of the mean intensities of the blood and myocardium tags: $\delta_{thresh}=(\mu_{blood}+\mu_{myo})/2$. We have found that this threshold selection method compares well with thresholds selected manually by selecting an intensity at a valley between peaks in the histogram of the opened image. Moreover the intensity inhomogeneity correction step described in the previous section makes the intensities of tissues within each volume more uniform and improves the results of thresholding the opened images using a threshold from the mid ventricular slice. Once we have thresholded the opened volume we compute the most *spatially and temporally* consistent binary region pair in the slices of each volumes processed thus far and attach the regions in the superior and inferior slices as described above. Since the base moves toward the apex, the mid-ventricular slice can change over time. By using both temporal consistency and spatial consistency we are able to update the mid-ventricular slice to be the slice that contains the pair of regions that change the least over time and throughout the imaged volume. The results for several times are shown in Fig. 5.

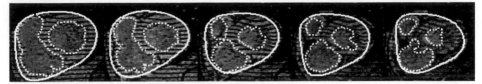

Fig. 5. All endocardium contours (dashed) and epicardium contours (solid) over time 2 through end ES (end systole) for a particular slice near the base

4   Epicardium Segmentation

We are interested in finding a contour on each slice that defines the epicardium of the heart, which is the boundary between the myocardium and the tissues that surround the heart. The epicardium is typically harder to segment than the endocardium because there is little contrast between the myocardium and surrounding tagged structures, such as the liver and the chest wall. Fat often appears as a partial ring of tissue surrounding the heart and is particularly challenging to handle since the ring is narrow. Fat is often included in the myocardium in methods that attempt to segment the endocardium in tagged MR images. Here we present an automatic method that largely overcomes this problem by expanding a physics-based deformable model known as an active contour [17] from the interior of the heart towards the exterior edge of the myocardium so that it will stop when it gets to the dark pixels between the myocardium and fat.

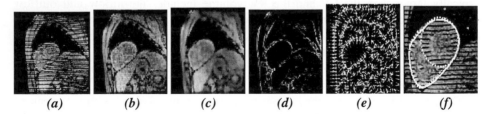

(a)   (b)   (c)   (d)   (e)   (f)

Fig. 6. Epicardium segmentation steps: (a) original image (b) grayscale closing (c) adaptive Wiener filtering (d) edge map (e) gradient vector flow field (f) Segmented LV-RV epicardium (single *solid* line) and separate, manual RV and LV epicardium (*dotted* lines)

We fill the tags in each slice at each time with a linear structuring element whose width is equal to the tag width. In our images the structuring element is 4 pixels and the filled images are shown in Fig. 6(b). This fills in all the tags while leaving most borders intact. Next we adaptively Wiener filter the filled images to smooth the intensities of the myocardium while preserving edges. We apply less filtering where the local intensity variance is large and greater filtering where the local variance is small. Fig. 6(c) shows the result, which we will refer to as $f(x, y)$. The magnitude of the gradient of this image, with edges in the endocardium regions found in section 3 suppressed, is shown Fig. 6(d). We compute a gradient vector flow (GVF) [18] field (see Fig 6(e)) from ∇f to provide forces for the deformable model. The GVF field captures object boundaries from either side and consists of a 2D vector field $\bar{v}(x, y) = (u(x, y), v(x, y))^T$ that minimizes the energy in eqn 7a. The PDE (eqn 7b) that minimizes this functional is found through the calculus of variations and the equilibrium solution to this equation defines the flow field.

(a) $E(\bar{v}) = \iint \mu\left(u_x^2 + u_y^2 + v_x^2 + v_y^2\right) + |\nabla f|^2 |\bar{v} - \nabla f|^2 dxdy$ (7)

(b) $\bar{v}_t = \mu\nabla^2\bar{v} - |\nabla f|^2 (\bar{v} - \nabla f)$

(c) $u_t = \frac{1}{\Delta t}\left(u_{i,j}^{n+1} - u_{i,j}^n\right)$ $\nabla^2 u = \frac{1}{\Delta x \Delta y}\left(u_{i+1,j} + u_{i,j+1} + u_{i-1,j} + u_{i,j-1} - 4u_{i,j}\right)$

We favor strong fidelity of the GVF field to ∇f since there are weak edges between the heart and liver that we want to capture with the active contour. We have found that setting $\mu = 0.05$ works well to segment the epicardium. To form an initial epicardium contour for our physics-based deformable model we construct the convex hull of the RV and LV regions from the previous section. We have found that using discrete approximations shown in eqn. 7c to the partial derivatives in eqn. 7b with $\Delta t = \Delta x = \Delta y = 1$ and iterating a forward Euler finite difference scheme 50 times is sufficient to extend the capture range of the initial active contour to segment the epicardium.

Our physics-based deformable active contour, $X(s)$, is parameterized by arc length and deforms according to Newton's second law (eqn. 8a). To stop at weak edges we set the mass, m, of the contour to zero. The governing motion equation (eqn. 8b) is formed by defining the internal force from the stretching and bending of the semi-rigid contour and the external force from the gradient vector flow field, $\bar{v}$.

(a) $m\dfrac{\partial^2 X}{\partial t^2} = F_{dampening}(X) + F_{internal}(X) + F_{external}(X)$ (8)

(b) $\underbrace{\omega_d \dfrac{\partial X}{\partial t}}_{-F_{dampening}} = \underbrace{\dfrac{\partial}{\partial s}\left(\omega_s \dfrac{\partial X}{\partial s}\right) + \dfrac{\partial^2}{\partial s^2}\left(\omega_r \dfrac{\partial^2 X}{\partial s^2}\right)}_{F_{internal}} + \underbrace{\omega_e \bar{v}(X)}_{F_{external}}$

The parameters used to control the deformable model are: elasticity $\omega_s = 0.5$, rigidity $\omega_r = 350$, viscosity $\omega_d = 1$ and external force field weight $\omega_e = 0.6$. We have found these values work well on all of our tests for both normal and diseased hearts. We approximate the derivatives with finite differences and iterate a forward Euler finite difference scheme until the contour converges. We define convergence to occur when the contour area has not changed appreciably (1 pixel area) over the last 10 iterations. In all our tests convergence occurs within 85 iterations. In Fig 7(a)-(e) we see that our approach has avoided classifying the ring of fat which appears near the top of the epicardium as myocardium. In Fig. 7(a),(c) the triangular shaped fat region which appears near the bottom left corner of the epicardium has also been excluded from the myocardium.

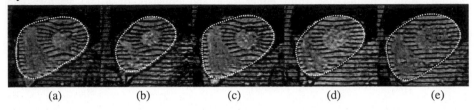

(a)   (b)   (c)   (d)   (e)

Fig. 7. The expansion of an initial active contour from inside the heart avoids classifying a surrounding layer of fat as myocardium

5   Results

Our method finds the bi-ventricular boundaries throughout the volume of the heart and over time during contraction, starting at end-diastole. We have a database of over 15 subjects with diseases affecting the left and right ventricles and normal subjects. We explain the analysis results on 3 of these subjects, two of whom are normal and one has right ventricular hypertrophy. Below we provide both qualitative and quantitative evidence of the accuracy and robustness of our tracking method.

For qualitative validation we compare the segmented bi-ventricular boundaries to those drawn by expert cardiologists (see Fig. 8a-d). These boundaries are shown for several slices at time 2 and time ES. By superimposing both boundaries over the images and enlarging them we find convincing evidence of the accuracy of our algorithm. We have also discovered cases (see Fig. 8e) in which the cardiologists have found our algorithm to be more accurate than those drawn by hand, causing us to have the anatomists revise the ground truth contours.

For quantitative validation we compute the distance between each segmented contour A and the corresponding contour, B, drawn by the expert anatomist by computing the distance $d(a, B) = \min_{b \in B} \|a - b\|$ for all points a on the automatic contour. We also compute $d(b, A)$ for the points, b on the expert contours. Fig. 9 shows the cumulative distribution of these error distances for the contour points over all slices in all volumes from ED (end diastole) to ES (end systole) for the normal and diseased subjects comprising over 175 images. To validate the segmented RV endocardium we use the full manually drawn RV endocardium and the portion of the LV epicardium that delineates the septum. Likewise during validation of the segmented single epicardium contour we use the full manual RV epicardium contour and the portion of the LV epicardium corresponding to the non-septum boundary. It can be seen (Fig. 9) that on the average the distance error of our segmented epicardium contour is less than 1.2 pixels and that 90% of the time the error is less than 4.1 pixels. The endocardium contours are still quite accurate although our contours include the papillary muscle in the myocardium while the manually drawn contours have excluded them, thus the "error" distance is larger. For the RV endocardium we still find though that on the average the distances are less than 2.3 pixels and 90% of the time the segmented contour is within 6.5 pixels of the expert's contour.

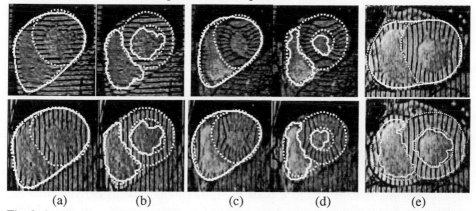

(a)   (b)   (c)   (d)   (e)

Fig. 8. Qualitative validation: segmented contours (solid lines), manual contours (dotted lines). Epicardium (a) and endocardium (b) contours from two slices at time 2. Epicardium (c) and endocardium (d) contours from the same two slices at time ES. Note that our algorithm finds one epicardium contour while two manual contours (LV and RV epicardium contours have been drawn). Also our algorithm includes papillary muscle in the myocardium while the manual contour excludes it. Shown in (e) top row is a case in which our *algorithm was more accurate* than manual contours along the RV. Bottom row: endocardium contours segmenting the papillary muscle

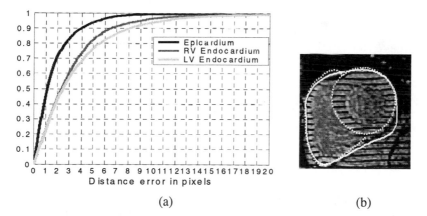

(a)   (b)

Fig. 9. (a) Cumulative distribution of distances errors between the corresponding portions of the expert manual contours and the segmented contours from all slices, in all volumes, from ED through ES. (b) Occasionally the *epicardium boundary* is too weak after the tags are filled via the morphological closing. Then the active contour can expand beyond the myocardium, so we are developing ways to correct this case (see text)

There is still room for improvement. Our quantitative results *include* time 1 (end-diastole). For this volume the tags have not washed away completely so we have used the endocardium contours from time 2 and used them to initialize our active contour that *locates* the epicardium at time 1. Using an active contour for both the endocardium segmentation (using the grayscale opened images) and the epicardium segmentation will enable us to estimate the velocity of the endocardium contour relative to the epicardium contour. Inverting the motion will give us an *improved* endocardium estimate for time 1. We are also experimenting with improved edge sensitivity that can handle the occasional leakage (see Fig 9b) of the epicardium contour into the liver.

6   Conclusions

We have presented a method that dramatically reduces the most significant portion of the analysis time required to process SPAMM data. All of the steps in our algorithm are completely automated, requiring no user input. The contours can be used to measure ejection fraction and as a basis to register motion fields derived from tag tracking algorithms which enables effective inter-subject comparison of motion data. The algorithm removes background intensity variation throughout each imaged volume using a new scale based intensity correction method and implements a novel region-based segmentation technique to segment the ventricular blood filled volumes and the LV and RV endocardium contours. We have also located the inflow and outflow tracts of the right ventricle automatically and obtained excellent epicardium results through a combination of adaptive local statistics-based image filtering, a gradient vector flow field and physics-based active contours.

References

1. L. Axel, L. Dougherty, "Heart wall motion: improved method of spatial modulation of magnetization for MR imaging", Radiology, 172, 349-350
2. E. Zerhouni, D. Parish, W. Rogers, et al, "Human heart: tagging with MR imaging-a method for non-invasive assessment of myocardial motion", Radiology, 169, 59-63
3. D. Kraitchman, A. Young, C. Chang, L. Axel, "Semi-automated tracking of myocardial motion in MR tagged images", IEEE Transactions on Medical Imaging, 14, 422-433, 1995
4. Young, "Model Tags: Direct 3D tracking of heart wall motion from tagged magnetic resonance images." Medical Image Analysis. 3:361-372, 1999
5. T. Denney, Jr., "Estimation and Detection of Myocardial Tags in MR images without User Defined Myocardial Contours", IEEE Transactions on Medical Imaging, 1999
6. N. Osman, W. Kerwin, E. McVeigh, and J. Prince, "Cardiac Motion Tracking Using CINE Harmonic Phase (HARP) Magnetic Resonance Imaging" Technical Report JHU/ECE 99-3, Electrical and Computer Eng., Johns Hopkins Univ.

7. W. Kerwin, N. Osman, J. Prince, "Ch 24: Image Processing and Analysis in Tagged Cardiac MRI", Handbook of Medical Imaging: Processing and Analysis, Editor-in-chief I. Bankman, 2000

8. Y. Chen, A. Amini, "A MAP Framework for Tag Line Detection in SPAMM Data Using Markov Random Fields on the B-Spline Solid", IEEE Workshop on Mathematical Methods in Biomedical Image Analysis, Dec 2001

9. Haber, "Three-dimensional motion reconstruction and analysis of the right ventricle from planar tagged MRI", Univ. of Penn. PhD Thesis, 2000

10. J.Park, D.Metaxas, A. Young, L. Axel, "Deformable models with Parameter Functions for Cardiac Motion Analysis" IEEE Transactions on Medical Imaging, Vol. 15, No 3, June 1996

11. J. Declerck, N. Ayache, E. McVeigh, "Use of a 4d Planispheric Transformation for the Tracking and Analysis of LV Motion with Tagged MR Images", 1999

12. Ozturk C, E. McVeigh, "Four Dimensional B-spline Based Motion Analysis of Tagged Cardiac MR Images", Proc. SPIE Medical Imaging 99, San Diego, CA, Feb 1999.

13. M. Guttman, J. Prince, E. McVeigh, "Tag and Contour Detection in Tagged MR Images of the Left Ventricle", IEEE transactions on Medical Imaging, 13(1): 74-88, 1994

14. J. Goutsias, S. Batman, "Ch 4: Morphological Methods for Biomedical Image Analysis", Editors M. Sonka, J Fitzpatrick, Handbook of Medical Imaging, Vol. 2. Medical Imaging Processing and Analysis, pp 255-263, SPIE, 2000

15. Y. Zhuge, J. Udupa, J. Liu, P. Saha, T. Iwanaga, "A Scale-Based Method for Correcting Background Intensity Variation in Acquired Images", SPIE Proceedings, 2002

16. R. Dann, J. Hoford, S. Kovacic, M. Reivich, R. Bajcsy, "Evaluation of Elastic Matching System for Anatomic (CT, MR) and Functional (PET) Cerebral Images", J. of Computer Assisted Tomography, 13(4) 603-611 July/August, 1989

17. M. Kass, A. Witkin, D. Terzopoulos, "Snakes: Active contour models", International Journal of Computer Vision, 2:321-331, 1988

18. Xu, J. Prince, "Generalized Gradient Vector Flow External Forces for Active Contours", Signal Processing 71, pp 131-139, 1998

Stochastic Finite Element Framework for Cardiac Kinematics Function and Material Property Analysis

Pengcheng Shi and Huafeng Liu

Biomedical Research Laboratory
Department of Electrical and Electronic Engineering
Hong Kong University of Science and Technology
Clear Water Bay, Kowloon, Hong Kong
{pengcheng.shi,eeliuhf}@ust.hk

Abstract. A stochastic finite element method (SFEM) based framework is proposed for the simultaneous estimation of cardiac kinematics functions and material model parameters. While existing biomechanics studies of myocardial material constitutive laws have assumed known kinematics, and image analyses of cardiac kinematics have relied on chosen constraining models (mathematical or mechanical), we believe that a probabilistic strategy is needed to achieve robust and optimal estimates of kinematics functions and material parameters at the same time. For a particular *a priori* patient-dependent constraining material model with uncertain parameters and *a posteriori* noisy observations, stochastic differential equations are combined with the finite element method. The material parameters and the imaging/image-derived data are treated as random variables with known prior statistics in the dynamic system equations of the heart. In our current implementation, extended Kalman filter (EKF) procedures are adopted to linearize the equations and to provide the joint estimates. Because of the periodic nature of the cardiac dynamics, we conclude experimentally that it is possible to adopt this physical-model based optimal estimation approach to achieve converged estimates. Results from canine MR phase contrast images with linear elastic model are presented.

1 Introduction

Myocardial dynamics can be stated by the following material parameter dependent differential equation:

$$\Phi(q, u(q)) = \Pi(u(q)) \tag{1}$$

with constraining mechanical model parameters q, kinematics states $u(q)$, system differential operators Φ, and loads Π. With this dynamic system, finite element method (FEM) has been used as a natural framework for the biomechanics studies of myocardium material constitutive laws with observations/measurements on the kinematics states [4, 6], and physically motivated image analyses of cardiac kinematics properties with assumed mechanical models [2, 9].

T. Dohi and R. Kikinis (Eds.): MICCAI 2002, LNCS 2488, pp. 634–641, 2002.

In biomechanics studies, the kinematics of the heart tissues is assumed known from implanted markers or imaging means. The issue is then to use these kinematics observations to estimate material parameters of the constitutive laws. While most works deal with regional finite deformations measured at isolated locations [4], MR tagging has been used more recently for the *in vivo* study of the mechanics of the entire heart. In [6], unknown material parameters were determined for an exponential strain energy function that maximized the agreement between observed (from MR tagging) and predicted (from FEM modeling) regional wall strains. However, it is well recognized that the recovery of kinematics from MR tagging or other imaging techniques is not a solved problem yet, and constraining models of mechanical nature may be needed to for the kinematics recovery in the first place [2].

In image-based analyses of cardiac kinematics functions, assumptions must be made about the myocardial behavior in order to constrain the ill-posed problem for a unique solution [2]. These constraining models could be either mathematically motivated regularization such as in [7], or continuum mechanics based energy minimization such as in [9]. Conjugate to biomechanics efforts, image analysis works are based on the premise that material or other model properties are known as prior information, and the issue is to use these models to estimate kinematics parameters in some optimal sense. The selection of an appropriate model with proper parameters largely determines the quality of the analysis results. Yet, for any given data, the precise or even reasonable material/mathematical models and parameters are usually not readily known *a priori*.

In this paper, we present a stochastic finite element framework for the simultaneous estimation of the cardiac kinematics functions and the material constitutive parameters from image sequence. Given the uncertainty of the material properties for a particular patient and the noisy nature of the imaging data, we believe that a probabilistic strategy is needed to achieve robust and optimal estimates for a particular *a priori* constraining model with uncertain parameters and *a posteriori* noisy observations. Coupling stochastic modeling of the myocardium with finite element method, we can now deal with noisy imaging/imaging-derived data and uncertain constraining material parameters in a coordinated effort. Because of the periodic nature of the cardiac behavior, we will show experimentally that it is possible to adopt this physical model based statistical estimation approach to achieve converged estimates.

2   Methodology

2.1   Stochastic Finite Element Method

Stochastic finite element method (SFEM) has been used for structural dynamics analyses in probabilistic frameworks [1]. In SFEM, structural material properties are described by random fields, possibly with known prior statistics, and the observations and loads are corrupted by noises. Hence, stochastic differential dynamics equations are combined with the finite element method to study the dynamic structures with uncertainty in their parameters and measurements.

2.2   Stochastic Dynamic Equation

For computational feasibility, our current implementation assumes temporally constant linear elasticity of the myocardium with varying spatial distributions of the Young's modulus and the Poisson's ratio. We derive the myocardial dynamics equation within a finite element framework to be:

$$M\ddot{U} + C\dot{U} + KU = R \tag{2}$$

with M, C and K the mass, damping and stiffness matrices, R the load vector, and U the displacement vector. M is a known function of material density and is temporally and spatially constant. K is a function of the material constitutive law (the strain-stress relationship), and is related to the material-specific Young's modulus E and Poisson's ratio ν, which can vary temporally and spatially. In our framework, these two local parameters are treated as random variables with known a *priori* statistics for any given data, and are needed to be estimated along with the kinematics functions (in this paper, we do not consider the temporal dependency of the material parameters). C is frequency dependent, and we assume Rayleigh damping with $C = \alpha M + \beta K$. Equation (2) is a stochastic differential equation in nature per Ito's calculus.

2.3   State Space Model

The above dynamics equation can be transformed into a state-space representation of a continuous-time linear stochastic system:

$$\dot{x}(t) = A_c(\theta)x(t) + B_c w(t) \tag{3}$$

where the material parameter vector θ, the state vector x, the system matrices A_c and B_c, and the control (input) term w are:

$$\theta = \begin{bmatrix} E \\ \nu \end{bmatrix}, \quad x(t) = \begin{bmatrix} U(t) \\ \dot{U}(t) \end{bmatrix}, \quad w(t) = \begin{bmatrix} 0 \\ R \end{bmatrix},$$

$$A_c = \begin{bmatrix} 0 & I \\ -M^{-1}K & -M^{-1}C \end{bmatrix}, \quad B_c = \begin{bmatrix} 0 & 0 \\ 0 & M^{-1} \end{bmatrix}$$

Meanwhile, the observed imaging/imaging-derived data $y(t)$ can be expressed in the measurement equation:

$$y(t) = Dx(t) + e(t) \tag{4}$$

where D is a known measurement matrix, and $e(t)$ is the measurement noise which is additive, zero mean, and white ($E[e(t)] = 0, E[e(t)e(s)'] = R_e(t)\delta_{ts}$).

In our case, Equations (3) and (4) describe a continuous-time system with discrete-time measurements (the imaging/imaging-derived data), or a so-called sampled data system. The input is computed from the system equation, and is piecewise constant over the sampling interval T. Thus, we arrive at the system equations [3]:

$$x((k+1)T) = Ax(kT) + Bw(kT) \tag{5}$$

$$A = e^{A_c T}, \quad B = A_c^{-1}(e^{A_c T} - I)B_c \tag{6}$$

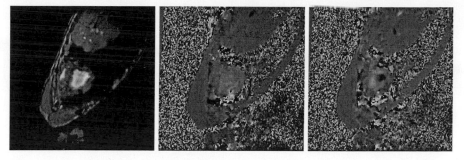

Fig. 1. Canine MR phase contrast images: magnitude (left), x-velocity (middle), and y-velocity (right).

For general continuous-time system with discrete-time measurements, including the additive, zero-mean, white process noise v ($E[v(t)] = 0, E[v(t)v(s)'] = Q_v(t)\delta_{ts}$, independent of $e(t)$), we have the following state equation:

$$x(t+1) = A(\theta)x(t) + B(\theta)w(t) + v(t) \tag{7}$$

2.4 Extended Kalman Filter for Joint State and Parameter Identification

We can then augment the state vector x by the material parameter vector θ to form the new state vector $z = [x \ \theta]^T$, and from Equations (4) and (7) we have the following pair of augmented state/measurement equations:

$$z(t+1) = \begin{bmatrix} A(\theta)x(t) + B(\theta)w(t) \\ \theta \end{bmatrix} + \begin{bmatrix} v(t) \\ 0 \end{bmatrix} = f(z(t), w(t)) + \begin{bmatrix} v(t) \\ 0 \end{bmatrix} \tag{8}$$

$$y(t) = \begin{bmatrix} D \ 0 \end{bmatrix} \begin{bmatrix} x(t) \\ \theta(t) \end{bmatrix} + \begin{bmatrix} e(t) \\ 0 \end{bmatrix} = h(z(t)) + \begin{bmatrix} e(t) \\ 0 \end{bmatrix} \tag{9}$$

The joint state and parameter estimation problem can be understood as a state estimation problem for a nonlinear system, and this form of formulation leads to a solution of the filtering problem based on continuous-system-discrete-measurement extended Kalman filter (EKF) framework, which is based on linearization of the augmented state equations at each time step. A recursive procedure with natural block structure is used to perform the joint state (kinematics) and parameter (material) estimation, and a general analysis of the convergence of the algorithm can be found in [5]:

$$\hat{x}(t+1) = A(\hat{\theta}(t))\hat{x}(t) + B(\hat{\theta}(t))w(t) + L(t)\left[y(t) - D\hat{x}(t)\right] \tag{10}$$

$$\hat{\theta}(t+1) = \hat{\theta}(t) + G(t)\left[y(t) - D\hat{x}(t)\right] \tag{11}$$

$$\hat{x}(0) = \hat{x}_0, \quad \hat{\theta}(0) = \hat{\theta}_0 \tag{12}$$

where

$$L(t) = \left[A(\hat{\theta}(t))P_1(t)D^T + M_t P_2^T(t)D^T\right] S^{-1}(t)$$

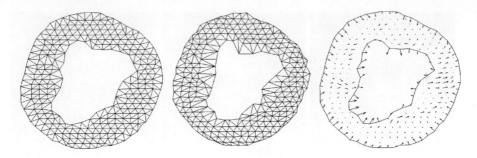

Fig. 2. Finite element meshes of the left ventricle: original (left, end-diastole), deformed (middle, end-systole), and ED to ES displacement map (right).

$$G(t) = P_2^T(t)D^T S^{-1}(t)$$

$$P_1(t+1) = A(\hat{\theta}(t)) \left[P_1(t)A^T(\hat{\theta}(t)) + P_2(t)M_t^T \right]$$
$$+ M_t \left[P_2^T(t)A^T(\theta(t)) + P_3(t)M_t^T \right] + Q_v - L(t)S(t)L^T(t)$$

$$P_2(t+1) = A(\hat{\theta}(t))P_2(t) + M_t P_3(t) - L(t)S(t)G^T(t)$$

$$P_3(t+1) = P_3(t) - G(t)S(t)G^T(t)$$

$$S(t) = DP_1(t)D^T + R_e$$

$$M_t = \frac{\partial}{\partial \theta}(A(\theta)\hat{x} + Bw(t))\Big|_{\theta=\hat{\theta}}$$

$$P(0) = \begin{bmatrix} P_1(0) & P_2(0) \\ P_2^T(0) & P_3(0) \end{bmatrix}$$

2.5 Computational Considerations

In our current 2D implementation, the left ventricle is Delaunay triangulated from the sampled end-diastolic myocardial points. Using the linear elastic model with uncertain parameters, the stiffness, mass, damping, and load matrices for each element and the entire ventricle are constructed and the SFEM framework is formed. Imaging and imaging-derived data are incorporated as the initial and boundary conditions, and are used in the optimization process.

Initial conditions: the use of the EKF algorithm for joint state and parameter estimation requires initial values for both the augmented state vector and the augmented state error covariance matrix $P(0)$, whose values are proportional to the expected errors in the corresponding parameters to ensure smooth convergence. As pointed in [8], if the covariance matrix expresses the errors in 1σ (stand deviation) format, then the actual errors of the estimates will be within $\pm 3\sigma$. For accuracy and computation considerations, we set the initial values of the covariance matrix for the displacements as 0.1, for the Poisson ratio as 0.001, and for the Young's modulus as 2000 in our current experiment. In addition, we model the process noise Q_v and measurement noise R_e as diagonal matrix, and for this paper we use fixed values for both. Specifically, let i be the frame

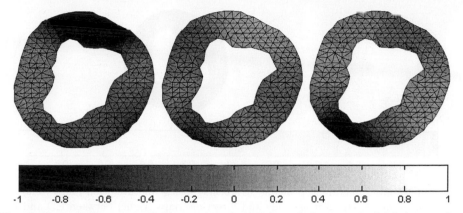

Fig. 3. Estimated x-strain (left), y-strain (middle), and shear strain (right) maps between ED and ES.

number, and j be the loop number (because the periodic nature of the cardiac dynamics, we can loop through the image sequence until convergence):

- If $j = 1$ and $i = 1$, the initial displacements are zero. Otherwise, the initial displacements are the estimates from previous frames/loops up to j^{th} loop, $(i - 1)^{th}$ frame.
- MR phase contrast velocity images at i^{th} frame, if available, provide the x- and y- components of the instantaneous velocities for the mid-wall points. For all other points, we use the estimated velocity from the previous frames up to j^{th} loop, $(i - 1)^{th}$ frame.
- The initial accelerations of all points are estimates from the previous frames up to j^{th} loop, $(i - 1)^{th}$ frame.
- If $j = 1$ and $i = 1$, the initial Young's modulus and Poisson's ratio are set to 75000 *Pascal* and 0.47 respectively [12]. Otherwise, we use the estimates from the previous frames up to j^{th} loop, $(i - 1)^{th}$ frame.
- The initial equivalent total loads are computed from the governing equations using the other initial condition.

Boundary conditions: the system equations are modified to account for the boundary conditions of the dynamic system. If the displacement of an arbitrary nodal point is known to be $U_b = b$, say from MR tagging images or shape-based boundary tracking [10], the constraint $kU_b = kb$ is added to the system governing equation, where k is related to the confidence on the displacement.

Error measures of the estimation process: the filtering process is optimized by minimizing a set of error residuals, based on the differences between experimentally measured imaging and image-derived data, i.e. mid-wall MR phase contrast velocity and MR tagging/shape-tracked displacement, and those estimated by EKF framework. With our definition of state vector and incomplete image data, the matrix D of Equation (4) should be properly chosen for all image frames, i.e. identity matrix where measurements are available and zero matrix for others.

After setting up all the initial and boundary conditions, the kinematics and material parameters can be estimated using the EKF strategy described earlier.

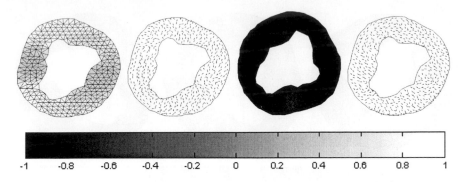

Fig. 4. Estimated maximum principle strain magnitude and direction maps (left) and minimum principle strain magnitude and direction maps (right) between ED and ES.

The estimation results at time t will be used as input for time $t+1$. The estimation process needs to loop through all image frames in the cardiac cycle several times until convergence.

3   Experiment

Imaging/imaging-derived data: sixteen canine MR phase contrast velocity and magnitude images are acquired over the heart cycle, with imaging parameters flip angle $= 30^o$, $TE = 34msec$, $TR = 34msec$, $FOV = 28cm$, $5mm$ skip 0, matrix 256x128, 4 nex, venc $= 15cm/sec$. The image resolution is $1.09mm/pixel$, and the velocity intensity ranges from $-150mm/sec$ to $150mm/sec$, with the signs indicating the directions. Fig.1 shows the images at end-diastole. Endocardial and epicardial boundaries are extracted using velocity field constrained levelset strategy [11], and boundary displacements between consecutive frames are detected based on locating and matching geometric landmarks and a local coherent smoothness model [10].

Experimental results: the framework is implemented in Matlab, and all presented results are acquired after running through the image sequence six times, which takes about 40 minute on a Pentium 4 1.8GHZ computer. Fig. 2 shows the left ventricular meshes at end-diastole (ED) and end-systole (ES), as well as the displacement map between these two frames. Fig. 3 shows the x-, y- direction normal strain and shear strain distributions and mapping scale between ED and ES. The principle strains and their directions are shown in Fig.4. The final converged estimates of the Young's modulus and Poisson's ratio distributions and mapping scales are in Fig.5. Spatially, the Young's modulus varies from 72000 to $81000Pascal$, and the Poisson ratio varies from 0.40 to 0.50. Analysis and interpretation of the results, as well as additional experiments, are underway.

4   Conclusions

We have developed a SFEM framework that can estimate left ventricular kinematics and material parameters simultaneously. We believe that this is the first

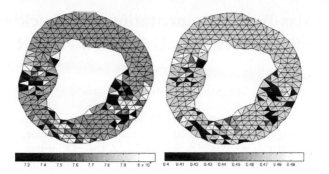

Fig. 5. Estimated Young's modulus (left) and Poisson's ratio (right) maps.

attempt in image analysis that incorporates uncertain constraining models in the ill-posed recovery problems, and the initial results are promising. We are working on issues related to robust estimation, numerical stability, realistic mechanical models, experiment validation, and extension to 3D.

This work is supported in part by the Hong Kong CERG HKUST6057/00E, and by a HKUST Postdoctoral Fellowship Matching Fund.

References

1. Contreras, H.: The stochastic finite element method. Computer and Structure **12** (1980) 341–348
2. Frangi, A.J., Niessen, W.J., Viergever, M.A.: Three-dimensional modeling for functional analysis of cardiac images. IEEE Trans. Med. Imag. **20(1)** (2001) 2–25
3. Glad T, T., Ljung, L.: Control Theory. Taylor & Francis (2000) London
4. Hunter, P.J., Smaill, B.H.: The analysis of cardiac function: a continuum approach. Progress in Biophysics and Molecular Biology **52** (1989) 101–164
5. Ljung, L.: Asymptotic behavior of the extended Kalman filter as a parameter estimator for linear system. IEEE Trans. on Auto. Control **AC24(1)** (1979) 36–50
6. Moulton, M.J., Creswell, L.L., Actis, R.L., Myers, K.W., Vannier, M.W., Szabo, B.A., Pasque, M.K.: An inverse approach to determining myocardial material properties. Journal of Biomechanics **28(8)** (1995) 935-948
7. Park, J., Metaxas, D.N., Axel, L.: Analysis of left ventricular wall motion based on volumetric deformable models and MRI-SPAMM. Medical Image Analysis **1(1)** (1996) 53–71
8. Rao, S.K.: Comments on "Optimal guidance of proportional navigation". IEEE Transactions on Aerospace and Electronic systems **34(3)** (1998) 981–982
9. Shi, P., Sinusas, A.J., Constable, R.T., Duncan, J.S.: Volumetric deformation analysis using mechanics-based data fusion: application in cardiac motion recovery. International Journal of Computer Vision **35(1)** (1999) 87–107
10. Shi, P., Sinusas, A.J., Constable, R.T., Duncan, J.S.: Point–tracked quantitative analysis of left ventricular motion from 3D image sequences. IEEE Transactions on Medical Imaging **19(1)** (2000) 36–50
11. Wong, L.N., Shi, P.: Velocity field constrained front propagation for segmentation of cardiac images. submitted to IEEE Workshop on Application of Computer Vision
12. Yamada, H.: Strength of Biological Material. Williams and Wilkins (1970)

Atlas-Based Segmentation and Tracking of 3D Cardiac MR Images Using Non-rigid Registration

M. Lorenzo-Valdés[1], G.I. Sanchez-Ortiz[1], R. Mohiaddin[2], and D. Rueckert[1]

[1] Visual Information Processing Group, Department of Computing,
Imperial College of Science, Technology, and Medicine,
180 Queen's Gate, London SW7 2BZ, United Kingdom
[2] Royal Bromptom and Harefield NHS Trust, Sydney Street,
London, United Kingdom

Abstract. We propose a novel method for fully automated segmentation and tracking of the myocardium and left and right ventricles (LV and RV) using 4D MR images. The method uses non-rigid registration to elastically deform a cardiac atlas built automatically from 14 normal subjects. The registration yields robust performance and is particularly suitable for processing a sequence of 3D images in a cardiac cycle. Transformations are calculated to obtain the deformations between images in a sequence. The registration algorithm aligns the cardiac atlas to a subject specific atlas of the sequence generated with the transformations. The method relates images spatially and temporally and is suitable for measuring regional motion and deformation, as well as for labelling and tracking specific regions of the heart. In this work experiments for the registration, segmentation and tracking of a cardiac cycle are presented on nine MRI data sets. Validation against manual segmentations and computation of the correlation between manual and automatic tracking and segmentation on 141 3D volumes were calculated. Results show that the procedure can accurately track the left ventricle (r=0.99), myocardium (r=0.98) and right ventricle (r=0.96). Results for segmentation are also obtained for left ventricle (r=0.92), myocardium (r=0.82) and right ventricle (r=0.90).

1 Introduction

The diagnosis and treatment monitoring of cardiac malfunction has improved with the advent of cardiac imaging techniques that provide 4D images of the heart by acquiring a sequence of 3D images throughout the cardiac cycle. An accurate identification of the borders of the structures to be analysed is needed in order to extract physiologically meaningful quantitative information from the images. Applications of cardiac segmentation include the calculation of volume and mass, blood ejection fraction, analysis of contraction and wall motion as well as the 3D visualisation of cardiac anatomy [1]. Segmentation needs to be automated in order to be clinically valuable, because when done manually it is very time consuming and partly subjective.

While good results for wall motion and left ventricular (LV) function have been shown in imaging modalities like SPECT or 3D echocardiography [2, 3], segmentation and tracking of other important anatomical structures like the right ventricle (RV) and myocardium are limited by the imaging methodologies, and the low contrast and signal

T. Dohi and R. Kikinis (Eds.): MICCAI 2002, LNCS 2488, pp. 642–650, 2002.

to noise ratio of the images. Recently, steady state free precession cine MR imaging with balanced gradients, known as TrueFISP [4], has been shown to be less susceptible to artifacts caused by slow flow and to provide significantly enhanced blood-myocardial contrast in comparison with conventional gradient echo image sequences. These True-FISP sequences allow a better delineation of the cardiac borders and have led to an increased interest in automatic segmentation techniques for 4D MR images.

Several approaches have been proposed for the automatic segmentation of cardiac structures in MR images (for a review see [5]). Recently, a number of techniques which are based on the use of a model or an atlas have been proposed [6, 7]. In these approaches the atlas is used to incorporate a-priori information which enables the use of both intensity and spatial information during the segmentation process. In particular active shape and appearance models [8] have shown promising results, where segmentation is achieved by minimisation of the difference in appearance between the model and the object of interest [9]. Most of these techniques work only for 2D even though extensions to 3D have been recently proposed [10]. A common problem of these techniques is the fact that the applicability of active appearance models is limited to the MR imaging sequence used for training since the intensity appearance is an explicit part of the statistical model. In addition, they do not exploit the relationship between time frames.

In this paper we propose a fully automated method for segmentation and tracking of the myocardium and ventricles which uses a non-rigid registration algorithm based on free-form deformations (FFDs) to register a model in the form of a cardiac atlas to a cine sequence of 3D MR volumes. Our approach to segmentation and tracking is registration-based and therefore fundamentally different from previous approaches to tracking of the heart using FFDs [11]. Registration-based segmentation is often used in brain segmentation [12]. In this work we are using registration to align an atlas of the heart with 3D cardiac MR images taking advantage of the spatial and temporal correlation of the images in a cardiac sequence. In the following we explain the registration algorithm, the construction of the atlas, and developed methodology in detail. Results are assessed by comparing to manual segmentations on nine subjects.

2   Non-rigid Registration

The purpose of image registration is to map points in one image to their corresponding point in another image [13]. In our case we are interested in finding corresponding points between a 3D atlas of the heart and 3D MR image as well as between different time frames in a sequence of 3D MR images. Figure 1 illustrates deformations of a 3D atlas after it has been registered to a cardiac MR image. To model these deformations we are using a non-rigid registration technique which has been previously used for a number of different applications [14, 15]. This algorithm uses a combined transformation model that consists of a global and local transformation:

$$\mathbf{T}(x, y, z) = \mathbf{T}_{global}(x, y, z) + \mathbf{T}_{local}(x, y, z) \tag{1}$$

The global motion can be described by an affine transformation which allows scaling, translation, rotation and shearing of the shape. The local deformations are represented using a free-form deformation (FFD) model based on B-splines. The basic idea of FFDs is to deform an object by manipulating an underlying mesh of control points. The resulting

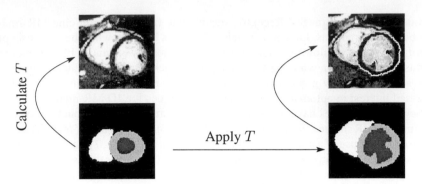

Fig. 1. Registration of a 3D cardiac atlas in form of a labelled image to a 3D MR image of the heart.

deformation controls the shape of the 3D object and can be written as the 3D tensor product of the familiar 1D cubic B-splines,

$$\mathbf{T}_{local}(x, y, z) = \sum_{t=0}^{3} \sum_{m=0}^{3} \sum_{n=0}^{3} B_l(u) B_m(v) B_n(w) \phi_{i+l, j+m, k+n} \qquad (2)$$

where ϕ denotes the control points which parameterise the transformation; u, v and w denote the lattice coordinates of x, y and z and B_l is the l-th B-spline basis function.

To relate the 3D cardiac atlas in form of a labelled image with a cardiac MR image, a measure of alignment between them is necessary. Information-theoretic similarity measures such as mutual information and normalised mutual information have been frequently used for the registration of multi-modal images. Since normalised mutual information only measures the statistical dependencies between the intensity distributions in both images but not the dependencies between the intensities directly, it can be used to align binary or labelled images (e.g. a cardiac atlas) with intensity images (e.g. cardiac MR images). For this reason we use normalised mutual information [16] as a measure of alignment between the 3D cardiac atlas and the cardiac MR image. For two images A and B, normalised mutual information I is defined as:

$$I(A, B) = \frac{H(A) + H(B)}{H(A, B)} \qquad (3)$$

where $H(A), H(B)$ are the marginal entropies of images A, B and $H(A, B)$ denotes the joint entropy between images A and B.

3   Atlas-Based Segmentation of the Heart

The key idea of the proposed technique is to reduce the problem of segmentation of the entire sequence of 3D MR images to the one of segmenting the end-diastolic time frame of this sequence (in our case the end-diastolic frame corresponds to the first frame of the sequence). In this section we describe how an automatic segmentation of the heart in the end-diastolic time frame can be obtained by non-rigid registration of a population-specific atlas to a subject-specific atlas corresponding to the end-diastolic time frame.

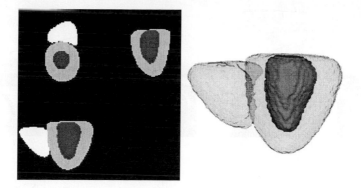

Fig. 2. The orthogonal views of the cardiac atlas (left) and the corresponding surfaces of the myocardium, left and right ventricle (right). The atlas has been constructed from 14 volunteers as described in [17, 18].

In the following we describe the construction of the population- and subject-specific atlases.

3.1 Construction of a Population-Specific Atlas

Fourteen normal adults were scanned on a 1.5 Tesla MR scanner (Philips ACS-NT, Pow-erTrak 6000 Gradient System) using an ECG-triggered Echo Planar Imaging (FFE-EPI) sequence. Cine acquisitions consisting of eight to ten short-axis slices of the heart and eighteen to twenty phases of the cardiac cycle were performed. From the acquired temporal sequence of each volunteer, the end diastolic frame was manually segmented. Using these segmented images we have constructed a labelled 3D atlas [17, 18] containing the myocardium and the left and right ventricles. Figure 2 shows the labelled atlas and the corresponding epi- and endocardial surfaces. It is important to note that the subjects used for the construction of the atlas are different from the subjects used for the validation of the proposed segmentation technique.

3.2 Construction of a Subject-Specific Atlas

As mentioned previously, a segmentation of the end-diastolic time frame is achieved by performing non-rigid registration between the population-specific atlas and the end-diastolic time frame of the 3D MR image sequence. The accurate and robust segmentation of this frame is crucial in order to allow the propagation of this segmentation throughout the entire sequence of 3D MR images. In order to reduce noise and obtain better contrast between the anatomical structures we have constructed a subject-specific intensity atlas of the heart corresponding to the end-diastolic time frame. This atlas has been calculated by registering all time frames to the end-diastolic time frame. This can be achieved by using the transformations as illustrated in the diagram of Fig. 3. After applying these transformations **T** the transformed images were averaged to produce an average intensity atlas which describes the cardiac anatomy at end diastole. Note the improved contrast and definition of the borders of the average intensity atlas compared to the original MR image.

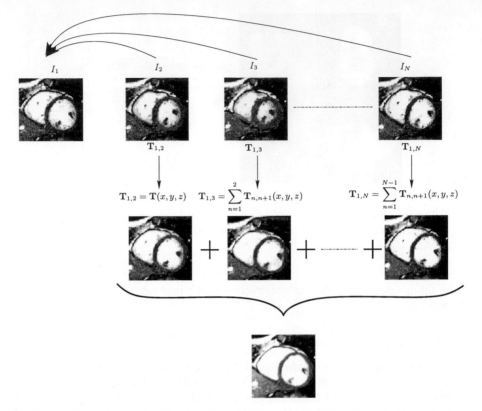

Fig. 3. Procedure to obtain a subject-specific atlas. I_n is the 3D MR volume at time n and $\mathbf{T}_{1,n}$ is the transformation that maps a point in the cardiac anatomy at time n into the corresponding point at time 1. The intensities are averaged to obtain the atlas.

4   Atlas-Based Tracking of the Heart

If the correspondences between the end-diastolic frame and all subsequent time frames are known, we can propagate the segmentation of the end-diastolic frame through the entire cardiac cycle. To calculate the correspondences within this sequence we are using an extension of the non-rigid registration technique to multi-level FFDs proposed by Schnabel *et al.* [19]. In this model the deformation between two consecutive time frames n and $n+1$ is represented as a single-resolution FFD, $\mathbf{T}_{n+1,n}$ and is defined by the local transformation of eq. (2) which maps a point in time frame n into the corresponding point in time frame $n+1$. The deformation between the end-diastolic time frame ($n = 1$) and time frame N is defined by a multi-level FFD, $\mathbf{T}_{N,1}$, which is the sum of the local deformations throughout the sequence, i.e.:

$$\mathbf{T}_{N,1}(x, y, z) = \sum_{n=1}^{N-1} \mathbf{T}_{n+1,n}(x, y, z) \tag{4}$$

Each non-rigid registration between the end-diastolic time frame and time frame N yields a transformation $\mathbf{T}_{N,1}$ that was used as initial transformation estimate $\mathbf{T}_{N+1,1}$ for the

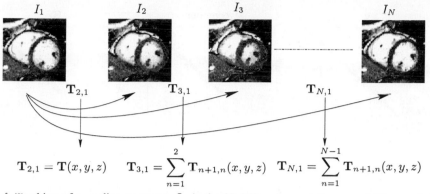

$$\mathbf{T}_{2,1} = \mathbf{T}(x, y, z) \qquad \mathbf{T}_{3,1} = \sum_{n=1}^{2} \mathbf{T}_{n+1,n}(x, y, z) \qquad \mathbf{T}_{N,1} = \sum_{n=1}^{N-1} \mathbf{T}_{n+1,n}(x, y, z)$$

Fig. 4. Tracking of a cardiac sequence. I_n is the 3D MR volume at time n and $\mathbf{T}_{n+1,n}$ is the transformation that maps a point in the cardiac anatomy at time n into the corresponding point at time $n + 1$.

registration of time frame $N + 1$. Therefore, The resulting transformations contained an accumulation of the transformations obtained starting from the end-diastolic frame and thus allowing to track the heart through the entire cardiac sequence (see Figure 4).

5   Results and Discussion

In order to assess the performance of the automatic segmentation method, results were compared against those obtained by manually segmenting nine 3D image sequences for the left ventricle (LV), right ventricle (RV) and myocardium. The images were acquired at the Royal Brompton Hospital, London, UK from nine healthy volunteers. Each image sequence comprises between 10 and 17 time frames, involving a total of 141 volumetric images. The images were acquired using a Siemens Sonata 1.5T scanner, with a TrueFisp sequence and $256 \times 256 \times 10$ voxels. The field of view ranged between 300-350 mm and thickness of slices was 10mm.

The volumes of the ventricles and myocardium were calculated and linear regression analysis was used to compare the manually and the automatically segmented images. Two different experiments were performed: The first experiment assessed the tracking of the heart in a cardiac sequence while the second experiment evaluated the fully automatic segmentation and tracking of the heart using the atlas. To assess the tracking, the transformations between different time frames were applied to the manual segmentation of the end-diastolic frame instead of the atlas. The volumes of the LV, myocardium and RV were calculated. Results in Figure 5 yield a very good correlation for all the structures (LV=0.99, myocardium=0.98, RV=0.96). In the second experiment the end-diastolic time frame has been segmented by deforming the population-specific atlas to the subject-specific atlas (corresponding to the end-diastolic time frame). Results in Figure 6 show the correlation between manual and automatic segmentation (LV=0.94, myocardium=0.83, RV=0.92).An example of automatic segmentation is shown in Figure 7, where the original image and its corresponding automatic segmentation are displayed.

6   Conclusions and Future Work

The presented approach enables the automatic segmentation of 4D cardiac MR images taking advantage of the temporal relation between images in order to identify the main

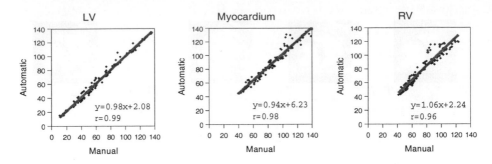

Fig. 5. Comparison of the volumes obtained by manual and automatic segmentation using the manual segmentation of the end-diastolic time frame to assess the tracking throughout the sequence (volumes are given in cm^3).

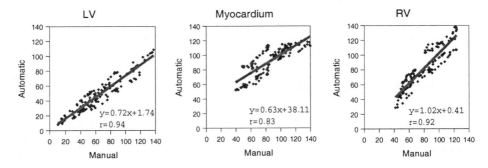

Fig. 6. Comparison of the volumes obtained by manual and automatic segmentation using the atlas-based segmentation of the end-diastolic time frame to assess the tracking throughout the sequence (volumes are given in cm^3).

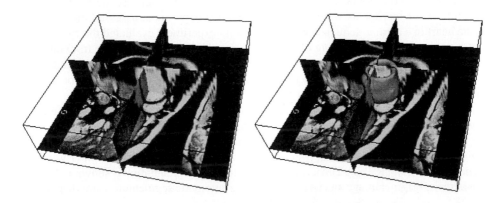

Fig. 7. Atlas-based segmentation of the end-diastolic time frame. An end-diastolic MR volume (shown on the left) with the deformed atlas (shown on the right as a green surface). An animated version of an entire cine sequence can be found at
http://www.doc.ic.ac.uk/~dr/projects/animations/MICCAI02.

structures of the heart. Since the proposed method is atlas based it enables the accurate and robust segmentation and tracking not only of the LV, but also of the RV and myocardium. In addition, it is independent of the image intensities in the MR images and can be applied to images acquired with other sequences (e.g. black-blood studies). The method has a major limitation, since the segmentation of the end-diastolic frame is still prone to errors, especially the segmentation of the myocardium where the contrast within other tissues is too low and might be underestimated or overestimated. These errors are propagated and they may even increase in subsequent time frames. This was reflected in the results where there were clusters corresponding to the different cardiac image sequences.

Future work will involve two essential aspects of the method presented. First, the spatial and temporal transformations computed by the registration algorithm provide the information necessary to assess regional motion and deformation, which are essential for the detection of various types of cardiac malfunction (e.g. ischaemia). Secondly, the registration of the atlas to the images also makes the method suitable for monitoring regions of interest (e.g. the septum). This can be achieved using a generic atlas for labelling specific regions of the heart and tracking them during the cardiac cycle.

Acknowledgements

M. Lorenzo-Valdés is funded by a grant from CONACyT, México. G. I. Sanchez-Ortiz is funded by EPSRC grant no. GR/R41002/01.

References

1. A. F. Frangi, W. J. Niessen, and M. A. Viergever. Three-dimensional modeling for functional analysis of cardiac images: A review. *IEEE Transactions on Medical Imaging*, 20(1):26–35, 2001.
2. J.P. Thirion and S. Benayoun. MyoTrack:A 3D deformation field method to measure cardiac motion from gated SPECT. In *Medical Image Computing and Computer-Assisted Intervention*, Lecture Notes in Computer Science, pages 697–706, Pittsburgh, USA, Oct 2000.
3. G.I. Sanchez-Ortiz, J. Declerck, J.A. Noble, and M. Mulet-Parada. Automating 3D Echocardiographic Image Analysis. In *Medical Image Computing and Computer-Assisted Intervention*, Lecture Notes in Computer Science, pages 687–696, Pittsburgh, USA, Oct 2000.
4. S. Plein, T.N. Bloomer, J.P. Ridgway, T.R. Jones, G.J. Bainbridge, and M.U. Sivananthan. Steady-state free precession magnetic resonance imaging of the heart: Comparison with segmented k-space gradient-echo imaging. *Journal of Magnetic Resonance Imaging*, 14(3):230–236, 2001.
5. J. S. Suri. Computer vision, pattern recognition and image processing in left ventricle segmentation: The last 50 years. *Pattern Analysis and Applications*, 3(3):209–242, 2002.
6. F. Vincent, P. Clarysse, P. Croiselle, and I. Magnin. Segmentation of the heart from MR image sequences using a 3D active model. *Annals of Biomedical Engineering*, 28(1):S–42, 2000.
7. B.P.F. Lelieveldt, R.J. Van der Geest, R.M. Ramze, J.G. Bosch, and J.H.C. Reiber. Anatomical model matching with fuzzy implicit surfaces for segmentation of thoracic volume scans. *IEEE Transactions on Medica Imaging*, 18(3):218–230, 1999.
8. T. F. Cootes, G. J. Edwards, and C. J. Taylor. Active appearance models. In *Proc. 5th European Conference on Computer Vision (ECCV'98)*, volume 2, pages 484–498, 1998.

9. S.C. Mitchell, B.P.F. Lelieveldt, R.J. Van Der Geest, H. G. Bosch, J.H.C. Reiber, and M. Sonka. Multistage hybrid active appearance model matching: Segmentation of left and right ventricles in cardiac MR images. *IEEE Transactions on Medical Imaging*, 20:415–423, 2001.

10. S.C. Mitchell, B.P.F. Lelieveldt, J. G. Bosch, R. Van Der Geest, J.H.C. Reiber, and M. Sonka. Segmentation of cardiac MR volume data using 3D active appearance models. In *SPIE Conference on Medical Imaging, Image Processing*, page In press, 2002.

11. E. Bardinet, L. D. Cohen, and N. Ayache. Tracking and motion analysis of the left ventricle with deformable superquadratics. *Medical Image Analysis*, 1(2):129–149, 1996.

12. D. L. Collins, A. C. Evans, C. Holmes, and T. M. Peters. Automatic 3D segmentation of neuro-anatomical structures from MRI. In Y. Bizais et al., editor, *Information Processing in Medical Imaging*, pages 139–152. Kluwer Academic Publishers, 1995.

13. J. M. Fitzpatrick, D. L. G. Hill, and C. R. Maurer, Jr. Image registration. In Milan Sonka and J. Michael Fitzpatrick, editors, *Handbook of Medical Imaging*, volume 2, pages 447–513. SPIE Press, 2000.

14. D. Rueckert, L.I. Sonoda, C. Hayes, D.L.G. Hill, M.O. Leach, and D.J. Hawkes. Non-rigid registration using free-form deformations: Application to breast CT images. *IEEE Transactions on Medical Imaging*, 18(8):712–721, 1999.

15. C. R. Maurer, Jr., D. L. G. Hill, A. J. Martin, H. Liu, M. McCue, D. Rueckert, D. Lloret, W. A. Hall, R. E. Maxwell, D. J. Hawkes, and C. L. Truwit. Investigation of intraoperative brain deformation using a 1.5T interventional MR system: preliminary results. *IEEE Transactions on Medical Imaging*, 17(5):817–825, 1998.

16. C. Studholme, D.L.G. Hill, and D.J. Hawkes. Automated three-dimensional regisration of magnetic resonance and positron emission tomography brain images by multiresolution optimization of voxel similarity measures. *Medical Physics*, 24(1):71–86, 1997.

17. A. F. Frangi, D. Rueckert, J. A. Schnabel, and W. J. Niessen. Automatic 3D ASM construction via atlas-based landmarking and volumetric elastic registration. In *Information Processing in Medical Imaging: Proc. 17th International Conference (IPMI'01)*, pages 78–91, Davis, CA, July 2001.

18. A. F. Frangi, D. Rueckert, J. A. Schnabel, and W. J. Niessen. Automatic construction of multiple-object three-dimensional statistical shape models: Application to cardiac modeling. *IEEE Transactions on Medical Imaging*, 2001. Submitted.

19. J.A. Schnabel, D. Rueckert, M. Quist, J.M. Blackall, A.D. Castellano-Smith, T. Hartkens, G.P. Penney, W.A. Hall, H. Liu, C.L. Truwit, F.A. Gerritsen, D.L.G. Hill, and D.J. Hawkes. A generic framework for non-rigid registration based on non-uniform multi-level free-form deformations. In *Medical image computing and computed-assisted intervention - MICCAI*, pages 573–581, 2001.

Myocardial Delineation via Registration in a Polar Coordinate System

Nicholas M.I. Noble[1], Derek L.G. Hill[1], Marcel Breeuwer[2], Julia A. Schnabel[1], David J. Hawkes[1], Frans A. Gerritsen[2], and Reza Razavi[1]

[1] Computer Imaging Science Group, Guy's Hospital, Kings College London, UK
[2] Philips Medical Systems, Medical Imaging Information Technology - Advanced Development

Abstract. This paper describes a technique for automatic analysis of dynamic magnetic resonance images of the left ventricle using a non-rigid registration algorithm. Short axis cine images were re-sampled into polar coordinates before all the time frames were aligned using a non-rigid registration algorithm. An manually delineated contour of a single phase was propagated through the dynamic sequence. Two variants of this approach were investigated and compared with manual delineation of all phases, and with the commercially available automatic MASS package. The results showed good correlation with manual delineation and produced fewer erroneous results than the commercial package.

1 Introduction

Cardiac magnetic resonance imaging (MRI) can now provide high quality images of the heart, including myocardial contraction, perfusion and with late enhancement, information on myocardial viability. A major obstacle to the widespread clinical use of cardiac MRI, however, is the difficulty in analysing the images produced [1]. To combine all of this information into a "one-stop-shop" assessment of patients with ischeamic heart disease requires a great deal of analysis, which when performed manually, is very time consuming. A rapid automated method of deriving information from these images would greatly facilitate their use. This paper addresses the problem of automatic analysis of short axis cine MR images in order to assess left ventricular function. The technique is potentially extendible to the analysis of data from an entire cardiac MR examination.

Quantitative measures of global left ventricular function (eg: ejection fraction and ventricular mass) and regional left ventricular function (eg: wall motion, wall thickness and wall thickening) can be calculated from segmented surfaces of the epicardium and endocardium. In our experience, current techniques for automatically delineating these surfaces from MR images are insufficiently robust for routine clinical use. Automatic techniques tend to fail around the papillary muscle or where pathology is present. As a consequence, the analysis of ventricular function currently requires substantial input from a skilled operator to perform manual delineation or manual correction of contours.

Segmentation techniques that are solely image driven, such as those based on image gradients alone, are unable to extract reliable myocardial surfaces [2], especially: in the presence of the papillary muscles and near the apex. Model based techniques that incorporate *a priori* knowledge into the segmentation process [3] [4] show good

T. Dohi and R. Kikinis (Eds.): MICCAI 2002, LNCS 2488, pp. 651–658, 2002.

promise, however the substantial variation in size and shape of pathological myocardium makes a comprehensive model hard to construct.

We, therefore, propose an alternative approach based on non-rigid image registration. In our current implementation, we assume that the endocardial and epicardial surfaces have been manually segmented at a single phase; end-diastole.

The intrinsic radial motion of the myocardium, suggests that registration algorithms optimised in Cartesian coordinate systems, may not be the optimal way in which to perform myocardial registration. Conventional short axis images were hence re-sampled into a polar coordinate system, and registered in that coordinate system before contour propagation was performed. The technique is compared with manual delineation and a commercial software package on a group of 10 patients.

2 Data

Short axis ECG triggered steady state free precession images with SENSE factor 2 (Figure 1, top row) were obtained in 10 patients undergoing cardiac MRI for the investigation of coronary artery disease. Three slices (corresponding to approximately basal, mid and apical positions) were selected from 8 - 9 contiguous slices, imaged with: slice thickness 8 - 10 mm, field of view 350×344 - 390×390 mm, image size 256×256, 20-25 phases in the cardiac cycle, flip angle 50 - 55°, TE 1.56 - 1.68 ms and TR 3.11 - 3.37 ms. The images were acquired on a Philips Gyroscan Intera 1.5 T with master gradients, using a 5 element cardiac synergy coil and vector ECG.

3 Methods

3.1 Technique 1: Manual Delineation

Clinical opinion is divided regarding the correct manual delineation of endocardial boundaries. In particular, different centres use different criteria for the inclusion of papiliary muscles. The manual delineation in our centre excluded papiliary muscles unless they were completely incorporated into the myocardial wall.

For every phase of each selected slice of each image set, both the epi- and endocardial contours were manually delineated in the original coordinate system. The volumes contained by the epi- and endocardial delineations were then calculated (area contained by contour × slice thickness) at each phase and for each selected slice of each image set.

3.2 Technique 2: All-to-One Registration

A centre of area (COA) of the left ventricular blood pool was calculated from the voxels enclosed by the manual endocardial delineation at end diastole (from technique 1) as per equation 1, where (x_i, y_i) are the coordinates of the ith voxel enclosed by the delineation and n is the total number of whole voxels contained within the delineation.

$$\text{COA} = \left(\frac{\sum_{i=1}^{n} x_i}{n}, \frac{\sum_{i=1}^{n} y_i}{n} \right) . \tag{1}$$

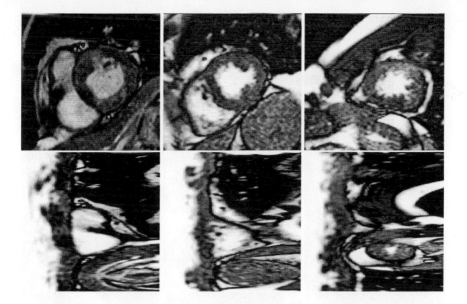

Fig. 1. Original (*top row*) and re-sampled images (*bottom row*) with intensity values for theta on the y-axis plotted *versus* radial distance from the origin on the x-axis, for basal, (*left*) mid (*centre*) and apical (*right*) slices. The bottom row images show from their left side; firstly the left ventricular blood pool, followed by the left ventricular myocardium

For each slice, every phase was then re-sampled in a polar fashion about the calculated COA for that slice, using bilinear interpolation with 256 eqi-spaced radial spokes, and 165 radial steps with a radial step size of 0.4 voxels.

The re-sampled images (Figure 1, second row) were then registered together in an all-to-one manner (phase 1 - phase 2, phase 1 - phase 3, phase 1 - phase 4 ...), using two dimensional non-rigid registration (based on [5]) with normalised mutual information [6] employed as the similarity measure. The epi- and endocardial manual delineations at phase 1 were then re-sampled into the polar coordinate system, and warped according to the results of the registrations, in an all-to-one fashion, the resultant warped contours were then re-sampled into the original Cartesian coordinate system (Figure 2, top row), and the epi- and endocardial volumes were calculated at each phase and for each selected slice of each image set as per section 3.1.

3.3   Technique 3: Piecewise Registration

Radial re-sampling was performed as per section 3.2. The images were then registered in a piecewise manner (phase 1 - phase 2, phase 2 - phase 3, phase 3 - phase 4 ...), using the same non-rigid registration algorithm employed in section 3.2. The epi- and endocardial manual delineations at end-diastole were then propagated and processed as per section 3.2, except that this time the delineations were warped in a piecewise manner (Figure 2, middle row).

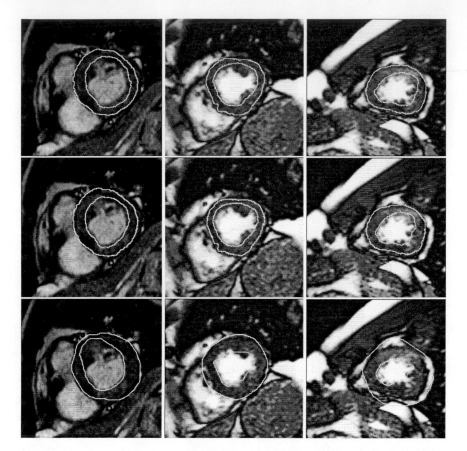

Fig. 2. Original images with overlaid delineations for techniques: 2 (*top row*), 3 (*middle row*) and 4 (*bottom row*), for basal (*left*), mid (*centre*) and apical (*right*) slices

3.4   Technique 4: Segmentation Using Commercial Software

Contours were automatically detected in the original coordinate system using the commercially available MASS package (Version 4.2, Medis, Leiden, the Netherlands),as described by Van der Geest et al. [7] (Figure 2, bottom row). The epi- and endocardial volumes were calculated at each phase and for each selected slice of each image set, as per section 3.1.

4   Results

The correlation coefficients between epi- and endocardial volumes (Figure 3) produced from manual delineations and techniques 2, 3 and 4 were calculated. These values are shown for all ten patients in figure 4.

For all three slices, the mean value of the correlation coefficient for the endocardial volume is higher for techniques 2 and 3 than for technique 4. For the apical and basal slices, this difference is significant at the 5% level (paired t-test). There is however no significant difference between technique 4 and either of techniques 2 and 3 for the epicardial boundary.

It is also interesting to assess which variant of the novel technique performs best. We found no significant difference for the endocardial boundaries. However, for the epicardial boundaries, technique 3 (piecewise) had a higher correlation coefficient than technique 2 (significant at the 5% level).

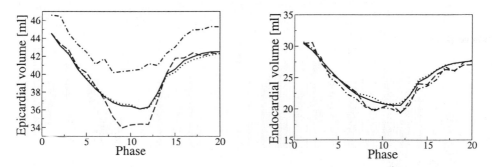

Fig. 3. Example of the epicardial (*left*) and endocardial (*right*) volumes plotted against phase in the cardiac cycle for techniques: 1 (*dashed line*), 2 (*dotted line*), 3 (*solid line*) and 4 (*dot-dashed line*) for the basal slice of a single patient

The quality of the delineations produced by the three methods was also assessed qualitatively. Each delineation was manually classified as either requiring a correction (a failure) or being plausible. The mean percentage of images per selected slice per patient (to normalise for non-uniform numbers of images per scan), that failed was calculated for techniques: 2, 3 and 4 for both epi- and endocardial contours at each selected slice (Figure 5). It can be seen from figure 5 that techniques 2 and 3 required significantly fewer manual corrections than technique 4 when detecting the endocardial contour for all slices. Figure 5 also shows that whilst techniques 2 and 3 required very little manual correction when detecting the epicardial contour, technique 4 required manual correction in 90 - 95% of contours detected.

5   Discussion

We have described a new technique for analysis of left ventricular function from short axis cine cardiac MR images. The technique delineates the epicardial and endocardial boundaries by non-rigid registration of the images across the phases of the cardiac cycle, and propagation of manually delineated boundaries at one phase using the calculated deformation field.

Manual problems. Although the results in this paper have been compared to manual delineation, this is by no means a 'gold standard' given the inherent human error in such delineations and the different techniques used especially in inclusion or exclusion

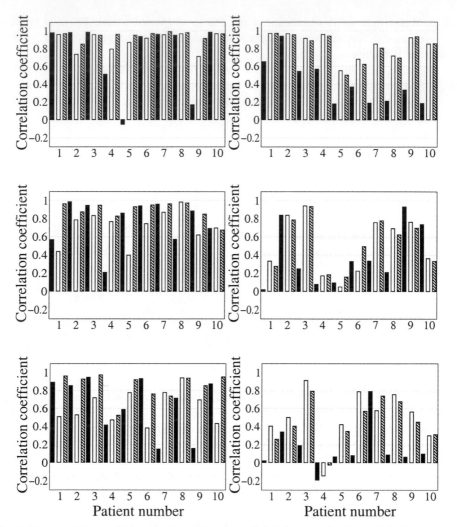

Fig. 4. Charts of the correlation of: epicardial volume (*left column*) and endocardial volume (*right column*) between manual delineation and techniques 2 (*light bar*), 3 (*striped bar*) and 4 (*dark bar*), for basal (*top row*), mid (*centre row*) and apical (*bottom row*) slices for each patient. *NB* techniques 2, 3 and 4 failed in all phases to correctly detect the endocardial contour of the apical slice of patient 4

of papiliary muscles. Also, the sensitivity of techniques 2 and 3 to the initial contour mean that the end result is only as good as the original delineation with which they are supplied.

Endocardial contour. Propagation of the end-diastole contour used in these techniques does not take into account the papiliary muscles which can form part of the myocardial mass especially in mid slices of the ventricle at end-systole. There is therefore discrep-

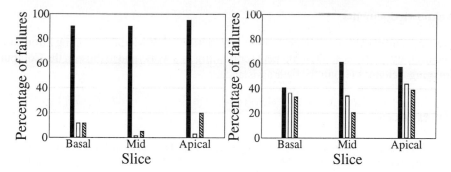

Fig. 5. Charts showing the mean percentage of images per selected slice per patient that required manual correction of the contour, for techniques: 2 (*light bar*), 3 (*striped bar*) and 4 (*dark bar*), for: epicardial (*left*) and endocardial (*right*) contours

ancy between techniques 2, 3 and technique 1, with techniques 2 and 3 overestimating the endocardial volume.

Through-slice motion. Throughout the cardiac cycle, papilliary muscles are constantly moving into and out-of the imaging plane. This complicates the alignment for techniques 2 and 3 as the registration algorithm attempts to align objects that are not present in both the source and target images. Manual observation of technique 3 shows that it manages to cope with such motion better than technique 2, the gradual warping of the contour making it easier to follow the endocardial contour. This problem could be solved by extending this two dimensional technique to a full three dimensional method.

Radial continuity. A lack of continuity at the edge of the re-sampled images means that two contour points which are adjacent in the original coordinate system could be warped to quite different positions after registration. Potential solutions to this could be: to wrap the registration b-splines around at the edge of the image, or to avoid the use of re-sampled images and the subsequent interpolation errors and instead implement a polar or radial control point spacing within the registration algorithm.

Quantitative comparison techniques. The validation experiments that we have performed could be complemented by a measure that incorporates the local distance between compared contours. Future work will incorporate such a technique.

6   Conclusion

A novel approach to the registration of cardiac magnetic resonance images has been introduced. Ten sets of patient images were re-sampled into a polar coordinate system and two registration strategies were investigated (all-to-one and piecewise). The resulting propagated contours were then compared with contours automatically created by MASS and with manual delineations. The piecewise technique correlated with manual delineation better than the all-to-one and MASS detected techniques, and also required fewer manual interactions to correct erroneously detected contours than MASS.

Acknowledgements

We are grateful to Philips Medical Systems Nederland B.V. Medical Imaging Information Technology - Advanced Development for funding this work, and to those at the Computer Imaging Sciences Group for their assistance.

References

1. A.F. Frangi, W.J. Niessen, and M.A. Viergever. Three-Dimensional Modeling for Functional Analysis of Cardiac Images: A Review. *IEEE Trans. Med. Imaging*, 20(1):2–25, 2001.
2. W.J. Niessen, B.M. ter Haar Romeny, and M.A. Viergever. Geodesic Deformable Models for Medical Image Analysis. *IEEE Trans. Med. Imaging*, 17(4):634–641, 1998.
3. S.C. Mitchell, P.F. Lelieveldt, R.J. van der Geest, H.G. Bosch, J.H.C. Reiber, and M. Sonka. Multistage Hybrid Active Appearance Model Matching: Segmentation of Left and Right Ventricles in Cardiac MR Images. *IEEE Trans. Med. Imaging*, 20(5):415–423, 2001.
4. L.H. Staib and J.S. Duncan. Model-Based Deformable Surface Finding for Medical Images. *IEEE Trans. Med. Imaging*, 15(5):720–731, 1996.
5. J.A. Schnabel, D. Rueckert, M. Quist, J.M. Blackall, A.D. Castellano-Smith, T. Hartkins, G.P. Penney, W.A. Hall, H. Liu, C.L. Truwit, F.A. Gerritsen, D.L.G. Hill, and D.J. Hawkes. A Generic Framework for Non-rigid Registration Based on Non-uniform Multi-level Free-form Deformations. In *Medical Image Computing and Computer Assisted Intervention (MICCAI)*, pages 573–581, 2001.
6. C. Studholme, D.L.G. Hill, and D.J. Hawkes. An Overlap Invariant Entropy Measure of 3D Medical Image Alignment. *Pattern Recognition*, 32:71–86, 1999.
7. R.J. van der Geest, V.G.M. Buller, E. Jansen, H.J. Lamb, L.H. Baur, E.E. van der Wall, A. de Roos, and J.H.C. Reiber. Comparison Between Manual and Semiautomated Analysis of Left Ventricular Volume Parameters from Short-Axis MR Images. *J. Comput. Assist. Tomogr.*, 21(5):756–765, 1997.

Integrated Image Registration for Cardiac MR Perfusion Data

Ravi Bansal[1] and Gareth Funka-Lea[1]

Department of Imaging and Visualization, Siemens Corporate Research, Inc.
Princeton, NJ 08540

Abstract. In this paper we present an integrated image registration algorithm for segmenting the heart muscle, the myocardium (MC). A sequence of magnetic resonance (MR) images of heart are acquired after injection of a contrast agent. An analysis of the perfusion of the contrast agent into myocardium is utilized to study its viability. Such a study requires segmentation of MC in each of the images acquired which is a difficult task due to rapidly changing contrast image the images. In this paper we present an information theoretic registration framework which integrates two channels of information, the pixel intensities and the local gradient information, to reliably and accurately segment the myocardium. In our framework, the physician hand draws contours representing the inner (the endocardium) and the outer (the epicardium) boundaries of the myocardium. These hand drawn contours are then propagated to the other images in the sequence of images acquired to segment the MC.

1 Introduction

Ischemic heart disease, the obstruction of blood flow to the heart, results due to excess fat or plaque deposits which narrows the veins that supply oxygenated blood to the heart. The reduced blood supply to the heart is typically manifested as reduced blood perfusion to the myocardium (MC), the heart muscle. Clinically, the myocardial perfusion measurements are routinely performed with single–photon emission computed tomography (SPECT) or with positron emission tomography (PET) images [1]. Some of the major drawbacks of these techniques are the low spatial resolution, attenuation artifacts of SPECT and limited availability of PET [11, 12]. Authors in [8, 15] show possibility of myocardial perfusion analysis with magnetic resonance images (MRIs) which also permits quantitative analysis of blood flow.

In MR perfusion analysis study, usually about 60 to 100 short axis 2D MR images of the heart are acquired after injecting contrast agent into the blood. As the heart is beating, the contrast in the acquired MR images is rapidly changing. The contrast agent passes through right ventricle (RV) to left ventricle (LV) and then perfuses into the myocardium. To do the perfusion analysis, it is necessary to segment the myocardium in all the MR images acquired in a perfusion scan. This is a tedious job, given that there are 60 to 100 images in each scan. The

T. Dohi and R. Kikinis (Eds.): MICCAI 2002, LNCS 2488, pp. 659–666, 2002.

problem gets compounded due to the fact that the contrast in the images is rapidly changing. When the contrast agent is in LV, the blood pool brighten ups and makes it easy to segment the inner wall of the myocardium, the endocardium. However, when there is no contrast agent in LV, it is very difficult to segment the endocardium. Segmentation of the outer boundary of the heart, the epicardium, remains difficult throughout the images acquired in the scan. In addition to the changing contrast, there could also be gross motion due to patient breathing and changes in heart shape as it is beating. Only recently there has been some published work [2, 13] in the medical image processing literature to address these issues.

2   Our Approach

In this paper we pose the myocardium segmentation problem as an image registration problem. Segmentation is achieved by template matching. In our registration framework, a physician hand draws contours, denoting the epicardium and endocardium, on one of the 2D MR images in the sequence. These contours are used to define a region of interest (ROI) locally around the hand drawn contours. This ROI, or the template, is then correlated with other images in the sequence to best estimate the myocardium.

As the image contrast is changing rapidly, we decided to utilize mutual information (MI) based match criteria [3, 14] for template matching while assuming only *whole* pixel shifts. However, in the images, there could be sub-pixel shifts which can quickly add up to a large motion if we utilize only gray scale information. Thus, there was a necessity to incorporate edge information within the registration framework to better estimate the registration parameters. Due to rapidly changing contrast in the images, sometimes the epicardium and the endocardium are not visible. In these cases then in order to keep propagating the contours properly, it is essential to utilize gray scale information. In this paper we present an example where while trying to achieve sub–pixel accuracy, in MI based approach, by doing bilinear interpolation leads to worse estimate of the registration parameters. Thus, we decided to limit estimation of the registration parameters to *whole* pixel shifts only while achieving further accuracy using the edge information. A number of methods have been proposed within image registration literature [5, 9, 10] which also combine gray scale with edge information to better estimate registration parameters. However, we feel that while these methods represent significant advances, they remain ad-hoc in their approach.

2.1   Mathematical Formulation

In our registration framework, the image on which the contours are hand drawn, or where the contours are estimated in the previous iteration, is called the *template image*. The image where the contours are being currently propagated to is called the *current image*. Our registration framework consists of two steps. In the first step we estimate the probability of each pixel, in the *current image*, being an edge as a function of local gradient and location of the contours at the current estimate of the registration parameters. These estimated edge probabilities are then utilized in the second step to estimate the registration parameters. These two steps are repeated till convergence. In our current formulation, we do not address the problem of changing heart shape, an issue that we plan to address in our future work.

Estimating Edge Probabilities. To estimate the edge probabilities in the *current image*, we model the current image as a 2D MRF (*Markov random field*) [4, 7] with discontinuities.

Let $S = \{1, \ldots, m\}$ denote the discrete set of m sites on a 2D grid of the *current image*. Let $N = \{N_i | \forall i \in S\}$ denote the neighborhood system with the properties (1) $i \notin N_i$ and (2) $i \in N_{i'} \Leftrightarrow i' \in N_i$. Let the set of first order C_1 and the set of second order C_2 cliques be defined as $C_1 = \{i | \forall i \in S\}$ and $C_2 = \{\{i, i'\} | \forall i \in S, i' \in N_i\}$. Let $F = \{F_1, \ldots, F_m\}$ be a family of random variables which are defined on S and let $f = \{f_1, \ldots, f_m\}$ be a realization of F. Define an *energy function* $U(f)$ as a function of the clique potentials $V_c(f)$ to be $U(f) = \sum_{c \in C} V_c(f)$.

Then the Gibbs distribution of the random field F is defined as $P(f) = \frac{1}{Z} \exp(-\beta U(f))$ which is also probability density function (pdf) on the MRF [4, 7]. Z, also called the *partition function*, is a normalization constant. Let $e^2_{ii'}$ be a random variable denoting an edge between sites i and i' and let $\mathcal{E}_2 = \{e^2_{ii'} | \forall i \in S, i' \in N_i\}$ denote the set of edges. Let $d = \{d_i | \forall i \in S\}$ denote the observed data. Let σ denote the standard deviation of the noise in the observed data d. Let $g^2_{ii'}$ denote the local intensity gradient in the *current image* at the site i. Let $\mathcal{E}_1 = \{c^1_i | e^1_i \bowtie e^2_{ii'}, \forall i' \in N_i, e^1_i \in C\}$ denote the set of corresponding edges, e^1_i, on the contours C in the *template image*. The symbol $\bowtie$ is used to denote the corresponding edges on the contours C. In our formulation, corresponding edges are the edges with the shortest Euclidean distance. Let us denote the distance between the corresponding edges, e^1_i and $e^2_{ii'}$ by s^1_i. Finally, let $\mathcal{L}(g^2_{ii'}, s^1_i)$ denote the likelihood of an edge $e^2_{ii'}$ which is a function of local image gradient and distance to the corresponding edge on the contours C.

Using these notations, the energy function, for a second order neighborhood, under given information is written as:

$$E(f, \mathcal{E}_2) = U(f, \mathcal{E}_2 | d, \mathcal{E}_1)$$
$$= \sum_{i=1}^{m} (f_i - d_i)^2 / (2\sigma^2) + \sum_i \sum_{i' \in N_i} \left\{ \mathcal{L}(g^2_{ii'}, s^1_i)(1 - e^2_{ii'}) + \alpha e^2_{ii'} \right\}$$
$$= \sum_{i=1}^{m} (f_i - d_i)^2 + \lambda \sum_i \sum_{i' \in N_i} \left\{ \mathcal{L}(g^2_{ii'}, s^1_i)(1 - e^2_{ii'}) + \alpha e^2_{ii'} \right\}.$$

The likelihood term $\mathcal{L}(g^2_{ii'}, s^1_i)$ is evaluated as:

$$\mathcal{L}(g^2_{ii'}, s^1_i) = P(e^1_i, g^2_{ii'} | e^2_{ii'} = 1) = P(e^1_i | e^2_{ii'} = 1) \ P(g^2_{ii'} | e^2_{ii'} = 1),$$

where we assume that e^1_i and $g^2_{ii'}$ are conditionally independent random variables and $P(e^1_i | e^2_{ii'} = 1)$ is evaluated as a function of s^1_i. The Gibbs distribution of the random field is then given as $P^{Gb}(E(f, \mathcal{E}_2)) = \frac{1}{Z} \exp\{-\beta E(f, \mathcal{E}_2)\}$.

The energy $E(f, \mathcal{E}_2)$ can then be optimized to estimate the MAP (*maximum a-posteriori*) estimate of the random field. However, this is a classical optimization problem which involved both discrete and continuous random variables. To overcome this problem, $\mathcal{E}_2$ are usually approximated with continuous variables [6, 16]. However, in this paper we propose to *integrate–out* the edge variables. In the process of integrating–out the edge variables, a new set of variables, $l_{ii'}$, appear which can be shown to be probability of not observing an edge given all the information. That is, $P^{Gb}(E(f)) = \sum_{\mathcal{E}_2} P^{Gb}(E(f, \mathcal{E}_2))$, where after few steps it can be shown that

$$E(f) = \sum_{i=1}^{m}(f_i - d_i)^2 + \lambda \ \sum_i \sum_{i' \in N_i} \left\{ \mathcal{L}(g_{ii'}^2, s_i^1) + \ln l_{ii'} \right\}$$

with $l_{ii'} = \frac{1}{1+\exp\{-\beta\lambda(\mathcal{L}(g_{ii'}^2, s_i^1)-\alpha)\}} = P(e_{ii'}^2 = 0|f, \mathcal{E}_2)$. The estimated $l_{ii'}$ are then utilized on the next step to better estimate the registration parameters.

Estimating Registration Parameters. Let $Y = \{Y_1, \ldots, Y_m\}$ be a random field denoting pixel intensities of the *template image*. Let $y = \{y_1, \ldots, y_m\}$ be a particular realization. Let T denote the two translation parameters that are being estimated. Then the optimal registration parameters, $\hat{T}$, are being estimated as minimization of the joint conditional entropy

$$\hat{T} = \arg\min_T H(F, \mathcal{E}_2|Y, \mathcal{E}_1, T) = \arg\min_T H(F, \mathcal{E}_2|Y(T), \mathcal{E}_1(T))$$
$$= \arg\min_T [H(F|\mathcal{E}_2, Y(T), \mathcal{E}_1(T)) + H(\mathcal{E}_2|Y(T), \mathcal{E}_1(T))]$$
$$\leq \arg\min_T [H(F|Y(T)) + H(\mathcal{E}_2|\mathcal{E}_1(T))] = \arg\min_T [H(F|Y(T)) + H(\mathcal{E}_2, \mathcal{E}_1(T))],$$

where $H(\mathcal{E}_1, T)$ is assumed to be a constant and $H(x) = -\sum p(x) \log p(x)$ is the Shannon's entropy. The first term in the equation above is the conditional entropy which is similar to the gray scale conditional entropy term in the mutual information formulation. The second term minimizes the entropy of the estimated edges in the *current image* and the edges on the contours in the *template image*. Thus, the above formulation integrates the two channels of information to better estimate the registration parameters.

To formulate the problem within the entropy framework, joint entropy between $\mathcal{E}_2$ and $\mathcal{E}_1$ is approximated as a joint entropy between $\mathcal{E}_2$ and the distance transform $S(T)$ of $\mathcal{E}_1$. This assumption is based on the intuition that when the two images are registered, the entropy of the distribution of the distances under $\mathcal{E}_2$ will be minimal. Thus, we evaluate $H(\mathcal{E}_2, \mathcal{E}_1(T)) = H(\mathcal{E}_2, S(T))$.

We assume the each pixel is independently distributed and hence write the joint distribution $p(\mathcal{E}_2, S(T))$ as:

$$p(\mathcal{E}_2, S(T)) = \prod_i \prod_{i' \in N_i} p(e_{ii'}^2, s_i) = \prod_i \prod_{i' \in N_i} P(e_{ii'}^2) \, p(s_i|e_{ii'}^2).$$

Thus, the joint entropy $H(\mathcal{E}_2, S(T))$ can be written as

$$H(\mathcal{E}_2, S(T)) = \sum_i \sum_{i' \in N_i} P(e_{ii'}^2 = 1)H_{i1}(s) + \sum_i \sum_{i' \in N_i} P(e_{ii'}^2 = 0)H_{i0}(s)$$

where $H_{i1}(s) = -\sum p(s_i|e_{ii'}^2 = 1) \, \log p(s_i|e_{ii'}^2 = 1)$. Further assuming that $H_{i1}(s)$ is identically distributed for each i and assuming that $H_{i0}(s)$ is almost constant, the joint entropy $H(\mathcal{E}_2, S(T))$ is further approximated to be

$$H(\mathcal{E}_2, S(T)) = \sum_i \sum_{i' \in N_i} P(e_{ii'}^2 = 1)H_{i1}(s) = H_1(s) \sum_i \sum_{i' \in N_i} P(e_{ii'}^2 = 1)$$
$$= N \, H_1(s)\frac{\sum_i \sum_{i' \in N_i} P(e_{ii'}^2 = 1)}{N} = N <\bar{e}> H_1(s)$$

Thus, finally, under the i.i.d. assumption, the optimal transformation parameters are estimated as

$$\hat{T} = \arg\min_T [H(F|Y(T)) + H(\mathcal{E}_2, \mathcal{E}_1(T))]$$
$$= \arg\min_T [mH(f|y(T)) + N <\bar{e}> H_1(s)]$$

2.2   Current Implementation

In our current implementation we further assume that the edges are localized at the pixels rather that between two pixels. Under this simplifying assumption, the two steps are

Estimating Edge Probabilities.

$$l_i = \frac{1}{1 + \exp\{-\beta\lambda(\mathcal{L}(g_i^2, s_i^1) - \alpha)\}}, \tag{1}$$

where g_i^2 denotes the local gradient magnitude at the site i and l_i denotes the probability of no edge at site i.

Estimating the Registration Parameters. Once the edge probabilities are estimated in the previous step, the optimal registration parameters $\hat{T}$ are estimated as

$$\hat{T} = \arg\min_T \left[H(f|y) + <\bar{e}> H_1(s) \right], \tag{2}$$

where $<\bar{e}> = \frac{\sum_i P(e_i^2 = 1)}{m}$.

The algorithm is initialized with all edge probabilities set to zero and initialize the temperature $1/\beta$ to a high value. Then the algorithm estimates the registration parameters (eq. (2)), updates the edge probabilities (eq. (1)), decreases the temperature and repeats till convergence.

3   Results

In this section we present the results of our integrated registration framework. In the results presented in this paper, we are estimating only two translation parameters. Thus, we are assuming that there is no rotation. Also, we assume that there are no sub–pixel shifts. This assumption is not true and might lead to drifts in estimated registration as the sub–pixel shifts add–up.

Fig. 1 shows few frames from a sequence of frames of synthetic data where, in addition to rapidly changing pixel intensities, there is a sub–pixel shift to the right. First row of images show the results obtained using mutual information [14, 3] based template matching where we assume no sub–pixel shifts. The registration is being done using pixel intensities only and the hand drawn contours are utilized to specify the ROI only. Notice that under this assumption the sub–pixel drifts quickly add up leading to noticeably shift towards the end of sequence.

Fig.2 shows results obtained for the MR perfusion study for a heavily sedated dog. As the dog is heavily sedated, no motion is expected. The first row of images in Fig.2 show the results obtained using pixel intensity based mutual information based registration algorithm. Again we are estimating only *whole* pixel shifts. Even though we are estimating only *whole* pixel shifts, we see that visually the mutual information based strategy accurately localized the myocardium.

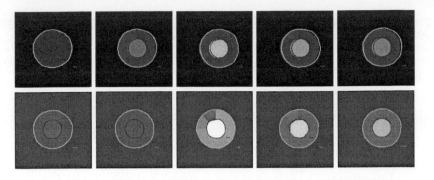

Fig. 1. Selected images from a sequence of synthetic data with sub–pixel shifts, in addition to rapidly changing pixel intensities. First row of images show results obtained using gray scale based mutual information only assuming no sub–pixel shifts. The second row of images show the results obtained using our proposed algorithm while estimating only *whole* pixel shifts.

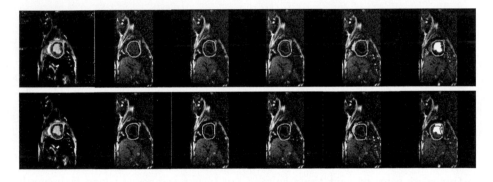

Fig. 2. Time sequence of MR perfusion obtained for a heavily sedated dog. The first row of images show the result obtained using pixel intensity based MI algorithm. For these results only *whole* pixel shifts are being estimated. The second row of images shows the results obtained using MI based strategy with sub–pixel accuracy.

However, results from Fig.1 showed that sub–pixel shifts might add–up for a big drifts. Therefore we implemented mutual information based strategy where we are estimating sub–pixel shifts. The second row of images in Fig.2 show the results obtained where we are estimating sub–pixel shifts. Note that while estimating the sub–pixel shifts lead to drifts in the estimated myocardium. This happens due to the fact that mutual information $I(f,y)$ between two random variables f and y, given by $I(f,y) = H(f) + H(y) - H(f,y)$ is while trying to minimize the joint entropy $H(f,y)$ is also trying to maximize the marginal entropy $H(y)$. For estimating sub–pixel shifts, interpolation of the pixel intensities is required. Interpolation is effectively smoothing the image and hence reduces the marginal entropy $H(y)$. To compensate for the reduction of marginal entropy due to smoothing, the algorithm shifts the optimal position where there is more

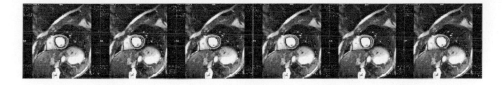

Fig. 3. Results obtained using our proposed integrated registration algorithm on a real patient MR perfusion sequence. Note again we are estimating only *whole* pixel shifts.

variations in pixel intensities. This conclusion was supported by the fact that we noticed shifts of the contours only when there was no contrast in the images. When there was contrast in the images, and hence already high marginal entropy $H(y)$, there were no spurious shifts of the contours. Since estimating sub–pixel shifts can lead to spurious drifts in the data where contrast is rapidly changing, we decided to estimate only *whole* pixel shifts. However, to account for drifts due to sub–pixel shifts, we incorporated a second channel of information in the form of edge information to pull the contours to myocardium.

The second row of images in Fig.1 shows the results obtained using our combined strategy. Notice that while we are estimating only the *whole* pixel shifts, the edge information in our registration framework pulls the contours every few frames to the right position so that the sub–pixel shifts do not add up.

Fig.3 shows results obtained using our integrated registration approach on the MR perfusion sequence of a real patient. Notice that using our integrated approach, we are able to segment the myocardium reliably in the complete sequence. An important point to make is that we cannot just use the edge information in the template correlation due to rapidly changing contrast in the MR perfusion sequence. In the sequence of images

4   Discussion

Results from Fig.1 showed that the registration results obtained while estimating only *whole* pixel shifts might not be sufficient if sub–pixel shifts are present in the image sequence. However, estimation of sub–pixel shifts can lead to spurious drifts in the sequence of images if there are images in the sequence with very low contrast, as shown in Fig.2. These spurious drifts occur due to the fact the while estimating sub–pixel shifts, the interpolation reduces the marginal entropy. Thus we devised a strategy, which while estimating only *whole* pixel shifts can account for sub–pixel shifts. To do this we proposed an integrated registration framework which integrated two channels of information, the pixel intensities and the local gradient, in one unifying registration framework. Notice that since we are estimating only *whole* pixel shifts, there will be sub–pixel errors in the estimated myocardial position but the edge term will pull the contours to the right location ever so often in the sequence such that the sub–pixel shifts do not add up. Our results seem to bring out explicitly the fact that care should be taken while trying to estimate sub–pixel shifts using MI based registration strategy.

As was mentioned earlier in the paper, while every effort is made during acquisition of MR perfusion sequence to obtain each image during the phase in the heart cycle, the shape of the heart changes locally. This is an issue which was not addressed in this paper. As a future work we plan to apply local deformations to the estimated contours to more accurately segment the changing heart shape.

References

1. N. Al-Saadi et al. Noninvasive detection of myocardial ischemia from perfusion reserve based on cardiovascular magnetic resonance. *Circulation*, 101, 2000.
2. M. Breeuwer et al. Automatic detection of the myocardial boundaries of the right and left ventricle in MR cardio perfusion scans. *Proc. SPIE Med. Imag.*, Feb. 2001.
3. A. Collignon, F. Maes, et al. Automated multimodality image registration using information theory. *Info. Proc. in Med. Imag. (IPMI)*, pages 263–274, 1995.
4. S. Geman and D. Geman. Stochastic relaxation, gibbs distributions and the bayesian restoration of images. *IEEE Trans. PAMI*, 6(6):721–741, Nov. 1984.
5. A. Hamadeh et al. A unified approach to 3D-2D registration and 2D images segmentation. *In H. U. Lemke, K. Inamura, C. C. Jaffe, and M. W. Vannier, editors, Computer assisted radiology*, pages 1191–1196, 1995. Springer-Verlag.
6. J.J. Hopfield. Neurons with graded response have computational properties like those of two–state neurons. *Proc. Natl. Acad. Sci.*, 81:3088–3092, 1984.
7. S.Z. Li. *Markov Random Field Modeling in Computer Vision*. Springer, 1995.
8. Jerosch H. M. et al. MR first pass imaging: quantitative assessment of transmural perfusion and collateral flow. *Int. J. Card. Imaging*, 13:205–218, 1997.
9. J. Pluim et al. Image registration by maximization of combined mutual information and gradient information. *IEEE Trans. Med. Imag.*, 19(8), 2000.
10. Alexis Roche et al. Rigid registration of 3D ultrasound with MR images: a new approach combining intensity and gradient information. *IEEE TMI*, 2001.
11. Go RT et al. A prospective comparison of rubidium 82 PET and thallium 201 SPECT myocardial perfusion imaging utilizing a single dipyridamole stress in the diagnosis of coronary artery disease. *J. Nucl. Med.*, 31:1899–1905, 1990.
12. M. Schwaiger. Myocardial perfusion imaging with PET. *J. Nucl. Med.*, 35:693–698, 1994.
13. L. Spreeuwers et al. Automatic detection of myocardial boundaries in MR cardio perfusion images. *MICCAI*, 2001. M88.
14. P. Viola and W. M. Wells. Alignment by maximization of mutual information. *Fifth Int. Conf. on Computer Vision*, pages 16–23, 1995.
15. N. Wilke et al. Myocardial perfusion reserve: assessment with multisection, quantitative, first pass MR imaging. *Radiology*, 204:373–384, 1997.
16. A. Yullie. Energy functions for early vision and analog networks. *Biol. Cybern*, 61:115–124, 1989.

4D Active Surfaces for Cardiac Analysis

Anthony Yezzi[1] and Allen Tannenbaum[2]

[1] Dept. of Electrical & Computer Eng., Georgia Tech, Atlanta, GA 30332-0250
[2] Depts. of Electrical & Computer and Biomedical Eng., Georgia Tech, Atlanta,
GA 30332-0250; and Dept. of EE, Technion, Haifa, Israel

Abstract. In this note, we employ the geometric active contour models
formulated in [5, 11, 19] for edge detection and segmentation to temporal MR cardiac images. The method is based on defining feature-based
metrics on a given image which leads to a snake paradigm in which the
feature of interest may be as the steady state of a curvature driven gradient flow. The implementation of the flow is done *without level sets*. This
allow us to segment 4D sets directly, i.e., not as a series of 2D slices or
a temporal series of 3D volumes.

1 Introduction

The technique of *active contours* or *snakes* has been employed for a number of
purposes in medical imaging. Snakes are based upon the utilization of deformable
contours which conform to various object shapes and motions. They have been
used for edge and curve detection, segmentation, shape modelling, and visual
tracking. A key application has been in medical imaging, in particular, the segmentation of endocardial heart boundary as a prerequisite from which such vital
information such as ejection-fraction ratio, heart output, and ventricular volume
ratio can be computed. See [6, 9, 16] and the references therein.

Ideally, one would want to segment 4D cardiac imagery directly as a 4D data
set; see [20] and the references therein. Because of problems in speed and accuracy, to the best of our knowledge such data sets have been segmented either as
sequence of 2D slices or a times series of 3D volumes. In this note, because of
conformal snake algorithms based on the [5, 11, 19], and certain discretizations
motivated partially by the work of Brakke [3], we feel that we can present practical algorithms for segmenting 4D MR cardiac data *as a 4D data set*. Geometric
active contour models involving curve evolution equations for segmentation were
earlier proposed in [4, 13]. Briefly, the 4D conformal method is based on considering the gradient direction in which the 3D boundary of a 4D dimensional volume
is shrinking as fast as possible relative to a conformal Euclidean metric. Thus, we
multiply the Euclidean 3D area by a function tailored to the features of interest
to which we want to flow, and compute resulting gradient evolution equations.
This will be explicated in the next section.

Besides the application to 4D segmentation, we believe that the methods in
this paper may have independent interest for various segmentation tasks in medical imaging, especially those involving geometric partial differential equations
defined as gradient flows from the minimization of energies based on geometric
properties (length, area, volume, etc.). Indeed, all the gradient snake segmentations performed in this paper, were done *without level sets*. This is important

T. Dohi and R. Kikinis (Eds.): MICCAI 2002, LNCS 2488, pp. 667–673, 2002.
© Springer-Verlag Berlin Heidelberg 2002

since we were able to perform our 4D segmentations very quickly: we tested 4 data sets each $256 \times 256 \times 18 \times 12$ (the last being the time parameter), with each segmentation taking about 25 seconds on a standard Sun Ultrasparc 60. More details will be given below.

Of course, we do not propose this methodology as a replacement for level sets [15], which have a number of attractive properties (including perhaps the best method for interface tracking), but rather as a complementary technique for certain specific problems such as that sketched in this paper.

We now briefly outline the contents of this paper. In Section 2, we describe the gradient (geodesic) active contour framework in 4D. In Section 3, we then discuss our discrete model of this evolution equation, and then in Section 4 we apply it to 4D cardiac MR imagery. Finally, we draw some conclusions in Section 5.

2   4D Gradient Snakes

In this section, we formally derive the 4D conformal active contour model based on a modified mean curvature flow.

Indeed, let $\phi : \Omega \to \mathbf{R}$ be a positive differentiable function defined on some open subset of $\mathbf{R}^4$. The function $\phi(x, y, z, w)$ will play the role of a "stopping" function, and so depends on the given grey-level image. Explicitly, the term $\phi(x, y, z, w)$ may chosen to be small near a 4D edge, and so acts to stop the evolution when the 3D contour reaches the edge. A standard choice would be

$$\phi := \frac{1}{1 + \|\nabla G_\sigma * I\|^2}, \tag{1}$$

where $I = I(x, y, z, w)$ is the (grey-scale) volumetric image and G_σ is a Gaussian (smoothing) filter.

The basic idea for 4D active contours is to replace the Euclidean surface area by a modified (conformal) area depending on ϕ namely,

$$dS_\phi := \phi dS.$$

Indeed, for a family of surfaces (with parameter t), consider the ϕ-area functional

$$A_\phi(t) := \int \int_S dS_\phi.$$

Then taking the first variation and using a simple integration by parts argument, we get that gradient flow is given by

$$\frac{\partial S}{\partial t} = (\phi H - \nabla \phi \cdot \mathcal{N}) \mathcal{N}, \tag{2}$$

where H denotes the mean curvature (sum of the principle curvatures; see [8]) and $\mathcal{N}$ the unit normal. Notice that Euclidean conformal area dS_ϕ is small near an edge. Thus we would expect and initial 4D contour to flow to the potential well indicated by the evolution (2). As in [4, 13], a constant inflation term ν may be added to give the model

$$\frac{\partial S}{\partial t} = (\phi(H + \nu) - \nabla \phi \cdot \mathcal{N}) \mathcal{N}. \tag{3}$$

This inflationary constant may be taken to be either positive (inward evolution) or negative in which case it would have an outward or expanding effect.

The flow from the inflationary constant in fact also can be derived as a gradient flow, this time one minimizing conformally weighted volume; see, e.g., [21].

3   Discrete Implementation

Level set methods introduced by Osher and Sethian [15] are powerful engines for evolving interfaces. In our case, one would have to evolve 4D surfaces in $\mathbf{R}^5$ in which the 3D active surfaces in which we are interested would be the zero level sets. There are methods based on taking narrow bands to handle such problems ([18]), and there is fast marching for the inflationary part of the flow [18, 22] which would make level sets more practical in our case. Because of noise in the image, we have found that one needs the curvature part throughout the evolution and so we cannot use fast marching, and the narrow band methods were difficult to implement because of the complicated 4D topology and the frequent need for re-initialization.

We therefore decided to use a discretization method based on ideas on Ken Brakke for directly minimizing the underlying energy functional, and using some elementary ideas in discrete geometry [3]. Essentially, we minimize the conformal functional using a conjugate gradient method.

In order to make our procedure fast and reliable we need corresponding algorithms to compute the mean curvature and normal vectors. For simplicity and for ease of visualization we explain the method in 3D. The extension to 4D (and even n-D) is immediate.

The basic geometric elements we use are vertices, edges, faces, and bodies. These elements are referred to by identifiers which also contain an orientation for each element. Controlling surface topology is essential in our method since we want to be able to include automatic merging and breaking of contours. When one starts from the growth of a single or several seeds in capturing a given structure, there may be a number of topological changes that must be automatically be built into the algorithm. In the methodology we employ, the surface topology is gotten by cross-references among the elements. In our case, each face-edge is in two double-linked list, one of face-edges around the edge, and another of face-edges around the face. Every edge points to its two endpoints, and to one face-edge loop around it. Each face points to one face-edge in the face-edge loop around it, and to the two bodies on its two sides. Each body points to one face-edge on its boundary. This allows us to keep track of the evolving surface and also to apply simple logical rules for splitting and merging. In doing this, we employ both global and local information.

At each point on an n-dimensional (hyper)surface, there are n principal curvatures, the eigenvalues of the shape operator. The *mean curvature* is then given by their sum. The mean curvature vector $H\mathcal{N}$ has a very simple geometric characterization which makes it easy to compute. Indeed, as alluded to above it gives the direction in which the surface area is shrinking as fast as possible using only local information. Therefore, we can find the mean curvature vector on a triangulated surface by taking the direction in which the the area will be decreasing most rapidly, and then given the length of this vector, we can compute the normal direction.

This leads to the following procedure for computing mean curvature on a triangulated surface. Let v be a vertex. Each vertex has a star of faces around it of area A_v. The force due to the surface tension on the vertex is given by

$$F_v = -\frac{\partial A_v}{\partial v}.$$

Since each face has three vertices, the area associated with v is $A_v/3$. Thus the (average) mean curvature at v is

$$h_v = \frac{3}{2}\frac{F_v}{A_v}.$$

We also use the Gaussian curvature (the product of the principal curvatures). At a vertex of a triangulated surface, this is very easy to compute as

$$\left(\sum_i \theta_i\right) - \pi,$$

where the sum is taken over the adjacent angles to a given vertex. This allows one to decide whether the surface is convex or concave at a given point (convex means that the about quantity will be $< \pi$, and concave $> \pi$). We should note that for hypersurfaces in 4D (the case of interest in our cardiac segmentation), we also compute the curvature defined by taking the sum of the products of the principal curvatures taken two at a time. In this case, these curvatures allow us to classify points as elliptic, hyperbolic, or parabolic.

Full details of our discrete implementation of the 4D conformal snakes will be reported in a forthcoming publication.

4   Smoothing the Gradient

For noisy images, some type of smoothing of the data may be necessary. This could be accomplished by using various types of anisotropic filters.

We also used a nice method reported in [25] . One can deal with the problem on which the nD snake may get caught by smoothing the gradient term $\nabla\phi$ in the following manner. (We work out the general case here. For the 4D cardiac, one can take $n = 4$.) Let

$$v(x_1, \ldots, x_n) = (v_1(x_1, \ldots, x_n), \ldots, v_n(x_1, \ldots, x_n)),$$

be the desired smoothed vector field. Then $v(x_1, \ldots, x_n)$ is derived as the minimal energy solution of the following variational problem:

$$\int\int 2\alpha \sum_{i=0}^{n} \|\nabla v_i\| + \|\nabla\phi\|^2\|v - \nabla\phi\|^2 dx_1 \ldots dx_n.$$

This minimization problem may be solved using gradient descent associated Euler-Lagrange equations:

$$\alpha\mathrm{div}(\frac{v_i}{\|v_i\|}) - (v_i - \nabla\phi)\|\nabla\phi\|^2 = 0, \quad i = 1, \ldots, n. \tag{4}$$

Note that for a function $f : \mathbf{R}^n \to \mathbf{R}$ we set

$$\mathrm{div} f := \sum_{i=0}^{n} \frac{\partial f}{\partial x_i}.$$

Here α acts as a scale space parameter: the larger the α the more the smoothing effect on the gradient vector field.

5   Endocardium Segmentation Results

We now describe the results applied to temporal 3D cardiac imagery. A cardiac data set was acquired consisting of 12 time points and 18 spatial locations on a normal volunteer in a 1.5 T MR imaging system using a segmented k-space sequence. The short axis slices were 5 mm thick and the field of view was 32 cm with a data matrix of 256×256. A body coil was used to provide a uniform signal intensity. The left hand blocks of Figures 1 and 2 indicate original data slices. The vertical columns are the time series, and the horizontal indicate the change in volumetric spatial location. The corresponding endocardial contours are indicated in the right hand blocks of Figures 1 and 2.

Only one initial contour on a single 2D slice was necessary to initialize this process. The total time for the segmentation took about 25 seconds on an Ultrasparc 60 machine. Note that some portions of the detected contours (which are really cross sections of a single 4 dimensional active surface) appear thicker than in other places. These correspond to regions in which the 4D surface runs tangentially to the plane of the 2D images. We notice the benefit the full spatial and temporal coherency, that is automatically ensured by using a single 4D surface rather than multiple 2D curves, particularly well by observing the results in the lower left 2D image of the sequence near the base of the heart. In this image we can see the dark mitrovalve in the middle of the bright blood pool. Furthermore, the edge of the endocardial wall is very weak near the bottom of the image. However, the final contour is not confused by the dark mitrovalve and successfully detects even the weak portions of the endocardial boundary.

6   Conclusions

In this paper, we indicated that with fast geometric contour based methods one can derive an efficient procedure for the segmentation of the endocardium from MR 4D data, and thus a very quick way of computing the ejection fraction.

We employed the gradient snake model of [5, 11, 19] but did not use the standard level set implementation. Instead of evolving a four dimensional hypersurface in $\mathbf{R}^5$, we instead used a method that did not increase the dimensionality of the problem. Our methodology was strongly motivated by the direct energy minimization ideas as described in [3].

For 4D MR endocardium segmentation, this approach seems to present an attractive alternative to the standard level set framework. Complete details about our algorithm will be presented in an upcoming publication.

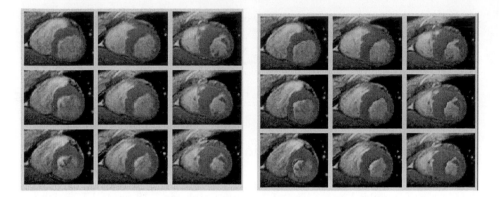

Fig. 1. Original Sequence Near Base of Heart (left) and Segmentation (right). This is a color image.

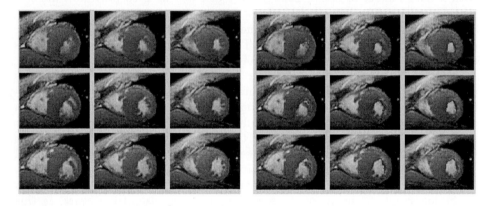

Fig. 2. Original Sequence Near Apex of Heart (left) and Segmentation (right). This is a color image.

References

1. A. Blake and A. Yuille, *Active Vision*, MIT Press, Cambridge, Mass., 1992.
2. K. Brakke, *Motion of a Surface by its Mean Curvature*, Princeton University Press, Princeton, NJ, 1978.
3. K. Brakke, *Surface Evolver Manual*, Research Report GCC 17, Geometry Center, University of MInnesota, 1990.
4. V. Caselles, F. Catte, T. Coll, and F. Dibos, "A geometric model for active contours in image processing," *Numerische Mathematik* **66**, pp. 1-31, 1993.
5. Caselles, R. Kimmel, and G. Sapiro, , "Geodesic snakes," *International Journal of Computer Vision*, 1997.
6. H. Cline, R. Hartley, and R. Curwen, *Fourth ISMRM Conference*, p. 1623, 1996.
7. L. D. Cohen, "On active contour models and balloons," *CVGIP: Image Understanding* **53**, pp. 211-218, 1991.
8. M. P. Do Carmo, *Differential Geometry of Curves and Surfaces*, Prentice-Hall, Inc., New Jersey, 1976.

9. A. Gupta, L. von Kurowski, A. Singh, D. Geiger, C. Liang, M. Chiu, P. Adler, M. Haacke, and D. Wilson, "Cardiac MRI analysis: segmentation of myocardial boundaries using deformable models," Technical Report, Siemens Corporate Research, Princeton, NJ, 1995.
10. M. Kass, A. Witkin, and D. Terzopoulos, "Snakes: active contour models," 'Int. Journal of Computer Vision 1, pp. 321-331. 1987.
11. S. Kichenassamy, P. Olver, A. Tannenbaum, and A. Yezzi, "Conformal curvature flows: from phase transitions to active vision," Archive of Rational Mechanics and Analysis 134 pp. 275-301, 1996.
12. B. B. Kimia, A. Tannenbaum, and S. W. Zucker, "On the evolution of curves via a function of curvature, I: the classical case," J. of Math. Analysis and Applications 163, pp. 438-458, 1992.
13. R. Malladi, J. Sethian, and B. Vemuri, Shape modeling with front propagation: a level set approach, IEEE Trans. Pattern Anal. Machine Intell. 17, pp. 158-175, 1995.
14. S. Osher, "Riemann solvers, the entropy condition, and difference approximations," SIAM J. Numer. Anal. 21, pp. 217-235, 1984.
15. S. J. Osher and J. A. Sethian, "Fronts propagation with curvature dependent speed: Algorithms based on Hamilton-Jacobi formulations," Journal of Computational Physics 79, pp. 12-49, 1988.
16. S. Raganath, "Contour extraction from cardiac MRI studies using snakes," IEEE Trans. on Medical Imaging 14, pp. 328-338, 1995.
17. G. Sapiro and A. Tannenbaum, "On invariant curve evolution and image analysis," Indiana Univ. Journal of Math. 42, 1993, pp. 985–1009.
18. J. A. Sethian, Level Set Methods and Fast Marching Methods, Cambridge Press, Cambridge, 1999.
19. J. Shah, "Recovery of shapes by evolution of zero-crossings," Technical Report, Dept. of Mathematics, Northeastern University, Boston, MA, 1995.
20. P. Shi, G. Robinson, A. Chakraborty, L. Staib, R. T. Constable, A. Sinusas, and J. Duncan, "A unified framework to assess myocardial function from 4D Images," Lecture Notes in Computer Science: First International Conference on Computer Vision, Virtual Reality, and Robotics in Medicine (1995), pp. 327-337.
21. Y. Lauzier, K. Siddiqi, A. Tannenbaum, and S. Zucker, "Area and length minimizing flows for segmentation," IEEE Trans. Image Processing 7 (1998), pp. 433-444.
22. J. Tsitsiklis, "Efficient algorithms for globally optimal trajectories," IEEE Trans. Aut. Control 40 (1995), pp. 1528-1538.
23. H. Tek and B. Kimia, "Deformable bubbles in the reaction-diffusion space," Technical Report 138, LEMS, Brown University, 1995.
24. A. Yezzi, S. Kichenesamy, A. Kumar, P. Olver, and A. Tannenbaum, "Geometric active contours for segmentation of medical imagery," IEEE Trans. Medical Imaging 16 (1997), pp. 199–209.
25. C. Xu and J. Prince, "Snakes, Shapes, and Gradient Vector Flow," IEEE Trans. Image Processing 7 (1998), pp. 359-369.

A Computer Diagnosing System of Dementia Using Smooth Pursuit Oculogyration

Ichiro Fukumoto

Institute of Biomedical Engineering, Nagaoka University of Technology
Kamitomioka 1603, Nagaoka, Niigata, Japan
ichiro@vos.nagaokaut.ac.jp
http://bio.nagaokaut.ac.jp/~fukumoto/

Abstract. Human smooth pursuit eye movement has been studied aiming to develop a new dementia diagnosing system. The glass-type measuring unit was installed with a small LCD monitor and a CCD digital camera as well as a built-in image-processing unit. The subjects are 19 demented patients, 18 normal elders and 7 healthy young volunteers. The adopted velocities of pursuing target are 300, 400 and 500 pixel/s. As diagnosing parameters, we have adopted the switching time of internal & external rectus muscles, max velocities and peaks of oculogyration. As a conclusion, the real-time measurement of human oculogyration seems to become a new diagnosing method of the dementia because the smooth pursuit of the demented patients has presented clear deviations from the healthy elders. Especially the pursuit velocity, peak value, switching time and correlation coefficient seems to be very useful to discriminate the demented patients from the healthy elder subjects objectively.

1 Introduction

Human beings use eye movement (oculogyration) not only to change his surrounding view but also to construct the information base of his conduct. It is widely admitted that aging may degrade the accommodating ability of internal eye muscles and the driving system for the external eye muscles' mobility. In 1980-1984 the abnormality of patients' oculogyration with Alzheimer type dementia were successively found out, that had opened a new panorama of dementia research based on physiological phenomena.[1, 2] There are two different types of oculogyration, namely saccade eye movement and smooth pursuit eye movement. Most of the traditional researches are mainly concerned to the former, but the results of many researchers are not consistent.[3–5] On the other hand, the latter is rather difficult in measuring as well as extracting useful parameters, partly because of the wave complexity overlapping with inevitable overwhelming saccades and partly because of its physiological ambiguity. We have since 1996 studied the dementia diagnosing system using the displacements of accommodative ability such as light reflexes. [6–8] The developed system was installed as a prototype set and it could get the preliminary results with discriminating accuracy of 90.5%. In order to improve the system further, we have tried to apply the

T. Dohi and R. Kikinis (Eds.): MICCAI 2002, LNCS 2488, pp. 674–681, 2002.

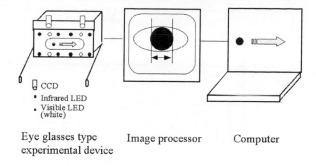

CCD
* Infrared LED
. Visible LED
(white)

Eye glasses type   Image processor   Computer
experimental device

Fig. 1. A block diagram of the measuring system for eye movement.

oculogyration phenomena for the compensational physiological data to evaluate the grade of dementia with further reliability. As diagnosing parameters in this study, we have adopted the switching time of internal & external rectus muscles, max velocities and peaks of oculogyration during pursuing a target presented in a small LCD display.

2   The Subjects and the Method

The subjects are 19 demented patients; AD (75.1±5.9 years old, HDS-R=11.3±7.7), 18 normal elders; EC (79.5±7.4 years old, HDS-R=27.9±3.4) and 7 healthy young volunteers; YC (24.9±4.8 years old, HDS-R=30.0). Subjects are instructed to wear a glass-type attachment that includes a small LCD monitor and a CCD digital camera. They are also instructed to track a small black dot running on a horizontal line in the LCD monitor from the right to left and vice versa randomly. The velocities of pursuing target are 300, 400 and 500 pixel/s. The location of an eye's pupil center is automatically calculated using cornea light reflex method by a built-in processing unit in the system through the CCD camera. Each five measured data of three types of the subject are adjusted by initial values and are rendered to visible curves by summation-averaging method. The adopted summation-averaging technique could successfully eliminate randomly inserting saccade that used to be annoying noises for the detection of the smooth pursuit eye movement. The oculogyration responses are calculated from the pupil center data afterward and are visualized as simple time versus eye-location curves in an off line batch process of connected another desktop type personal computer. As diagnosing parameters, we have adopted the switching time of internal and external rectus muscles, velocities, peak values, the averaged difference between the patient and the normal.

3   Results and Discussions

The measuring system is composed of three parts. (Fig.1) The first part is a glass type visual stimulating & observing system including a LCD display and

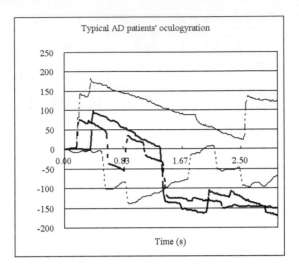

Fig. 2. Some examples of unprocessed raw data of demented patients' eye movements.

a CCD camera. Each subject is asked to wear the glass-type attachment during the measurement. A small black dot as a pursuing target runs randomly on a horizontal line in the small LCD display. The CCD camera detects the eye movement and records it time-sequentially. The second part of the system is a image-processor, which can recognize the outline of pupil from the eye image and automatically find its center. The processor calculates the eye movement that is defined as the deviation of the pupil center from the initial location during target pursuing. As is shown in Fig.2, original curves of the eye movements usually include not only smooth pursuit but also saccades. Therefore, their raw data should be processed before visualization of the desirable smooth pursuit eye movement. (Fig.2) The finally processed data of the three kinds of subjects are visualized in three graphs of different target velocities. (Fig.3, Fig.4 and Fig.5) The graphs show that the averaging is successful and that all the saccades are almost eliminated out, comparing Fig.2. From the observation of the eye movement curves, the typical patterns of smooth pursuit model of the demented, the healthy elders and the healthy young subjects are reconstructed as a simple template. (Fig.6) As far as our measured data, though we could not find any meaningful differences in delay time among the three subjects groups, we have noticed that "the switching time " shows a clear negative correlation with the delay time. (Fig.7) We have here defined the peak time as "the switching time" of two rectus eye muscles. Additionally we have found the following remarks by observing the Fig.3, Fig.4 and Fig.5.

1. The tracking velocity has a tendency that the AD patients' tracking speed is slower than the normal elders', which is further slower than the normal young subjects'. (Fig.8)

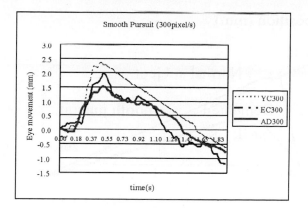

Fig. 3. The averaged smooth pursuit in 300 pixels/s target velocity.

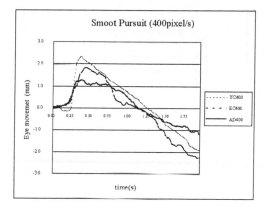

Fig. 4. The averaged smooth pursuit in 400 pixels/s target velocity.

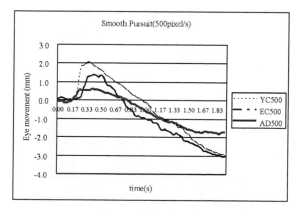

Fig. 5. The averaged smooth pursuit in 500 pixels/s target velocity.

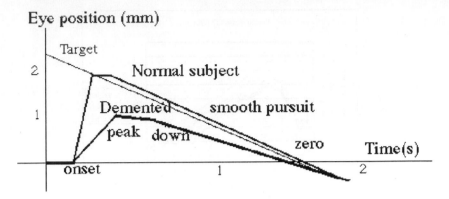

Fig. 6. A simplified pattern of smooth pursuit model from AD, EC and YC.

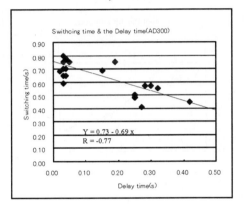

Fig. 7. A negative correlation between switching time and the delay time.

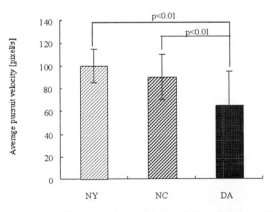

Fig. 8. Comparison of averaged tracking velocity (= pursuit velocity)

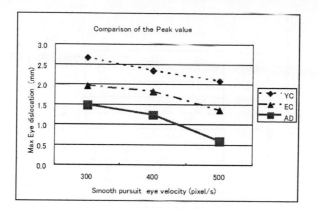

Fig. 9. Peak values of the subjects.

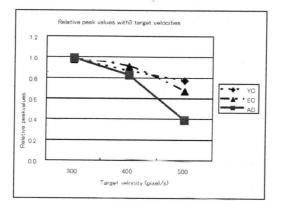

Fig. 10. The relative peak values.

2. The peak values of the eye locations have the same order as the velocities, namely $AD < EC < YC$. The gpeak valueh here means the maximum eye movement at the switching time point of internal and external rectus muscles. The peak values decrease naturally because the distances for eye to meet the target become shorter in proportion to the target velocities. But the rates of decreasing are not same in the three types of subjects but they are clearly different and line up in the order, namely $AD > EC > YC$. (Fig.9)

3. The relative peak value drastically falls down especially in AD patients with target velocity of 500 pixels/s. (Fig.10) It suggest that the eye controlling mechanism in AD patient can not catch up the speed of the target probably because of brain degeneration.

4. A correlation coefficient between the target movement and the eye movement is also smallest in the AD patient with target velocity of 300 pixels/s. (Fig.11) It is interesting this time that the difference between AD and other

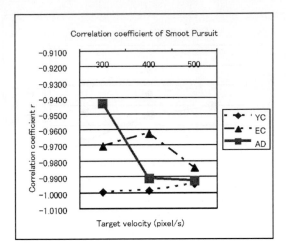

Fig. 11. Correlation coefficient of Smoot Pursuit.

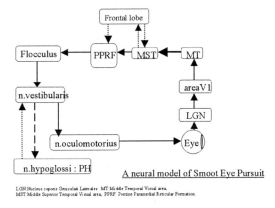

Fig. 12. A neural model of smooth pursuit eye movement.

subject groups becomes most clear in the slowest target velocity. The phenomena may be caused by the demented patients' difficulty to concentrate his attention during slow pursuing problem.

4   A Neural Model of the Smooth Pursuit

From a viewpoint of brain anatomy and neuron physiology, the mechanism of smooth pursuit eye movement is not clear yet. [4] As many study on several animal experiments have given us some standpoints as is shown in Fig.12. This figure indicates that the most part of the neural network of smooth pursuit are included in the just deteriorated part of the demented brain such as frontal lobe and parietal lobe. Considering the participation of widely spread neural network for the smooth pursuit, it seems not astonishing that the demented patients show the deviated response in oculogyration including smooth pursuit. (Fig.12)

5   Conclusions

Human oculogyration may become a new diagnosing method for the Alzheimer type dementia because the smooth pursuit of the demented patients has shown clear deviations from the healthy elders. Especially the pursuit velocity, peak value, switching time and correlation coefficient seems to be useful to discriminate the demented patients from the healthy subjects.

Acknowledgment

We extend sincere thanks to Dr. Shogo Fukushima in Matsushita Denko who has developed the measuring system and Dr. Xue Ming Shi who has executed the clinical experiments supervising other postgraduate students in our institute. We would like to thank also many patients and volunteers who have kindly participated in the study.

References

1. A.Jones, R.P.Friedland, B.Koss, L.Stark and B.A.Thompkins-Ober: Saccadic intrusions in Alzheimer-type dementia, J.Neurol, Vol.229, pp189-194, 1983.
2. Hutton JT, Nagel JA, Loewenson RB: Eye tracking dysfunction in Alzheimer-type dementia, Neurology vol.34,pp99-102,1984.
3. Robinson, D.A., Gordon, J. L. and Gordon, S. E.: A model of the smooth pursuit eye movement system,Biological Cybernetics, vol.55, pp43-57. 1988.
4. Lisberger, S.G., Morris, E.J. and Tychsen. L.: Visual motion processing and sensory-motor integration for smooth pursuit eye movements. Annual Review Neuro-science, vol.10, pp97-129. 1987.
5. G.Zaccara, P.F.Gangemi, G.C.Muscas, M.Paganini, S.Pallanti, A.Parigi, A.Messori and G.Arnetoli: Smooth-pursuit eye movements: alterations in Alzheimer's disease, J.Neurological Sciences, Vol.112, pp81-89, 1992
6. Ichiro FUKUMOTO:A computer simulation of the new diagnosing method by human eye light-reflexes,Proceedings of IEEE-EMBS Asia-Pacific Conference on Biomedical Engineering(APBME2000), pp624-625, 2000.9.26
7. Ichiro FUKUMOTO:A basic study for the new dementia diagnostic system using human eye light reflex, Proceeding, International Workshop Gerontechnology-Age-Related Change in Human Factors and Application Technology, 2001.3.13Tue.-16Fri.
8. Ichiro Fukumoto: A basic study of new dementia diagnosing methods by neuro physiological measurement and computer aided parameter visualizing technique, IEICE TRANS.FUNDAMENTALS, Vol.E82-, No.1 2001.6

Combinative Multi-scale Level Set Framework for Echocardiographic Image Segmentation

Ning Lin[1], Weichuan Yu[2], and James S. Duncan[1,2]

[1] Department of Electrical Engineering, Yale University
[2] Department of Diagnostic Radiology, Yale University
PO Box 208042, New Haven, CT 06520-8042, USA
{James.Duncan,ning.lin}@yale.edu, weichuan@noodle.med.yale.edu

Abstract. In the automatic segmentation of echocardiographic images, *a priori* shape knowledge is used to compensate poor features in ultrasound images. The shape knowledge is often learned via off-line training process, which requires tedious human effort and is unavoidably expertise-dependent. More importantly, a learned shape template can only be used to segment a specific class of images with similar boundary shapes.

In this paper, we present a multi-scale level set framework for echo image segmentation. We extract echo image boundaries automatically at a very coarse scale. These boundaries are then not only used as boundary initials at finer scales, but also as an external constraint to guide contour evolutions. This constraint functions similar to a traditional shape prior. Experimental results validate this combinative framework.

1 Introduction

Echocardiography is a widely used imaging technique in clinical diagnosis of heart disease. In order to improve the diagnosis performance and to reduce the dependency of human expertise, it is desired to automatically estimate important indices such as left ventricle (LV) deformation from echo images directly. This requires a reliable, automatic segmentation of LV boundary. However, the ultrasound images are always accompanied with degradations including intensity inhomogeneity [1], distortion, and speckle noise [2] which cause the failure of simple image feature-based thresholding methods. Currently, reasonable segmentation results are obtained mainly using tedious, interactive methodology. Automatic segmentation of echo images still remains a challenging topic.

Some groups have attacked this topic by modeling the physical principle of ultrasound imaging degradations. Different filtering methods and statistic models are presented to correct the intensity inhomogeneity [1] and reduce speckle noise [3–5]. It has been shown that the performance of image feature-based thresholding methods will be improved after the correction and de-noising. But the evaluation of these physical and statistic models still needs to be addressed.

Some other groups proposed to segment original echo images directly. They used sophisticated algorithms to combine *a priori* shape knowledge [6], texture information [7], spatio-temporal continuity of neighboring images [8,9], and motion information

T. Dohi and R. Kikinis (Eds.): MICCAI 2002, LNCS 2488, pp. 682–689, 2002.

[10]. Among these features, *a priori* shape knowledge has been proven to be a powerful constraint in the segmentation of noisy images [11]. Usually, the shape knowledge is learned via interactive training process. Though training process can take place off-line, a lot of expertise effort is still needed. More importantly, a learned shape template can only be used to segment a specific class of images with similar boundary shapes.

The main contributions of this paper are: 1. we demonstrate that a region- and edge-based level set method can be used to segment echo images at a coarse scale. 2. The boundary shape is used in a multi-scale analysis framework **not only** as boundary initials at finer scales, **but also** as an additional constraint to guide contour evolutions. Note that the term *boundary shape* here does not mean a probabilistic template prior. Rather, it is the form of a deterministic boundary.

The rest of the paper is organized as follows: Section 2 explains our combinative multi-scale level set framework in detail. Section 3 presents validation and comparison experiments. Section 4 concludes the paper.

2 Combinative Multi-scale Level Set Framework

Before we describe our method, it is worth reviewing the state-of-the-practice of echo imaging technique for a better understanding of our motivation. 3D echo (3DE) imaging was introduced to provide 3D volume and surface information of the heart with greater accuracy than 2D echo (2DE) imaging [5]. Though the newest 3DE system uses a linear-array transducer to get a 3D volume which consists of almost parallel image planes, the popular imaging system nowadays uses a transducer rotating around a fixed axis to get a set of 2DE planes at different angles. When we use a rotating transducer, we have to face the problem of reconstructing 3D volume or surface from a set of 2D image planes. As simple interpolation methods either introduce artifacts or leave the gap between two neighboring planes unfilled (specially at some distance from the rotating axis), it would be logical to segment 2D image planes at first and then construct a 3D boundary surface or a 3D volume using 2D boundaries [12]. At the same time, it is worth mentioning that automatic segmentation of 2DE images is still an unsolved problem. Based on this thought and the available data, we focus on 2DE segmentation in this paper, though it would be straightforward to extend our method to 3DE segmentation once the linear-array transducer is available.

In the following, we list our algorithm and then explain each step in detail.

1. For each 2DE image, construct a Gaussian pyramid.
2. Initialize the level set inside the LV chamber at the coarsest scale level of the Gaussian pyramid.
3. Apply region homogeneity and edge-based level set method to find out the LV chamber boundary.
4. Interpolate the boundary to a finer scale level. Use edge-based level set constrained by boundary similarity to refine the contour.
5. If the finest scale level has been reached, stop.
   Otherwise, go to step 4.

2.1   Intensity Distribution in Gaussian Pyramid

The intensity distribution of echo images is not clear yet, but it is definitely not Gaussian. This explains why additive Gaussian noise model performs poorly in the segmentation of echo images. This situation changes, however, at higher levels of Gaussian pyramid (the reader is referred to [13] for details about Gaussian pyramid). The high-frequency noise is smoothed out with the increase of pyramid level. Besides, the neighboring pixels at higher levels are more likely to be independent as subsampling reduces their correlation. According to Central Limit Theorem, the gray values of these pixels after Gaussian smoothing may be approximated as a Gaussian distribution. Therefore, we may use the additive Gaussian noise model at the highest pyramid level to extract boundaries. At lower pyramid levels, though the additive Gaussian noise model is not valid, the boundary shapes remain similar, as shown in figure 1. In the next subsection, we will use this shape similarity as an additional constraint in the level set methods.

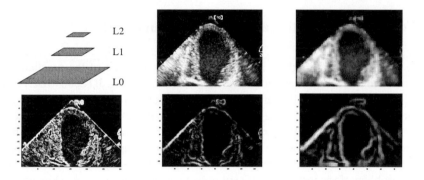

Fig. 1. Top: The principle of Gaussian pyramid algorithm (left). The original image (middle) is denoted as level L0. A 5 × 5 2D Gaussian kernel is used for smoothing before subsampling the image. The expanded image L2 (right) is smoother than the original image, while the boundary shapes are similar at both L0 and L2. **Bottom:** The derivative amplitudes of L0 (left), of L1 (middle), and of L2 (right). The disturbance of speckle noise decreases with the increase of pyramid level. At the same time, the boundary of the LV chamber is blurred as well.

2.2   Level Set Methods at Different Scale Levels

In this subsection, we explain the reason of using different level set methods at step 3 and step 4 in our algorithm. We also give the details of the level set implementation.

Finding a contour can be described as an energy minimization problem. For example, finding a 2D contour C in an image $I(x, y)$ using edge information is equivalent to minimizing the following energy function

$$F_1 = \int_0^1 g(I(C(q)))|C'(q)|dq, \tag{1}$$

here $g(I) = \frac{1}{1+|\nabla I|^2}$ is a monotonously decreasing function of image gradients and $|\mathcal{C}'(q)|dq$ denotes the unit length of the contour (see [14] for details).

For echo images at different pyramid levels, solely edge-based detection techniques may not work due to weak edges (cf northeast direction of L2 in figure 1). Thus, we need additional constraints to guide the segmentation. The *Active Contour without Edge* method [15] shows promising results in segmenting images with weak edges. This method is based on the Gaussian noise assumption and is therefore an appropriate constraint for echo images at very coarse scales, as we mentioned in section 2.1.

In an image $I(x,y)$ satisfying the Gaussian noise model, assume that we have a foreground object and a background with intensity mean values c_1 and c_2, respectively. According to [15], the object contour $\mathcal{C}$ can be found by minimizing

$$F_2 = \frac{1}{2\sigma_1^2} \iint_{inside(\mathcal{C})} |I(x,y) - c_1|^2 \, dxdy + \frac{1}{2\sigma_2^2} \iint_{outside(\mathcal{C})} |I(x,y) - c_2|^2 \, dxdy. \quad (2)$$

Here σ_1 and σ_2 denote the standard deviations of gray values inside and outside the contour, respectively. It is worth mentioning that c_i and σ_i ($i = 1,2$) are normally independent, while in echo images we have an extra relation: $c_1/\sigma_1 \approx c_2/\sigma_2$ [16]. This relation actually simplifies the evaluation of F_2, since we can replace σ_2 with $\sigma_1 c_2/c_1$.

Recently, Paragios and Deriche [17] further unified boundary and region-based information for tracking purpose. This combination increases the robustness of the level set method. Here we adopt their method for echo image segmentation, yielding the following minimization framework

$$\min_{\mathcal{C}}\{F_1 + \lambda_1 F_2\}. \quad (3)$$

Here λ_1 is a weighting coefficient to adjust the relative importance of region information with respect to edge information.

After extracting boundaries at the coarsest scale level, we gradually interpolate them to finer levels as initial contours and refine them using local image features. In the refining process, the *active contour without edge* method (cf equation (2)) can no longer be used because the gray value distribution at lower levels of the pyramid cannot be approximated as a Gaussian. If we use simple edge-based level set methods without further constraint, the active contours may easily collapse due to noisier image features, even when the contour initials are very close to the real boundaries.

When we check the traditional multi-scale framework closely, we will find that the boundary shape at the highest pyramid level is used **only** as a initial contour at a lower pyramid level, while the shape similarity of boundaries at different scale levels is not used. Thus, we propose to add the boundary shape similarity as an additional constraint to guide the contour evolution at lower pyramid levels. Correspondingly, the minimization framework is modified as

$$\min_{\mathcal{C}}\{F_1 + \lambda_2 F_3\} \quad (4)$$

with the boundary similarity function F_3 defined as

$$F_3 = \int_0^1 D[\mu \mathcal{C}^*(q), \mathcal{C}(q)]|\mathcal{C}'(q)| \, dq. \quad (5)$$

In equation (5), μ is a scaling factor which interpolates C^* to the next finer scale level, and D is the distance of the corresponding points between contours μC^* and C. The parameter $\lambda_2 > 0$ in equation (4) is used to adjust the relative importance of boundary similarity function.

The above energy minimization problems can be viewed in a more general Geometric Variational Framework and can be solved using level set methods. The basic idea of 2D level set methods is to embed a 2D curve C as the zeroth level set of a hyperplanar function $\phi(x, y)$ and convert the propagation of C into the temporal evolution of $\phi(x, y)$. Concretely, we use a Heaviside function

$$H(z) = \begin{cases} 1 & z \geq 0 \\ 0 & z < 0 \end{cases} \tag{6}$$

and a 1D Dirac function $\delta(z) = \frac{d}{dz} H(z)$ to reformulate equations (1), (2), and (5) in the Euclidean space as:

$$E_1(\phi) = \int_x \int_y g(I(x,y))\delta(\phi)|\nabla\phi|dxdy \tag{7}$$

$$E_2(\phi) = \int_x \int_y \frac{1}{2\sigma_1^2}|I(x,y) - c_1|^2 H(\phi) + \frac{1}{2\sigma_2^2}|I(x,y) - c_2|^2[1 - H(\phi)]\, dxdy \tag{8}$$

$$E_3(\phi) = \int_x \int_y D[\mu\delta(\phi^*), \delta(\phi)]\, \delta(\phi)|\nabla\phi|dxdy \tag{9}$$

By replacing F_1, F_2, and F_3 with E_1, E_2, and E_3 in equations (3) and (4) and then solving their Euler-Lagrange equations with respect to ϕ, we obtain two level set evolution equations of equations (3) and (4), respectively:

$$\frac{\partial\phi}{\partial t} = |\nabla\phi|\, \delta(\phi)\, \{[g(-)\kappa + \nabla g \cdot \frac{\nabla\phi}{|\nabla\phi|}]$$
$$- \frac{\lambda_1}{2\sigma_1^2}[|I(x,y) - c_1|^2 + \frac{c_1^2}{c_2^2}|I(x,y) - c_2|^2]\}, \tag{10}$$

$$\frac{\partial\phi}{\partial t} = |\nabla\phi|\, \delta(\phi)\, \{[g(-)\,\kappa + \nabla g \cdot \frac{\nabla\phi}{|\nabla\phi|}]$$
$$+ \lambda_2\, [D(\mu\phi_0^*, \phi_0)\,\kappa + \nabla D(\mu\phi_0^*, \phi_0) \cdot \frac{\nabla\phi}{|\nabla\phi|}]\}. \tag{11}$$

Here the variables of the function D are represented as $\mu\phi_0^* = \{(\mu x, \mu y)|\phi^* = 0\}$ and $\phi_0 = \{(x, y)|\phi = 0\}$. For a point A on contour $\mu\phi_0^*$, a point B on ϕ_0 is defined as its corresponding point if the vector $\boldsymbol{AB}$ is normal to contour $\mu\phi_0^*$.

3   Experiment

The experimental images are obtained using HP Sonos 5500 imaging system with 3D omniprobe transducer. Each 3D+T data set has 13 to 17 frames between end-diastole

(full expansion) and end-systole (full contraction). The rotation interval of the transducer is 5 degrees per slice. In the experiments, only 2DE images with closed LV
boundaries are chosen to simplify the implementation of level set methods. Image intensities, gradients, and boundary similarity measures are equally normalized to the interval [0,1] in order to simplify the setting of weighting parameters. We set $\lambda_1/2\sigma_1^2 = 1$
and $\lambda_2 = 0.2$ for all experiments.

For validation, we use 24 2DE images with closed boundary contours from five different sequences in four different 3D+T datasets. They cover different slice angles and
different frames between end-diastole and end-systole. As no gold standard is available, three experienced observers are asked to manually segment the LV boundary in
each 2DE image. These results are used as reference to judge if the performance of our
automatic segmentation algorithm is within the variation range of manual segmentation
results. Here we use the mean absolute distance (MAD) (cf [18] for details) to compare
the shape difference between two contours. For each 2DE image, the MADs of every
two manual contours and the MADs between the automatic contour and each manual
contour are estimated. Thus, we have three manual MADs and three automatic-manual
MADs for each 2DE image. Then, we choose five 2DE images from one sequence with
the best quality (sequence 1 in table 1) and six 2DE images from one other sequence
with the worst quality (sequence 2 in table 1) as two testing groups. The mean values
and the standard deviations of manual MADs and of automatic-manual MADs are separately calculated in each group, as shown in the first two rows in table 1. The same
process takes place for all 24 2DE images. Table 1 shows that the standard deviation
of MADs using automatic segmentation is in the same range of that using manual segmentation. One exception is the MAD comparison of the good sequence (row 1), where
the standard deviation of MADs using automatic segmentation is larger than that using
manual segmentation. This indicates that the importance of shape constraint is reduced
when the image quality is adequately good. But in general, the results in table 1 validate
that the performance of our framework is comparable to that of manual segmentation.

Table 1. The performance comparison between manual segmentation results and the results using combinative multi-scale level set framework. *Manual MADs* describes the shape distance of
different manual contours, while *Automatic-Manual MADs* denotes the difference between our
automatic segmentation results and manual ones.

	Manual MADs	Automatic-Manual MADs
sequence 1 (mean/deviation [pixel])	1.447 / 0.199	1.302 / 0.242
sequence 2 (mean/deviation [pixel])	2.370 / 0.794	1.958 / 0.683
all sequences (mean/deviation [pixel])	1.859 / 0.672	1.643 / 0.503

In images at the coarsest scale, the combinative level set method using both region
and edge information is superior to the edge-based level set (figure 2). The edge-based
active contour model cannot stop at the blurred boundary, while the combinative framework can.

In figure 3, we pass the boundary shapes from level 1 back to original images as
contour initials. Traditional multi-scale analysis frameworks (such as solely edge-based

level set method) do not use the boundary shape constraint and they do not get reasonable results, even when the initial contours are very close to the true ones. The performance of the level set method is improved after using boundary shape constraint, which restricts the evolution region of the active contour and therefore guarantees the correct convergence of the level set method.

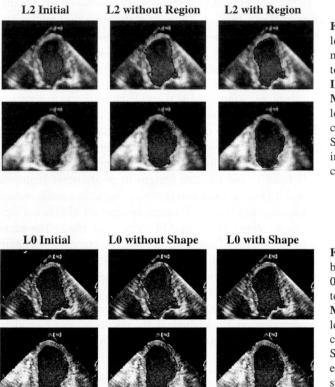

L2 Initial   **L2 without Region**   **L2 with Region**

Fig. 2. Performance of the level set method at pyramid level 2. The active contours are marked in black. **Left:** The initial level set. **Middle:** Solely edge-based level set cannot provide accurate boundaries. **Right:** Segmentation results using edge and region-based combinative level set.

L0 Initial   **L0 without Shape**   **L0 with Shape**

Fig. 3. **Left:** Interpolated boundary initials at level 0. They are very close to the actual boundaries. **Middle:** Solely edge-based level set cannot provide accurate boundaries. **Right:** Segmentation results using edge level set method constrained by boundary similarity.

4   Conclusion and Future Work

In shape-based approaches, the shape information has been learned via off-line training. In our approach, the boundary information is extracted automatically at the highest scale level of the pyramid. No interactive effort is needed, except the initialization step of the level set algorithm. In our algorithm, we use the boundary shape **not only** as initial contours at finer scales, **but also** as additional constraint to guide contour evolutions.

One limitation of the level set method is that it assumes a boundary is a closed curve or surface, while some long-axis echo images may not have a closed contour. The relaxation of this assumption needs to be studied in the future work. We also plan to extend our algorithm to 3D surface segmentation for real 3D echo volume data.

References

1. Xiao, G., Brady, M., Noble, J., Zhang, Y.: Segmentation of Ultrasound B-Mode images with intensity inhomogeneity correction. IEEE Trans. Medical Imaging 21(1) (2002) 48–57
2. Dias, J., Leitão, J.: Wall position and thickness estimation from sequences of echocardiographic images. IEEE Trans. Medical Imaging 15(1) (1996) 25–38
3. Evans, A., Nixon, M.: Biased motion-adaptive temporal filtering for speckle reduction in echocardiography. IEEE Trans. Medical Imaging 15(1) (1996) 39–50
4. Zong, X., Laine, A., Geiser, E.: Speckle reduction and contrast enhancement of echocardiograms via multiscale nonlinear processing. IEEE Trans. Medical Imaging 17(4) (1998) 532–540
5. Angelini, E.D., Laine, A.F., Takuma, S., Holmes, J.W., Homma, S.: LV volume quantification via spatiotemporal analysis of real-time 3-d echocardiography. IEEE Trans. Medical Imaging 20 (2001) 457–469
6. Bosch, J., Mitchell, S., Lelieveldt, B., Nijland, F., Kamp, O., Sonka, M., Reiber, J.: Automatic segmentation of echocardiographic sequences by active appearance motion models. IEEE Trans. Medical Imaging (2001)
7. Hao, X., Bruce, C., Pislaru, C., Greenleaf, J.: Segmenting high-frequency intracardiac ultrasound images of myocardium into infarcted, ischemic, and normal regions. IEEE Trans. Medical Imaging 20(12) (2001) 1373–1383
8. Mulet-Parada, M., Noble, J.: 2D+T acoustic boundary detection in echocardiography. In: Medical Image Computing and Computer-Assisted Intervention (LNCS 1496), Cambridge, MA, USA, October 11-13, Springer Verlag (1998) 806–813
9. Brandt, E., Wigström, L., Wranne, B.: Segmentation of echocardiographic image sequences using spatio-temporal information. In: Medical Image Computing and Computer-Assisted Intervention (LNCS 1496), Cambridge, UK, September 19-22, Springer Verlag (1999) 410–419
10. Mikić, I., Krucinski, S., Thomas, J.: Segmentation and tracking in echocardiographic sequences: Active contours guided by optical flow estimates. IEEE Trans. Medical Imaging 17(2) (1998) 274–284
11. Chen, Y., Thiruvenkadam, S., Tagare, H., Huang, F., Wilson, D., Geiser, E.: On the incorporation of shape priors into gemetric active contours. IEEE Workshop on Variational and Level Set Methods in Computer Vision 1 (2001)
12. Rohling, R., Gee, A., Berman, L.: A comparison of freehand three-dimensional ultrasound reconstruction techniques. Medical Image Analysis 3(4) (1999) 339–359
13. Burt, P.J., Adelson, E.H.: The Laplacian pyramid as a compact image code. IEEE Transactions on Communications 31 (1983) 532–540
14. Caselles, V., Kimmel, R., Sapiro, G.: Geodesic active contours. International Journal of Computer Vision 22(1) (1997) 61–79
15. Chan, T., Vese, L.: Active contours without edges. IEEE Trans. Image Processing 10(2) (2001) 266–277
16. Tao, Z., Beaty, J., Jaffe, C., Tagare, H.: Gray level models for segmenting myocardium and blood in cardiac ultrasound images. Technical report, Department of Diagnostic Radiology, Yale University (2002)
17. Paragios, N., Deriche, R.: Unifying boundary and region-based information for geodesic active tracking. In: IEEE Conf. Computer Vision and Pattern Recognition. Volume II., Fort Collins, CO, June 23-25 (1999) 300–305
18. Chalana, V., Linker, D., Haynor, D., Kim, Y.: A multiple active contour model for cardiac boundary detection on echocardiographic sequences. IEEE Trans. Medical Imaging 15(3) (1996) 290–298

Automatic Hybrid Segmentation of Dual Contrast Cardiac MR Data

A. Pednekar[1], I.A. Kakadiaris[1], V. Zavaletta[1], R. Muthupillai[2], and S. Flamm[3]

[1] Visual Computing Lab, Department of Computer Science, University of Houston,
Houston, TX 77204-3010 {vedamol,ioannisk,vzavalet}@cs.uh.edu
[2] Philips Medical Systems North America, Bothell, WA Rmuthup@aol.com
[3] Dept. of Radiology, St. Luke's Ep. Hospital, Houston, TX 77030 sflamm@sleh.com

Abstract. Manual tracing of the blood pool from short axis cine MR images is routinely used to compute ejection fraction (EF) in clinical practice. The manual segmentation process is cumbersome, time consuming, and operator dependent. In this paper, we present an algorithm for the automatic computation of the EF that is based on segmenting the left ventricle by combining the fuzzy connectedness and deformable model frameworks. Our contributions are the following: 1) we automatically estimate a seed point and sample region for the fuzzy connectedness estimates, 2) we extend the fuzzy connectedness method to use adaptive weights for the homogeneity and the gradient energy functions that are computed dynamically, and 3) we extend the hybrid segmentation framework to allow forces from dual contrast and fuzzy connectedness data integrated, with shape constraints. Finally, we compare our method against manual delineation performed by experienced radiologists on the data from nine asymptomatic volunteers with very encouraging results.

1 Introduction

With the rapid development of cardiovascular MR, it is feasible to image the entire ventricle using 3D cine images. 3D cine imaging allows building a patient specific model of the ventricle for investigating the cardiac morphology and dynamics. However, the use of cine multi-slice or 3D techniques involves the delineation of structures on a large number of images. Manual tracing is labor intensive and can involve considerable inter- and intra-observer variations [7].

These limitations have motivated the development of automated segmentation techniques for more accurate and more reproducible left ventricle (LV) segmentation. Significant research has been performed in the last 20 years towards the analysis of medical images in general [2], and in automating the contour delineation process [13, 11, 15]. The most widely used active contour/surface model delineation technique [14, 10, 8] relies on user interaction for the initialization of the initial shape and location of cardiac boundaries. Research is ongoing in developing hybrid segmentation methods combining edge, region, and shape information [1, 3, 4]. Recently, statistics-based techniques following the active appearance-based model (AAM) have emerged showing improved results in terms of reliability and consistency [6]. However, these methods require an extensive training set.

T. Dohi and R. Kikinis (Eds.): MICCAI 2002, LNCS 2488, pp. 690–697, 2002.
© Springer-Verlag Berlin Heidelberg 2002

In parallel with the research efforts for more reliable segmentation techniques, researchers are working towards improved imaging sequences. Recent developments in cine imaging using steady state free precession sequences (balanced FFE) provide high intrinsic myocardial and blood pool contrast. However, this high contrast by itself is not sufficient for appropriate segmentation of the three primary tissues (i.e., myocardium, blood, and fat). We propose a multi-spectral approach, where we choose two sequences that intrinsically have high contrast difference for the blood signal, i.e., double inversion black blood sequences (dual IR TSE), and the recently described bFFE for bright blood. In this paper, we present a new hybrid approach for the automatic computation of the EF (ratio of the stroke volume to the diastolic volume) of the LV from dual contrast short axis cardiac MR data, that combines the fuzzy connectedness region-based segmentation method with the deformable-model-based boundary segmentation method.

Our work is inspired by the work of Metaxas' and Udupa's research groups [16, 5, 12, 3]. The most closely related work is [5]. Our approach differs from that work in the following: a) our algorithm does not need any manually selected seed area for the fuzzy connectedness; b) we employ adaptive weights for the fuzzy segmentation; d) we have developed a new class of forces derived from multi-valued data and fuzzy connectedness data; and d) segmentation of multi-valued as opposed to segmentation of scalar data is performed. Our contributions are the following: 1) we automatically estimate a seed point and sample region for the LV for the fuzzy connectedness estimates, 2) we extend the fuzzy connectedness method to compute dynamically changing weights for the homogeneity and the gradient energy functions, and 3) we extend the hybrid segmentation framework to allow forces from dual contrast and fuzzy connectedness data.

2   Methods

2.1   Adaptive Dual Contrast Fuzzy Connectedness

The Fuzzy Connected Image Segmentation framework developed by Udupa and his collaborators [16, 12] assigns fuzzy affinities between two given pixels or voxels in an image or a volume based on a weighted function of the degree of coordinate space adjacency, degree of intensity space adjacency, and degree of intensity gradient space adjacency to the corresponding target object features. Specifically, the membership function of the fuzzy spel affinity is defined as: follows: $\mu_k(c, d) = \mu_\alpha(c, d)[\omega_1 h_1(I(c), I(d)) + \omega_2 h_2(I(c), I(d))]$, if $c \neq d$ and $\mu_k(c, c) = 1$, where $\mu_\alpha(c, d)$ is the membership function of the spatial adjacency between spels c and d, I denotes the intensity values, and ω_1 and ω_2 are free parameters satisfying: $\omega_1 + \omega_2 = 1$. For a dual contrast neighborhood, we used the functions as suggested in [16]:

$$h_1 = \frac{1}{(2\pi)^{\frac{r}{2}}|\mathbf{S}_1|^{\frac{1}{2}}} e^{-\frac{1}{2}[\frac{1}{2}(\mathbf{I}(c)+\mathbf{I}(d))-\mathbf{m}_1]^\top \mathbf{S}_1^{-1}[\frac{1}{2}(\mathbf{I}(c)+\mathbf{I}(d))-\mathbf{m}_1]}$$
$$h_2 = \frac{1}{(2\pi)^{\frac{r}{2}}|\mathbf{S}_2|^{\frac{1}{2}}} e^{-\frac{1}{2}[|\mathbf{I}(c)-\mathbf{I}(d)|-\mathbf{m}_2]^\top \mathbf{S}_2^{-1}[|\mathbf{I}(c)-\mathbf{I}(d)|-\mathbf{m}_2]} \tag{1}$$

where $\mathbf{I}(c) = (I_{bFFE}(c), I_{TSE}(c))^\top$ is the two component intensity vector, $\mathbf{m}_1$ and $\mathbf{S}_1$ are the mean vector and covariance matrix of spels in the intensity space, $\mathbf{m}_2$ and $\mathbf{S}_2$ are the mean vector and covariance matrix of spels in the gradient magnitude space. With ω_1 and ω_2 kept as free parameters, the results obtained from fuzzy connectedness remain highly sensitive to the selection of the sample region. To overcome this problem, we compute ω_1 and ω_2 as adaptive parameters depending on the ratio of homogeneity and gradient function values at each spel location as follows: $\omega_1 = \frac{h_1}{(h_1+h_2)}$ and $\omega_2 = 1 - \omega_1$. This method of weight assignment takes advantage of the fact that when the spels are closer to the center of the target object, then the degree of intensity space adjacency will be higher than when a spel is near the boundary of the target. As a spel moves towards the boundary, automatically more weight is given to the degree of adjacency in intensity gradient space, thus enabling more accurate boundary definition. In particular, this method enhances the difference in affinities attached to the pixels on either side of the boundary, and thus gives better defined fuzzy objects without involving a user to adjust the values of these parameters to find the best possible combination of ω_1 and ω_2. To improve the accuracy of the boundary information, we incorporate information from both the imaging spectra to compute the fuzzy affinities. In Fig. 2 we present our results showing the improvements achieved by these extensions and modifications. Since our refined fuzzy connectedness attaches much higher affinities to the target object relative to rest of the image, the need for a complex algorithm to determine the appropriate threshold to segment the membership scene is eliminated. In addition, the edges of fuzzy affinity images are pronounced which is crucial for the integration with the deformable model.

2.2   Deformable Model

To extract and reconstruct the LV surface from the 3D dual contrast MR data, we employ an elastically adaptive deformable model [9]. We have defined a new class of forces derived from multi-valued volume data that localize salient data features. In order to attract our model towards significant 3D gradients of the multi-spectral data $\mathbf{I}(x,y,z) = (I_{bFFE}(x,y,z), I_{TSE}(x,y,z))^\top$ and of the volume fuzzy connectedness data $\mathbf{F}$ derived with the techniques explained in the previous section, we construct a 3D potential function as follows: $\mathbf{P}(x,y,z) = \lambda_1 \|D_{MD} * \mathbf{I}\| + \lambda_2 \|D_{MD} * \mathbf{F}\|$, whose potential minima coincides with the LV surface. The 3D Monga-Deriche (MD) operator is applied to the multi-valued data and the fuzzy connectedness data to produce two gradient fields. A weighted combination of these terms is formed to force the model to drop into the deeper valleys and lock onto the LV surface boundary. Then, the following force distribution can be derived from this potential function: $\mathbf{f}(x,y,z) = c \frac{\nabla \mathbf{P}(x,y,z)}{\|\nabla \mathbf{P}(x,y,z)\|}$, where the variable c controls the strength of the force. Once the model converges towards the LV boundary, the smoothing effect of the model will allow it to ignore the data from the papillary muscle. Computation of the forces at any model point is achieved using tri-linear interpolation.

2.3   Ejection Fraction Computation Algorithm

Step 1 - Acquire and pre-process the data: Studies were performed in nine subjects (7m/2f) with normal sinus rhythm, with consent. Contiguous 10mm short axis slices were obtained to cover the left ventricle (LV) from the apex of the ventricle to the mitral valve annulus within a breath-hold. For this study, it was assumed that respiratory motion with the breath-hold would be negligible. Scans were acquired using a dual IR black-blood sequence (TE/TR/TSE factor: 80/2hb/23, a single diastolic phase), and cine bFFE sequence (TE/TR/flip: 3.2/1.6/55 deg; 38-40 msec temporal resolution) using VCG gating at 1.5T. A TSE scan can be performed in just a single additional breath-hold and thus does not have any significant effect on the total scan time. All the images were stored in standard DICOM format. Figs. 1(a,b) depict the data from the 6th bFFE and TSE slice (subject-1). The data were analyzed manually by experienced radiologists and using the automated analysis in a post-processing workstation. 3D registration of the diastolic bFFE and TSE volumes is achieved using the Normalized Mutual Information algorithm. Figs. 3(a-h) illustrate a sample set of diastolic bFFE and TSE images from the apex to the base of the LV.

Step 2 - Construct spatio-dual-intensity 4D vector space: The promise of dual contrast acquisition is that the dimensionally expanded measurement space will allow differentiations about the different tissues to be made, which are impossible in any of the component images. To that end, we construct a four dimensional measurement space, which combines the spatial and dual contrast intensity information. The basis components of our 4D vector are the (x,y) Euclidean coordinates of the pixels and their signal intensities in bFFE and TSE scans. Tissue types due to their signal intensity responses (Fig. 1(c)) and organs due to their spatial adjacency (Fig. 1(d)) form 4D clusters in this measurement space, thus providing clues for tissue and organ classification.

Step 3   Estimate the cluster center and the corresponding region for the LV: The three major tissue types present in the MR scans are blood, myocardium, and fat. For example in Fig. 1(c), we do observe a distinct cluster for blood, a number of clusters where the myocardium cluster is expected, and a cluster due to background. In this specific case, fat being almost negligible doesn't appear as a distinct cluster. We employ a conventional Fuzzy C-means clustering to estimate these clusters. Figs. 1(c,d) depict the results of estimating these clusters. Having identified the blood cluster (Fig. 1(e)) we can easily classify the blood in the scan (Fig. 1(f)) as the projection of the blood cluster on the spatial (x-y) plane. Since the LV contains the more oxygenated blood, it appears brighter compared to RV blood in the bFFE. This fact is used to split the blood cluster into two clusters - one for the LV and one for the RV (Fig. 1(g)). The cluster to the right on the bFFE-TSE plane corresponds to the LV. Projections of these clusters on the spatial (x-y) plane give the centroids and regions for LV and RV (Fig. 1(h)). Once the LV is identified this estimation is further rectified by using region growing to keep only the LV region and then we recompute its centroid. Fig. 3(x) depicts the estimated centroids for nine subjects mapped on a normalized circle fitted to the LVs. Note that the LVs of all the nine subjects were identified correctly with the estimated centroids always well within the LV blood pool.

Step 4 -Perform Fuzzy Connected LV blood pool segmentation: The estimated LV centroid and region are used as seed and sample statistics for our

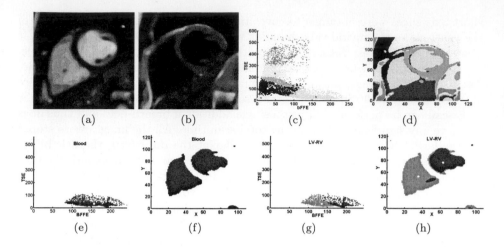

Fig. 1. (a,b) Slice 6 from the bFFE and TSE scans of Subject-1, (c) projection of the 4D measurement space on bFFE-TSE, and (d) x-y planes, respectively. Projection of the identified blood cluster on the (e) TSE-bFFE and (f) x-y planes, respectively. Projection of the identified LV and RV clusters and centroids on the (g) TSE-bFFE and (h) x-y planes, respectively.

3D adaptive dual contrast fuzzy connectedness algorithm. The average intensity of the LV blood pool drops off as we move towards the apex of the heart, due to coil intensity fall off (Fig. 3(y)). We begin with the central slice and FCM-based LV estimation followed by LV segmentation; then we use the same statistics for the next slice and update the seed (centroid), the threshold of the membership scene, and the intensity and gradient statistics to refine the segmentation. The new threshold for the scene membership is computed as:

$$expoI = \frac{(prevSliceMeanLVIntensity - currSliceMeanLVIntensity)}{prevSliceMeanLVIntensity},$$
$$thresh = thresh \times e^{-\sqrt{expoI}}.$$

(2)

In this way, we adaptively propagate the LV blood pool segmentation along the volume and time.

Step 5 - Fit a Deformable Model: An elastically adaptive LV deformable model [9] is fitted to the fuzzy connectedness and dual contrast data using shape constraints. The domain specific prior knowledge that LV boundary is non-intersecting, closed and includes the papillary is incorporated to optimize fitting of deformable model to LV boundary (Fig. 3(q-w)). The elasticity parameters of the deformable model are changed adaptively depending on the gradient values allowing us to overcome spurious boundaries.

Step 6 - Compute the EF: Compute the EF by computing the volumes of the fitted deformable models at the end of systolic and diastolic phase.

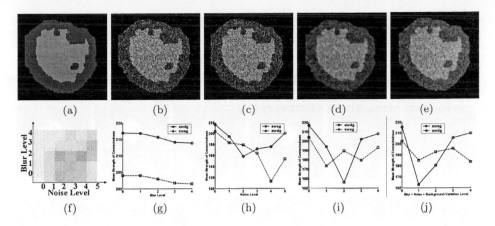

Fig. 2. Images from a phantom data set. (a) Synthetic image and (b-e) synthetic image contaminated with blur, noise, blur + noise, and blur + noise + background variation, respectively. (f) Robustness of adaptive fuzzy connectedness over noise and blur variations with the mean intensity values of the segmented region of interest mapped to gray scale (0-255). Plots (g-j) depict the results of a comparative study between the adaptive and the conventional fuzzy connectedness with $w_1 = w_2 = 0.5$ for various levels of: (g) blur, (h) noise, (i) blur + noise, and (j) blur + noise + background variation.

3   Results, Discussion and Conclusion

We have performed a number of experiments to assess the accuracy, limitations and advantages of our approach. The processing time on an Intel Pentium III 900Mz workstation with 0.5GB RAM ranged from 30-45s for each dual contrast dataset comprised of 20 images.

For the first experiment, we designed a number of synthetic 3D dual contrast datasets with different levels of noise, blurring, and gradual intensity change effects (Fig. 2), in order to assess the benefits from adapting the weights for fuzzy connectedness dynamically. The membership scene for spels belonging to the target object is defined as the square region of 100 pixels in the target of the central $c_1 c_2$ slice. We use the mean values of strength of connectedness attached to the ground truth as metric to compare the performance of adaptive fuzzy connectedness-based segmentation with respect to the conventional fuzzy connectedness-based segmentation. Fig. 2 depicts the results of the comparison study of the two methods on a phantom dataset.

Next, we present the results from the segmentation of the data acquired from Subject-1. Figs. 3(a-h) illustrate a sample set of diastolic short-axis bFFE and TSE images. Corresponding FCM based LV region and centroid estimates are shown in Figs. 3(i-l). The segmentation results using adaptively weighted Fuzzy Connectedness for the LV blood pool are depicted in Fig. 3(m-p). Figs. 3(q-t) depict projections of the fitted elastically adaptive shape-constrained deformable model on the corresponding slices. Figs. 3(u-w) depict the fitted deformable models for subjects 1, 4, and 9, respectively.

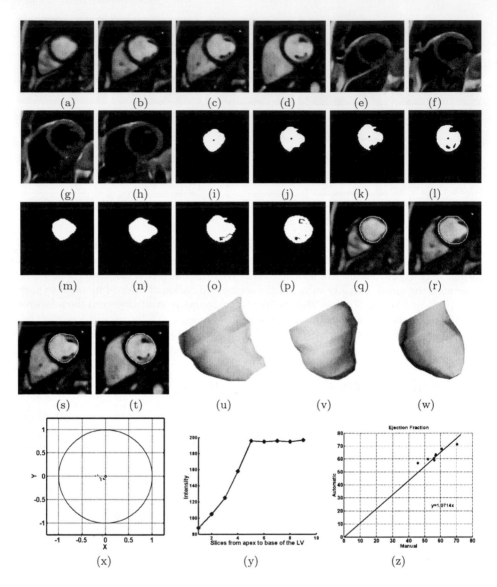

Fig. 3. Slices for the diastolic dataset from a single-breath-hold multi-slice cine (subject-1), acquired with (a-d) bFFE, and (e-h) TSE MR imaging. (i-l) FCM-based LV estimation with centroid and (m-p) resulting Fuzzy connectedness data. (q-t) Projection of the fitted elastically adaptive deformable model. Fitted deformable models of the LV blood pool for (u) Subject-1, (v) Subject-4, (w) Subject-9,respectively. (x) Estimated centroids for nine subjects mapped on a normalized circle fitted to the LVs obtained manually, (y) coil intensity fall off in MR, and (z) EFs for nine subjects using manual and automatic methods.

The EFs computed for nine volunteers using the manual method and automated blood segmentation method are shown in Fig. 3(z). Our initial validation results demonstrate the feasibility of using bFFE/TSE for automated segmentation of the LV.

References

1. A. Chakraborty and J. Duncan. Game-theoretic integration for image segmentation. *PAMI*, 21(1):12–30, January 1999.
2. J. Duncan and N. Ayache. Medical image analysis: Progress over two decades and the chanllenges ahead. *IEEE T-PAMI*, 22(1):85–106, 2000.
3. C. Imielinska, D. Metaxas, J. Udupa, Y. Jin, and T. Chen. Hybrid segmentation of anatomical data. In *Proceedings of the 4th MICCAI*, pages 1048–1057, Utrecht, The Netherlands, October 2001. Springer-Verlag.
4. M. Jolly. Combining edge, region, and shape information to segment the left ventricle in cardiac MR images. In *Proceedings of the 4th MICCAI*, pages 482–490, Utrecht, The Netherlands, October 2001. Springer-Verlag.
5. T. N. Jones and D. N. Metaxas. Automated 3D segmentation using deformable models and fuzzy affinity. In J. Duncan and G. Gindi, editors, *Proceedings of the XVth International Conference on Image Processing in Medical Imaging*, volume 1230, pages 113–126, Poultney, Vermont, 1997. Springer.
6. B. Lelieveldt, R. van der Geest, S. Mitchell, M. Sonka, and J. Reiber. Fully automatic detection of right- and left ventricular contours in short-axis cardiac mr images using active appearance models. In *Annual Meeting of the Society for Cardiovascular MR*, page 65, Atlanta, 2001.
7. N. Matheijssen, L. Baur, J. Reiber, E. V. der Velde, P. V. Dijkman, R. V. der Geest, A. de Ross, and E. V. der Wall. Assessment of left ventricular volume and mass by cine magnetic resonance imaging in patients with anterior myocardial infarction: Intra-observer and inter-observer variability on contour detection. *International Journal of Cardiac Imaging*, 12:11–19, 1996.
8. T. McInerney and D. Terzopoulos. Deformable models in medical image analysis: A survey. *Medical Image Analysis*, 1(2):91–108, 1996.
9. D. Metaxas and I. Kakadiaris. Elastically adaptive deformable models. *IEEE T-PAMI*, October 2002. (In Press).
10. D. Metaxas and D. Terzopoulos. Shape and nonrigid motion estimation through physics-based synthesis. *IEEE T-PAMI*, 15(6):580–591, June 1993.
11. J. Park, D. Metaxas, A. Young, and L. Axel. Deformable models with parameter functions for cardiac motion analysis from tagged MRI data. *IEEE Trans. Medical Imaging*, 15:278–289, 1996.
12. P. K. Saha and J. K. Udupa. Fuzzy connected object delineation: Axiomatic path strength definition and the case of mulitiple seeds. *CVIU*, 83:275–295, 2001.
13. L. Staib and J. Duncan. Model-based deformable surface finding for medical images. *IEEE Transactions on Medical Imaging*, 15:720–731, 1996.
14. D. Terzopoulos and D. Metaxas. Dynamic 3D models with local and global deformations: Deformable superquadrics. *IEEE T-PAMI*, 13(7):703–714, 1991.
15. D. Thendens. Rapid left ventricular border detector with a multi-resolution graph searching approach. In *Proc. Intl. Soc. Mag. Reson. Med*, 9, page 601, 2001.
16. J. Udupa and S. Samarasekera. Fuzzy connectedness and object definition: theory, algorithms, and applications in image segmentation. *Graphical Models and Image Processing*, 58(3):246–261, 1996.

Efficient Partial Volume Tissue Classification in MRI Scans

Aljaž Noe[1] and James C. Gee[2]

[1] Faculty of Electrical Engineering, University of Ljubljana
[2] Department of Radiology, University of Pennsylvania

Abstract. A probabilistic tissue classification algorithm is described for robust MR brain image segmentation in the presence of partial volume averaging. Our algorithm estimates the fractions of all tissue classes present in every voxel of an image. In this work, we discretize the fractional content of tissues in *partial volume voxels*, to obtain a finite number of mixtures. Every mixture has a label assigned to it, and the algorithm searches for the labeling that maximizes the posterior probability of the labeled image. A prior is defined to favor spatially continuous regions while taking into an account different tissue mixtures. We show that this extension of an existing partial volume clustering algorithm, [8], improves the quality of segmentation, without increasing the complexity of the procedure. The final result is the estimated fractional amount of each tissue type present within a voxel in addition to the label assigned to the voxel.

1 Introduction

In this work, we consider the problem of segmenting magnetic resonance (MR) images, which is made difficult by the existence of partial volume (PV) averaging and intensity shading artifacts due to limited spatial resolution of the scanner and RF field inhomogeneity, respectively. To improve the quantitative precision of segmentation, we develop a method for determining the fractional content of each tissue class for so-called partial volume voxels of mixed tissue type, taking into account shading artifacts. Of specific interest in the current work are the primary tissue constituents of the brain: gray (GM) and white matter (WM) as well as cerebrospinal fluid (CSF).

Two general approaches have been applied to address the problem of partial volume (PV) segmentation. In [2, 7], a *mixel model*, assumes that every voxel in an image is a PV voxel, consisting of a mixture of pure tissue classes. Because of the number of parameters that must be estimated, either multi-channel data and/or additional constraints are required to obtain the segmentation solution. A second approach, [8, 5, 9] to dealing with PV voxels is to marginalize over the variables describing the fractional portions of each *pure tissue class*. This produces an additional, new set of *partial volume classes*, with which each image voxel may be associated. However, an additional estimation step is necessary to obtain the fractional amount of different tissues in each voxel.

T. Dohi and R. Kikinis (Eds.): MICCAI 2002, LNCS 2488, pp. 698–705, 2002.

In the current work we develop a method that shares aspects of both approaches. In the mixel-model approach, noise in the image limits the precision with which the fractional tissue content in PV voxels can be estimated from the image. This in turn results in either a noisy or over smoothed final segmentation. The marginalization approach identifies PV voxels, but does not provide an estimate of the tissue fractions for these voxels. Moreover, both approaches are computationally expensive. The mixel model entails a large number on unknowns, whereas the marginalization requires numeric integration to obtain a distribution function of PV classes.

We propose to use only a *finite* number of mixtures for a given pair of tissue classes to model the PV averaging effect. In this way, marginalization is not required and the fractional tissue content of PV voxels is directly provided by the mixture label. The precision of the fractional tissue estimates can be controlled through the appropriate discretization of the continuous mixture.

While this approach can and should also be used within the implementation of the clustering procedure for the estimation of class probability paramaters, we choose to treat it separately to be able to obtain unbiased evaluation of its functionality.

2   Image Model

Let $\mathbf{y}_i = (y_{i,1}, y_{i,2}, \ldots y_{i,M})^T$ be the M-channel observation at the i-th voxel of an input image. At each voxel we assume there exists a mixture of several different tissue types. The contribution of a specific tissue type to the voxel measurement is weighted by its fractional ammount in the voxel. Tissues are modeled by voxel classes that are assumed to have Gaussian probability distribution of the intensity. This type of image model was also used by several other authors [2, 7] and in part also by [5, 9]. Measurement at each voxel is modeled as a linear combination of Gaussian random variables:

$$\mathbf{y}_i = \sum_{k \in \mathcal{K}} t_{i,k} \mathbf{N}(\boldsymbol{\mu}_k(i), \boldsymbol{\Sigma}_k), \quad \sum_{k \in \mathcal{K}} t_{i,k} = 1, \quad 0 \le t_{i,k} \le 1, \tag{1}$$

where $\mathbf{N}(\boldsymbol{\mu}_k, \boldsymbol{\Sigma}_k)$ represents a multivariate Gaussian random variable with $\boldsymbol{\mu}_k = (\mu_{k,1}, \ldots, \mu_{k,M})^T$ the vector of mean intensity values (M channels), and $\boldsymbol{\Sigma}_k$ is the associated M-by-M covariance matrix for the M-channel observation. Each tissue class k can have different mean and variance, where $\mathcal{K}$ is the set of permissible tissue types. Note that mean vector $\boldsymbol{\mu}_k(i)$ is also a function of voxel location i, which allows us to take into account intensity inhomogeneities that may be present in the data.

$t_{i,k}$ represents the fraction of pure tissue class k that is present at the i-th voxel. The goal of the partial volume segmentation is to estimate $t_{i,k}, \forall k \in \mathcal{K}$ for each voxel i in the image. In order to do that, we can solve (1) for each i. Since we have in general more than one unknown variable per equation and there is also noise present in an image, the problem is severely under constrained. Additional constraints must therefore be introduced on the image model.

In [6] the PV effect is assumed to be caused by downsampling a high resolution image. We use this idea and constrain the image model in (1) in two ways. First, we assume the number of different tissue types in a voxel is limited to two, which in practice introduces negligible error in the image model. Second, we discretize the continuous mixture variable and consider only a finite number of mixture possibilities:

$$t_{i,k} \in \mathcal{T},$$
$$\mathcal{T} = \{\tau_1, \tau_2, \ldots, \tau_T\}, \quad \tau_i \neq \tau_j. \tag{2}$$

The motivation for the latter constraint is that the presence of image noise may limit the precission with which the fractional tissue content can be estimated. This constraint, on the other hand, makes the problem of estimating fractions of pure tissue classes much easier.

In practical applications the number of specific mixtures T is chosen to obtain a compromise between the amount of partial volume voxels in the image, required precision of segmentation and the computational time. We then consider these mixtures as additional voxel classes in our image—*mixture classes*. Since the measurement of each mixture class is defined by a linear combination of two Gaussian random variables, the distribution of mixtures is again a Gaussian distribution, with the following mean and variance:

$$\boldsymbol{\mu}_{t,k_1,k_2} = \boldsymbol{\mu}_{k_1} + (1-t)\boldsymbol{\mu}_{k_2}$$
$$\boldsymbol{\Sigma}_{t,k_1,k_2} = t^2\boldsymbol{\Sigma}_{k_1} + (1-t)^2\boldsymbol{\Sigma}_{k_2}, \tag{3}$$

where $t \in \mathcal{T}$ is the specific mixture ratio between tissue classes k_1 and k_2. When segmenting MR images of the brain, we define two sets of mixtures: one modeling PV voxels containing CSF and GM, and the other modeling the voxels containing GM and WM. A different label λ is assigned to every mixture class—one for each (t, k_1, k_2) triplet.

2.1 Bayesian Formulation of Segmentation Problem

The posterior probability of the classification $\boldsymbol{\Lambda}$ given the data $\mathbf{Y}$ is defined as:

$$P(\boldsymbol{\Lambda}|\mathbf{Y}) = \frac{P(\mathbf{Y}|\boldsymbol{\Lambda})P(\boldsymbol{\Lambda})}{P(\mathbf{Y})}, \tag{4}$$

where $P(\mathbf{Y}|\boldsymbol{\Lambda})$ is our observation/image model and $P(\boldsymbol{\Lambda})$ is a prior on the label field. As in [9], we use a Potts model for the prior to penalize the granualities in the labeling,

$$P(\boldsymbol{\Lambda}) = \frac{1}{Z} \exp\left[-\beta \sum_i \sum_{j \in \mathcal{N}_i} \delta(\lambda_i, \lambda_j)\right], \tag{5}$$

where β is a constant that controls the strength of a prior, $\mathcal{N}_i$ is the set of voxels in some neighborhood of voxel i and Z is a scaling constant. $\delta(\lambda_i, \lambda_i)$ defines the "similarity" between mixture classes λ_i and λ_j. Specifically $\delta(\lambda_i, \lambda_j) = \frac{o}{d(i,j)}$,

Table 1. Tissue overlap between different mixture classes. First three columns/rows correspond to pure classes, and the rest are different PV mixtures—here we have 4 different PV mixture ratios. Column labels are identical to rows labels but are partially omited to save space. By changing the values in this table, different mixture classes can be favored.

mixture class	CSF	GM	WM	.	.	.	.	.	.	.	.
CSF	1.0	0.0	0.0	0.8	0.6	0.4	0.2	0.0	0.0	0.0	0.0
GM	0.0	1.0	0.0	0.2	0.4	0.6	0.8	0.8	0.6	0.4	0.2
WM	0.0	0.0	1.0	0.0	0.0	0.0	0.0	0.2	0.4	0.6	0.8
0.8CSF, 0.2GM	0.8	0.2	0.0	1.0	0.8	0.6	0.4	0.2	0.2	0.2	0.2
0.6CSF, 0.4GM	0.6	0.4	0.0	0.8	1.0	0.8	0.6	0.4	0.4	0.4	0.2
0.4CSF, 0.6GM	0.4	0.6	0.0	0.6	0.8	1.0	0.8	0.6	0.6	0.4	0.2
0.2CSF, 0.8GM	0.2	0.8	0.0	0.4	0.6	0.8	1.0	0.8	0.6	0.4	0.2
0.8GM, 0.2WM	0.0	0.8	0.2	0.2	0.4	0.6	0.8	1.0	0.8	0.6	0.4
0.6GM, 0.4WM	0.0	0.6	0.4	0.2	0.4	0.6	0.6	0.8	1.0	0.8	0.6
0.4GM, 0.6WM	0.0	0.4	0.6	0.2	0.4	0.4	0.4	0.6	0.8	1.0	0.8
0.2GM, 0.8WM	0.0	0.2	0.8	0.2	0.2	0.2	0.2	0.4	0.6	0.8	1.0

where $0 \leq o \leq 1$ is the amount of "tissue overlap" between the two mixture classes λ_i and λ_j and $d(i,j)$ is the distance between voxels i and j. Overlap values are shown in table 1. This definition favors smooth transition of estimated fractions between regions of pure tissue type.

We find the labeling Λ that maximizes the posterior probability $P(\Lambda|Y)$:

$$\Lambda = \arg\max_{\Lambda} P(\Lambda|Y). \tag{6}$$

3 Implementation

We use the ICM algorithm [1] to maximize the posterior probability (4):

$$\lambda_i^{n+1} = \arg\max_{\lambda} \left[\log P(\mathbf{y}_i|\lambda) - \beta \sum_{j \in \mathcal{N}_i} \delta(\lambda, \lambda_j^n) \right], \tag{7}$$

where $P(\mathbf{y}_i|\lambda)$ is the conditional probability density function for observing $\mathbf{y}$ at voxel i given mixture class λ, and λ_i^n is the mixture label for voxel i computed at n-th iteration.

In order to evaluate $P(\mathbf{y}_i|\lambda)$, its parameters $\boldsymbol{\mu}_k$ and $\boldsymbol{\Sigma}_k$, must be estimated from the image prior to the classification. We use maximum likelihood mixture model clustering [8] to estimate these parameters externally without affecting the classifier. The expectation maximization algorithm is used to iteratively update the class parameters:

$$\boldsymbol{\mu}_k = \frac{\sum_{i=1}^{N} P(k|\mathbf{y}_i) \cdot \mathbf{y}_i}{h_k}; \quad \boldsymbol{\Sigma}_k = \frac{\sum_{i=1}^{N} P(k|\mathbf{y}_i) \cdot \mathbf{y}_i \cdot \mathbf{y}_i^T}{h_k} - \boldsymbol{\mu}_k \cdot \boldsymbol{\mu}_k^T; \tag{8}$$

$$h_k = \sum_{i=1}^{N} P(k|\mathbf{y}_i), \quad k \in \mathcal{K}.$$

The clustering algorithm also takes into account any PV averaging that may be present in the image and in addition estimates the intensity nonuniformity field, thus obtaining the class mean intensity value for each voxel in the image $\mu_k(i)$. This implies that probability density functions $P(\mathbf{y}_i|k)$ are also spatially dependent. The mean values and variances of a specific mixture class can then be computed for any i using (3).

4   Experiments and Discussion

In order to evaluate the segmentation accuracy of the proposed method we require a test image for which a ground truth partial volume information is available. Manual segmentations of real MR data do not provide such information. We must therefore resort to the use of simulated MR images. Specifically we used the 1 mm T1, BrainWeb[3, 4] phantom images produced by the McConnell Brain Imaging Centre at the Montreal Neurological Institute. For each simulated image, true fraction of the gray and white matter and cerebrospinal fluid is known at every voxel in an image. Parameter β was set to 0.4 and 4 ICM iterations were used.

To estimate the disparity between the segmentation results and ground truth, we calculated the mean squared difference between the estimated and true fractional values over the entire image for each tissue type. Images with various amounts of noise were segmented into 3 pure tissue classes (GM, WM, CSF) and 2 PV classes (GM/WM, GM/CSF) with 9 different mixtures each. This gives a total of 21 different classes into which each image voxel can be segmented. The mean square differences averaged over all tissue types were 0.0182, 0.0086 and 0.0048 for BrainWeb images containing 9%, 3% and 0% noise respectively. Results of the evaluation are presented in Fig. 1.

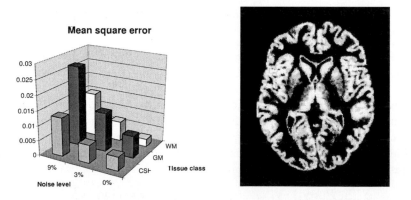

Fig. 1. Segmentation results for BrainWeb phantom. (Left) Mean square error in estimation of tissue fractions. (Right): Example gray matter segmentation.

We found slight difference between the current results of our BrainWeb seg-mentation and those obtained using a marginalization approach [8] in favor of the former. This is in part due to relatively small amount of partial volume artifact present in the data. Although the spatial prior reduces noise in the seg-mented image, it also introduces smoothing, which is manifested as errors in segmentation.

Since the number of partial volume voxels is small in comparison to the size of the BrainWeb image, changing the number of mixture classes has little effect on the segmentation results. To further explore the relationship between the amount of noise in the image, number of mixture classes and the quality of segmentation, we performed a series of tests on a synthetic images of a square, exhibiting different amounts of noise and partial volume averaging artifact.

We constructed a square, 300-by-300, image and subdivided the image into 3 regions, each separated by a vertical boundary. The left and right most regions were considered pure "tissues" and their image values were drawn from normal distributions with the following mean and variance values, respectively: $\mu_1 = 70$, $\Sigma_1 = 100$ and $\mu_2 = 150$, $\Sigma_2 = 400$. The middle strip of the image, 100 pixels wide, contained partial volume pixels, which modeled a smooth linear transition between the two pure classes. The synthetic image is shown in Fig. 2.

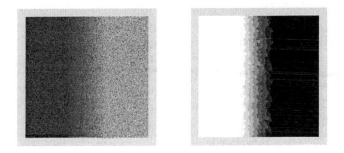

Fig. 2. Synthetic data. (Left) Test image used in evaluation. (Right) Segmentation result for using 8 PV mixtures, where the intensity reflects the fractional content—white indicates 100%, black 0%.

In Fig. 3, we show the mean square error in segmentation as a function of the number of mixtures. We can clearly observe the inverse relationship between these two parameters. We can see that increasing the number of mixture classes beyond a certain number only minimally improves the segmentation. This en-ables considerable savings in computational time compared to the marginaliza-tion approach for PV segmentation, by avoiding numerical integration required to obtain PV distribution. This holds for both the clustering step, where class parameters are estimated, as well as during the voxel classification procedure. We have also observed that the number of steps required for the ICM algorithm to converge increases with the number of mixture classes. It however remains manageble, and we never had to use more than 15 steps to achieve convergence.

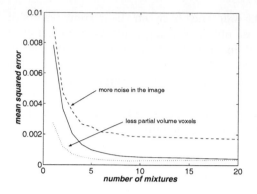

Fig. 3. Relationship between the mean square error in segmentation of the synthetic image of a square and number of PV mixture classes used in the segmentation. Solid line shows the error for image as defined above, dashed line represents error for the image that contained three times the amount of noise and dotted line is for the image that contained only one third of the partial volume effect.

We observed minimal changes in the above relationship as a result of different noise levels in the image. The difference in image noise is directly related to the segmentation error and does not affect the ratio between number of mixtures and error. The amount of PV voxels in the image, however, clearly affects this ratio and thereby defines the optimal number of mixtures. This allows us to efficiently segment images with various amounts of PV averaging, by simply changing the number of mixture classes accordingly.

Although this is not clearly visible in the graph, we have also observed a slight increase in error when number of mixture classes was too large. Error when using 20 mixture classes was for example larger than it was when only 10 mixtures were used. While this error could be contributed to the fact that the ICM algorithem simply did not finish in the minimum, there nevertheless clearly exists a number of mixture classes, that provides an optimal balance between segmentation error and numeric complexity.

5   Summary

We presented a method for partial volume segmentation of MR images. The method represents an intermediate approach between the estimation of continuous tissue fractions in the image model (1) and the addition of a single class with which all partial volume voxels of a certain tissue combination are labeled regardless of the mixture ratio of the combination. The modeling of multiple mixture ratios in the current work enables a more efficient implementation than the latter approach in which a marginalization must be numerically evaluated. Furthermore, our method's small number of unknown parameters in comparison to mixel model based-methods results in a more stable algorithms. At the same time, in preliminary evaluations, we found little degradation in partial volume segmentation accuracy as a consequence of using only a discrete range of mixture ratios. This remains to be validated on a more comprehensive data set, which is planned for the future.

References

1. Julian Besag. On the Statistical Analysis of Dirty Pictures. *Journal of the Royal Statistical Society, Series B*, 48(3):259–302, 1986.
2. Hwan Soo Choi, David R. Haynor, and Yongmin Kim. Partial volume tissue classification of multichannel magnetic resonance images - a mixel model. *IEEE Transactions on Medical Imaging*, 10(3):395–407, September 1991.
3. http://www.bic.mni.mcgill.ca/brainweb/.
4. R.K.-S. Kwan, A.C. Evans, and G. B. Pike. *An Extensible MRI Simulator for Post-Processing Evaluation*, volume 1131 of *Lecture Notes in Computer Science*, pages 135–140. Springer-Verlag, May 1996.
5. David H. Laidlaw, Kurt W. Flescher, and Alan H. Barr. Partial-volume bayesian classification of material mixtures in MR volume data using voxel histograms. *IEEE Transactions on Medical Imaging*, 17(1):74–86, February 1998.
6. Koen Van Leemput and Paul Suetens Frederik Maes, Dirk Vandermeulen. A statistical framework for partial volume segmentation. In *Proceedings 4th international conference on medical image computing and computer-assisted intervention - MICCAI2001*, volume 2208 of *Lecture Notes in Computer Science*, pages 204–212, October 2001.
7. Lucien Nocera and James C. Gee. Robust partial volume tissue classification of cerebral MRI scans. In K. M. Hanson, editor, *SPIE Medical Imaging*, volume 3034, pages 312–322, February 1997.
8. Aljaž Noe, Stanislav Kovačič, and James C. Gee. Segmentation of Cerebral MRI Scans Using a Partial Volume Model, Shading Correction, and an Anatomical Prior. In *Proceedings of the SPIE Symposium on Medical Imaging 2001: Image Processing*, volume 4322, pages 1466–1477, San Diego, California, USA, February 2001.
9. David W. Shattuck, Stephanie R. Sandor-Leahy, Kirt A. Schaper, David A. Rottenberg, and Richard M. Leahy. Magnetic resonance image tissue classification using a partial volume model. *NeuroImage*, 13(5):856–876, May 2001.

In-vivo Strain and Stress Estimation of the Left Ventricle from MRI Images

Zhenhua Hu[1], Dimitris Metaxas[2], and Leon Axel[3]

[1] Department of Computer and Information Science
University of Pennsylvania, Philadelphia, PA 19104, USA
zhhu@seas.upenn.edu
[2] The Center of Computational Biomedical, Imaging and Modeling
Rutgers University, New Brunswick, NJ 08854-8019, USA
dnm@cs.rutgers.edu
[3] Department of Radiology
New York University, New York City, NY 10016, USA
Leon.axel@rad.nyu.edu

Abstract. Little information is known about in-vivo heart strain and stress distribution. In this paper, we present a novel statistical model to estimate the in-vivo material properties and strain and stress distribution in the left ventricle. The displacements of the heart wall are reconstructed in previous work of our group by using MRI-SPAMM tagging technique and deformable model. Based on the reconstructed displacements, we developed the statistical model to estimate strain and stress by using EM algorithm. Two normal hearts and two hearts with right-ventricular hypertrophy are studied. We find noticeable differences in the strain and stress estimated for normal and abnormal hearts.

1 Introduction

To better understand cardiac diseases, we need to get more information about cardiac motion. Among the factors characterizing heart's motion, stress and strain are two of the most important determinants of various aspects of cardiac physiology and pathophysiology [1]. Stress and strain in the heart depends on not only the structure and material properties of heart but also the active force generated by the heart muscle and the blood pressure on the heart wall. To fully understand it, we need clear pictures on all these issues. The structure of heart has been intensively investigated in the last four decades. It's known that myocardium consists of locally parallel muscle fibers, a complex vascular network, and a dense plexus of connective tissue[1]. Systematic measurements of muscle fiber orientations were carried out by Streeter [10]. His main finding was that fiber directions generally vary in a continuous manner from +60° on the endocardium to -60° on the epicardium. The material properties of heart wall were initially based on uniaxial tests mostly performed with papillary muscles [17,18]. Then the biaxial tests were carried out [19,20] and the constitutive relations were proposed [21,22], which has shown that the myocardium is anisotropic. The active force was modeled in [13] and the blood pressure can be referred in [23]. In the last few years, some experiments were carried out on in-vitro left ventricle strain and stress [2]. But little in-vivo cardiac stress and strain has been estimated. This is because any invasive method will change the heart's material property and non-invasive method is not yet possible to measure these parameters. Some other experiments estimated in-

T. Dohi and R. Kikinis (Eds.): MICCAI 2002, LNCS 2488, pp. 706–713, 2002.
© Springer-Verlag Berlin Heidelberg 2002

vivo strain by using echocardiography [5,24]. But echocardio-graphy doesn't have accurate spatial resolution compared to MRI.

In this paper, the displacements of the left ventricle are reconstructed by using MRI-SPAMM tagging [3] and physics-based deformable model [4] based on previous work of Haber [14,25]. First we present a novel statistical model to estimate the material properties of left ventricle. Second we use the statistical model to compute the strain and stress distribution in different time intervals between the end of diastole and the end of systole.

2   Mechanical Model

2.1   Geometrical Model

The geometrical model is chosen the same as given in [14,25]. We added the fiber direction into each element. The left ventricle is divided into two layers circumferentially, we assume the fiber is +60° on the endocardium and -60° on the epicardium.

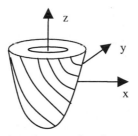

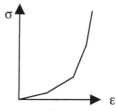

Fig. 1. Fiber orientation on epicardium of left ventricle

Fig. 2. Piece-wise linearity of Young's modulus E_1 and E_2

2.2   Strain-Stress Relationship

Myocyte is the main structural components of myocardium, which normally occupies 70% of ventricular wall volume. Myocytes look like cylinders and are embedded in a complex matrix of collagen, elastin, etc [1]. In recent work [5,6], transversely isotropic linear material model were used in the estimation of cardiac motion. Unlike in [5,6], we model the myocardium as transversely isotropic material with symmetric stiffness matrix and piece-wise linear elasticity. The stress-strain relationship is given by [8]:

$$\underline{\varepsilon} = \begin{bmatrix} 1/E_1 & -v_{12}/E_1 & -v_{12}/E_1 & 0 & 0 & 0 \\ -v_{12}/E_1 & 1/E_2 & -v_{23}/E_2 & 0 & 0 & 0 \\ -v_{12}/E_1 & -v_{23}/E_2 & 1/E_2 & 0 & 0 & 0 \\ 0 & 0 & 0 & 2(1+v_{23})/E_2 & 0 & 0 \\ 0 & 0 & 0 & 0 & 1/G_{12} & 0 \\ 0 & 0 & 0 & 0 & 0 & 1/G_{12} \end{bmatrix} \underline{\sigma} \qquad (1)$$

where E_1 is the Young's modulus along fiber direction, E_2 is the Young's modulus along cross-fiber direction, v_{12} and v_{23} are the corresponding Poisson ratios, and G_{12} is the Shear Modulus. Since the myocardium is approximately incompressible, the Poisson ratios are both set to 0.4 [9]. Both Young's modulus are assumed piece-wise linear, which are shown qualitatively in Fig 2.

2.3   Coordinates Transformation Relation

Since the myofiber direction varies in different parts of the left ventricle [10], we need to transform the local fiber coordinates into global element coordinate when implementing finite element method. For coordinates shown in Fig. 3, the stress in local fiber coordinate $(1,2,3)$ can be transformation into global element coordinate (x,y,z) by [8]:

$$
\begin{bmatrix} \sigma_1 \\ \sigma_2 \\ \sigma_3 \\ \tau_{23} \\ \tau_{31} \\ \tau_{12} \end{bmatrix} = \begin{bmatrix} \cos^2\theta & \sin^2\theta & 0 & 0 & 0 & 2\sin\theta\cos\theta \\ \sin^2\theta & \cos^2\theta & 0 & 0 & 0 & -2\sin\theta\cos\theta \\ 0 & 0 & 1 & 0 & 0 & 0 \\ 0 & 0 & 0 & \cos\theta & -\sin\theta & 0 \\ 0 & 0 & 0 & \sin\theta & \cos\theta & 0 \\ -\sin\theta\cos\theta & \sin\theta\cos\theta & 0 & 0 & 0 & \cos^2\theta-\sin^2\theta \end{bmatrix} \begin{bmatrix} \sigma_x \\ \sigma_y \\ \sigma_z \\ \tau_{yx} \\ \tau_{zx} \\ \tau_{xy} \end{bmatrix} \tag{2}
$$

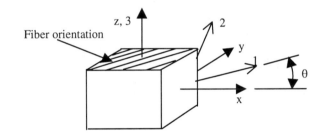

Fig. 3. Coordinate transformation between local and global coordinates

2.4   Model Dynamics

Using the energy minimization and variational formulation [11], we derived the finite element equation:

$$\dot{q} + Kq = P \tag{3}$$

where q represents the displacement, K is the stiffness matrix and:

$$K = \sum_e (\int_{V^e} B^T DB dV) , \quad P = P_p + P_a = \sum_e (\int_{S^e} N^T f_p dS + \int_{V^e} N^T f_a dV) \tag{4}$$

where f_p is the boundary force mainly generated by the blood, and f_a is the active force generated by the myofiber. D is the stress-strain matrix that relates nodal stress, σ, to nodal strain, ε, as $\sigma = D\varepsilon$. B is the strain-displacement matrix that relates nodal strain, ε, to nodal displacements, q, as $\varepsilon = Bq$. N is the shape function for interpolation.

3   Statistical Estimation of K and f_a

In equation 3, stiffness matrix K and active force f_a are unknown. We need to estimate them before the calculation of strain and stress. The in-vitro stiffness parameters were measured through experiments carried on canine heart [13], we'll use the data as the initial state based on similarity between human and canine hearts. The Expectation/Maximization (EM) algorithm is used for the estimation.

3.1   Expectation/Maximization (EM) Algorithm

EM algorithm [15] is typically used to compute maximum likelihood estimates given incomplete samples. Define $J(\theta|\theta_0)$ as:

$$J(\theta \mid \theta_0) \equiv E_{\theta_0} \left(\log \frac{p(X, \theta)}{p(X, \theta_0)} \bigg| S(X) = s \right) \tag{5}$$

where X is the random variable, θ is the parameter to be estimated, S(X) is the sufficient statistics on X, p(X, θ) is the probability density function. The EM algorithm works as following:

1. Initialize $\theta_{old} = \theta_0$
2. Compute $J(\theta|\theta_{old})$ for as many values of θ as possible
3. Maximize $J(\theta|\theta_{old})$ as a function of θ
4. Set $\theta_{new} = \arg \max J(\theta|\theta_{old})$, if $\theta_{old} \neq \theta_{new}$, set $\theta_{old} = \theta_{new}$ and go to step 2, otherwise, return $\theta = \theta_{new}$.

where Step 2 is often referred to as the expectation step and Step 3 is called the maximization step.

3.2   Implementation

In our experiment, $\theta = (E_1, F_2, f_a)$. Since we don't have explicit form of probability density function p(X, θ), we use the following way to construct it. We define the displacement divergence as:

$$d(x, \hat{\theta}) = \frac{1}{n} \sum_{i=1}^{n} \left[(x_i - x_{it})^2 + (y_i - y_{it})^2 + (z_i - z_{it})^2 \right] \tag{6}$$

where (x_i, y_i, z_i) is the computed displacement based on estimation $\theta = \hat{\theta}$ and (x_{it}, y_{it}, z_{it}) is the reconstructed displacement from MRI tagging. Since the smaller the displacement divergence, the better the estimation is, we put more weight on estimation with less displacement divergence. Then the normalized density function is defined as:

$$p(x, \hat{\theta}) = \frac{1 / d(x, \hat{\theta})}{\sum_{\theta \in \Theta} (1 / d(x, \theta))} \tag{7}$$

As shown in Fig. 2, E_1 and E_2 are stepwise linear, so we need to estimate θ in each time interval. We assume E_1 and E_2 are linearly related. The implementation algorithm is:

1. Initialize t = 1
2. In the t th time interval, calculate d(θ) and p(x, θ) for all $\theta \in \Theta$

3. Initialize $(E_{1,old}, E_{2,old}) = (E_{1,0}, E_{2,0})$, where $E_{1,0}$ and $E_{2,0}$ are calculated from the experiments' data given in [13]
4. Fix $(E_{1,old}, E_{2,old})$, using the EM algorithm to get estimation $f_{a,new}$
5. Fix $f_{a,new}$, using the EM algorithm to get estimation $(E_{1,new}, E_{2,new})$
6. If $(E_{1,old}, E_{2,old}) \neq (E_{1,new}, E_{2,new})$, set $(E_{1,old}, E_{2,old}) = (E_{1,new}, E_{2,new})$, go to step 4, otherwise, return $(E_1, E_2) = (E_{1,new}, E_{2,new})$, $f_a = f_{a,new}$
7. $t = t+1$, if $t < nt$, go to step 2, otherwise, stop.

where nt is the number of time steps.

4   Results

We did experiments for two normal hearts and two abnormal hearts with right ventricular hypertrophy. The blood pressures were set to average clinical measurements as shown in Table 1. The procedure from the end of diastole to the end of systole was divided into 4 time intervals. Time 1 corresponds to the end of diastole and time 5 corresponds to the end of systole. The Young's modulus in each time interval were set initially as shown in Table 2, which is computed from the data given in [13].

Table 1. Blood Pressures in left and right ventricles

	LV Blood Pressure	RV Blood Pressure
Normal Heart	120 mmHg	30 mmHg
RVH Heart	120 mmHg	80 mmHg

Table 2. Initial Young's modulus in each time interval

	Time Interval	1-2	2-3	3-4	4-5
Normal	E_1 (Pa)	50,000.0	60,000.0	70,000.0	80,000.0
	E_2 (Pa)	15,000.0	18,000.0	20,000.0	22,000.0
Abnormal	E_1 (Pa)	60,000.0	70,000.0	80,000.0	90,000.0
	E_2 (Pa)	18,000.0	20,000.0	22,000.0	25,000.0

Using the statistical method, we get the estimation of Young's modulus in each time interval as shown in Table 3:

Table 3. Final estimation of Young's modulus in each time interval

	Time Interval	1-2	2-3	3-4	4-5
Normal	E_1 (Pa)	48,320.0	59,780.0	71,230.0	77,590.0
	E_2 (Pa)	14,210.0	16,700.0	20,980.0	20,810.0
Abnormal	E_1 (Pa)	61,700.0	73,560.0	82,370.0	95,770.0
	E_2 (Pa)	23,550.0	24,350.0	33,360.0	36,790.0

The largest principal strain and stress in the free wall are shown in Fig. 4 and Fig. 5 respectively. From the figures, we know that the largest principal strain and stress get larger from the end of diastole to the end of systole in both normal and abnormal heart. Both normal heart and abnormal heart have larger strain and stress in the apex than in the base. Quantitatively, normal heart has smoother distribution of strain and stress than abnormal heart in the free wall. In addition, normal heart has larger strain than the abnormal heart although the stress has no much difference between normal heart and abnormal heart. This means the normal heart deforms more than the abnormal heart, but their stresses are similar because the normal heart has smaller Young's modulus.

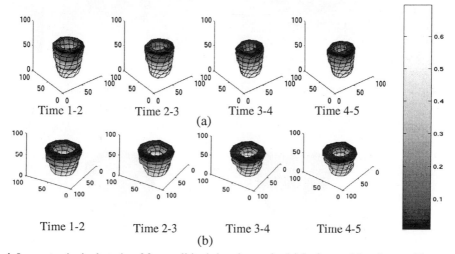

Fig. 4. Largest principal strain of free wall in 4 time intervals: (a) Left ventricle of normal heart (b) Left ventricle of abnormal heart with right ventricle hypertrophy

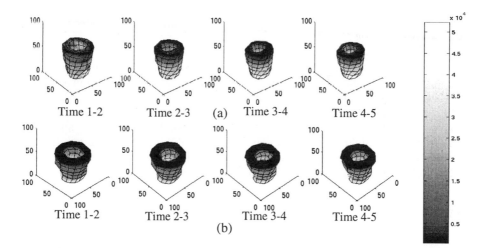

Fig. 5. Largest principal stress of free wall in 4 time intervals: (a) Left ventricle of normal heart (b) Left ventricle of abnormal heart with right ventricle hypertrophy

Comparisons between septum and free wall are also made as shown in Fig. 6 and Fig. 7. It shows that the normal heart has larger stress in the septum than in the free wall. For the abnormal heart, it has no much difference between septum and free wall. This is because the higher pressure in the right ventricle prevents the left ventricle of abnormal heart deforming as much as that of normal heart.

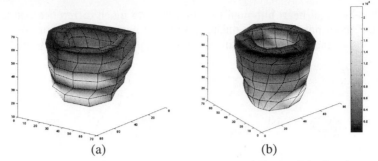

Fig. 6. Largest principal stress of normal heart: (a) Septum (b) Free wall in time interval 1-2

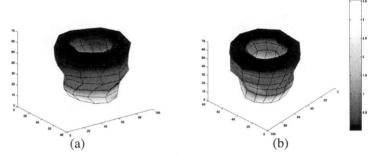

Fig. 7. Largest principal stress of left ventricle of abnormal heart: (a) Septum (b) Free wall in time interval 1-2

5   Conclusions

In-vivo strain and stress estimation is an intrinsically difficult problem. We developed a novel statistical method to compute the strain and stress by using accurate displacements reconstructed from MRI-SPAMM tagging and deformable model. Some interesting differences were found between abnormal hearts' left ventricle and normal hearts' left ventricle. The difference between septum and free wall were also found in the same left ventricle. The results may be used in the future clinical practice. More human hearts need to be studied to validate our model and our next goal is to compute strain and stress in right ventricle as well as left ventricle.

Acknowledgements

This research has been funded by grants from the NIH.

References

1. L. Glass, P. Hunter, A. McCulloch. Theory of Heart: Biomechanics, Biophysics, and Non-linear Dynamics of Cardiac Function. Springer-Verlag, 1991.
2. K. Costa. The Structural Basis of Three-Dimensional Ventricular Mechanics, Ph.D. Dissertation, University of California, San Diego, CA, 1996.

3. L. Axel, L. Dougherty. Heart wall motion: Improved method of spatial modulation of magnetization for MR imaging. Radiology, 272:349-50, 1989.
4. D. N. Metaxas. Physics-based deformable models: applications to computer vision, graphics, and medical imaging. Kluwer Academic Publishers, Cambridge, 1996.
5. X. Papademetris, A. Sinusas, D. P. Dione, J. S. Duncan. Estimation of 3D left ventricular deformation from echocardiography. Medical Image Analysis, 5:17-28, 2001.
6. M. Sermesant, Y. Coudiere, H. Delingette, N. Ayache, J. A. Desideri. An Electro-Mechanical Model of the Heart for Cardiac Image Analysis. In Medical Image Computing and Computer-Assisted Intervention (MICCAI'01), 2001.
7. Y. C. Fung. Biomechanics: mechanical properties of living tissues, 2nd ed. Springer-Verlag, 1993.
8. M. W. Hyer. Stress Analysis of Fiber-Reinforced Composite Materials. McGraw-Hill, 1998.
9. A. Amini, Y. Chen, R. W. Curwen, V. Manu, J. Sun. Coupled B-Snake grides and constrained thin-plate splines for analysis of 2D tissue deformations from tagged MRI. IEEE Transaction on Medical Imaging 17(3),344-356, 1998.
10. D. D. Streeter Jr., W. T. Hanna. Engineering mechanics for successive states in canine left ventricular myocardium: I. Cavity and wall geometry. Circulation Research, 33:639-655, 1973.
11. K. Bathe. Finite element procedures in engineering analysis. Prentice Hall, 1982.
12. O. C. Zienkiewicz, R. L. Taylor. The finite element method. McGraw-Hill, 1989.
13. T. P. Usyk, R. Mazhari, A. D. McCulloch. Effect of laminar orthotropic myofiber architecture on regional stress and strain in the canine left ventricle. Journal of Elasticity, 61, 2000.
14. Haber, D. N. Metaxas, L. Axel. Three-dimensional motion reconstruction and analysis of the right ventricle using tagged MRI. Medical Image Analysis, 4, 2000.
15. P. J. Bickel, K. A. Doksum. Mathematical statistics: basic ideas and selected topics, Vol. I. Prentice Hall, 2001.
16. Y. C. Fung. A first course in continuum mechanics: for physical and biological engineers and scientists, 3rd ed. Prentice Hall, 1994.
17. J. G. Pinto, Y. C. Fung. Mechanical properties of the heart muscle in the passive state. Journal of Biomechanics, 6:597-616,1973.
18. Y. C. Pao, G. K. Nagendra, R. Padiyar, E. L. Ritman. Derivation of myocardial fiber stiffness equation on theory of laminated composite. Journal of Biomechanical Engineering, 102:252-257, 1980.
19. L. L. Demer, F.C.P. Yin. Passive biaxial properties of isolated canine myocardium. Journal of Physiology, 339:615-630, 1983.
20. F.C.P. Yin, R. K. Strumpf, P.H. Chew, S.L. Zeger. Quantification of the mechanical properties of non-contracting myocardium. Journal of Biomechanics, 20:577-589, 1987.
21. J.D. Humphrey, F.C.P. Yin. Biomechanical experiments on excised myocardium: Theoretical considerations. Journal of Biomechanics, 22:377-383, 1989.
22. J.D. Humphery, F.C.P. Yin. On constitutive relations and finite deformations of passive cardiac tissue: I. A pseudostrain-energy function. Journal of Biomechanical Engineering, 109:298-304, 1987.
23. C. Guyton, J. E. Hall. Textbook of Medical Physiology, 10th ed. W.B. Sauders Company, 2000.
24. X. Papademetris. Estimation of 3D left ventricular deformation from medical images using biomechanical models, Ph.D. Dissertation, Yale University, New Haven, CT, May 2000.
25. Haber. Three dimensional motion reconstruction and analysis of the right ventricle from planar tagged MRI. Ph.D. Dissertation, University of Pennsylvania, Philadelphia, PA, 2000.
26. Haber, D. Metaxas, L. Axel. Motion analysis of the right ventricle from MRI images. In Medical Image Computing and Computer-Assisted Intervention (MICCAI'98), 1998.

Biomechanical Model Construction from Different Modalities: Application to Cardiac Images

M. Sermesant*, C. Forest, X. Pennec, H. Delingette, and N. Ayache

Epidaure Research Project, INRIA Sophia Antipolis
2004 route des Lucioles, 06902 Sophia Antipolis, France
*Corresponding author: Maxime.Sermesant@inria.fr

Abstract. This article describes a process to include in a volumetric model various anatomical and mechanical information provided by different sources. Three stages are described, namely a mesh construction, the non-rigid deformation of the tetrahedral mesh into various volumetric images, and the rasterization procedure allowing the transfer of properties from a voxel grid to a tetrahedral mesh. The method is experimented on various imaging modalities, demonstrating its feasibility. By using a biomechanical model, we include physically-based *a priori* knowledge which should allow to better recover the cardiac motion from images.

1 Introduction

In a previous publication [19], we presented an active electro-mechanical model of the heart triggered by the electrocardiogram. The future objective of this model is the automatic segmentation of temporal sequences of cardiac images and the automatic extraction of functional parameters useful for the diagnosis and for patient's follow up [1]. This work was initially motivated by the seminal work of McCulloch *et al.* on the construction of electro-mechanical models of the heart [11] and the use of myocardium mechanical properties in a segmentation process by Papademetris and Duncan [15].

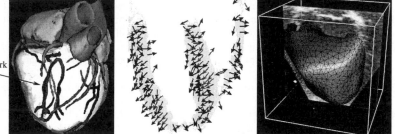

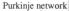
Purkinje network

Fig. 1. Left: isosurfaces extracted from the segmented heart of the Visible Human Project. Middle: diffusion tensor image to define fiber directions. Right: the electro-mechanical model of the heart in a 3D ultrasound image.

An intermediate stage to reach this objective is the ability to include in the model various anatomical and mechanical information provided by different

T. Dohi and R. Kikinis (Eds.): MICCAI 2002, LNCS 2488, pp. 714–721, 2002.

sources. An example is the introduction of the precise location of the Purkinje network, which provides important information on the sources of the electrical impulse in the myocardium. Another example is the knowledge of the fiber directions, which create dramatic mechanical and electrical local anisotropy. A last example is the knowledge of interactions between the organ and nearby structures, which can be modeled by fixed points at specific locations for instance.

Once the model is equipped with the required attributes, it is then possible to use a subset (or all) of these properties to guide its deformation in the images of a studied patient. This last stage is different but connected to other approaches, which also propose to use biomechanically controled meshes to compute deformations [6, 9, 2, 5].

The process of building a biomechanical heart model can be decomposed into three independent tasks. First, a geometric mesh consisting of a set of tetrahedra is created from a volumetric image or from any other dataset. Second, this mesh must be registered to a given image modality (such as Diffusion Tensor Imaging, MR Imaging or histology reconstruction). Finally, the third stage consists in retrieving the information of interest (fiber directions, anatomical regions,...) from the volumetric image to the volumetric mesh. Since, we are using different image modalities, several registration and information retrieval tasks may be performed. The next three sections detail each of these three stages.

2   Volumetric Mesh Creation

We created a volumetric mesh of the heart that includes both right and left ventricles. Indeed, many image modalities have a field of view large enough to include both ventricles. Furthermore, the right ventricle motion provides also information that are relevant clinically. We have chosen to use a geometric representation based on tetrahedra rather than hexahedra (as proposed in [11]) in order to better capture the important geometric details of the RV and LV during the image segmentation stage. Moreover, tetrahedral meshes allow to perform local mesh refinement in a straightforward manner, whereas one must use more sophisticated hierarchical adaptive refinement of basis functions for achieving the same results on hexahedral meshes. However, it is widely accepted that hexahedral finite elements are better suited than tetrahedral elements for the deformation computation of incompressible materials.

When creating a tetrahedral mesh, one must take into account two parameters. First the mesh size should be small enough in order to keep the computation time compatible with user interaction. Second, the shape quality of tetrahedra must be high enough in order to produce accurate results. Our approach has been to create a triangular mesh of the ventricles as the result of a several low-level tasks: image segmentation, morphological operations, image smoothing, connected component extraction, isosurfacing and mesh decimation. The quality of triangular elements and their sampling (increased at parts of high curvature) was controlled visually. The tetrahedral mesh was generated with this triangular shell using the commercial software GHS3D[1] developed at INRIA. The resulting mesh has 2000 vertices and 10000 tetrahedra.

---

[1] http://www-rocq.inria.fr/gamma/ghs3d/ghs.html

3   Registering the Mesh to a Given Image Modality

The registration of our biomechanical heart model to a given image modality is necessary in order to fuse multiple information in the same volumetric model. Furthermore, this stage is also a prerequisite before performing the segmentation and tracking in a image modality (MR, 3D US or functional imaging) used clinically. For this reason, this registration stage must be robust but also fairly efficient since it is part of interactive segmentation software.

To achieve the non-rigid registration, we rely on a coarse-to-fine approach proposed by Montagnat *et al.* [12] that smoothly combines registration and deformable model framework. At a coarse scale, an Iterative Closest Point [3] type of algorithm is applied with successively a rigid, similarity and affine transformations (see section 3.2). At a fine scale, the minimization of an internal and external energy allows to obtain more local deformations (see section 3.3). For both methods, it is necessary to determine the closest boundary point to each mesh vertex.

3.1   Computation of the Closest Boundary Points

Few authors [7] have previously proposed to segment myocardium images based on a volumetric model. They often rely on interactive segmentation [15] or pre-computed distance maps [17] to define the boundary attracting force driving their models. In our approach, the computation of this force at a surface vertex depends not only on the vertex location but also on its normal direction. Different type of forces may be applied depending on the image modality. We have chosen to combine intensity and gradient information with a region-based approach [13] applied to the intensity profile extracted at each vertex in its normal direction. It consists in defining a region with a range of intensity values and then finding its boundary by looking at the voxels of high gradient value. The extent of the intensity profile is decreased in the coarse-to-fine process.

Since there are often occlusions or very noisy parts (for instance, the right ventricle may not be visible or may be greatly biased), we can set the extent of the image interaction (external force) to different values depending on the anatomical regions of our model (determined in section 4): parts which are not seen in the image do not contribute to the external energy.

3.2   Computation of the Global Transformation

In our case the initial alignment is simply given by the correspondence of the image and model axes and the rough super-imposition of the ventricles. Then, we iteratively estimate the point matches and the transformation in an Iterative Closest Point-like loop. A rigid transformation is first estimated, then a similarity and finally an affine transformation.

The problem we had with standard least-square similarity and affine estimations in such an iterative loop with real data (like MRI) is that a global minimum is obtained if all model points are matched to the same image point, in which case the transformation is singular (null determinant of the linear part) but the error is null (thus minimized!). In practice, we observed that the least-square estimation was biased toward singular transformations and that the ICP loop often lead to collapse the model into a single voxel.

To avoid this problem, we use a new affine registration criterion C which is symmetric and forbids singular transformations (x_i and y_i are the matched model and image points, A the affine transformation and t the translation):

$$C(A,t) = \sum_i (A.x_i + t - y_i)^t.(\mathrm{Id} + A^t.A).(A.x_i + t - y_i)$$

This criterion can be derived from a statistical formulation and has a closed form solution, detailed in [16]. The scale estimation is different from the least-squares and the Procrustes ones: it is symmetric (like the Procrustes method [8]) but takes into account the individual matches and not only global properties of the point sets.

The use of this criterion allowed to initialize well the model with a global transformation even in biased images, before fitting the model with a better accuracy using local deformations.

3.3   Computation of the Local Deformation

At this stage, our biomechanical model evolves under both the influences of an *Internal Energy* computed from the physical properties of the organ and an *External Energy* computed from the image, as defined in the deformable model framework.

Internal Energy. The internal energy is computed with linear elasticity using the Tensor-Mass model [4]. We use the Finite Element Method with linear tetrahedral elements and mass-lumping in a Newtonian differential equation with an explicit time integration scheme. If we want to fit a model built from a heart to an image from another heart, there is no physical basis to the deformation, so we use isotropic elasticity with small Lamé constants to allow greater deformations. But if we want to adapt a model to another image of the same heart, we use anisotropic linear elasticity with Lamé constants, as it physically corresponds to a deformation of the myocardium. And we can also use the anatomical regions to better control the internal energy as we can include different regions (like fat, ischemic zones,...) modeled with different Lamé constants.

External Energy. At each step of the deformation, we apply forces on the surface nodes of the model along the normal which are proportional to the distance to the match point. The *a priori* information used is the fact that the points of the mesh we want to match with the image are on the surface of the model and that we know the intensity profile of the boundaries we want to match on these points.

3.4   Results of the Fitting of the Model to a 3D Image

We first experimented this method by fitting a canine heart model from dtMRI to the human heart of the VHP (see fig. 2). We used this segmented VHP heart image to define the anatomical regions in the mesh. Although the rotation between the initial mesh and the data was quite important and we were fitting a canine heart mesh to a human image, the rigid to affine to local transformation sequence allowed us to register the model to the image and gave a qualitatively good segmentation of the myocardium.

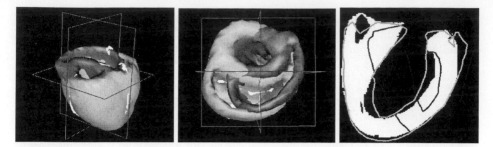

Fig. 2. Fitting of a canine heart model to the Visible Human heart image. dark: before deformation, light: after deformation

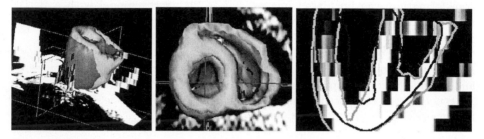

Fig. 3. Fitting of a canine heart model to a human MRI. dark: initial mesh, light: after deformation

Before the transfer of the regions from the image to the mesh by the described rasterization process, we built distance maps from the anatomical image: it allows to assign regions to the parts of the mesh which are not included in the anatomical image due to the limitations of the fitting.

Another experiment was the fitting of the same canine model to a human cardiac MRI. The similarity and the affine transformations could not be computed with the classical least-squares criterion and we had to use the new criterion presented in 3.2. As the right ventricle is very noisy in this image, we only used regions where the myocardium was visible to compute the external forces. MR Images are biased, and a consequence is that the intensity is higher in the apex than around the base. Automatic segmentation of the myocardium in MRI is rather difficult and the presented method gave qualitatively good results (cf. fig. 3).

The fitting of the model in a 3D image takes around 30 s on a standard PC with a 10 000 tetrahedra mesh (due to the anisotropy of the MRI voxels, a finer mesh would not be useful). It is fast enough to be visually controled and interactive.

4   Assignment of Anatomical Properties

Our objective is to store several informations originating from different image modalities inside the same volumetric mesh. This information may be quantitative in the case of Diffusion Tensor Magnetic Resonance Imaging (dtMRI) where fiber directions of the myocardium [10]) are extracted. But it can also

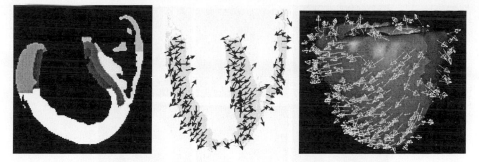

Fig. 4. Left: segmented heart image of the VHP to define anatomical regions. Middle: dtMRI vectorial image to define fiber directions. Right: dorsobasal left epicardial ventricle zone and anisotropy displayed on the final biomechanical model.

be qualitative (semantic) when extracted from precisely segmented anatomical atlases built from the Visible Human Project (VHP) [18] or histology [14]. This information may be stored at the vertex or tetrahedron level.

If we assume that the mesh has been precisely registered with a given image modality, we need to find for each tetrahedron (resp. vertex) of the mesh, its corresponding voxels in the volumetric image: this is called the rasterization stage. If the information is to be stored at a vertex, we estimate the attribute with a trilinear or nearest-neighbor interpolation depending if it is a quantitative or qualitative parameter. However, when the information is to be stored at a tetrahedron, we first find the image voxels whose center points are located inside this tetrahedron and then assign either the median or average value depending of the signal to noise ratio.

This set of voxels is found by performing a cascading set of 1D drawing operations. First, the highest and the lowest horizontal planes intersecting the tetrahedron is determined. Then we find the analytical intersection of its six edges for each intermediate horizontal planes spaced by one voxel height. Thus, we define for each plane, an intersected convex polygon (triangle or quadrilateral) for which we must again find all inside voxels. The same algorithm is applied for filling this polygon by selecting all parallel planes orthogonal to the X direction for instance. A more complex algorithm would consist in taking into account the partial volume effect by weighting each voxel by its amount of inclusion inside a tetrahedron. However, considering that the size of tetrahedra is larger that the size of a voxel, we think this level of accuracy is not necessary. A result of this process is a biomechanical model of the heart for cardiac image analysis (fig. 4).

5   Conclusion and Perspectives

We presented an efficient process to build biomechanical models using a fast volumetric deformation method to fit these models to 3D images. Using a biomechanical model ensures a strong topology constraint and allows to easily include many anatomical and mechanical properties. The deformable model framework is efficient to link biomechanical models and medical images as the image inter-

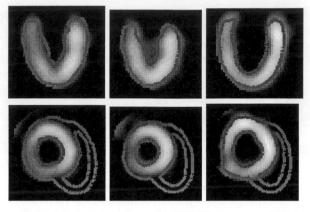

Fig. 5. Tracking of the left ventricle in a 4D SPECT sequence (8*64 × 64 × 64). The right ventricle regions have no interaction with the image as they do not appear in it.

acts as a boundary condition in the model evolution. Additional videos can be found on the web[2].

A near perspective is to segment sequences of cardiac images by propagating the fitting result obtained a time t as the initialization in the image at time $t + 1$. Preliminary results were obtained on a cardiac SPECT sequence of the left ventricle (fig. 5). The evolution of the wall thickness was well represented by this segmentation.

Future work will couple this with the electro-mechanical model presented in [19] to propose a spatiotemporal segmentation process for cardiac images based on a dynamic model of the heart. By using a biomechanical model with an electro-mechanical internal energy, we include *a priori* knowledge on the geometry *and* the motion, and we believe it should allow to better recover the cardiac motion from cardiac images.

Acknowledgements: The authors would like to thank Céline Fouard for the distance maps, Prof. Karl Heinz Höhne and his group for the segmented heart data, Dr. Edward Hsu for the Diffusion Tensor images and Philips Research France for the cardiac MRI. This work is a part of the Collaborative Research Action ICEMA[3].

References

1. N. Ayache, D. Chapelle, F. Clément, Y. Coudière, H. Delingette, J.A. Désidéri, M. Sermesant, M. Sorine, and J. Urquiza. Towards model-based estimation of the cardiac electro-mechanical activity from ECG signals and ultrasound images. In *Functional Imaging and Modelling of the Heart (FIMH'01)*, number 2230 in Lecture Notes in Computer Science (LNCS), pages 120–127. Springer, 2001.
2. F. Azar, D. Metaxas, and M. Schnall. Methods for modeling and predicting mechanical deformations of the breast under external perturbations. *Medical Image Analysis*, 6(1):1–27, 2002.

---

[2] http://www-sop.inria.fr/epidaure/personnel/Maxime.Sermesant/gallery.php
[3] http://www-rocq.inria.fr/who/Frederique.Clement/icema.html

3. P.J. Besl and N.D. McKay. A method for registration of 3D shapes. *IEEE transactions on Pattern Analysis and Machine Intelligence*, 14(2):239–256, 1992.
4. S. Cotin, H. Delingette, and N. Ayache. A hybrid elastic model allowing real-time cutting, deformations and force-feedback for surgery training and simulation. *The Visual Computer*, 16(8):437–452, 2000.
5. C. Davatzikos. Nonlinear registration of brain images using deformable models. In *IEEE Workshop on Math. Methods in Biomedical Image Analysis*, pages 94–103, 1996.
6. M. Ferrant, S. Warfield, C. Guttmann, R. Mulkern, F. Jolesz, and R. Kikinis. Registration of 3D intraoperative MR images of the brain using a finite element biomechanical model. In *MICCAI'00*, volume 1935 of *Lecture Notes in Computer Science (LNCS)*, pages 19–28. Springer, 2000.
7. A.F. Frangi, W.J. Niessen, and M.A. Viergever. Three-dimensional modeling for functional analysis of cardiac images: A review. *IEEE Trans. on Medical Imaging*, 1(20):2–25, 2001.
8. C.R. Goodall. Procrustes methods in the statistical analysis of shape (with discussion). *J. Roy. Statist. Soc. Ser. B*, 53:285–339, 1991.
9. A. Hagemann, K. Rohr, and H.S. Stiehl. Biomechanically based simulation of brain deformations for intraoperative image correction: coupling of elastic and fluid models. In *Medical Imaging 2000 - Image Processing (MI'00)*, pages 658–667. K. M. Hanson, 2000.
10. E.W. Hsu and C.S. Henriquez. Myocardial fiber orientation mapping using reduced encoding diffusion tensor imaging. *Journal of Cardiovascular Magnetic Resonance*, 3:325–333, 2001.
11. A. McCulloch, J.B. Bassingthwaighte, P.J. Hunter, D. Noble, T.L. Blundell, and T. Pawson. Computational biology of the heart: From structure to function. *Progress in Biophysics & Molecular Biology*, 69(2/3):151–559, 1998.
12. J. Montagnat and H. Delingette. Globally constrained deformable models for 3D object reconstruction. *Signal Processing*, 71(2):173–186, 1998.
13. J. Montagnat, M. Sermesant, H. Delingette, G. Malandain, and N. Ayache. Anisotropic filtering for model based segmentation of 4D cylindrical echocardiographic images. *Pattern Recognition Letters (in press)*, 2001.
14. S. Ourselin, E. Bardinet, D. Dormont, G. Malandain, A. Roche, N. Ayache, D. Tande, K. Parain, and J. Yelnik. Fusion of histological sections and mr images: towards the construction of an atlas of the human basal ganglia. In *MICCAI'01*, volume 2208 of *LNCS*, pages 743–751, Utrecht, The Netherlands, October 2001.
15. X. Papademetris, A. J. Sinusas, D. P. Dione, and J. S. Duncan. Estimation of 3D left ventricle deformation from echocardiography. *Medical Image Analysis*, 5(1):17–28, 2001.
16. X. Pennec. Statistical criterions for the rigid, similarity and affine registration of multiple point sets: shape estimation. Research report, INRIA, 2002. To appear.
17. Q.C. Pham, F. Vincent, P. Clarysse, P. Croisille, and I. Magnin. A FEM-based deformable model for the 3D segmentation and tracking of the heart in cardiac MRI. In *Image and Signal Processing and Analysis (ISPA'01)*, 2001.
18. A. Pommert, K.H. Höhne, B. Pflesser, E. Richter, M. Riemer, T. Schiemann, R. Schubert, U. Schumacher, and U. Tiede. Creating a high-resolution spatial/symbolic model of the inner organs based on the visible human. *Medical Image Analysis*, 5(3):221–228, 2001.
19. M. Sermesant, Y. Coudière, H. Delingette, N. Ayache, and J.A. Désidéri. An electro-mechanical model of the heart for cardiac image analysis, as in [14].

Comparison of Cardiac Motion Across Subjects Using Non-rigid Registration

A. Rao[1], G.I. Sanchez-Ortiz[1], R. Chandrashekara[1], M. Lorenzo-Valdés[1], R. Mohiaddin[2], and D. Rueckert[1]

[1] Visual Information Processing Group, Department of Computing,
Imperial College of Science, Technology, and Medicine,
180 Queen's Gate, London SW7 2BZ, United Kingdom
[2] Royal Bromptom and Harefield NHS Trust, Sydney Street,
London, United Kingdom

Abstract. We present a novel technique that enables a direct quantitative comparison of cardiac motion derived from 4D MR image sequences to be made either within or across patients. This is achieved by registering the images that describe the anatomy of both subjects and then using the computed transformation to map the motion fields of each subject into the same coordinate system. The motion fields are calculated by registering each of the frames in a sequence of tagged short-axis MRI images to the end-diastolic frame using a non-rigid registration technique based on multi-level free-form deformations. The end-diastolic untagged short-axis images acquired shortly after the tagged images were obtained are registered using non-rigid registration to determine an inter-subject mapping, which is used to transform the motion fields of one of the subjects into the coordinate system of the other, which is thus our reference coordinate system. The results show the transformed myocardial motion fields of a series of volunteers, and clearly demonstrate the potential of the proposed technique.

1 Introduction

Despite the advent of increasingly sophisticated cardiac imaging and surgery techniques, cardiovascular disease remains the leading cause of death in the western world [1]. It most frequently appears as coronary heart disease, in which an atherosclerosis of the coronary arteries reduces the oxygen supply to the muscles of the heart, causing them to become ischemic. This leads to a loss of function of the heart and a reduced contractility. Tagged MRI imaging [2, 3] provides a means to investigate the deformations that the heart undergoes through the cardiac cycle, and is thus a potential tool for coronary heart disease diagnosis. It relies on the perturbation of magnetisation in the myocardium in a specified spatial pattern at end-diastole. These appear as dark stripes or grids when imaged immediately after the application of the tag pattern, and, since the myocardial tissue retains this perturbation, the dark stripes or grids deform with the heart as it contracts, allowing local deformation parameters to be estimated.

Many of the techniques for the analysis of tagged MR images are based on deformable models [4–9] or optical flow [10, 11]. More recently, Chandrashekar et al. [12] described a fully automated method for tracking the cardiac motion in a sequence of tagged MRI images using non-rigid registration. In this algorithm, a sequence of free-form deformations is used to represent myocardial motion and the motion field is extracted by maximising the mutual information between images in the cine sequence.

T. Dohi and R. Kikinis (Eds.): MICCAI 2002, LNCS 2488, pp. 722–729, 2002.
© Springer-Verlag Berlin Heidelberg 2002

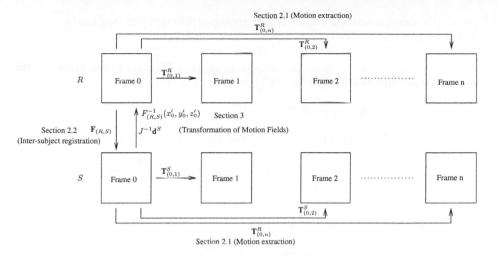

Fig. 1. Overview of proposed technique for mapping cardiac motion between subjects

The result of this algorithm is a set of motion fields for each time frame relative to an end-diastolic reference image. It would be extremely useful if we could compare the motion fields of two different image sequences obtained using this technique. There are two principal reasons for this: Firstly it would enable us to compare the motion fields of a single subject obtained at different times. This would, for example, facilitate an assessment of the cardiac function of a subject before and after undergoing pharmacological or surgical interventions. Secondly, it would enable a comparison to be made of the cardiac function of two different subjects. Unfortunately, we cannot make our comparison of the two sets of motion fields as they stand, because they are defined with respect to the coordinate systems of the end-diastolic images used to calculate them, which in general will be different.

In this paper we present a novel technique to map the myocardial motion fields that describe the cardiac motion of a subject S into the coordinate system of a reference subject R to facilitate comparisons between the cardiac function of each of the subjects. The original (unmapped) myocardial motion fields are calculated using both short-axis and long-axis tagged MRI sequences as described by [12], while the corresponding untagged MRI sequences are used to determine the mapping of anatomical information between subjects. This inter-subject transformation facilitates the final mapping of myocardial motion fields into the reference coordinate system. An overview of the various operations required by our method along with the section in which their calculation is described, is given in Figure 1.

In the next section we explain the non-rigid registration algorithm we used to determine the original myocardial motion fields and calculate the inter-subject mapping. We go on to describe in detail each of the stages of our technique, before showing results with four subjects in section 4.

2   Non-rigid Registration

Image registration entails the determination of a transformation that maps points within one image to their corresponding points in another image. For our purposes we will require the mappings between corresponding points at different time frames of a sequence of MR images taken of a single subject, as well as the mappings between corresponding points of two MR images of different subjects. We model the transformations using the non-rigid registration technique of Rueckert et al. [13]. This algorithm expresses the required transformation as the sum of a global and local component:

$$\mathbf{T}(x, y, z) = \mathbf{T}_{global}(x, y, z) + \mathbf{T}_{local}(x, y, z)$$

$\mathbf{T}_{global}$ is modelled by an affine transformation that incorporates scaling, shearing, rotation and translation. $\mathbf{T}_{local}$, the local deformations, are modelled using a free-form deformation (FFD) model based on B-splines that manipulates an underlying mesh of control points ϕ, thus changing the shape of the object. The resulting deformation can be expressed as the 3D tensor product of the standard 1D cubic B splines

$$\mathbf{T}_{local}(x, y, z) = \sum_{l=0}^{3} \sum_{m=0}^{3} \sum_{n=0}^{3} B_l(u) B_m(v) B_n(w) \phi_{i+1, j+m, k+n}$$

where B_l denotes the l-th B-spline basis function. In our algorithm the optimal transformation $\mathbf{T}$ is found by maximising a voxel-based similarity measure, normalised mutual information [14], which measures the degree of alignment between images. The normalised mutual information of two images A and B is defined as

$$I(A, B) = \frac{H(A) + H(B)}{H(A, B)}$$

where $H(A), H(B)$ are the marginal entropies of images A and B, and $H(A, B)$ denotes the joint entropy of the combined images A, B. We are using normalised mutual information as a similarity measure because it only measures the statistical dependencies between the intensity distributions in both images and therefore can be used in tagged MR images where the image intensities can change as a result of tag fading.

2.1   Motion Modelling from Tagged MR Using Non-rigid Registration

The first step in our process requires the calculation of the myocardial motion fields for the subject S that we will later map into the coordinate system of R, the reference subject. To facilitate this we must first choose an image in our tagged image sequence S_i, $i = 0, ..., n$, to be our temporal reference point, i.e. the one in whose coordinate system all calculated motion fields of S will be expressed and will be relative to. We choose the end-diastolic image S_0 to be this reference because cardiac motion is minimal at this time, and we denote its coordinate system as the triple (x', y', z'). Similarly, we define the end-diastolic image of subject R, R_0, to be the analogous reference point for this subject, denoting its coordinate system as (x, y, z). This makes (x, y, z) the coordinate system to which we ultimately would like to map the myocardial motion fields of S.

To calculate the myocardial motion fields we are using an extension of the free-form deformation (FFD) model described in the previous section. In this extension a number of single-level FFDs are combined in a multi-level FFD framework [15]. This approach has been previously applied successfully for myocardial motion tracking in tagged MR images [12]. The estimation of the motion field proceeds in a sequence of registration

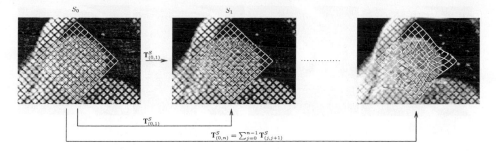

Fig. 2. Extraction of cardiac motion parameters for Subject S: A virtual tag grid which has been aligned with the tag pattern at time $t = 0$ is overlaid on different time frames of the tagged MR sequence to illustrate the tag tracking with non-rigid registration. As time progresses the virtual tag grid is deformed by the MFFD and follows the underlying tag pattern in the images. An animated colour version of this figure can be found at
http://www.doc.ic.ac.uk/~dr/projects/animations/MICCAI02.

steps as shown in Figure 1: After registering the image S_1 to S_0 we obtain a multi-level FFD (MFFD) consisting of a single FFD representing the motion of the myocardium at time $t = 1$. To register volume S_2 to S_0 a second level is added to the sequence of FFDs and then optimised to yield the transformation at time $t = 2$. This process continues until all the volumes in the sequence are registered, allowing us to relate any point in the myocardium at time $t = 0$ to its corresponding point throughout the sequence. The transformation between the end-diastolic time frame S_0 and the image S_i at time frame $t = i$ is then given by:

$$\mathbf{T}^S_{(0,i)}(x', y', z') = \sum_{j=0}^{i-1} \mathbf{T}^S_{(j,j+1)}(x', y', z')$$

Figure 2 shows the short axis tagged images of a subject taken at different time frames overlayed with a virtual grid which has been aligned with the tag pattern of the end-diastolic frame. As time progresses, the virtual tag grid is deformed by the calculated MFFD and is seen to follow the underlying tag pattern in the images. This demonstrates the success of the tracking algorithm used.

The actual myocardial motion fields $\mathbf{D}^S_{(0,i)}(x', y', z')$ that we require are given by

$$\mathbf{D}^S_{(0,i)}(x', y', z') = \mathbf{T}^S_{(0,i)}(x', y', z') - (x', y', z')$$

Using the same approach we can calculate the myocardial motion fields $\mathbf{D}^R_{(0,i)}(x, y, z)$ for subject R.

2.2 Non-rigid Registration of Untagged MR between Subjects

We now need to calculate a mapping between the end-diastolic MR images of subject and reference, S_0 and R_0, so that we can map the myocardial motion fields $\mathbf{D}^S_{(0,i)}$ into the coordinate system of R, (x, y, z). Since the untagged images are obtained shortly after the tagged images, the end-diastolic untagged frames of each subject are already aligned with the end-diastolic tagged frames of each subject that were used to define the

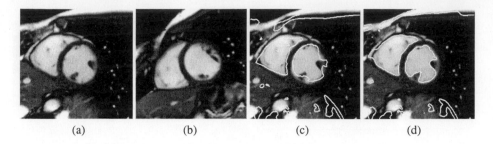

(a)　　　　　　　(b)　　　　　　　(c)　　　　　　　(d)

Fig. 3. This figure illustrates the short axis views of a reference end-diastolic image (a), a subject end-diastolic image (b), the subject image after global registration (c), and non-rigid registration (d)

co-ordinate systems of R and S. This means that we can use the end-diastolic untagged images of each subject to calculate the inter-subject co-ordinate system mapping. The transformation between subjects R and S is determined using the non-rigid registration algorithm described in the introduction of section 2, giving a mapping $\mathbf{F}_{(R,S)}$ between coordinate systems (x, y, z) and (x', y', z'):

$$\mathbf{F}_{(R,S)} : (x, y, z) \longmapsto (x'(x, y, z), y'(x, y, z), z'(x, y, z))$$

In this case there will be a non-zero global component as we are registering between subjects. Note that here the registration algorithm is being used to calculate a transformation of co-ordinates of the reference anatomy that aligns it with the subject anatomy, in contrast to its use in section 2.1 where it was used to calculate the motion of the heart in a fixed co-ordinate system.

Figure 3 shows the short-axis end-diastolic image of a reference subject (a), and of a second subject (b). In Figure 3(c) we see the overlayed anatomy contours of the second subject on the reference subject anatomy if we register the images using only the affine global component, while figure 3(d) shows the contours if we include the local deformations in the registration. It is clear that the anatomies are much better aligned when we include local deformations in our registration.

3   Transformation of Myocardial Motion Fields

We are now in a position to transform the motion fields $\mathbf{D}_{(0,i)}^{S}(x', y', z')$ $i = 1, ...n$ into the coordinate system of R, (x, y, z). If the motion vector at a point P with positional coordinate (x'_0, y'_0, z'_0) in the coordinate system of S is equal to $\mathbf{d}^S$, this transforms to the vector $\tilde{\mathbf{d}}^S$ at the location (x_0, y_0, z_0) in the coordinate system of R, where

$$(x_0, y_0, z_0) = \mathbf{F}_{(R,S)}^{-1}(x'_0, y'_0, z'_0) \quad \text{and} \quad \tilde{\mathbf{d}}^S = J^{-1}\mathbf{d}^S$$

Here, J is the Jacobian matrix of the transformation $\mathbf{F}_{(R,S)}$ evaluated at P:

$$J = \left.\begin{bmatrix} \frac{\partial x'(x,y,z)}{\partial x} & \frac{\partial x'(x,y,z)}{\partial y} & \frac{\partial x'(x,y,z)}{\partial z} \\ \frac{\partial y'(x,y,z)}{\partial x} & \frac{\partial y'(x,y,z)}{\partial y} & \frac{\partial y'(x,y,z)}{\partial z} \\ \frac{\partial z'(x,y,z)}{\partial x} & \frac{\partial z'(x,y,z)}{\partial y} & \frac{\partial z'(x,y,z)}{\partial z} \end{bmatrix}\right|_{(x,y,z)=(x_0,y_0,z_0)}$$

which can be determined analytically. Transforming the vectors of each of the $\mathbf{D}^S_{(0,i)}$ (x', y', z') in the above manner yields the transformed myocardial motion fields for S, $\tilde{\mathbf{D}}^S_{(0,i)}(x, y, z)$

4   Results and Discussion

We applied and evaluated our technique on sets of untagged and tagged short-axis images of four healthy volunteers. The untagged and tagged MR images have been acquired shortly after each other to minimise any motion between the image acquisitions. All images were acquired using a Siemens Sonata 1.5T scanner. For the tagged sequences, a cine breath-hold sequence with a SPAMM tag pattern was used to acquire ten short-axis slices covering the entire LV. For the untagged images a cine breath-hold TrueFisp sequence was used to acquire ten slices in the same anatomical planes as the tagged imaging planes. In both cases the images have a resolution of 256 x 256 pixels with a field of view ranging between 300 and 350mm depending on the subject and a slice thickness of 10mm. In both cases imaging was done at the end of expiration and all images have been visually assessed for motion between the acquisitions.

Firstly, the myocardial motion fields of each subject relative to the end-diastolic frame in their respective sequence, were calculated using the tagged image sequences. Our previous experiments [12] have shown that the non-rigid registration algorithm is able to track the myocardial motion with an RMS of less than 0.5mm in simulated data and with an RMS error between 1 and 2mm on tagged MR images. One of the four subjects was designated a reference subject, and the untagged end-diastolic images of the other were registered to this one. The calculated transformations were then used to map the myocardial motion fields of each of these three subjects into the co-ordinate system of the reference subject.

In figure 4 we show the transformed myocardial motion fields describing cardiac motion between end-diastole and end-systole for each of the four subjects. We chose to show the motion fields at end-systole because this is when the deformation of the heart is greatest. The field in the top left of the figure shows the myocardial motion field of the reference subject, while the other fields show the transformed myocardial motion fields of the three other subjects when mapped into the correct anatomical location of the reference. Vector magnitude is indicated by the length of the arrows. For clarity, we show only the motion fields for the middle short-axis slice and have projected the motion fields onto this plane, even though we had also obtained long-axis tagged and untagged images. It is clear that the transformed motion fields of the three subjects bear a high degree of similarity to that of the reference, and the mapping allows us to make comparisons of the cardiac motion of each subject.

5   Conclusions and Future Work

In this paper we have developed a non-rigid registration based technique to compare cardiac motion patterns derived from tagged MR images within patients and across patients. The comparison of cardiac motion patterns within subjects has a number of potential applications, including the comparison in changes of the cardiac function over time in patients as a result of pharmacological or surgical interventions. In these patients the effect of pharmacological or surgical interventions could be assessed by comparing

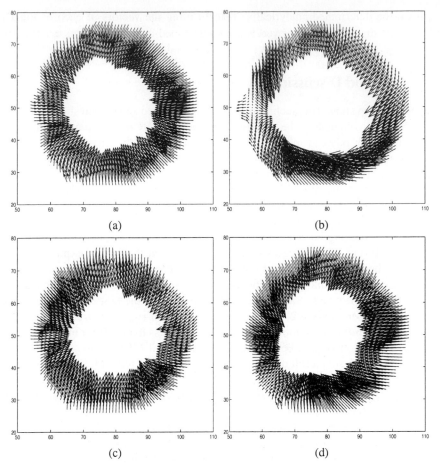

(a)   (b)

(c)   (d)

Fig. 4. The myocardial motion field of a chosen reference subject between end-diastole and end-systole is shown in (a). Images (b)-(d) shows the transformed myocardial motion fields of 3 other subjects placed at the correct anatomical location of the reference subject. Colour versions of these fields can be found at
`http://www.doc.ic.ac.uk/~dr/projects/animations/MICCAI02`.

images acquired before and after the intervention. By mapping images acquired after intervention into the same spatial frame of reference as images acquired before the intervention, one can study in detail the effect of the intervention on the cardiovascular physiology. It is likely that the same methodology will be applicable to other clinical scenarios in which changes in cardiovascular morphology and function over time need to be assessed. In particular, it may be possible to assess cardiac and vascular remodelling as a result of ischemia, infarction and other pathologies.

Future work will focus primarily on the temporal normalisation of image sequences. Even if the temporal resolution of the acquired cine MR images remains constant the variability of the heart beat rate within a single subject (i.e. in rest and stress) and across subjects will necessitate a temporal normalisation of the acquired images. In addition, future work will focus on the construction of a subject-independent reference space in which to perform comparisons on cardiac anatomy and function. Ideally, such a reference space should not be based on a single individual subject, but rather correspond to the space which minimises any patient-specific spatial and temporal variability of anatomical and functional landmarks as a result of differences in position, orientation, size and heart rate during the image acquisition.

References

1. American Heart Association. Heart and stroke statistical update. http://www.americanheart.org/, 2002.
2. E. A. Zerhouni, D. M. Parish, W. J. Rogers, A. Yang, and E. P. Shapiro. Human heart: Tagging with MR imaging – a method for noninvasive assessment of myocardial motion. *Radiology*, 169(1):59–63, 1988.
3. L. Axel and L. Dougherty. MR imaging of motion with spatial modulation of magnetization. *Radiology*, 171(3):841–845, 1989.
4. A. A. Amini, Y. Chen, R. W. Curwen, V. Mani, and J. Sun. Coupled B-snake grids and constrained thin-plate splines for analysis of 2D tissue deformations from tagged MRI. *IEEE Transactions on Medical Imaging*, 17(3):344–356, June 1998.
5. A. A. Amini, Y. Chen, M. Elayyadi, and P. Radeva. Tag surface reconstruction and tracking of myocardial beads from SPAMM-MRI with parametric B-spline surfaces. *IEEE Transactions on Medical Imaging*, 20(2):94–103, February 2001.
6. Alistair A. Young, Dara L. Kraitchman, Lawerence Dougherty, and Leon Axel. Tracking and finite element analysis of stripe deformation in magnetic resonance tagging. *IEEE Transactions on Medical Imaging*, 14(3):413–421, September 1995.
7. J. Park, D. Metaxas, and L. Axel. Analysis of left ventricular wall motion based on volumetric deformable models and MRI-SPAMM. *Medical Image Analysis*, 1(1):53–71, 1996.
8. S. Kumar and D. Goldgof. Automatic tracking of SPAMM grid and the estimation of deformation parameters from cardiac MR images. *IEEE Transactions on Medical Imaging*, 13(1):122–132, March 1994.
9. J. Huang, D. Abendschein, V. G. Dávila-Román, and A. A. Amini. Spatio-temporal tracking of myocardial deformations with a 4-D B-spline model from tagged MRI. *IEEE Transactions on Medical Imaging*, 18(10):957–972, October 1999.
10. J. L. Prince and E. R. McVeigh. Motion estimation from tagged MR images. *IEEE Transactions on Medical Imaging*, 11(2):238–249, June 1992.
11. L. Dougherty, J. C. Asmuth, A. S. Blom, L. Axel, and R. Kumar. Validation of an optical flow method for tag displacement estimation. *IEEE Transactions on Medical Imaging*, 18(4):359–363, April 1999.
12. R. Chandrashekara, R. H. Mohiaddin, and D. Rueckert. Analysis of myocardial motion in tagged MR images using non-rigid image registration. In *Proc. SPIE Medical Imaging 2002: Image Processing*, San Diego, CA, February 2002. In press.
13. D. Rueckert, L. I. Sonoda, C. Hayes, D. L. G. Hill, M. O. Leach, and D. J. Hawkes. Non-rigid registration using free-form deformations: Application to breast MR images. *IEEE Transactions on Medical Imaging*, 18(8):712–721, August 1999.
14. C. Studholme, D. L. G. Hill, and D. J. Hawkes. An overlap invariant entropy measure of 3D medical image alignment. *Pattern Recognition*, 32(1):71–86, 1998.
15. J. A. Schnabel, D. Rueckert, M. Quist, J. M. Blackall, A. D. Castellano Smith, T. Hartkens, G. P. Penney, W. A. Hall, H. Liu, C. L. Truwit, F. A. Gerritsen, D. L. G. Hill, and D. J. Hawkes. A generic framework for non-rigid registration based on non-uniform multi-level free-form deformations. In *Fourth Int. Conf. on Medical Image Computing and Computer-Assisted Intervention (MICCAI '01)*, pages 573–581, Utrecht, NL, October 2001.

From Colour to Tissue Histology: Physics Based Interpretation of Images of Pigmented Skin Lesions

Ela Claridge[1], Symon Cotton[2], Per Hall[3], and Marc Moncrieff[4]

[1] School of Computer Science, The University of Birmingham, Birmingham B15 2TT, U.K.
[2] Astron Clinica, The Mount, Toft, Cambridge CB3 7RL, U.K.
[3] Addenbrooke's Hospital, Cambridge CB2 2QQ, U.K.
[4] West Norwich Hospital, Norwich NR2 3TU, U.K.

Abstract. Through an understanding of the image formation process, diagnostically important facts about the internal structure and composition of the skin lesions can be derived from their colour images. A physics-based model of tissue colouration provides a cross-reference between image colours and the underlying histological parameters. This approach was successfully applied to the analysis of images of pigmented skin lesions. Histological parametric maps showing the concentration of dermal and epidermal melanin, blood and collagen thickness across the imaged skin have been used to aid early detection of melanoma. A clinical study on a set of 348 pigmented lesions showed 80.1% sensitivity and 82.7% specificity.

1 Introduction

Colour is an important sign in the clinical diagnosis of many conditions. In the computer analysis of medical images colour also plays an important role, for example in segmentation and classification. These and similar operations utilise colour as one of the *image features*, but the question "why a particular colour is associated with a particular medical condition" is not frequently asked. How do the colours that we see on the surface arise? Light emitted by a source interacts with the surface and the interior of an object and through these interactions (mainly absorption and scatter) the spectral composition of light is altered. The changes reflect the structure and optical properties of the materials constituting the object and in this sense the light remitted from the object "encodes" its properties. If this encoding is understood, it should be possible to deduce the structure and composition of the object from its colour image.

In this paper we show how the understanding of the image formation process enables us to derive diagnostically important facts about the internal structure and composition of the skin lesions from their colour[1] images. This information is then used for diagnosis of pigmented skin lesions to aid the detection of melanoma.

2 Outline of the Method

The key to the interpretation of image colours in terms of the underlying histological parameters is a *model of tissue colouration* which provides a cross-reference between the colour and the histology. This model is constructed by computing the spectral composition of light remitted from the skin given parameters specifying its structure

---

[1] In the remainder of the paper "colour" is taken to be a vector of n primaries. For example, a standard colour image is represented by 3 primaries: red, green and blue, i.e. a vector $[r\ g\ b]$.

T. Dohi and R. Kikinis (Eds.): MICCAI 2002, LNCS 2488, pp. 730–738, 2002.
© Springer-Verlag Berlin Heidelberg 2002

and optical properties. This step needs to be carried out only once. As the mapping between the colours and the parameters is unique for the skin [1], each colour corresponds to one specific set of histological parameters. For each derived parameter a *parametric image* is then created which shows the magnitude of a given parameter at each pixel location. In comparison with traditional methods, this approach to image interpretation requires two additional inputs. One is the set of parameters which characterise a given tissue by specifying its components, their optical properties, their quantities, and their geometry. The other is a method for computing the remitted spectra from the given parameters; in physics terminology "a model of light transport".

Our group has successfully applied this approach to the analysis of images of pigmented skin lesions [2]. Histological parametric maps showing the concentration of dermal and epidermal melanin, blood and collagen thickness across the imaged skin (see Fig. 3) have shown to aid early detection of melanoma [3].

3   Structure and Optical Properties of the Normal Skin

The skin consists of a number of layers with distinct function and distinct optical properties (Fig. 1). White light shone onto the skin penetrates superficial skin layers and whilst some of it is absorbed, much is remitted back and can be registered by a camera.

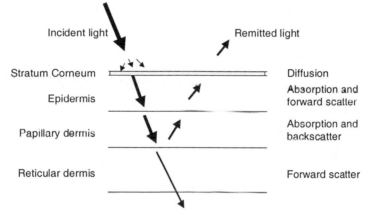

Fig. 1. A schematic representation of the skin layers (names on the left) and their optical properties (on the right). The arrows indicate the path of light through the skin tissues

The stratum corneum is a protective layer consisting of the keratin-impregnated cells and it varies considerably in thickness. Apart from scattering the light, it is optically neutral.

The epidermis is largely composed of connective tissue. It also contains the melanin producing cells, the melanocytes, and their product, melanin. Melanin is a pigment which strongly absorbs light in the blue part of the visible spectrum and in ultraviolet. In this way it acts as a filter which protects the deeper layers of the skin from harmful effects of UV radiation. Within the epidermal layer there is very little scattering, with the small amount that occurs being forward directed. The result of this is that all light not absorbed by melanin can be considered to pass into the dermis.

The dermis is made of collagen fibres and, in contrast to the epidermis, it contains sensors, receptors, blood vessels and nerve ends. Haemoglobin, present in blood vessels across the whole dermis, acts a selective absorber of light. Dermis consists of two structurally different layers, papillary and reticular, which differ principally by the size of collagen fibres. The small size of the collagen fibres in the papillary dermis (diameter of an order of magnitude less than the incident visible light) makes this layer highly back-scattering; i.e. any incoming light is directed back towards the skin surface. The scatter is greatest at the red end of the spectrum and increases even further in near infrared (nir). As absorption by melanin and blood is negligible in infrared, this part of the spectrum is optimal for assessing thickness of the papillary dermis.

Within the reticular dermis, the large size of collagen fibre bundles causes highly forward-directed scattering. Thus any light which gets to this layer is passed on deeper into the skin and does not contribute to the spectrum remitted from the skin (Fig. 1).

4   Model of Colouration for Normal Skin

From the above analysis, the normal skin can be optically modelled as consisting of three layers:

- epidermis, characterised by the wavelength (λ) dependent set of absorption coefficients for melanin, $\mu_a^{m}(\lambda)$, and the melanin concentration, c^m;
- papillary dermis, characterised by the absorption coefficients for haemoglobin, $\mu_a^{h}(\lambda)$, the haemoglobin concentration, c^h, the scatter coefficient for collagen, μ_s^{pd}, and the thickness of the collagen layer, d^{pd};
- reticular dermis, characterised by the scatter coefficient, μ_s^{rd}, and the layer thickness, d^{rd}.

By supplying these parameters and the spectral composition of the incident light $E(\lambda)$ to a model of light transport, the spectral composition of the light remitted from the skin, $R(\lambda)$, can be computed:

$$R(\lambda) = Model\_of\_light\_transport(\ E(\lambda),\ \mu_a^{m}(\lambda),\ c^m,\ \mu_a^{h}(\lambda),\ c^h,\ \mu_s^{pd},\ d^{pd},\ \mu_s^{rd},\ d^{rd}\ )$$

In the final step a colour vector [$r\ g\ b\ nir$], is derived from the remitted spectrum $R(\lambda)$ by convolving it with suitable spectral response functions for the red, green, blue and near infrared primaries, $S_R(\lambda),\ S_G(\lambda),\ S_B(\lambda)$ and $S_{NIR}(\lambda)$:

$$r = \int_0^\infty R(\lambda)S_R(\lambda)d\lambda,\ g = \int_0^\infty R(\lambda)S_G(\lambda)d\lambda,\ b = \int_0^\infty R(\lambda)S_B(\lambda)d\lambda,\ nir = \int_0^\infty R(\lambda)S_{NIR}(\lambda)d\lambda$$

In this way we can compute the colour of light remitted from the skin's surface.

Parameters in the *Model_of_light_transport( )* above can be subdivided into those which characterise the entire tissue type and those which characterise a specific instance of the tissue. The absorption and scatter coefficients ($\mu_a^{m}(\lambda),\ c^m,\ \mu_a^{h}(\lambda),\ \mu_s^{pd}$, μ_s^{rd}) belong to the first group. The thickness of the reticular dermis can be assumed constant because due to its strong forward scattering properties even a thin layer will prevent any remission of light. The levels of melanin and blood concentration c^m and c^h, and thickness of the papillary dermis, d^{pd}, vary for different skin locations. The model captures this variability by computing a set of colour vectors for parameters spanning *the entire range* of histologically valid concentrations and thicknesses. In this way a cross-reference between histology and colour is formed. Expressed as a fragment of a pseudocode, the process of building of the model of colouration can be described as follows:

```
given
    incident light E(λ)
    absorption coefficients of melanin and blood, μ_a^m(λ), μ_a^h(λ)
    scatter coefficient of the papillary dermis, μ_s^{pd}
    scatter coefficient and thickness of the reticular dermis, μ_s^{rd}, d^{rd}
    spectral response functions for the red, green blue and nir
        primaries, S_R(λ), S_G(λ), S_B(λ) and S_{NIR}(λ)
for all valid concentrations of epidermal melanin, c^m
 for all valid concentrations of dermal blood, c^h
  for all valid thicknesses of papillary dermis, d^{pd}
   compute
    R(λ) = Model_of_light_transport( E(λ), μ_a^m(λ), c^m, μ_a^h(λ), c^h, μ_s^{pd}, d^{pd}, μ_s^{rd}, d^{rd} )
    colour vector [r g b nir]
```

This forward process computes explicitly tissue colour given a set of histological parameters. As the mapping between the histological parameters and the primaries is unique for the skin [1], the inverse mapping is possible: from the tissue colour to its histological parameters:

$$[r\ g\ b\ nir] \leftrightarrow [\,c^m\ c^h\ d^{pd}\,]$$

The quantities $[\,c^m\ c^h\ d^{pd}\,]$ are then used to construct parametric maps.

5   Model of Light Transport

The optical characteristics of the skin tissue are such that a number of different light transport models can be used. We have implemented a two-flux model [5] based on Kubelka-Munk theory [6]. It computes the remitted (R) and transmitted (T) light separately for each layer i: R_i and T_i. For an n layered system, values for $R_{12...n}$ and $T_{12...n}$ are computed recursively [7]:

$$R_{12...n} = R_{12...n-1} + \frac{T^2_{12...n-1}R_n}{1 - R_{12...n-1}R_n}$$

and

$$T_{12...n} = \frac{T_{12...n-1}T_n}{1 - R_{12...n-1}R_n}$$

The model for the normal skin has three layers, corresponding to epidermis, upper papillary dermis (with prevalence of blood) and lower papillary dermis. All the absorption and scatter coefficients are based on the published data (e.g. [4]). The range of wavelengths, from $\lambda = 400$ to 1200 nm, covers the whole visible spectrum and a small range of near infrared radiation. The wavelengths used for computations are taken at equal intervals of 30nm, giving 30 discrete points for each spectrum. The incident light is "white", i.e. it has equal contributions from each discrete wavelength. The [r g b nir] vectors are derived from the computed spectra using a set of response functions equivalent to physical filters used by a camera. Figure 2 represents schematically the relationship between the two reference systems: colour, [r g b];

and histological parameters: melanin concentration, blood concentration and thickness of the papillary dermis, [c^m c^h d^{pd}].

Recently the model has been verified by comparing its output to the output generated by a stochastic Monte-Carlo method using a public domain implementation by Prahl *et al* [8].

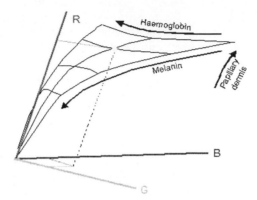

Fig. 2. Schematic relationship between two reference systems: colour system, with axes R, G and B; and histological parameter system, with axes Haemoglobin, Melanin and Papillary Dermis

6   Abnormal Skin

The model above has been constructed for skin which has a normal structure. Skin colouration associated with abnormal conditions does not necessarily have to conform to this model and this has been found to be true for some classes of pigmented skin lesions. We shall review briefly the characteristics of common lesions and discuss the implications of their structure on the model of colouration.

Pigmented skin lesions appear as patches of darker colour on the skin. In most cases the cause is excessive melanin concentration in the skin. In benign lesions (e.g. common naevi) melanin deposits are normally found in epidermis. Excessive pigmentation can also occur as the result of the papillary dermis becoming thin (light instead of being back-scattered is absorbed by structures beyond the reticular dermis). Sometimes small deposits of blood or large concentrations of small blood vessels can take the appearance similar to a pigmented skin lesion. All these types of lesions conform to the "normal" skin model, frequently at the high end of pigment concentration ranges or low end of the thickness range.

Malignant melanoma occurs when melanocytes reproduce at the high, abnormal rate. Whilst they (and their associated melanin) remain in the epidermis, melanoma is termed "in situ". At this stage it is not life-threatening and its optical properties make it conform to the "normal" model of colouration. When malignant melanocytes have penetrated into the dermis, they leave melanin deposits there, changing the nature of skin colouration. The likelihood of metastases increases with the depth of penetration and patient prognosis becomes increasingly worse. Sometimes dermal melanin is found also in benign lesions (e.g. junctional naevus and blue naevus).

The colour of the skin with melanin deposits in the dermis no longer fits the model of normal colouration. This non-conformance to the model marks it as being "abnormal" and provides a highly sensitive diagnostic sign. Such abnormal colours are marked on a fourth parametric map which shows the presence of melanin in the dermis.

The presence of melanin in the dermis is the most significant sign of melanoma. However, it cannot be used as a sole diagnostic criterion because *in situ* melanomas do not have dermal melanin; moreover, some naevi have dermal deposits (although their spatial patterns tend to be more regular than in melanoma). Other signs, some of which can be indicative of melanoma *in situ*, are thickening of the collagen fibres in the papillary dermis (fibrosis); increased blood supply at the lesion periphery (erythematous reaction); and lack of blood within the lesion, in the areas destroyed by cancer. All these signs can be captured in the parametric maps. Figure 3 shows an image of a lesion (a melanoma) and the four parametric maps.

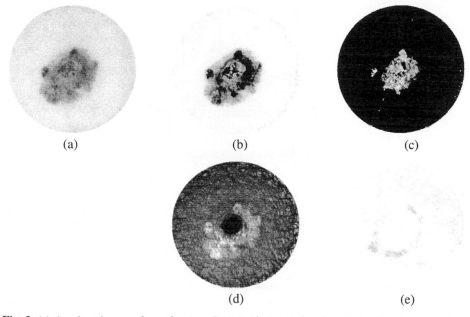

(a)   (b)   (c)

(d)   (e)

Fig. 3. (a) A colour image of a melanoma; Parametric maps showing (b) total melanin; (c) dermal melanin (note that dermal melanin is present); (d) thickness of the papillary dermis (note the increased amount on the periphery and also a "collage hole" in the centre of the lesion where collagen was displaced by melanin); (e) blood (note the absence of blood in the centre of the lesion - white area - and increased amount of blood on a periphery - an erythematous reaction)

7   Clinical Evaluation

This method was evaluated in a clinical study at the Addenbrooke's Hospital, Cambridge, and at the Norwich Hospital. The objective of the study was to see whether the histological features which can be directly observed in parametric maps improve diagnosis of melanoma in comparison to standard clinical examination.

A set of 348 lesion images was collected inspecialized dermatology clinics in Cambridge and Norwich using a SIAscope [9], see figure 4. Lesions were scored according to a revised seven-point checklist [10] – a standard method in clinical assessment of lesions. Each imaged lesion was then excised and sent for histolopathological analysis. Histology reports (melanoma vs. non-melanoma) were taken to be the ground truth. The set included 52 melanomas of various sub-types and at various stages of development. Most of the non-melanomas were benign naevi. Factual and clinical information was also recorded, including gender, location on the body, diameter, symmetry and others.

The parametric maps of the lesions, together with their clinical information and colour images, were examined visually by an experienced clinician. This preliminary analysis [3] identified the features listed in Table 1 as being most strongly associated with melanoma. The table lists also sensitivity and specificity of the individual features.

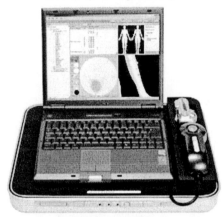

Fig. 4. SIAscope – a certified commercial device developed using the model of skin colouration described in this paper

Table 1. Diagnostic features associated with the parametric maps, and sensitivity and specificity of the individual features in melanoma classification

Diagnostic feature	Parametric map	Sensitivity (%)	Specificity (%)
Presence of dermal melanin	Dermal melanin	96.2	56.8
Areas within the lesion with no blood present ("blood displacement")	Dermal blood	75.0	70.3
Increase in blood level on the lesion periphery ("erythematous blush")	Dermal blood	75.0	65.5
Areas within the lesion with no collagen present ("collagen holes")	Collagen thickness	78.8	74.0
Asymmetry	Total melanin	76.9	62.2

The subsequent logistic regression analysis identified the combinations of the features which result in the best overall classification of melanoma [3]. Figure 5 shows ROC curves for two best combinations. A curve for a clinical diagnosis based on a revised seven-point checklist is included for comparison.

8   Discussion and Conclusions

The classification results of 80.1% sensitivity and 82.7% specificity compare very well with other diagnostic methods (clinical diagnosis [10] and dermatoscopy [11]). This can be attributed to the fact that the parametric maps provide a clinician with information which can be easily understood and interpreted because it is directly related to histology.

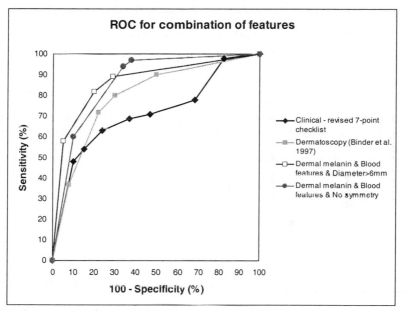

Fig. 5. Receiver-operator characteristic (ROC) curves for combinations of features, compared with clinical assessment and dermatoscopy

Traditional computer based techniques for the analysis of pigmented skin lesions all aim to correlate the lesion's appearance with its diagnosis. Visual features are usually based on the published "checklists " [12] [13], and include colour, pigmentation, pigment variation, border irregularity, asymmetry, size etc. The methods differ in the way that the measurements of these features are derived from digital images and the way that they are correlated with diagnosis ([14]-[18]). However, they lack explanatory power and in most instances act as "black boxes" which take in the images and output either numerical parameters or a putative diagnosis. Systems of this nature are not well accepted by practicing clinicians.

Our approach is fundamentally different in two ways. First, it does not concentrate on *image* patterns and *image* features, but through a physics-based interpretation of image colours it makes explicit the underlying *histology*. Second, by generating images showing relative magnitudes of the histological entities, the lesion appearance can be correlated with its structure, thus providing an *explanation* as to why various skin diseases manifest themselves through particular visual signs. The model of normal skin colouration is representative of *all* the normal skins, irrespective of racial origin, age or gender [5]. The structure remains the same, and the only differences are in the magnitudes of the parameters c^m, c^h, and d^{pd}.

Colour changes of many body tissues are used for diagnosing diseases. Most tissues have regular laminar structure, collagenous framework and contain a small number of pigments. The colour interpretation method presented in this paper can be clearly extended to other tissues and in some cases it may be an attractive alternative to biopsy.

References

1. Cotton SD (1998) *A non-invasive imaging system for assisting in diagnosis of malignant melanoma*. PhD Thesis, School of Computer Science, The University of Birmingham.
2. Cotton SD, Claridge E, Hall PN (1997) Noninvasive skin imaging, *Information Processing in Medical Imaging* (Springer-Verlag, LNCS 1230), 501-507.
3. Moncrieff M, Cotton S, Claridge E and Hall PN (2002) Spectrophotometric Intracutaneous Analysis: a new technique for imaging pigmented skin lesions. *British Journal of Dermatology* 146(3), 448-457.
4. Anderson R, Parrish BS, Parrish J (1981) The optics of human skin. The Journal of Investigative Dermatology 77(1), 13-19.
5. Cotton SD, Claridge E (1996) Developing a predictive model of human skin colouring, Vanmetter RL, Beutel J Eds., *Proceedings of the SPIE Medical Imaging 1996* vol. 2708, 814-825.
6. Egan WG, Hilgeman TW (1979) *Optical Properties of Inhomogeneous Materials*: Academic Press.
7. Spiegel MR (1962) *Theory and Practice of Advanced Calculus*: McGraw-Hill.
8. Prahl S A, Keijzer M, Jacques S L and Welch A J 1989 A Monte Carlo Model of Light Propagation in Tissue *SPIE Institue Series IS* **5** 102-11.
9. http://www.siascope.com
10. Morton CA, MacKie RM (1998) Clinical accuracy of the diagnosis of cutaneous malignant melanoma. *British Journal of Dermatology* 138, 283-287.
11. Binder M, Puespoeck-Schwarz M, Steiner A et al (1997) Epiluminescence microscopy of small pigmented skin lesions: short-term formal training improves the diagnostic performance of dermatologists. *Journal of the American Academy of Dermatology* 36, 197-202.
12. MacKie R (1985) *An illustrated guide to the recognition of early malignant melanoma*. University Department of Dermatology, Glasgow.
13. ABCDE system of the American Cancer Society - "Asymmetry, Border, Colour, Diameter and Elevation".
14. Ercal F, Chawla A, Stoecker W, *et al.* (1994) Neural network diagnosis of malignant melanoma from color images. *IEEE Transactions on Biomedical Engineering* **41**, 837-845.
15. Bono A, Tomatis S, *et al.* (1996) Invisible colours of melanoma. A telespectrophotometric diagnostic approach on pigmented skin lesions. *European Journal of Cancer* **32A**, 727-729.
16. Menzies S, Crook B, McCarthy W, *et al.* (1997) Automated instrumentation and diagnosis of invasive melanoma. *Melanoma Research* **7**, 13.
17. Ganster H, Pinz A, Kittler H, *et al.* (1997) Computer aided recognition of pigmented skin lesions. *Melanoma Research* **7**, 19.
18. Elbaum, M, Kopf AW, Rabinovitz HS et al (2001) Automatic differentiation of melanoma from melanocytic naevi with multispectral digital dermoscopy: A feasibility study. *Journal of the American Academy of Dermatology* 44(2) 207-218.

In-vivo Molecular Investigations of Live Tissues Using Diffracting Sources

Vasilis Ntziachristos, Jorge Ripoll, Edward Graves, and Ralph Weissleder

Center for Molecular Imaging Research
Massachusetts General Hospital and Harvard Medical School Boston MA
{vasilis, ripoll, graves, weissleder}@helix.mgh.harvard.edu

Abstract. We present novel technologies based on reconstructions employing diffracting sources in fluorescent mode that resolve molecular function in deep tissues. To facilitate time-efficient three-dimensional reconstructions we have employed fast analytical solutions of the diffusion equation to allow for close to real-time volumetric imaging of fluorescent near-infrared beacons that activate (fluoresce) with high specificity in the presence of specific molecular targets.

1 Introduction

Systematic efforts are under way to develop fluorescent markers and imaging systems that would allow in-vivo examinations of pathogenesis and of treatment at the molecular level [1]. The rationale for developing such technologies is a) to elucidate molecular mechanisms of disease in unperturbed environments over time, b) to allow earlier detection of disease based on molecular targets and c) to permit design of patient-specific treatments and monitor therapies on their molecular effect. Fluorescence imaging has recently seen significant growth due to its ability in assessing protein function and gene expression in-vivo [2]. Several elegant technologies that evolved to assess the fluorescence emitted from extrinsically administered fluorescent probes or markers or the expression of fluorescent proteins from engineered cells. Traditionally, fluorescence investigations have been performed by microscopic observations of surface or subsurface (0-500 μm) fluorescence using confocal microscopy and multi-photon microscopy. Both techniques have allowed unprecedented insights in in-vivo imaging biology at the cellular or subcellular level [3, 4]. A similar technology, evanescent wave microscopy, has also been used for fluorescent investigations of cell membranes [5]. However for clinical implementations it would be advantageous to develop technologies that could probe deeper in tissue and elucidate molecular function of tissues in-vivo based on highly specific fluorescent molecular probes.

Herein we present the implementation of three-dimensional fluorescence-mediated molecular tomography (FMT), a novel technique that is based on the general principles of tomography with diffracting sources [6, 7] and can probe molecular function deep in tissues (0.2- 12 cm). The technique shines light through tissue at different projections and concurrently utilizes intrinsic and fluorescence

T. Dohi and R. Kikinis (Eds.): MICCAI 2002, LNCS 2488, pp. 739–745, 2002.

measurements to provide quantitative images of fluorescent molecular probes. High molecular specificity and deep tissue penetrations can be achieved by capitalizing on activatable probes [8, 9] (molecular beacons) i.e. quenched (dark) probes that fluoresce only upon interaction with certain molecular targets offering great background signal suppression. Of particular importance are recent advances in quantitatively solving the inversion problem without need of additional measurements besides in-vivo measurements from the tissue of interest in fluorescent and intrinsic mode and the reduction of the computational expense in calculating complex boundaries. These two developments have facilitated the implementation of FMT systems in three-dimensional imaging schemes of murine models and could propagate in human applications as well.

In the following we discuss the algorithmic advances that allow the implementation of time-efficient forward problems and subsequent inversion and demonstrate the capacity of the technology to resolve protease activity in-vivo attaining inversion times of less than 3 minutes for the three-dimensional animal imaging problem.

2 Theory

Fluorescence-mediated tomography is based on a self-calibrated algorithm developed specifically for imaging fluorochrome distribution in-vivo [10]. The algorithm has been implemented into functional code using the Matlab software (Mathworks Inc) and combines a normalized-Born algorithm with the tangent-plane method, which is an analytical time-efficient approximation for solving the forward problem in the presence of complex boundaries. The algorithmic specifics are presented in the following:

2.1 Normalized-Born Expansion

In its general form, the forward problem can be written as an integral equation that related the unknown fluorochrome distribution $n(\vec{r})$ to a synthetic measurement $U_s(\vec{r}_s,\vec{r}_d)$ detected at position $\vec{r}_d$ due to a source at position $\vec{r}_s$, which is written as

$$U_s(\vec{r}_s,\vec{r}_d) = S_0 \cdot \frac{U_{fl}(\vec{r}_s,\vec{r}_d)-U_{bl}(\vec{r}_s,\vec{r}_d)}{U_{inc}(\vec{r}_s,\vec{r}_d)} =$$
$$= \frac{1}{U_0(\vec{r}_s,\vec{r}_d,k^{\lambda 1})} \int d^3r \cdot (U_0(\vec{r}_s-\vec{r},k^{\lambda 1})\cdot n(\vec{r})\cdot \frac{\upsilon}{D^{\lambda 2}} G(\vec{r}_d-\vec{r},k^{\lambda 2})$$

(1)

where $U_{fl}(\vec{r}_s,\vec{r}_d)$, $U_{inc}(\vec{r}_s,\vec{r}_d)$ are measurements at the emission and excitation wavelength respectively, $U_{bl}(\vec{r}_s,\vec{r}_d)=\Theta_f \cdot U_{inc}(\vec{r}_s,\vec{r}_d)$ is the bleed-through signal (i.e. intrinsic signal not perfectly filtered out by the fluorescence band-pass filters),

Θ_f is the band-pass filter attenuation factor, S_0 is a gain term that accounts for instrument gain differences at the excitation (λ_1) and emission (λ_2) wavelengths, $n(\vec{r})$, the fluorochrome distribution, is the product of the fluorochrome absorption coefficient and fluorescence quantum yield, $k^{\lambda 1}, k^{\lambda 2}$ are the wave propagation vectors at λ_1 and λ_2 respectively, υ is the speed of light into the medium, $D^{\lambda 2}$ is the diffusion coefficient at the λ_2, $U_0(\vec{r}_s - \vec{r}, k^{\lambda 1})$ is a term that theoretically describes the established photon field at position $\vec{r}$ into the medium at λ_1 and $G(\vec{r}_d - \vec{r}, k^{\lambda 2})$ is a term that describes the propagation of the emission photon wave from a fluorochrome at position $\vec{r}$ to the detector. The right-most part of Eq.1 reminds the formulation used in the Rytov approximation for DOT applications and attains similar imaging advantages over a standard Born expansion [7]. The terms U_0, G, also referred to as the "forward model" are calculated analytically or numerically depending on the complexity of the geometry imaged. Experimentally, we have found that the algorithm of Eq. 1 performs very accurately in phantom measurements [10] and heterogeneous real tissue (c.f. Fig. 2).

2.2 Fast Forward Model Generation

While Eq. 1 can be solved analytically for simple boundaries, such as an infinite slab or a cylinder, in-vivo applications require forward models for diffuse media with complex boundaries, typically obtained using numerical methods. Complex geometries are the air-tissue boundaries between diffuse and non-diffuse media and possibly mismatches between diffuse media. While numerical methods offer a convenient method to implement complex boundaries, three-dimensional solutions become impractical due to the large computation times required. Alternative solutions for modeling complex boundaries can be achieved using the tangent-plane method or Kirchoff approximation [11].

The method is simply explained if we assume a diffusive object of volume V surrounded by a non-diffuse medium. This object is delimited by a surface S, defined by a unit normal $\vec{n}(\vec{r})$ at each point of the interface. The Kirchhoff Approximation (KA) assumes that the surface is replaced at each point by its tangent plane. Therefore, the value of the total average intensity U at any point of the surface S is given by the sum of the homogeneous incident intensity U_{inc} and the wave reflected from the local plane defined by the surface normal $\vec{n}(\vec{r}_p)$ at that surface point. So as to obtain the expression for the reflected wave, the reflection coefficient for diffusive/non-diffusive interfaces is used [12]. Taking into account the boundary condition at a diffusive/non-diffusive interface [13], $U = -C_{nd} D \partial U / \partial n$, the total intensity measured inside volume V assuming a source at $\vec{r}_s$, and a detector at $\vec{r}_d$, is expressed as:

$$U^{KA}(\vec{\mathbf{r}}_d) = U^{(inc)}(\vec{\mathbf{r}}_s - \vec{\mathbf{r}}_d) +$$

$$+ \frac{\Delta S}{4\pi} \sum_{p=1}^{N} \left[C_{nd} D \frac{\partial g(\kappa \, | \, \vec{\mathbf{r}}_p - \vec{\mathbf{r}}_d \, |)}{\partial \vec{\mathbf{n}}_p} + g(\kappa \, | \, \vec{\mathbf{r}}_p - \vec{\mathbf{r}}_d \, |) \right] \frac{\partial U^{KA}(\vec{\mathbf{r}}_p)}{\partial \vec{\mathbf{n}}_p}. \qquad (2)$$

In Eq. (2), U^{KA} represents the total intensity given by the KA, g is the infinite homogeneous Green's function, D is the diffusion coefficient and C_{nd} is a constant that takes into account the index or refraction mismatch between the diffusive and the non-diffusive medium [13]. The surface values $\partial U^{KA}/\partial \vec{n}$ are given in terms of the local reflection coefficient R_{nd} and the incident intensity by:

$$\frac{\partial G^{KA}(\vec{r}_s, \vec{r}_p)}{\partial \hat{n}_p} = \int_{-\infty}^{+\infty} [1 - R_{ND}(\vec{K})] \frac{\partial \tilde{U}^{(inc)}(\vec{K}, \overline{Z})}{\partial \overline{Z}} \exp(i\vec{K} \cdot \overline{R}) d\vec{K}, \qquad (3)$$

where $(\overline{R}, \overline{z})$ are the coordinates of $\left| \vec{r}_s - \vec{r}_p \right|$ with respect to the plane defined by $\vec{n}(\vec{r}_p)$, namely $\overline{Z} = (\vec{r}_p - \vec{r}_p) \cdot [-\vec{n}(\vec{r}_p)]$, $\overline{R} = \overline{Z} - (\vec{r}_s - \vec{r}_p)$. An analogous expression to Eq. (2) can be found for diffusive/diffusive interfaces by means of the diffusive/diffusive reflection and transmission coefficients derived in Ref.[12].

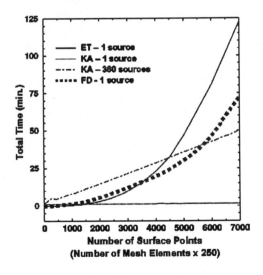

Fig. 1: Computation time of the KA method versus an exact solution using the extinction theorem (ET) and a finite-differences solution (FD).

Figure 1 shows the comparison of the KA method (for 1 and 360 sources) with a) an exact solution using the extinction theorem (ET) [11] and a single source and b) a finite-difference (FD) solution of the diffusion equation for a single source and identical geometrical parameters. The volume simulated was a 2cm diffuse cylinder with varying height (surface elements for KA and ET and mesh elements for FD) from 0 to 10cm. As the number of sources and cylinder height increases, the KA approximation becomes the only viable solution of the three methods for realistic implementations. FD and KA simulations were run to achieve accuracy within 2% of the exact solution.

2.3 Inverse Problem

For reconstruction purposes equation Eq. 1 was discretized into a number of volume elements (voxels), which yielded a set of coupled linear equations [10]. The terms U_0 and G were then calculated using Eq.2 for the appropriate boundary conditions and background optical properties at λ_1, λ_2 respectively. The resulting system of equations was then inverted for the unknown quantity $n(\vec{r})$ using the algebraic reconstruction technique with positive restriction (since no negative fluorescence concentration exists) [7]. There are several other ways to solve the inverse problem such as direct inversion, χ^2 - based minimization but we have found that the algebraic reconstruction techniques offer a time-efficient and robust approach.

3 Imaging Results

The above algorithms have been recently evaluated with phantom measurements [14]. In addition FMT has been recently used for imaging of cathepsin B activity in nude mice implanted with appropriate tumors known to up-regulate certain proteases [15]. Here we show the results obtained using Eq.1 –Eq.3 in imaging a cylindrical geometry containing an HT1080 tumor implanted in the mammary fat pad of a nude mouse. MR imaging on the same animal was also performed for data validation as well as immunohistochemistry and Western blotting in order to verify the FMT findings. To facilitate optimum photon coupling the animal was immersed in a cylindrical bore that was filled with water, TiO_2 particles and India Ink to match the optical properties of the mouse. Figure 2a depicts the correlative axial MR image obtained using a T1 weighted spin echo sequence (TR/TE 300 msec / 13 msec). The MR slice shown passes through the tumor region and demonstrates the geometry used. Here a single image is shown although volumetric imaging was performed. Figure 1b depicts an axial FMT image from the mouse examined using a cathepsin B sensitive NIR activatable probe [8]. Fig. 1b depicts an axial FMT image and Fig. 1c depicts a superposition of the MR and FMT images. The bright white spot shown in the left bottom quadrant of the MR image is a fiducial marker containing water and CuSO4 that was used for registration purposes. The tumor was well resolved by FMT and demonstrated significant cathepsin B over-expression. Western blotting and immunohistochemistry verified the increased cathepsin B concentration in the tumor of investigation (results not shown). The total time for a full three-dimensional reconstruction of 5 FMT planes (slices) was approximately 2 minutes on a Pentium 4 1.7Ghz processor. Currently other tumor models with smaller tumors and deeper implantation are investigated.

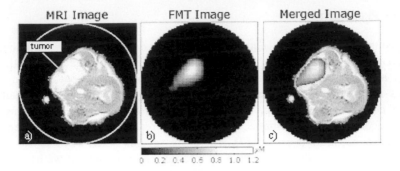

Fig. 2. In-vivo tomography of cathepsin B expression. **a)** MRI image passing through an HT1080 tumor implanted in the mammary fat pad of a nude mouse. **b)** Corresponding FMT image **c)** Superposition of a) and b).

4 Discussion and Conclusion

FMT offers a platform for interrogating targeted molecular events in tissue and offers unique features that are very attractive for animal research and clinical imaging. First, it can penetrate for several centimetres into tissue, therefore it is not limited to imaging surface events. It has been predicted recently that NIRF signals could propagate for more than 15 centimetres in breast tissue and lung and more than 5 cm in the adult brain [16]. Therefore the technique could be applied to imaging large organs. Second, it allows the quantification of NIRF probes, which translates into quantitative insights of enzymatic activity. Third, it offers excellent molecular specificity and target to background ratio by capitalizing on fluorescence dequenching of the employed NIRF probes. Fourth, it offers very sensitive photon detection (fempto-mole quantities for millimetre sized objects). Finally, it can be engineered to simultaneously target multiple specific molecular processes by imaging appropriate NIRF probes at different wavelengths and uses optical technology, which is inexpensive, easy to built, safe and does not use ionising radiation.

In this paper we demonstrated that time-efficient reconstructions can be achieved in three-dimensional problems and that the combination of Eq.1 – Eq.3 can yield accurate reconstruction results in in-vivo imaging of molecular function. A technique capable of imaging and quantifying enzymatic activity in deep tissues should prove to be a powerful diagnostic and treatment guidance tool in clinical medicine. It is expected that the propagation of fluorescent probes into clinical examinations, will be directly associated with the development of clinical FMT systems for diagnosis and treatment planning. The use of safe radiation and the cost-efficiency of the development also meet successfully the practical aspects of a clinical implementation. Therefore FMT could propagate quickly in research and perhaps the everyday clinical interrogation of basic functional and molecular processes.

Acknowledgements

V.N gratefully acknowledges support in-part from fellowship DRG-1638 of the Cancer Research Fund of the Damon Runyon-Walter Winchell Foundation and the US Army CDMRP BC995360 concept award. R.W. acknowledges support from the NIH P50 CA86355 grant.

References

1. Weissleder, R., A clearer vision for in vivo imaging. Nature Biotechnology, 2001. 19(4): p. 316-317.
2. Budinger, T.F., D.A. Benaron, and A.P. Koretsky, Imaging transgenic animals. Annual Review of Biomedical Engineering, 1999. 1: p. 611-648.
3. Korlach, J., et al., Characterization of lipid bilayer phases by confocal microscopy and fluorescence correlation spectroscopy. Proc Natl Acad Sci, 1999. 96(15): p. 8461-6.
4. Rajadhyaksha, M., et al., In vivo confocal scanning laser microscopy of human skin: melanin provides strong contrast. J Invest Dermatol, 1995. 104(6): p. 946-52.
5. Toomre, D. and D.J. Manstein, Lighting up the cell surface with evanescent wave microscopy. Trends in Cell Biology, 2001. 11(7): p. 298-303.
6. Arridge, S.R., Optical tomography in medical imaging. Inverse Problems, 1999. 15(2): p. R41-R93.
7. Kak, A. and M. Slaney, Principles of Computerized tomographic imaging. 1988, New York: IEEE Press.
8. Weissleder, R., et al., In vivo imaging of tumors with protease-activated near-infrared fluorescent probes. Nature Biotech, 1999. 17(4): p. 375-8.
9. Tyagi, S., S.A.E. Marras, and F.R. Kramer, Wavelength-shifting molecular beacons. Nature Biotechnology, 2000. 18(11): p. 1191-1196.
10. Ntziachristos, V. and R. Weissleder, Experimental three-dimensional fluorescence reconstruction of diffuse media using a normalized Born approximation. Optics Letters, 2001. 26(12): p. 893-895.
11. Ripoll, J., et al., Kirchhoff approximation for diffusive waves. Phys Rev E, 2001. 64(5 Pt 1): p. 051917.
12. Ripoll, J. and M. Nieto-Vesperinas, Reflection and transmission coefficients for diffuse photon density waves. Optics Letters, 1999. 24: p. 796-798.
13. Aronson, R., Boundary conditions for diffusion of light. J Opt Soc Am A, 1995. 12(11): p. 2532-9.
14. Ripoll, J., et al., A fast analytical method for optical tomography in diffusive media with arbitrary geometry. Optics Letters, 2002. 27(7), 527-529.
15. Ntziachristos, V., et al., Fluorescence-mediated tomography resolves protease activity in vivo. Nature Medicine, July 2002. in press.
16. Ntziachristos, V., J. Ripoll, and R. Weissleder, Would near-infrared fluorescence signals propagate through large human organs for clinical studies. Optics Letters, 2002. 27(5), 333 - 335.

Automatic Detection of Nodules Attached to Vessels in Lung CT by Volume Projection Analysis

Guo-Qing Wei, Li Fan, and JianZhong Qian

Intelligent Vision and Reasoning Department
Siemens Corporate Research, Inc.
755 College Road East, Princeton NJ 08536, USA

Abstract. Automatic detection of abnormalities or lesions that are attached to other anatomies in medical image analysis is always a very challenge problem, especially when the lesions are small. In this paper a novel method for the automatic detection of lung cancers or nodules attached to vessels in high-resolution multi-slice CT images is presented. We propose to use volume projection analysis to mimic physicians' practices in making diagnosis. The volume projection analysis is performed on 1-dimensional curves obtained from the 3-dimensional volume. A multi-scale detection framework is proposed to detect nodules of various sizes. A set of features for characterizing nodules is defined. Results of experimental evaluation of the method are presented.

1 Introduction

The use of low dose CT to detect early stage of lung cancer as a screening method has shown great promises [2]. The early detection and treatment of lung cancer is vitally important in improving the cure rate. However, the number of CT slices per patient produced by multi-detector CT systems is usually in the range of 300 to 600 or even more, and the number of screenings made yearly is increasing dramatically [3]. This high volume of patient data virtually makes the softcopy reading slice-by-slice very difficult or impossible in clinical practice. To mitigate the problem, a computer system, which can automatically detect nodules and provide assistance to physicians in the process of diagnostic decision making, is highly desirable.

Early work on computer aided nodule detection relied on 2D features in multiple slices to distinguish nodules from vessels. Giger et al. [8] used multi-level thresholding to binarize individual slices to extract features, such as compactness, circularity, and perimeters. A tree structure relating segmentations in neighboring slices is formed to analyze the 3D shape of the suspected region. Recent work on nodule detection has focused on the use of 3D features directly to perform the detection. Armato *et al* applied both intensity and 3D morphological features to classify nodules and non-nodules [4,5]. Kawata et al [6] employed 3D curvature, texture and moment features to characterize begin and malignant nodules. A major problem with existing nodule detection methods lies in the high false positive rate. With a sensitivity of around 80%, typical false positive

T. Dohi and R. Kikinis (Eds.): MICCAI 2002, LNCS 2488, pp. 746–752, 2002.

(FP) rate is in the range 1 to 3 per slice [5,1]. This amounts to a few hundred FPs per case for a 200-slice volume, which is too high to be acceptable in a clinical practice. Better results were achieved recently by using patient-specific models in follow-up, with a specificity of 11 FPs per case [9]. Although it is difficult to make a consistent comparison of the different methods because of the different data set used, the above numbers do reflect the current state of the art in CT lung nodule detection.

One of the reasons why current algorithms generate too many false positives is because of the similarities of the extracted features between nodules that are attached to vessels and vessels. For example, nodules attached to vessels have many common characteristics with vessel bifurcations to a computer. Nodules attached to vessels or with vessel-feeding patterns, however, are more likely to be lung cancers and have higher clinical significance. The detection of such nodules is thus very important. The usual way of handling nodules attached to vessels is to use morphological operations, such as opening, to detach nodules from vessels [3,4]. Vessel bifurcations, however, when repeatedly opened, may exhibit similar shapes as nodules, and thus cause false detection. Methods that do not try to detach nodules from vessels, but use some statistical measurement of the volume of interest [5,6] suffer from another problem: contributions from the vessel part cannot be separated well from those from the nodule. One has to lower the acceptance threshold in order to increase sensitivity, admitting also, at the same time, more non-nodule anatomies.

In this paper, we propose a novel approach to the detection of nodules attached to vessels. The method mimics physicians' practices in detection of nodules from CT studies in soft-copy reading process. When physicians are examining the CT slices, they often view the axial slices in alternating forward and backward directions along the body-long-axis, and use size change information and patterns of the object of interest to make judgment. We propose to use volume projection analysis to extract the same information the physicians are relying on. The volume projection analysis is based on the analysis of several 1-dimensional curves that are obtained as the projection of the volume from preferred directions. The preferred directions are automatically computed by eigen-value analysis of the volume of interest. To do quantitative shape analysis of the projection curves, Gaussian curve fitting is first conducted on the projection data. Then classification is made in the parameter space of the fitted curves.

2   Volume Projection Analysis (VPA) Method

2.1   Nodule Model

Most previous methods either implicitly or explicitly use a sphere as the nodule model. For example, the widely accepted spheracity measurement is based on the assumption of a spherical nodule shape, whereas other methods explicitly search for nodules by spherical templates [1]. In this paper an ellipsoidal model is proposed. The reason why ellipsoidal model was not adopted before is probably because of the complexity of the model in comparison with a spherical one.

Six parameters are involved in an ellipsoidal model instead of one for a spherical model. They are the lengths along the three major axes and the three orientation parameters of the ellipsoid. Without loss of generality, we express the ellipsoid in its own coordinate system (the nodule coordinate system) by

$$\frac{x^2}{a^2} + \frac{y^2}{b^2} + \frac{z^2}{c^2} = 1 \tag{1}$$

with the x,y,z axes coincident with the major axes, and a, b, c are the lengths of the major axes. The orientation of the nodule coordinate system with respect to the original volume coordinate system defines the orientation of the ellipsoid.

It is observed that solitary nodules tend to follow a Gaussian intensity distribution. The intensity has the highest value at the center of the nodule and drops off exponentially in the radial directions. For the ellipsoidal nodule model, the intensity profile can be approximated as

$$I(x, y, z) = \rho \, e^{-(\frac{x^2}{\sigma_a^2} + \frac{y^2}{\sigma_b^2} + \frac{z^2}{\sigma_c^2})} \tag{2}$$

where the Gaussian sizes $\sigma_a, \sigma_b, \sigma_c$ are linearly proportional to the lengths of the major axes of the ellipsoid.

2.2 Multiscale Smoothing

Due to image noises, it is necessary to smooth the volume. Furthermore, malignant nodules are often more irregular in shape than benign ones; star-like shapes are often to be seen for such nodules. Smoothing will help to reduce such shape irregularity. We use Gaussians of multiple scales for the smoothing

$$G_\sigma(x, y, z) = e^{-\frac{x^2 + y^2 + z^2}{\sigma^2}} \tag{3}$$

The smoothed volume is represented by

$$I_\sigma(x, y, z) = I(x, y, z) * G_\sigma(x, y, z) \tag{4}$$

where * represents convolution. It can be shown that the smoothed intensity distribution of a Gaussian model is still a Gaussian, with the new Gaussian sizes being

$$\sigma_x = \sqrt{\sigma^2 + \sigma_a^2}, \quad \sigma_y = \sqrt{\sigma^2 + \sigma_b^2}, \quad \sigma_z = \sqrt{\sigma^2 + \sigma_c^2} \tag{5}$$

2.3 Volume Projection

Volume projection is an operation that reduces the 3-dimensional (3D) data of the volume to a 1D curve. Given a projection direction vector v, the projection axis ζ is defined in the same direction as v, with the origin the same as the original volume of interest. Denote the coordinate on the projection axis by ζ, then the projection of volume $I_\sigma(x, y, z)$ on ζ can be expressed as

$$p_v(\zeta) = \sum_{(x,y,z) \in x | x \bullet v = \zeta} I_\sigma(x, y, z) \tag{6}$$

where $\mathbf{x} = (x, y, z)$. The meaning of (6) is to compute the total voxel intensity on the plane orthogonal to v and at a distance ζ from the origin. The projection operation possesses several nice features. The following two are essential in our nodule detection algorithm.

Property 1 (Invariance): The projection of a Gaussian-distributed volume I_σ (x, y, z) along any projection direction v is still a Gaussian.

Property 2 (Boundness): The size of the projected Gaussian is bounded by

$$\min(\sigma_x, \sigma_y, \sigma_z) < \sigma_\zeta < \max(\sigma_x, \sigma_y, \sigma_z) \tag{7}$$

The first property means that the Guassian shape is invariant under projection operation. This allows us to use lower dimensional data to identify the shape of a higher dimensional volume. Property two, when combined with equation (5), states that the measured shape in the lower dimensional space is quantitatively related to that in the higher dimensional space. Therefore it is feasible to use the projection data to infer the shape of the original volume. Note that by applying the volume projection, we have avoided doing the actual fitting in the original 3D space, which would be otherwise needed to extract the nodule shape and size information. When the projection axes are chosen as the three major axes of the ellipsoid, it is even possible to approximately *reconstruct* the 3D structure from the 1D measurements.

2.4   Computing the Projection Axes

The projection axes should be selected to best distinguish nodules from non-nodule structures. For nodules, the invariance and boundness properties should result in consistent measurements in any projection axes, whereas for non-nodule anatomies, such as vessels, measurements in the projection data will give inconsistent predictions about the 3D shape a nodule structure would exhibit. For example, when one projection axis is chosen as being along the vessel axis, and the other being orthogonal to the vessel axis, the two projection curves will not match any projection curves generated by a nodule. We compute the projection axes based on the eigenvector analysis of the volume of interest. The projection axes are selected corresponding to the dominant structures in the volume of interest.

2.5   Classification

To make quantitative analysis of the projected data, Gaussian fitting is conducted for each of the projected curves. Since the data is 1D, the fitting is much simplified in comparison with that in 3D. A Gaussian curve will take the following form

$$G(\zeta) = \rho_\zeta \, e^{-\frac{(\zeta - \zeta_0)^2}{\sigma_\zeta^2}} \tag{8}$$

where ρ_ζ, ζ_0 and σ_ζ^2 are the Gaussian parameters. A five dimensional feature vector is extracted from all the fittings. It consists of the maximum size, minimum size, maximum size ratio, maximum center offset, and maximum error of the fitting. A simple linear classifier is then used to make distinction between nodules and non-nodule structures.

After a nodule is detected, the center of the nodule in 3D can be estimated from the Gaussians' centers in 1D by the least squares method. Although the exact size of the nodule is difficult to estimate, we can compute a mean radius of the nodule by averaging the size estimates from the 1D projections. Alternatively, we can use ellipsoidal surface fitting to get more accurate shape information. Note that this is different from a fitting intended for nodule detection, since the volume of interest has already been identified as containing a nodule.

3   Experiments

3.1   Materials

We applied the proposed method to 10 CT screening studies of smokers. The data sets are all low dose multi-slice, high resolution CT images, with dosages from 20 to 40 mAs, in-plane resolutions from 0.57 to 0.67mm/pixel, slice thickness of 1.25mm with 0.25mm overlap. The image sizes are all 512*512 within cross section, with 280 to 300 slices in Z direction.

3.2   Preprocessing

First, the lung volume is pre-processed to remove the chest wall so that only the lung area remains as the volume of interest. This is performed by intensity thresholding and morphological operations.

3.3   Seed Points Generation

This step generates points of interest in the volume to examine. These points could be specified by scanning through the whole CT volume. To do this, only points whose intensities are greater than a certain threshold need to be considered. However, this is a rather time-consuming approach since the number of candidate points thus generated is huge. We use an intelligent seed point generation method [10] to speed up the detection.

If the nodule detection method is intended to work in an interactive way, the user can pick up seed points manually, e.g., by using a computer mouse to move to the suspicious point and to detect nodules on-line.

3.4   Ground Truth

Three chest radiologists first evaluated the patient studies on 7mm hard copies separately. Meanwhile, the proposed automatic detection is applied to thin slice multi-slice HR CT data. Finally, two experienced chest radiologists examined all the marks detected by both radiologists and computer, and determined ground truth by consensus.

3.5   Results

Preliminary results show that radiologists plus the automatic detection algorithm detected 34 nodules in total, two of which are ground glass nodules (GGNs) detected by radiologists. The radiologists combined together detected 25 nodules. Individual detection ranges from 14 to 21, with the sensitivities ranging

Table 1. Experimental results of the proposed lung nodule detection method.

	Nodules detected	Sensitivity %	Sensitivity with VPA * %	Overlap with computer	Overlap rate %
All nodules confirmed: 34					
Radiologist 1	21	61.8	97.1	11	52.4
Radiologist 2	17	50.0	85.3	11	64.7
Radiologist 3	14	41.2	88.2	7	50.0
Automatic detection	23	67.6	-	FPs/study: 6.2	
All nodules confirmed: 32					
	Nodules detected	Sensitivity %	Sensitivity with VPA * %	Overlap with computer	Overlap rate %
Radiologist 1	19	59.4	96.9	11	57.9
Radiologist 2	16	50.0	87.5	11	68.8
Radiologist 3	12	37.5	87.5	7	58.3
Automatic detection	23	71.9	-	FPs/study: 6.2	

*: *Sensitivity with VPA* refers to the sensitivities that radiologists can achieve with the help of the automatic nodule detection algorithm.

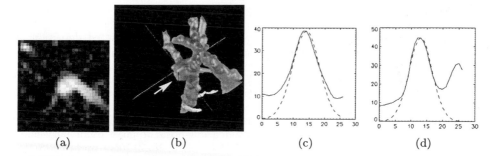

(a)   (b)   (c)   (d)

Fig. 1. Volume projection profiles and curve fitting for a nodule attached to vessel. (a) one slice of theVOI; (b) a shaded surface views of the VOI; the nodule position is indicated by the arrows; (c)-(d) the volume projection curves (solid lines) and fitted curves (dashed lines).

from 41.2% to 61.8%. The proposed automatic detection algorithm detected 23 nodules, achieving a sensitivity of 67.6% with a false positive rate of 6.2 FPs per case. The overlapping rate between the automatic detection and each individual radiologist's detection ranges from 50.0% to 64.7%. With the assistant of automatic detection, radiologists can detect an average of 80.7% more nodules than alone, and reach the sensitivities ranging from 88.2% to 97.1%. If excluding the GGNs, the radiologists combined together detected 23 nodules. Individual detection ranges from 12 to 19, with the sensitivities ranging from 37.5% to 59.4%. The proposed automatic detection algorithm detected 23 nodules, with a sensitivity of 71.9%. The overlapping rate between the automatic detection and each individual radiologist's detection ranges from 58.3% to 68.8%. With the assistant of automatic detection, radiologists can detect an average of 90.5% more nodules than alone, and reach the sensitivities ranging from 87.5% to 96.9%. The overall experimental results are listed in Table 1.

An example of the detection using volume projection data is shown in Fig.1.

4   Conclusions

In this paper, we have presented a novel detection method based on volume projection analysis for solving the problem of automatic detection of lesions that are attached to other anatomies in medical image analysis, especially when the lesions are small. The method projects the 3D volume data onto 1D space and extracts the 3D information from the reduced data space. An ellipsoidal nodule model is used to represent a nodule. Under the Gaussian intensity model, two fundamental properties of the projection are established and utilized to design the nodule detection algorithm. The method is able to detect both isolated nodules and nodules attached to vessels.

The method has been applied to 10 patient studies. A low false positive rate of 6.2 FPs per study is achieved, with a comparable sensitivity to existing methods. Experiments have shown that with the help of the proposed method, physicians can detect significantly more nodules than working without.

References

1. Y. Lee, T. Hara, H. Fujita, S. Itoh, and T. Ishigaki, "Automated detection of pulmonary nodules in helical CT images based on improved template-matching technique", IEEE Trans Medical Imaging, Vol,20, No.7, 2001, pp.595-604
2. C. I Henschke, D. I. McCauley, D. F. Yankelevitz, D. P. Naidich, G. McGuinness, O. S. Miettinen, D. M. Libby, M.W. Pasmantier, J. Koizumi, N. K. Altorki, J. P. Smith, "Early lung cancer action project: overall design and findings from baseline screening," *The Lancet*, Vol.354, July 10, 1999, pp.99-105
3. A.P. Reeves, W. J. Kostis, "Computer-aided diagnosis of small pulmonary nodules," *Seminars in Ultrasound, CT, and MRI*, Vol.20, No.2, 2000, pp.116-128
4. S.G. Armato III, M.L. Giger, J.T. Blackburn, K. Doi, H. MacMahon, "Three-dimensional approach to lung nodule detection in helical CT", *Proc. SPIE Medical Imaging*, pp.553-559, 1999
5. S.G. Armato III, M.L. Giger, K. Doi, U. Bick, H. MacMahon, "Computerized lung nodule detection: comparison of performance for low-dose and standard-dose helical Ct scans", *Proc. SPIE Medical Imaging*, pp.1449-1454, 2001
6. Y. Kawata, N. Niki, H. Ohmatsu, M. Kusumotot, R. Kakinuma, K. Mori, H. Nishiyama, K. Eguchi, M. Kaneko, N. Moriyama, "Curvature based characterization of shape and internal intensity structure for classification of pulmonary nodules using thin-section CT images", *Proc. SPIE Medical Imaging*, pp.541-552, 1999
7. J. Qian, L. Fan, G.-Q. Wei, C.L. Novak, B. Odry, H. Shen, L. Zhang, D.P. Naidich, J.P. Ko, A.N. Rubinowitz, G. McGuiness, G. Kohl, E. Klotz, "Knowledge-based automatic detection of multi-type lung nodules from multi-detector CT studies", *Proc. SPIE Medical Imaging*, 2002, to appear
8. M.L. Giger, K.T. Bae, H. MacMahon, "Computerizied detection of pulmonary nodules in computed tomography images", *Investigat. Radiol.*, Vol.29, pp.459-465, 1994
9. M.S. Brown, M.F. McNitt-Gray, J. G. Goldin, R.D. Suh, J.W. Sayre, D.R. Aberle, "Patient-specific models for lung nodule detectionand surveillance in CT images," *IEEE Trans Medical Imaging*, Vol.20, No.12, 2001, pp.1242-1250
10. L. Fan, J. Qian, G.Q. Wei, "Automatic Generation of Vessel-feeding Pulmonary Nodule Candidates from High-resolution Thin-slice CT Data", *US Patent,* pending, 2001

LV-RV Shape Modeling
Based on a Blended Parameterized Model

Kyoungju Park[1], Dimitris N. Metaxas[1,2], and Leon Axel[3]

[1] Department of Computer and Information Science
University of Pennsylvania, Philadelphia, PA 19104, USA
kypark@graphics.cis.upenn.edu
[2] CBIM Center, Computer Science Department and Bioengineering Department
Rutgers University, New Brunswick, NJ 08854, USA
dnm@cs.rutgers.edu
[3] Department of Radiology
New York University School of Medicine, New York, NY10016, USA

Abstract. Making a generic heart deformable model to be able to analyze normal and pathological hearts is important. Such a generic model gives more stability and accuracy for segmentation, analysis and classification. Due to the conflicting demands of shape generality and shape compactness, such a generic heart model is difficult to define. In order to be useful, a generic heart model should be defined with a few number of parameters. In all the previous work on the modeling of the LV-RV shape the deformable model is built from the given datasets. Therefore such methods have limitations that the quality of shape estimation are dependent on the quality of the datasets. In this paper, we introduce a blended deformable model approach with parameter functions which is generic enough to deal with the different heart shapes. Using a method we are able to model the 3D shape of the heart which include the left ventricle(LV) and the right ventricle(RV). We also include the inflow and outflow tract of the RV basal area, so that the full LV-RV shape can be estimated.

1   Introduction

Making a generic heart deformable model to be able to analyze normal and pathological hearts is important. We can estimate heart shape automatically with a generic model so that we do not have a problem with a tedious mesh generation process depending on segmented datasets. Also we can compare the different heart shapes based on a generic model. Such a generic model gives more stability and accuracy for segmentation, analysis and classification.

Due to the conflicting demands of shape generality and shape compactness, a generic heart model is difficult to define. In shape estimation and motion analysis, the various shapes, morphological changes and deformation over time should be covered.

On the other hand, a compact description is important. Features of the heart shape and motion should be represented quantitatively in terms of relatively few descriptors. Thus it is very easy to compare different heart shapes.

T. Dohi and R. Kikinis (Eds.): MICCAI 2002, LNCS 2488, pp. 753–761, 2002.

In this paper, we introduce a blended deformable model approach with parameter functions which are generic enough to deal with the different heart shapes. Using this method we are able to model the 3D shape of the heart which include the left ventricle(LV) and the right ventricle(RV).

This blending operation on deformable models allows the combination of two different shape primitives in one single model. The parameter functions describe the object with a few parameters while allowing variations by those parameter functions. In the past, the parameter functions are used to model the LV[9, 10]. Now we extend to the LV-RV model with a blended model. The blended shape is employed more to cover not only the LV but also the more complicated right ventricle(RV) and the up basal area.

The heart boundary datasets are extracted from our MRI-SPAMM imaging technique [1] which has been shown to be the best non-invasive in-vivo motion study tool. In shape estimation, we use the physics-based framework of Metaxas and Terzopoulos [7]. The heart shape model deforms due to forces exerted from the datasets.

Our method of a blended deformable model with parameter functions automatically generates the FEM meshes and is generic enough to deal with the normal and pathological hearts. Thus we can compare the different hearts based on the generic heart model.

In section 2 and 3, we will explain how to define a generic heart shape model and how to estimate the shape using physics-based framework. Then section 4 shows the reconstructed heart models of normal subjects and patient studies.

1.1   Related Work

Many approaches have been developed for making a heart model. Such models usually have a number of parameters to control the shape and pose of all or part of the model.

Park et al.[10, 9] used the parameter functions with the generalization of an ellipsoid primitive for LV motion analysis based on MRI-SPAMM. Similarly Young[11] build a heart model using the prolate spheroidal coordinates. This model is used to the direct motion traking from tagged images. Declerck et al.[3] use the 4D planispheric transformation for tracking and motion analysis of LV. Papademetris et al.[8] use the active elastic model for regional cardiac deformation from MR and the 3D Echocardiography. All these approaches, however, are applied only to the LV rather than the whole LV-RV.

Only a few approaches are made to build the LV-RV model. Haber et al.[4] reconstructed the LV-RV motion. It is the only model so far that constructed the RV motion. However, this heart model depends on the quality of the input data. For every dataset, the different meshes should be generated and that makes it difficult to compare the different hearts. It is therefore difficult to be used for analyzing, classifying and comparing large datasets.

2   Shape Modeling

We introduce the use of a blended model with parameter functions. Blended shapes and boolean operations have been used in geometric model and recently exploited in free-form solids[6] and deformable models[2].

2.1   Blended Deformable Shape Model

The blended shape is composed of several primitive parts by use of the blending function. The component primitives we pick are the deformable primitives with a small number of parameters. Examples are generalized cylinders, geons, superquadrics, hyperquadrics etc.

With the structured shape representation scheme, the single blended shape model can be thought of as the combination of two deformable primitive parts. Portions of component primitives are cut out, and the selected portions are joined together.

Our blended shape model combines portions from component primitives $s1$ and $s2$. The resulting created model, s, has a global single coordinate system (u, v) (latitude u, longitude v). Thus we can define s as the new class of deformable primitives.

For example, something shaped like a half-moon can be built from two ellipsoid like primitives. Firstly, we define underlying deformable primitives $s_1(u, v)$ and $s_2(u, v)$ as follows:

$$s_1(u,v) = \begin{pmatrix} r_{11}\cos u\cos v \\ r_{12}\cos u\sin v \\ r_{13}\sin u \end{pmatrix}, \; s_2(u,v) = \begin{pmatrix} r_{21}\cos u\cos v \\ r_{22}\cos u\sin v \\ r_{23}\sin u \end{pmatrix} \quad (1)$$

where $-\pi/2 \le u \le \pi/5, -\pi \le v < \pi$. The cut-and-paste operations on $s_1(u, v)$ and $s_2(u, v)$ are placed over the (u, v) coordinates level. This allows blended shape s to have global parameterization without reparameterizing. Our created blended shape s in Fig. 1 is defined as follows:

$$s(u,v) = \begin{cases} s1(u,v) & \text{if } 0 < v < \pi \\ s2(u,-v) & \text{if } -\pi < v < 0 \\ (s1(u,v) + s2(u,-v))/2 & \text{if } v = 0, v = -\pi \end{cases} \quad (2)$$

where $-\pi/2 \le u \le \pi/5, -\pi \le v < \pi$.

In addition to blending we allow further local variations on the underlying shape by replacing the parameters of deformable primitives with functions. This allows the flexibility of capturing specific variations while keeping the guidance of the generic model.

2.2   Heart Model Geometry

We apply the method of blending with parameter functions to build a LV-RV generic model. The heart is actually two separate pumps: a right heart and a

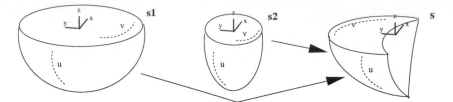

Fig. 1. Blended shape s from shape $s1$ and $s2$

left heart. Each of these hearts is a two-chamber pump composed of an atrium and a ventricle.

To build the whole ventricle including the LV and RV with the material coordinates $\mathbf{u} = (u, v, w)$, we define a heart shape model $x(\mathbf{u}) = \mathbf{c} + \mathbf{R}s(\mathbf{u})$ where $\mathbf{c}$ and $\mathbf{R}$ are the global translation and rotation of the model, and $s(\mathbf{u})$ is a blended model where $\mathbf{u}$ is taken from (u, v, w) coordinates representing longitude, latitude and number of primitives respectively. Therefore $\mathbf{s}(\mathbf{u})$, the blended model, presents the position of the points on the model relative to the model frame. The underlying deformable primitive $e(\mathbf{u})$ is a generalization of an ellipsoid primitive such that piecewise functions of $\mathbf{u}$ take the place of parameters, as follows:

$$
e(\mathbf{u}) = \begin{pmatrix} x \\ y \\ z \end{pmatrix} = sc \begin{pmatrix} r_1(\mathbf{u}) \cos u \cos v \\ r_2(\mathbf{u}) \cos u \sin v \\ r_3(\mathbf{u}) \sin u \end{pmatrix} \tag{3}
$$

where $-\pi/2 \leq u \leq \pi/5, -\pi \leq v < \pi, w > 0, r_1(\mathbf{u}), r_2(\mathbf{u}), r_3(\mathbf{u}) \geq 0$; sc is the scaling parameter for the model and $r_1(\mathbf{u}), r_2(\mathbf{u})$ and $r_3(\mathbf{u})$ are the x, y, z axial deformation parameters respectively.

Our heart shape model is composed of three layers($w = 1, 2, 3$); LV endocardium, epicardium and RV endocardium respectively. The origin of model frame is the center of LV. The principal axis (z-axis) of heart model is the line that connects the center of the LV apex and the center of the LV base and the y-axis is the line that connects the center of the the LV and the center of the RV.

The LV endocardium and epicardium are defined in (3). Each (r_1, r_2, r_3) has two values : positive direction parameter (r_{1+}, r_{2+}, r_{3+}) and negative direction parameter (r_{1-}, r_{2-}, r_{3-}) along x, y, z axes. The RV endocardium, unlike LV endocardium and epicardium, is a blended shape. As in (2), we create a blended model from two component primitives defined in (3). When shaping the RV endocardium, we cut-and-paste the selected portions of the above given deformable primitive e, as follows:

$$
s_1(u, v, 3) = \begin{cases} e(u, r_s(\mathbf{u})v + r_t(\mathbf{u}), 3) & \text{if } 0 \leq v < \pi \\ e(u, -r_s(\mathbf{u})v + r_t(\mathbf{u}), 4) & \text{if } -\pi \leq v < 0 \end{cases} \tag{4}
$$

where $0 < r_s(\mathbf{u}) < 1, 0 < r_t(\mathbf{u}) < \pi$; $r_s(\mathbf{u})$ is proportion(the arc length ratio of the septum) parameter function on xy-plane and $r_t(\mathbf{u})$ is the angle between the end of the septum and the x-axis on the xy-plane.

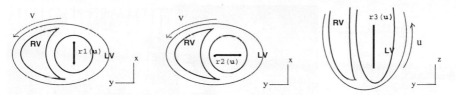

(a) Axial deformation parameters, r1(**u**), r2(**u**), r3(**u**) along x,y,z−axis respectively

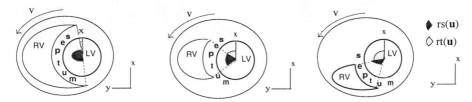

(b) Various septum aspect ratio rs(**u**) and septum rotation rt(**u**) parameters

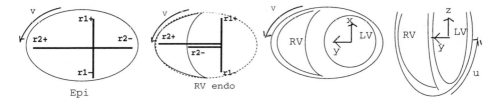

Fig. 2. Shape Model Parameters; Axial Deformation, Blending

Thus, the resulting volumetric blended heart shape model s is:

$$s(\mathbf{u}) = \begin{cases} s_1(\mathbf{u}) & \text{if } w = 3 \\ e(\mathbf{u}) & \text{if } w = 1, 2 \end{cases} \tag{5}$$

where $w = 1, 2, 3$ represent LV endocardium, epicardium and blended RV endocardium. Therefore the blended model parameter vector $\mathbf{q}_s$ is defined as

$$\mathbf{q}_s = (r_1(\mathbf{u}), r_2(\mathbf{u}), r_3(\mathbf{u}), r_s(\mathbf{u}), r_t(\mathbf{u}))$$

The deformable shape model parameters are $\mathbf{q} = (\mathbf{q}_c^T, \mathbf{q}_\theta^T, \mathbf{q}_s^T)^T$, where $\mathbf{q}_c = c$ is the global translation, and $\mathbf{q}_\theta$ is the quaternion that states global rotation matrix $\mathbf{R}$.

3   Fitting

With our heart model geometry, we fit the model to the boundary datasets from our MRI-SPAMM [1] imaging technique. The heart imaging is taken from 13 short-axis views and 9 long-axis views for 7 time frames during systole. In 2D images we segment the LV-RV boundary using the active contours, snakes [5]. Based on those boundary datapoints we build the 3D heart model.

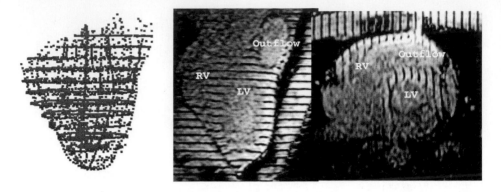

Fig. 3. Heart boundary data from MRI-SPAMM images

3.1   Heart Model Dynamics

The shape reconstruction process is done using the physics-based framework of
Metaxas and Terzopoulos [7] with the geometrically defined model. Using this
framework, a model deforms due to forces from datasets so as to minimize the
applied forces. We use data forces to esimate the model parameters.

Estimation of the parameters is based on the simplified version of the Lagrangian dynamics equation of motion given by:

$$\dot{\mathbf{q}} = \mathbf{f_q} \tag{6}$$

where $\mathbf{q}$ is the vector of shape parameters of the model and $\mathbf{f_q}$ is the parameter
forces which are determined from the 3D forces, $\mathbf{f}$ from datasets:

$$\mathbf{f_q} = \int \mathbf{L^T f} \tag{7}$$

The Jacobian matrix $\mathbf{L}$ converts the 3D data forces $\mathbf{f}$ into forces which directly
affect the parameters of the model[7]. The data forces, from each boundary point
to the corresponding model wall, are computed by distributing force weights to
the closest triangular element on the corresponding wall[10].

3.2   Shape Estimation Process

To fit the model to the data, the model is translated and rotated to the center
of the mass of boundary datasets. Then we approximate the global shape and
estimate the further local shape variations. With this hierarchical estimation,
we can capture LV-RV shape accurately with enough degrees of freedom.

Our heart model with material coordinates $\mathbf{u}=(u, v, w)$ estimates the shape
as follows:

1. initialize a heart model with material coordinates
2. compute global translation and rotation :
   translate model to the center of the boundary datapoints
   rotate model so that z-axis set to the principal axis of the heart and y-axis points toward the RV
3. estimate scaling parameter: sc
4. estimate axial parameters for each wall $w = 1, 2, 3$ and on positive and negative directions along xyz-axes:
   $r_{1+}, r_{1-}, r_{2+}, r_{2-}, r_{3+}, r_{3-}$ for LV endocardium, RV endocardium and epicardium
5. compute blending parameters along u for RV endocardium wrt model frame:
   the septum arc length ratio r_s and septum rotation parameter r_t
6. estimate the piecewise axial parameters along u, w :
   $r_{1+}, r_{1-}, r_{2+}, r_{2-}, r_{3+}, r_{3-}$
7. estimate the local variations on all the material coordinates (u, v, w):

4   Result

Our blended model approach with parameter functions describe the heart shape quantitatively with translation, rotation, scaling, axial deformation and blending parameters. These parameters allow enough DOFs to deal with normal and pathological hearts and therefore are good to compare the different heart shapes. We applied the methods to the two normals and one abnormal datasets and we can see the differences in shapes and parameters.

Table 1. Axial Deformation Parameters r1, r2, r3 (mm)

	r1+		r1-		r2+		r2-		r3
	apex	base	apex	base	apex	base	apex	base	
LV endo	9.23	11.70	10.07	12.32	7.87	10.69	9,83	11.12	64.07
RV endo	11.88	14.53	17.37	24.22	27.70	33.98	14.25	16.18	67.67
Epicardium	13.33	15.82	17.11	23.61	29.27	35.64	14.86	16.43	70.70

Table 1 is the typical parameters extracted from normal hearts. Figure 4 shows a reconstructed heart model at end-diastole phase of a normal subject. Figure 5 is RV hypertrophy patient model.

5   Conclusion

We have shown how to build a generic heart model including the RV and its outflow tract. Furthermore, the analysis of the shape parameters can be applied

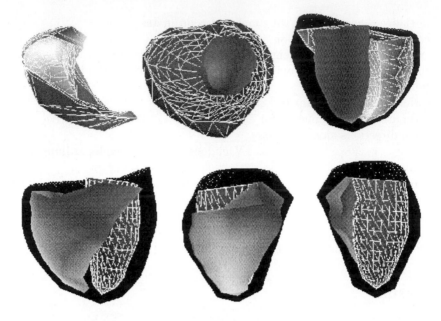

Fig. 4. LV-RV Heart Model at end-diastole

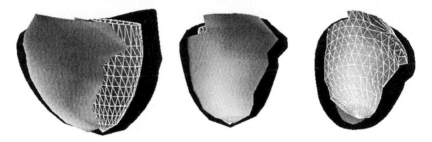

Fig. 5. RV Hypertrophy Model at end-diastole

to the morphological study of the shape. Future study will be the motion reconstruction and analysis of the heart from the MRI-SPAMM data. After a large number of experiments we will be able to define the parameters associated with normal motion and parameters associated with abnormal motion.

References

1. L. Axel and L. Dougherty. Heart wall motion: Improved method of spatial modulation of magnetization for mr imaging, 1989.
2. D. DeCarlo and D. Metaxas. Blended deformable models. In *Proceedings of the Conference on Computer Vision and Pattern Recognition*, pages 566–572, Los Alamitos, CA, USA, June 1994. IEEE Computer Society Press.

3. Jerome Declerck, Nicholas Ayache, and Elliot R. McVeigh. Use of a 4D plani-spheric transformation for the tracking and the analysis of LV motion with tagged MR images. Technical Report RR-3535, Inria, Institut National de Recherche en Informatique et en Automatique.

4. Edith Haber, Dimitris N. Metaxas, and Leon Axel. Motion analysis of the right ventricle from MRI images. *Lecture Notes in Computer Science*, 1496:177–??, 1998.

5. Michael Kass, Andrew Witkin, and Demetri Terzopoulos. Snakes: Active Contour Models . *Academic Publishers*, 1987.

6. Daniel Kristjansson, Henning Biermann, and Denis Zorin. Approximate boolean operations on free-form solids. In *Proceedings of ACM SIGGRAPH 2001*, Computer Graphics Proceedings, Annual Conference Series, pages 185–194. ACM Press / ACM SIGGRAPH, August 2001. ISBN 1-58113-292-1.

7. D. Metaxas and D. Terzopoulos. Shape and nonrigid motion estimation through physics-based synthesis, 1993.

8. X. Papademetris, A. J. Sinusas, D. P. Dione, and J. S. Duncan. Estimation of 3D left ventricular deformation from echocardiography. *Medical Image Analysis*, 2001.

9. J. Park, D. Metaxas, and L. Axel. Analysis of left ventricular wall motion based on volumetric deformable models and MRI-SPAMM. *Medical Image Analysis*, 1(1):53–71, 1996.

10. J. Park, D. Metaxas, A. Young, and L. Axel. Deformable models with parameter functions for cardiac motion analysis from tagged mri data. 1996.

11. Alistair A. Young. Model tags: Direct 3D tracking of heart wall motion from tagged MR images. *Lecture Notes in Computer Science*, 1496:92–101, 1998.

Characterization of Regional Pulmonary Mechanics from Serial MRI Data

James Gee, Tessa Sundaram, Ichiro Hasegawa,
Hidemasa Uematsu, and Hiroto Hatabu

University of Pennsylvania, Departments of Bioengineering and Radiology
3600 Market Street, Suite 370, Philadelphia, PA 19104, USA

Abstract. We describe a method for quantification of lung motion from
the registration of successive images in serial MR acquisitions during normal respiration. MR quantification of pulmonary motion enables in vivo
assessment of parenchymal mechanics within the lung in order to assist
disease diagnosis or treatment monitoring. Specifically, we obtain estimates of pulmonary motion by summing the normalized cross-correlation
over the lung images to identify corresponding locations between the images. The normalized correlation is robust to linear intensity distortions
in the image acquisition, which may occur as a consequence of changes in
average proton density resulting from changes in lung volume during the
respiratory cycle. The estimated motions correspond to deformations of
an elastic body and reflect to a first order approximation the true physical behavior of lung parenchyma. The method is validated on a serial
MRI study of the lung, for which breath-hold images were acquired of a
healthy volunteer at different phases of the respiratory cycle.

1 Introduction

The ability to quantify lung deformation is useful in characterizing the changes
brought on by pulmonary pathology. Diseases such as idiopathic pulmonary fibrosis (IPF) and chronic obstructive pulmonary disease (COPD) change the
structural properties of the lung parenchyma, and directly affect the lung's ability to normally expand and contract, [1, 2]. COPD (or emphysema) increases lung
compliance by promoting the destruction of the alveolar framework. Conversely,
IPF stiffens the lung via an idiopathic increase in parenchymal connective tissue.
It would be helpful to be able to observe and detect such morphologic changes
and their effects on normal lung motion using medical imaging techniques.

Surrogate measures based on the motion of chest wall and diaphragm, [3, 4],
have been reported. However, magnetic resonance (MR) grid-tagging techniques
allow the direct assessment of regional motion of moving structures in the human
body, [5–7]. The technique has recently been applied to evaluate local mechanical
properties of the lung with highly promising results, [8, 9]. However, there are
limitations due to (a) the relatively low spatial resolution of the estimated motion
fields, stemming from the coarse grid intervals that are currently practicable, (b)
fading of the grid by T1 decay time of the tissue, and (c) the difficulty of applying

T. Dohi and R. Kikinis (Eds.): MICCAI 2002, LNCS 2488, pp. 762–769, 2002.

the method in 3-D. Moreover, because the T1 decay time of lung parenchyma is much shorter than the duration of the respiratory cycle, the technique can only be applied to study certain respiratory phases and not the entire breathing cycle, [8].

In this work, a method is developed to determine a *dense* motion field—i.e., a displacement vector at every imaged point of the lung parenchyma—at each sampling time of a serial MR image sequence. The motion is estimated using the pulmonary vasculature and parenchymal structures as natural sources of spatial markers, *without* the requirement for explicit correspondence information, thus enabling the assessment and quantification of regional parenchymal deformation in the lungs over complete breathing cycles.

2   Methods

2.1   Quantification of Lung Motion via Image Registration

The goal of a registration algorithm is to find a spatial transformation or image warp that brings the features of one *source* image into alignment with those of a second, *target* image with similar content. Thus, registration algorithms can be used to determine the spatial locations of corresponding features in a sequence of MR pulmonary images. The computed correspondences immediately yield the displacement fields corresponding to the motion of the lung during the image sequence.

Many techniques for registration of MR images have been proposed, [10]. Simple methods assume that a rigid or affine transformation is sufficient to warp one image to another. Although such transformations may be sufficient to account for within-subject variation in rigid structures, to align features in lung images from different individuals or from the same individual acquired at different times, higher dimensional, non-rigid transformations are required in general.

A review of non-rigid registration techniques can be found in [11]. In previous work, [12, 13], we have developed a system in which an initial *global* affine registration of the source 3-D volume to the fixed target volume is performed to correct differences in object pose and location. This provides a starting point for an elastic registration algorithm, [12], which subsequently computes a *local* match, described by a dense displacement field **u** over the source image, that brings the detailed anatomy into register. The algorithm uses a finite element method iteratively to optimize an objective function π, which balances the pointwise *similarity* (or voxel-to-voxel correspondence) of the warped source and target images with the amount of *deformation* caused by **u**:

$$\pi = \lambda \cdot \text{deformation} - \alpha \cdot \text{similarity}, \tag{1}$$

where λ moderates the smoothness of the warps and α encodes the uncertainty in our image measurements, [12]. In this work, we obtain estimates of pulmonary motion by summing the *normalized cross-correlation* over the lung images to identify corresponding locations between the images, I_1, I_2, [10]:

$$\frac{\sum_{\mathbf{X}_i \in \mathcal{G}(\mathbf{X})} I_1(\mathbf{X}_i) I_2(\mathbf{X}_i)}{\left(\sum_{\mathbf{X}_i \in \mathcal{G}(\mathbf{X})} I_1(\mathbf{X}_i) I_1(\mathbf{X}_i) \sum_{\mathbf{X}_i \in \mathcal{G}(\mathbf{X})} I_2(\mathbf{X}_i) I_2(\mathbf{X}_i) \right)^{1/2}},$$

where $\mathcal{G}(\mathbf{X})$ is a neighborhood of voxels around the location $\mathbf{X}$ at which the images are being compared. By measuring the similarity over a neighborhood of each voxel and thus taking into account the voxel's *local image structure*, the normalized correlation should yield better results than pointwise measures such as the squared intensity difference. Moreover, unlike the latter measure which assumes that the intensity of any point tracked during motion is constant, [14], the normalized correlation is robust to linear intensity distortions in the image acquisition, which may occur in our studies as a consequence of changes in average proton density resulting from changes in lung volume during the respiratory cycle.

For the deformation term in (1), we use the linear elastic strain energy, [15]:

$$\frac{1}{2} \int_V \boldsymbol{\sigma} : \boldsymbol{\varepsilon} \, dV, \tag{2}$$

where $\boldsymbol{\sigma}$ and $\boldsymbol{\varepsilon}$ denote the stress and strain tensors, respectively [15]. Their elastic constitutive relation is given by the generalized Hooke's law: in indicial notation, $\sigma_{ij} = D_{ijkl} \, \varepsilon_{kl}$, where the elastic coefficients $D_{ijkl}(\mathbf{X})$ reduce to two constants known as the Lamé parameters for the homogeneous, isotropic material idealization used in the current work. The estimated motions thus correspond to deformations of an elastic body and reflect to a first order approximation the true physical behavior of lung parenchyma—the source image volume takes on the properties of an idealized elastic material under the influence of loads which act along the gradients in the similarity between the image and the target volume.

2.2   In Vivo Assessment of Regional Pulmonary Mechanics

From the calculated displacement field, $\mathbf{u}$, representing pulmonary motion, a quantitative description of the tissue deformation induced in the lung can be derived in the form of the *(finite) Lagrangian strain tensor*, $\boldsymbol{\varepsilon}^*$, [15]: $\boldsymbol{\varepsilon}^* = 1/2 \{ \nabla \mathbf{u} + (\nabla \mathbf{u})^\mathrm{T} + (\nabla \mathbf{u})^\mathrm{T} \cdot (\nabla \mathbf{u}) \}$, where $\nabla \mathbf{u}$, the second-order displacement gradient, can be numerically computed, [13]. When the displacement gradients are small, the product terms in $\boldsymbol{\varepsilon}^*$ can be neglected to obtain the *infinitesimal* or *small-deformation* strain tensor, $\boldsymbol{\varepsilon}$, whose components with respect to rectangular Cartesian coordinates $\mathbf{X}$ (in the undeformed configuration) are given by $\varepsilon_{ij} = 1/2(\partial u_i / \partial X_j + \partial u_j / \partial X_i)$.

Visualization and analysis of either strain tensor over the imaged anatomy can be accomplished by mapping pointwise various scalar indices derived from the tensors. Specifically, the *principal strains*, which include the maximum and minimum *normal* strains experienced at a point, are characterized by the tensor cigenvalues. Two frame-independent indices are the first and second moments of the distribution of tensor eigenvalues: the former represents the trace of the tensor or the sum of its eigenvalues and provides an overall measure of strain magnitude; and the second moment measures the variance of the eigenvalues, which indicates the degree of directional bias (or *anisotropy*) in the strain profile. The strain anisotropy can be further analyzed by examining the off-diagonal elements or *shear* strain components of ε^* or ε. The strain magnitude and anisotropy measures depend only on the tensor eigenvalues and not on the eigenvectors. The eigenvectors, however, also reveal important information about the observed deformation, particularly in regions of the lung where the strain anisotropy is the greatest. The eigenvectors are the directions along which the principal strains are experienced; thus, they characterize the *orientation* of the strain profile.

3   Experimental Results

Figures 1 and 2 demonstrate preliminary results obtained in an MRI study of simulated lung motion, [16]. Images were acquired of a young healthy male volunteer on a 1.5 T whole body MRI scanner (Signa Horizon, General Electric) using a two-dimensional true FISP sequence, with TR = 3.0 msec, TE = 1.5 msec and matrix size = 128×128, resulting in a total acquisition time of 0.4 sec per image. Other imaging parameters were as follows: flip angle = 35 degrees; field of view = 450 mm; and section thickness = 10 mm. Five sagittal images of the right lung were obtained with breath-holding at different phases of the respiratory cycle, spanning full inhalation (phase I) to full exhalation (phase V).

Each image was non-rigidly registered to the next image in the sequence. In Fig. 1, the registration transformation between the first two images in the sequence, represented as a field of displacement vectors, is shown superimposed on the first image, where the vectors indicate the corresponding locations in the second image and thus provide a direct, quantitative measure of the lung motion between the images. The associated finite strain tensor was computed over each displacement field and is visualized in Fig. 2 using an ellipse to depict each tensor, where the major and minor axes of the ellipse are directed along the tensor eigenvectors, respectively, and scaled by the corresponding principal strain values.

The dynamics of respiratory lung deformation was studied by examining the measurements over the image sequence, as exemplified by the series of motion and strain tensor maps depicted in Fig. 2. The diaphragm rises as the lung volume decreases from total lung capacity (TLC) to residual volume (RV). At the same time, the posterior portion of the lung displaces superiorly, whereas the anterior portion is displaced posteriorly and superiorly. Regional parenchymal strain appears oriented toward the pulmonary hilum, with strain magnitude maximal at the mid-cycle of the expiratory phase.

These preliminary data—specifically, the estimated lung motion between successive images—have been validated, [17]. The validation protocol was designed

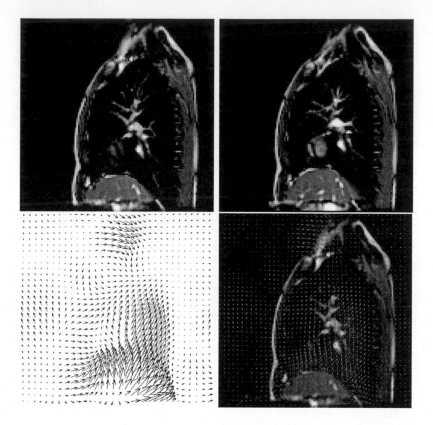

Fig. 1. Illustration of the estimated lung motion between two consecutive frames (top row) in a sequence of MR images. The registration transformation between the images, represented as a field of displacement vectors (bottom left), is shown superimposed on the first image (bottom right), where the vectors indicate the corresponding locations in the second image and thus provide a direct, quantitative measure of the lung motion between the images.

around the identification and tracking of 22 landmarks chosen at the bifurcations of pulmonary vasculature. Experts skilled at reading MR images independently identified the landmarks at each of the five phases. Three sets of expert data were then averaged to form a "ground truth" set of landmarks for the expiratory phase. The displacements of these truth landmarks were calculated and compared to the displacements determined by the registration algorithm at the landmark locations (Fig. 3). No significant difference was detected between the three sets of expert landmarks and the truth landmark set ($p > 0.9$), suggesting a minor contribution by user variation to the overall error. In addition, a significant difference was neither observed between the magnitudes ($p > 0.3$) nor the directions ($p > 0.4$) of the registration-derived and landmark-derived displacements. The average error between the endpoints of the displacement vectors was 1.14 ± 0.93 pixels.

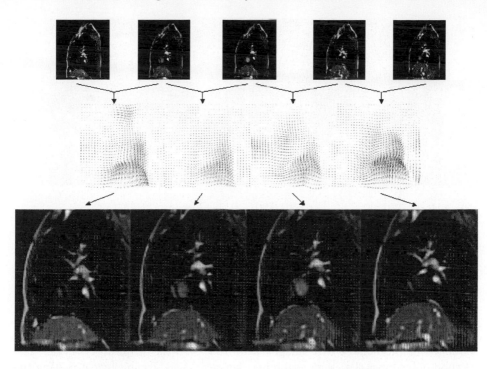

Fig. 2. Visualization of the dynamics of respiratory lung deformation. The calculated motion fields (middle row) between successive pairs of MR images (top row) over the expiratory phase of the respiratory cycle are shown along with the induced strain tensor fields (bottom row), where each tensor is depicted using an ellipse with major and minor axes directed along its eigenvectors, respectively, and scaled by the corresponding principal strain values.

4   Discussion

The recent development of fast MR imaging techniques has made possible detailed, non-invasive imaging of pulmonary parenchyma by overcoming the inherent difficulties associated with lung imaging, including low proton density, severe magnetic field susceptibility, and respiratory and cardiac motion artifacts. A gradient-echo sequence with ultra-short TE and a single-shot fast SE sequence can together provide a platform for MR imaging of the lung. Pulmonary perfusion can be assessed using a T1-weighted gradient-echo sequence with ultra-short TE and contrast agents. Regional pulmonary ventilation can also be evaluated by MR using molecular oxygen or laser-polarized Xe-129 and He-3. In the current work, we explore the use of fast MR imaging to study lung mechanics, which should provide a third, key diagnostic dimension in the assessment of pulmonary function, augmenting the information provided by studies of ventilation and perfusion. Specifically, the determination of regional biomechanical parameters in the lung has the potential to assist detection of early and/or localized pathological processes. Moreover, quantitative measurements of these

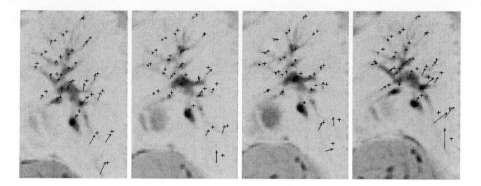

Fig. 3. Enlarged comparison of the landmark-based (arrows) and registration-derived (plus signs) displacements for each of the four motion fields. Only the endpoints of the registration-derived vectors are shown.

physical properties could provide an objective evaluation of therapeutic effects in various pulmonary disorders

The feasibility of a novel method is demonstrated here for quantifying lung motion (and, in turn, in vivo assessment of parenchymal deformation) from a sequence of pulmonary MR images acquired over the respiratory cycle. The method determines the lung motion between sequential frames by estimating the spatial transformation which brings the images into register. The approach has been verified over simulated motion data, but it remains to be tested on image sequences acquired without breath-holding, which is planned for the future.

References

1. Pratt, P. C.: Emphysema and Chronic Airways Disease. In: Dail, D., Hammar, S. (eds.): Pulmonary Pathology. Springer-Verlag, New York (1988) 654–659
2. Fulmer, J. D., Roberts, W. C., von Gal, E. R., Crystal, R. G.: Morphologic-Physiologic Correlates of the Severity of Fibrosis and Degree of Cellularity in Idiopathic Pulmonary Fibrosis. J. Clin. Invest. **63** (1979) 665–676
3. Suga, K., Tsukuda, T., Awaya, H., Takano, K., Koike, S., Matsunaga, N., Sugi, K., Esato, K.: Impaired Respiratory Mechanics in Pulmonary Emphysema: Evaluation With Dynamic Breathing MRI. J. Magn. Reson. Imaging **10** (1999) 510–520
4. Cluzel, P., Similowski, T., Chartrand-Lefebvre, C., Zelter, M., Derenne, J. P., Grenier, P. A.: Diaphragm and Chest Wall: Assessment of the Inspiratory Pump With MR Imaging-Preliminary Observations. Radiology **215** (2000) 574–583
5. Zerhouni, E. A., Parish, D. M., Rogers, W. J., Yang, A., Shapiro, E. P.: Human Heart Tagging With MR Imaging—A Method for Noninvasive Assessment of Myocardial Motion. Radiology **169** (1988) 59–63
6. Axel, L., Dougherty, L.: MR Imaging of Motion with Spatial Modulation of Magnetization. Radiology **171** (1989) 841–845
7. Axel, L., Dougherty, L.: Heart Wall Motion: Improved Method of Spatial Modulation of Magnetization for MR Imaging. Radiology **172** (1989) 349–350

8. Chen, Q., Mai, V. M., Bankier, A. A., Napadow, V. J., Gilbert, R. J., Edelman, R. R.: Ultrafast MR Grid-Tagging Sequence for Assessment of Local Mechanical Properties of the Lungs. Magn. Reson. Med. **45** (2001) 24–28
9. Napadow, V. J., Mai, V., Bankier, A., Gilbert, R. J., Edelman, R., Chen, Q.: Determination of Regional Pulmonary Parenchymal Strain During Normal Respiration Using Spin Inversion Tagged Magnetization MRI. J. Magn. Reson. Imag. **13** (2001) 467–474
10. Maintz, J. B. A., Viergever, M. A.: A Survey of Medical Image Registration. Medical Image Analysis **2** (1998) 1–31
11. Lester, H., Arridge, S. R.: A Survey of Hierarchical Non-Linear Medical Image Registration. Pattern Recognition **32** (1999) 129–149
12. Gee, J. C., Bajcsy, R. K.: Elastic Matching: Continuum Mechanical and Probabilistic Analysis. In: Toga, A. W. (ed.): Brain Warping. Academic Press, San Diego (1999) 183–197
13. Gee, J. C., Haynor, D. R.: Numerical Methods for High-Dimensional Warps. In: Toga, A. W. (ed.): Brain Warping. Academic Press, San Diego (1999) 101–113
14. Horn, B., Schunck, B.: Determining Optical Flow. Artif. Intell. **17** (1981) 185–203
15. Malvern, L. E.: Introduction to the Mechanics of a Continuous Medium. Prentice-Hall, Englewood Cliffs (1969)
16. Hatabu, H., Ohno, Y. Ucmatsu, H., Nakatsu, M., Song, H. K., Oshio, K., Gefter, W. B., Gee, J. C.: Lung Biomechanics Via Non-Rigid Registration of Serial MR Images. Proc. ISMRM 9th Scientific Meeting (2001) 2008
17. Sundaram, T. A., Gee, J.C., Hasegawa, I., Uematsu, H., Hatabu H.: Validation of A Registration Algorithm for Computing Lung Deformation From MR Images. Proc. ISMRM 10th Scientific Meeting (2002) in press

Using Voxel-Based Morphometry to Examine Atrophy-Behavior Correlates in Alzheimer's Disease and Frontotemporal Dementia

Michael P. Lin, Christian Devita, James C. Gee, and Murray Grossman

University of Pennsylvania
Departments of Radiology and Neurology
Philadelphia, PA 19104
gee@grasp.cis.upenn.edu

1 Background

Computational Morphometry With the advent of more sophisticated computer and medical imaging technology, computational morphometry of MRI images has become a standard tool in the statistical analysis of differences in brain structure between two groups of subjects. This comparative work represents an important advance in the diagnostic armamentarium for neurodegenerative diseases such as Alzheimer's disease (AD) and frontotemporal dementia (FTD), where no definitive diagnostic tests are available. This preliminary report describes morphometric analyses of MRI datasets of AD and FTD patients, and relates these to clinical measures. We will begin this paper by describing voxel based morphometry (VBM), a powerful, quantitative tool for analyzing structural brain images. We then describe our implementation of a fully automated, user-independent algorithm for morphometric analysis of structural MRI data.

Voxel-Based Morphometry (VBM) VBM is a voxel-wise comparison of gray matter intensity, where groups of images are normalized, segmented, smoothed, and then compared using voxel-wise statistical parametric tests. As opposed to label-based approaches to morphometry, where changes are measured over regions of interest (ROI) defined by the operator, VBM does not require the *a priori* selection of ROIs. This has three main potential advantages over label-based methods: (a) removal of operator bias in ROI definition (local bias), (b) quantification of subtle features easily missed by operator inspection, and (c) assessment of global structural changes in brain, unrestricted by the selection of specific ROIs (global bias). [1, 10, 19] One problem with VBM is differences detected due to the presence of mis-segmented, non-brain voxels. These errors become significant as study groups grow large, although algorithms have been developed to manage this problem. [11]

Alzheimer's Disease (AD) AD is perhaps the most common neurodegenerative disease. Yet there is no definitive clinical test for identifying this condition or distinguishing it from other conditions such as FTD. Patients suffering from AD tend to show symptoms of decreased language aptitude, such as deficits in

T. Dohi and R. Kikinis (Eds.): MICCAI 2002, LNCS 2488, pp. 770–776, 2002.

naming and semantic comprehension. [12] Areas of atrophy associated with AD may include the temporal-parietal, dorsolateral pre-frontal, and hippocampal regions, based largely on user defined ROI analyses. [17] These areas contribute to language, executive, and memory functioning. [12] It has been claimed that atrophy in the hippocampal formation is a marker for AD, and that this atrophy is related to memory loss. [7, 20] However, this distribution of atrophy may not be specific to AD, as it is also found in temporal lobe epilepsy, schizophrenia and FTD. [9]

Frontotemporal Dementia (FTD) Frontotemporal dementia, also known as frontotemporal lobar degeneration or Pick's disease, refers to one important form of non-Alzheimer's dementia. Behavioral studies have shown that patients suffering from FTD have cognitive difficulty, with aphasia (disorder of language), executive resource limitations such as poor working memory and impaired planning, and a disorder of behavior and social comportment. [17] ROI studies suggest that areas of atrophy associated with FTD may include orbitofrontal, dorsolateral pre-frontal, and anterior temporal regions, areas thought to contribute to language and executive resources. [9]

Hypothesis Comparative structural and behavioral studies of AD and FTD have been rare. In our study, we will first use VBM to examine the gray matter structure of FTD and AD patients to determine locations of significant cortical atrophy. Then we will use VBM to look for correlations between regional atrophy and performance on behavioral tests that measure specific cognitive functions. Our hypothesis is that certain types of clinically observable deficits in FTD and AD patients are due to specific areas of cortical atrophy in the brain, that these brain behavior relations can be identified through correlation analyses, and that different patterns of brain-behavior correlations in AD and FTD reflect distinct clinical impairments and the unique ways in which complex tasks such as naming can be compromised in different neurodegenerative diseases.

2   Methods

Subject Population We studied forty-five subjects in total belonging to one of the patient groups or to a healthy control group. Nine subjects were healthy, elderly controls. The 20 AD patients and 26 FTD patients were diagnosed by a board-certified neurologist using published criteria (see Table 1). All patients were mild to moderately impaired.

Behavioral Tests All of these subjects, in addition to being imaged, performed a battery of cognitive tasks designed to assess their mental ability. The test used to illustrate the correlation analysis in this study was a confrontation naming task known as the "Boston Naming Test" (BNT). The subject is presented with a line drawing of an object and the subject must say the appropriate name for the object.

Magnetic Resonance Imaging Imaging was performed using a GE Horizon Echospeed 1.5 T MRI scanner (GE Medical Systems, Milwaukee, WI). First, a

Table 1. Subject group breakdown.

Subject Group	Number	Mean Age (St. Dev)	Mean MMSE (St. Dev)	Disease Duration in Yrs (St. Dev)
Elderly Controls	9	66.75(10.53)	N/A	N/A
AD	20	72.19(6.43)	18.76(7.90)	4.9(3.1)
FTD	26	63.70(10.05)	19.91(6.67)	3.5(2.4)

rapid sagittal T1-weighted image was acquired to align the patient in the scanner. Then, a high resolution volumetric structural scan was obtained. The volumes are comprised of T1-weighted 3D spoiled gradient echo images, with a repetition time (TR) of 35 ms, echo time (TE) of 6 ms, flip angle of 30 degrees, matrix size of 128 x 256 and a rectangular field of view giving an in-plane resolution of 0.9 x 1.3 mm, and slice thickness of 1.5mm. The subjects spent a total of ten minutes in the scanner to acquire the anatomical images.

Image Analysis Morphometric analysis was performed on structural images from each group using the 1999 version of the Statistical Parametric Mapping (SPM) package (Wellcome Department of Cognitive Neurology). [1] The VBM analysis was carried out as follows. All of the images were first normalized to match the SPM T1-weighted template brain. Non-linear normalization was performed with the following parameters: bilinear interpolation, 7 x 8 x 7 basis functions with 12 iterations. Next, each voxel of the normalized image was classified into gray matter, white matter and cerebrospinal fluid using the SPM segmentation algorithm. Then, the segmented images were smoothed with a 12mm Gaussian kernel. Two kinds of statistical analyses were performed using only the smoothed gray matter segmented images. First, a two-sample t-test was carried out comparing each patient group to the control group. Then, using a regression analysis, we correlated gray matter density to cognitive test scores for each patient group. [1]

3 Results

Anatomical results We used a statistical threshold of $p < 0.0001$ uncorrected (equivalent to a Z-score of 3.82) and an extent threshold of 50 adjacent voxels. Anatomical results are summarized in Tables 2 and 3. A rendering of brain atrophy location for AD and FTD can be found in Figure 1. AD patients have significant atrophy that is most prominent in temporal cortex but also involves frontal cortex, and the atrophy is more evident in the right hemisphere than the left hemisphere. FTD patients show significant atrophy in frontal cortices, particularly in right inferior frontal and left superior frontal regions.

Atrophy-Behavior correlation results The rendered brains displaying the anatomic distribution of the correlations are found in Figure 2. In AD, performance accuracy on the confrontation naming task (54% mean correct) correlates

Table 2. Anatomic distribution of gray matter atrophy in AD compared to healthy control subjects.

Atrophy Locus (Brodmann Area)	Coordinates	Atrophy Extent (voxels)	Z-values
Right Middle Temporal, Superior Temporal(BA 21,22)	44 -30 20	7967	4.97
Left Middle Temporal, Superior Temporal(BA 21,22)	-64 -6 -16	2145	4.34
Right Precuneus(BA 7,31)	10 -50 38	118	4.30
Right Middle Frontal(BA 8)	34 38 48	66	4.21
Right Medial Frontal(BA 10)	16 50 2	178	4.21
Right Inferior Frontal(BA 6)	40 8 56	121	4.15
Right Middle Frontal(BA 46)	54 34 22	68	4.01
Left Inferior Frontal(BA 45)	-40 14 14	141	3.99
Left Medial Temporal(BA 25)	-8 0 -8	311	3.98
Left Fusiform(BA 20)	-50 -32 -24	354	3.87

Table 3. Anatomic distribution of gray matter atrophy in FTD compared to healthy control subjects.

Atrophy Locus (Brodmann Area)	Coordinates	Atrophy Extent (voxels)	Z-values
Right Inferior Frontal(BA 47)	54 32 -16	67	4.05
Left Parietal(BA 7)	-22 -50 48	57	3.88
Left Middle Frontal(BA 8)	-28 20 46	77	3.81

with atrophy in lateral aspects of the right temporal and parietal lobes as summarized in Table 4. Table 5 shows a correlation in FTD patients between confrontation naming accuracy (69% mean correct) and atrophy also in the right temporal region (superior and inferior), and in the left frontal and temporal regions.

4   Discussion

A statistical threshold of $p < 0.001$ uncorrected (equivalent to a Z-score of 3.1) and an extent threshold of 50 adjacent voxels was used in the correlation analyses. We implemented VBM analyses in a user-independent manner to quantify the anatomic distribution of atrophy in mild to moderate AD and FTD patients. We found bilateral temporal atrophy in AD, consistent with the known distribution of histopathological abnormalities in these patients. This is also consistent with previous ROI-based analyses of regional atrophy in AD. [4, 8] VBM analyses of FTD showed atrophy in a different anatomic distribution from AD. The FTD group had more atrophy in the left hemisphere with several isolated frontal regions. These findings are also consistent in part with previous ROI based analyses, and with the known distribution of pathology in FTD. [15, 13]

These different anatomic distributions of anatomy in distinct neurodegenerative diseases are thought to explain the different clinical presentations of these patients. We tested this expectation with correlations that can relate atrophy of

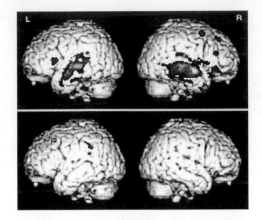

Fig. 1. Atrophy compared to control. (Top) AD. (Bottom) FTD.

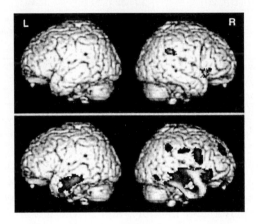

Fig. 2. Correlation of atrophy to BNT. (Top) AD. (Bottom) FTD.

these brain regions to common clinical difficulties in these patients. We examined impairments in naming to illustrate our method, though measures of semantic comprehension, executive functioning, and other cognitive measures also can be used.

In AD, we found correlations between naming accuracy and right inferior frontal and superior regions. These are homologues of left hemisphere regions often implicated in naming in functional imaging studies of healthy adults, and we and others have found compensator up regulation of ordinarily quiescent right hemisphere regions on functional neuroimaging studies of language tasks in AD. This correlation of naming with right hemisphere structural anatomy thus may reflect the brain regions contributing to residual naming success in AD.

In fMRI activation studies of FTD, we have also found compensatory activation of brain regions not ordinarily recruited in healthy subjects to help support language functioning. We found with our automated VBM technique, naming

Table 4. Atrophy-Behavior correlation results of AD subjects.

Correlation Locus (Brodmann Area)	Coordinates	Correlation Extent (voxels)	Z-values
Right Inferior Frontal(BA 47)	30 24 -8	309	3.22
Right Inferior Parietal(BA 39,40)	44 -18 28	230	3.13

Table 5. Atrophy-Behavior correlation results of FTD subjects.

Correlation Locus (Brodmann Area)	Coordinates	Correlation Extent (voxels)	Z-values
Right Anterior Temporal, Inferior Temporal(BA 12, 20)	60 10 -10	8453	4.95
Left Inferior Temporal, Middle Temporal(BA 20, 21)	-50 -24 -16	1308	4.50
Right Inferior Frontal(BA 44)	68 8 22	369	4.29
Left Middle Frontal, Inferior Frontal	-24 28 -8	195	3.78
Right Anterior Cingulate(BA 24)	8 8 26	304	3.48
Right Inferior Parietal(BA 40)	62 -44 40	132	3.30
Right Postcentral(BA 1,2,3)	68 -18 36	87	3.27
Right Orbital Frontal(BA 11)	6 56 -22	149	3.22
Left Superior Frontal(BA 8)	-2 42 48	256	3.18
Right Middle Frontal(BA 9)	22 50 34	169	3.15
Left Medial Temporal(BA 36)	-26 -32 -20	99	3.13
Right Inferior Temporal(BA 37)	58 -64 -10	92	3.12

accuracy correlates with bilateral temporal and right frontal and parietal cortices. While these areas of anatomic correlation do not necessarily correspond to the distribution of anatomic atrophy, it is likely that the connectivity pattern of cortical regions involved in naming links significantly atrophic areas with areas unusual to naming that may have less significant atrophy.

These preliminary results emphasize the feasibility of using computational morphometry to define regional gray matter atrophy in AD and FTD, and help us improve diagnostic accuracy and understand brain-behavior relationships in neurodegenerative diseases.

References

1. Ashburner J, Friston KJ. Voxel-based morphometry—The methods. Neuroimage 2000; 11:805-821.
2. Ashburner J, Friston KJ. Why voxel-based morphometry should be used. Neuroimage 2001; 14:1238-1243.
3. Baron JC, Chetelat G, Desgranges B, Perchey G, Landeau B, De la Sayette V, Eustache F. In vivo mapping of gray matter loss with voxel-based morphometry in mild Alzheimer's disease. Neuroimage 2001; 14:298-309.

4. Bierer L, Hof P, Purohit D, Carlin L, Schmeidler J, Davis K, Perl D. Neocortical neurofibrillary tangles correlate with dementia severity in Alzheimer's disease. Archives of Neurology 1995; 52(1):81-88.

5. Bookstein, FL. "Voxel-Based Morphometry" should not be used with imperfectly registered images. Neuroimage 2001; 14:1454-1462.

6. Bozeat S, Gregory CA, Ralph MAL, Hodges JR. Which neuropsychiatric and behavioral features distinguish frontal and temporal variants of frontotemporal dementia from Alzheimer's disease? Journal of Neurology, Neurosurgery, and Psychiatry 2000; 69(2):178-186.

7. Departments of Neurology and Neuropsychology, Department of Neuroanatomy, Department of Neuroradiology. Memory disorders in probable alzheimer's disease: The role of hippocampal atrophy as shown with MRI. Journal of Neurology, Neurosurgery, and Psychiatry 1995; 58(5):590-597.

8. Eberhard DA, Lopes MBS, Trugman JM, Brashear HR. Alzheimer's disease in a case of cortical basal ganglionic degeneration with severe dementia. Journal of Neurology, Neurosurgery, and Psychiatry 1996; 60(1):109-110.

9. Frisoni GB, Beltramello A, Geroldi C, Weiss C, Bianchetti A, Trabucchi M. Brain atrophy in frontotemporal dementia. Journal of Neurology, Neurosurgery & Psychiatry 1996; 61(2):157-165.

10. Gitelman DR, Ashburner J, Friston KJ, Tyler LK, Price CJ. Voxel-based morphometry of herpes simplex encephalitis. Neuroimage 2001; 13:623-631.

11. Good CD, Johnsrude IS, Ashburner J, Henson RNA, Friston KJ, Frackowiak RSJ. A voxel-based morphometric study of ageing in 465 normal adult human brains. Neuroimage 2001; 14:21-36.

12. Grossman M, Payer F, Onishi K, White-Devine T, Morrison D, D'Esposito M, Robinson K, Alavi A. Constraints on the cerebral basis for semantic processing from neuroimaging studies of Alzheimer's disease. Journal of Neurology, Neurosurgery, and Psychiatry 1997; 63(2):152-158.

13. Kertesz A, Munoz D. Pick's disease, frontotemporal dementia, and Pick complex: Emerging concepts. Archives of Neurology 1998; 55(3):302-304.

14. Levy M, Miller B, Cummings J, Fairbanks L, Craig A. Alzheimer disease and frontotemporal dementias: Behavioral distinctions. Archives of Neurology 1996; 53(7):687-690.

15. Lund and Manchester Groups. Clinical and neuropathological criteria for frontotemporal dementia. Journal of Neurology, Neurosurgery, and Psychiatry 1994; 57:416-418.

16. Mummery CJ, Patterson K, Wise RJS, Vandenbergh R, Price CJ, Hodges JR. Disrupted temporal lobe connections in semantic dementia. Brain 1999; 122:61-73.

17. Rozzini L, Lussignoli G, Padovani A, Bianchetti A, Trabucchi M. Alzheimer disease and frontotemporal dementia. Archives of Neurology 1997; 54(4):350-352.

18. Snowden JS, Bathgate D, Varma A, Blackshaw A, Gibbons ZC, Neary D. Distinct behavioral profiles in frontotemporal dementia and semantic dementia. Journal of Neurology, Neurosurgery, and Psychiatry 2001; 70(3):323-332.

19. Wilke M, Kaufmann C, Grabner A, Putz B, Wetter TC, Auer DP. Gray matter changes and correlates of disease severity in schizophrenia: A statistical parametric mapping study. Neuroimage 2001; 13:814-824.

20. Yamaguchi S, Meguro K, Itoh M, Hayasaka C, Shimada M, Yamazaki H, Yamadori A. Decreased cortical glucose metabolism correlates with hippocampal atrophy in Alzheimer's disease as shown by MRI and PET. Journal of Neurology, Neurosurgery, and Psychiatry 1997; 62(6):596-600.

Detecting Wedge Shaped Defects in Polarimetric Images of the Retinal Nerve Fiber Layer

Koen Vermeer[1], Frans Vos[1,3], Hans Lemij[2], and Albert Vossepoel[1]

[1] Pattern Recognition Group, Delft University of Technology
Lorentweg 1, 2628 JC Delft, The Netherlands
{koen,frans,albert}@ph.tn.tudelft.nl

[2] Rotterdam Eye Hospital, Schiedamsevest 180, 3011 BH Rotterdam, The Netherlands
lemij@wxs.nl

[3] Academic Medical Center, Department of Radiology
P.O. Box 22660, 1100 DD Amsterdam, The Netherlands

Abstract. Wedge shaped defects of the retinal nerve fiber layer (RNFL) may occur in glaucoma. Currently, automatic detection of wedge shaped defects in Scanning Laser Polarimetry images of the retinal nerve fiber layer is unavailable; an automatic classification is currently based only on global parameters, thereby ignoring important local information. Our method works by a modified dynamic programming technique that searches for locally strong edges with a preference for straight edges. These edges are initially classified based on their strength and then combined into wedge shaped defects. The results of our method on a limited set of 45 images yields a sensitivity of 88% and a specificity of 92%. More importantly, it shows that it is possible to automatically extract local RNFL defects such as wedges.

1 Introduction

Glaucoma is a fairly common eye disease that leads to thinning and loss of the retinal nerve fiber layer ((R)NFL). As a result, visual field defects develop. If untreated, the disease will lead to blindness. Many methods are available for diagnosis and screening of glaucoma, including Scanning Laser Polarimetry (SLP). In this method the thickness of the NFL is calculated by measuring the retardation of reflecting polarized light [1].

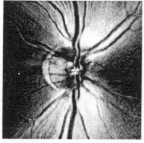
(a)

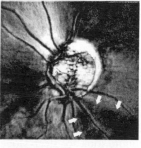
(b)

Fig. 1. Retardation images. (a) Healthy eye. (b) Wedge shaped defect, marked by white arrows.

T. Dohi and R. Kikinis (Eds.): MICCAI 2002, LNCS 2488, pp. 777–784, 2002.

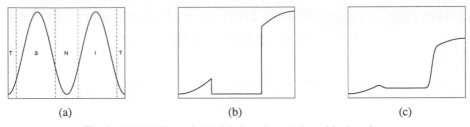

Fig. 2. (a) TSNIT-graph. (b) Ideal wedge. (c) Less ideal wedge.

A commercially available SLP based device is the GDx[1], which was used to acquire the images in this paper. Our version was a prototype that included a so-called variable cornea compensator. An example of a retardation image is shown in Fig. 1(a). All images in this paper are stretched to enhance the contrast. The circular object in the center of the image is the optic disc, where the NFL exits the eye.

Currently, parameters based on global properties of the retardation image are used for computer aided diagnosis. However, there is more information to the trained observer. An important local abnormality that is not detected by current computer algorithms is the *wedge shaped defect*. An example is given in Fig. 1(b) (located at 5 o'clock, marked by white arrows). A wedge shaped defect, which can precede visual field loss, is caused by localized loss of grouped nerve fibers. Wedges almost always signify an abnormality, although this may not always be glaucoma [2].

This paper aims to present a new detection scheme for wedge shaped defects, which can help in the diagnosis of glaucoma. To the best of our knowledge, no such automated wedge detection currently exists. Our method uses a polar representation of the retardation image and novel dynamic programming techniques. It opens a new way to interpret the information contained in these images.

2   Method

2.1   Model

A TSNIT-graph is a graph of the thickness of the RNFL at a certain distance from the optic disc at all angles, starting at the Temporal area, running through the Superior, Nasal, Inferior and again the Temporal area. The TSNIT-graph ideally looks like the double sinus of Fig. 2(a). Only the superior part of the temporal half will be displayed in the next figures, because clinically significant wedge defects mostly occur on the temporal side. Also, for the sake of argument, the superior and inferior sides can be considered similar. The ideal wedge shaped defect is modelled in Fig. 2(b). It is characterized by two opposing strong step edges.

The NFL of real eyes, however, is less ideal than this. The general NFL thickness can be much less, resulting in less contrast. Also, the detected NFL thickness inside a wedge can be significantly larger than zero and the step edges may be blurred. Figure 2(c) shows all these deviations. Therefore, when looking for the edges of a wedge, one should look for steep slopes.

---

[1] GDx Nerve Fiber Analyzer, Laser Diagnostic Technologies, Inc., San Diego, CA, http://www.laserdiagnostic.com

The wedges are modelled by two radially orientated, opposing edges. These edges start at the outside of the image, running approximately straight to the border of the optic disc. The edges can be observed most clearly at the outside of the image, because on these locations, they are less frequently occluded by blood vessels. By definition, wedge defects must extend to the border of the optic disc. Moreover, one of the edges will have a steeper slope and will thus be stronger than the other; the former one will be called 'strong', the latter 'weak'.

2.2 Outline

We will locate the wedges by applying the next scheme:

- Preprocessing.
- Edge detection.
- Matching edges.

The preprocessing step consists of the detection and removal of blood vessels and a transformation of the image coordinates. In the edge detection step, the locally strong edges are located. In the last step, the edges that have been found are classified based on their strength and corresponding edges are matched. In the following sections, each step is described thoroughly.

2.3 Preprocessing

Blood vessels show the same strong edges as do wedges. In addition, the NFL is occluded by them. Therefore, blood vessel detection is required. In Fig. 3(a), the result of our blood vessel detection scheme is shown. A comprehensive description is given in [3]. We estimate the NFL in areas occluded by the blood vessels by a Gaussian extrapolation of the surrounding neighborhood (see Fig. 3(b)).

Since the edges of the wedge are orientated radially, we introduce a polar representation of the NFL. The diameter of the optic disc in the center of the image, which is of no interest to us, is generally at least one quarter of the image. Therefore, a circle with a radius of one quarter of the image size is ignored. The coordinate transformation results in Fig. 4. The far left side of the polar representation corresponds to the 6 o'clock

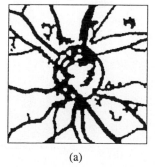

(a)

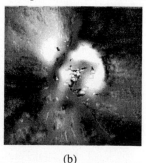

(b)

Fig. 3. Estimating the NFL. (a) Result of blood vessel detection. (b) Estimation of NFL at blood vessel areas.

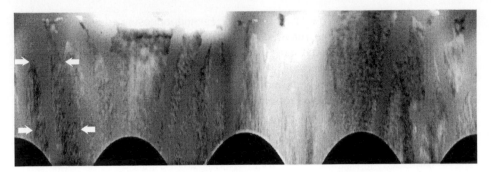

Fig. 4. Polar representation. The wedge shaped defect is marked by white arrows.

position in the original image. The positive x-direction of the polar image corresponds to an anti-clockwise rotation. In this polar image, the wedge is located on the left side of the image (marked by white arrows). Since wedges almost exclusively occur on the temporal half (97% according to [4]), we will focus only on the left half of the polar image.

2.4   Finding Edges

The procedure to identify edges consists of three steps:

1. Texture removal.
2. Differentiation.
3. Edge detection.

The image consists of both larger scale 'objects' such as the local thickness of the NFL and smaller ones that are superimposed (texture). To remove the ripple (texture) without removing the larger (objects) edges, the average of the closing and the opening operator (see [5]) is taken. Wedges, by definition, are larger than the blood vessels. Also, there is a need to retain spatial coherence in the vertical direction. Consequently, an ellipse-shaped structuring element of size 12x3 (hor. x vert.) pixels is used, resulting in Fig. 5(a).

Differentiating is done horizontally by calculating the central difference (see Fig. 5(b)).

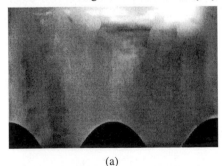   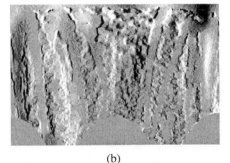

(a)   (b)

Fig. 5. (a) Image with texture removed. (b) Central difference in x direction. The white pixels have a large positive difference while the black pixels have a large negative difference.

The strongest edges, running across the whole image from top to bottom, are detected through a method inspired by dynamic programming (see [6], [7]). Dynamic programming is generally only used to find the single optimal solution to a problem with a specific cost function [8]. The need for locally optimal solutions calls for a new method. By searching for such solutions, a difference between forward and backward operation is introduced, that does not exist in the conventional dynamic programming approach ([8], p. 24-25).

In dynamic programming, the optimal solution to a problem corresponds to a specific path in a cost matrix. Starting at one end of the matrix gives the same result as starting at the other end. With locally optimal solutions, this is not the case.

To clarify this, take a look at the example cost matrix shown in Fig. 6(a). The value in a cell on the n-th row, i-th column will be denoted by c_n^i. A conventional cumulative cost function ϕ, taking into account the connectivity between pixels, would be

$$\phi_{n+1}^i = c_{n+1}^i + \max(\phi_n^{i-1}, \phi_n^i, \phi_n^{i+1}) \ .$$

However, we prefer solutions with as little side-steps as possible. Therefore, we pose a penalty on these side-steps, resulting in the cumulative cost function

$$\phi_{n+1}^i = c_{n+1}^i + \max(\phi_n^{i-1} - 1, \phi_n^i, \phi_n^{i+1} - 1) \ .$$

Starting at the top and working our way down, Fig. 6(b) results. We can now select all local maxima at the bottom row. For each of these maxima, we look at the three cells above it, and we select the one with the largest value. This way, we work our way up for all bottom row maxima. The paths found in this way are displayed in boldface.

Reversely, when calculating the cumulative cost function starting at the bottom, the function values for each cell are as shown in Fig. 6(c). Selecting the local maxima at the top and working our way back down, other locally optimal paths are found, again displayed in boldface. Note that the overall best solution is the same in both cases, but the local best solutions are different.

This procedure, starting at the local maxima and work our way back does not always give us the optimal path for the returned endpoints. For example, in Fig. 6(c), the first local maximum is 2. However, the fourth cell in the first row (italic in the figure) would also lead us towards the same endpoint (the fourth cell in the third row), and this route is better (i.e. has a higher cumulative cost function) than the first one. To handle this, we should try all cells in the row, determine their endpoint and, for each endpoint, find the cell that has the optimum cost for each endpoint.

The difference between forward and backward operation forces us to choose either method. Now, the solutions will be strongly influenced by the value of the cost function at the start of the algorithm.

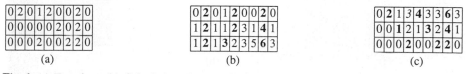

(a) (b) (c)

Fig. 6. (a) Test data. (b) Calculating the cumulative cost function from top to bottom, finding maxima from bottom to top. (c) Calculating the cumulative cost function from bottom to top, finding maxima from top to bottom.

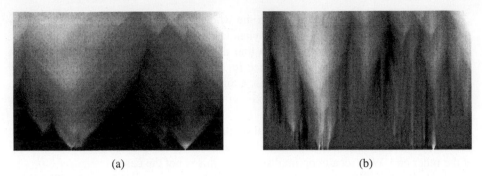

(a)	(b)

Fig. 7. Cumulative cost matrices. Each horizontal line is normalized. (a) Without penalty. (b) With penalty.

For our images, the bottom of the image is of most interest. This corresponds to the outside of the normal images, where less occlusion occurs and the edges of the wedge are better visible. We therefore calculate the cost function starting at the bottom, working our way up, and then select our paths starting at the top. The cumulative cost function used is similar to that of the example:

$$\phi_{n+1}^i = c_{n+1}^i + \max(\phi_n^{i-1} - \text{pen}, \phi_n^i, \phi_n^{i+1} - \text{pen}),$$

where pen is the penalty on a diagonal connection. If we omit the penalty, and apply the cost function to the example image, Fig. 7(a) results (for display purposes only, each horizontal line is normalized by dividing all pixels on a line by the maximum pixel value on that line). Introducing a penalty of, for example, 10 (about twice the largest pixel value in the differentiated image) gives better results, as can be seen in Fig. 7(b). High values are propagated less in horizontal direction, thereby favoring straight paths.

At last, we now calculate the route and the endpoint for each pixel in the top row and keep the best route for each endpoint, defining the detected edges. The same can be done for the edges in the opposing direction by negating our differentiated image and following the same procedure. The result is displayed in Fig. 8(a).

The strength $s(i)$ of a pixel on an edge, at distance i from the bottom, can be defined in two ways: Absolute (the value of the pixel in the differentiated image) or relative (the absolute difference divided by the maximum of the left and right pixel value in the original polar image). The average strength of a part of an edge with length l, starting

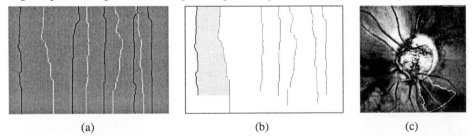

(a)	(b)	(c)

Fig. 8. (a) Located edges. White edges have a positive difference, black edges have a negative difference. (b) Matched edges (grey area). The black line (left from the grey area) is a strong edge, the other (grey) lines are weak edges. (c) Detected wedge shown overlayed on retardation image.

from the bottom is defined by $s_{avg}(l) = \frac{1}{l} \int_0^l s(i) \, di$. We now define the strength of the edge as $\max(s_{avg}(l))$ for $\frac{2}{3}L \leq l \leq L$, with L being the total length of the edge. The minimum length of $\frac{2}{3}L$ allows for optic disc diameters of up to half the image size.

By putting thresholds (θ) on the strength of the edge, we define two edges types: Strong edges (strength$\geq \theta_s$) and weak edges (strength$\geq \theta_w$), with $\theta_s > \theta_w$. Edges with a strength smaller than θ_w are ignored.

2.5   Matching Edges

For the image at hand, we now have both strong and weak edges, in both directions. Matching edges is done by starting at a strong edge and looking for an opposing weak edge that is located at the correct side of the strong edge within a distance of $60°$([4]).

The result for the example image is shown in Fig. 8(b). When drawn in the original retardation image, Fig. 8(c) results.

3   Results

The images recorded with the GDx are 256 x 256 pixels at a quantization of 8 bits per pixel. The viewing angle is $15°$; the sampling density is approximately 59 pixels/mm.

To show the usefulness of our detection scheme, we used a total of 45 images of both normal and glaucomatous eyes. Eight of these 45 images showed one or more wedges shaped defects, defined by a physician. Analysis of the edges of these wedges resulted in an relative threshold for the strong edges of 0.14. For the weak edges, both a relative threshold of 0.033 and an absolute threshold of 1.5 were found, which had to be satisfied both. The results of the detection scheme, presented in Table 1 are on a per image basis, meaning that if an eye had a wedge and the algorithm detected one, it was counted as a true positive. Consequently, eyes with more than one wedge were counted as one. The approach was chosen with a diagnosis setup in mind, where the eventual conclusion concerns the whole eye.

Of the 8 images with wedge shaped defects, 7 were detected. So, the sensitivity was 88%, but because of the small number of images with wedges in our set, the 95% confidence interval of the sensitivity was quite large (47%-99%). Three false positives resulted, giving a specificity of 92%, with a smaller 95% confidence interval of 77%-98%. By changing the parameters, such as the thresholds, these values can be adjusted.

Table 1. Results. (a) True positive, false positive, false negative and true negative results. (b) Sensitivity and specificity, including their estimated 95% confidence interval.

	Wedge visible	Wedge not visible	Totals
Wedge detected	7	3	10
Wedge not detected	1	34	35
Totals	8	37	45

(a)

	Estimated	95% confidence interval
Sensitivity	0.88	0.47-0.99
Specificity	0.92	0.77-0.98

(b)

4 Conclusion

By modelling wedge shaped defects and using a novel dynamic programming technique, it proved to be possible to automatically detect wedge shaped defects. While the detection scheme needs more testing, the preliminary results are promising. Our method combines good sensitivity with great specificity. It also shows that it is possible to extract more information from the retardation images in an automated way than is currently done. This can greatly help computer assisted diagnosis.

4.1 Discussion

The visibility of wedges in advanced glaucomatous eyes can be much worse than in eyes in which the NFL is still (largely) unaffected [4]. Current methods can detect glaucomatous eyes quite well, but perform worse in cases of early glaucoma. Therefore, application of this automated wedge detection will be most beneficial in cases where conventional methods do not classify an eye as glaucomatous.

With a prevalence of glaucoma of approximately 2% in the general Caucasian population, screening for the disease requires a high specificity, at the expense of sensitivity, to avoid an unacceptably high overcalling by any diagnostic tool. By adjusting the threshold values, our algorithm can be tuned to the specific needs of the setting in which it is used.

References

1. Andreas W. Dreher and Klaus Reiter. Scanning laser polarimetry of the retinal nerve fiber layer. *In Polarization Analysis and Measurement,* volume 1746 of *Proc. SPIE,* pages 34–41, 1992.
2. Jost B. Jonas and Albert Dichtl. Evaluation of the retinal nerve fiber layer. *Surv Ophthalmology,* 40(5):369–378, Mar-Apr 1996.
3. K.A. Vermeer, F.M. Vos, H.G. Lemij, and A.M. Vossepoel. A model based method for retinal blood vessel detection. Internal report.
4. Jost B. Jonas and Dennis Schiro. Localised wedge shaped defects of the retinal nerve fibre layer in glaucoma. *Br J Ophthalmology,* 78(4):285–290, Apr 1994.
5. P.W. Verbeek, H.A. Vrooman, and L.J. van Vliet. Low-level image processing by min-max filters. *Signal Processing,* 15(3):249–258, 1988.
6. J. J. Gerbrands. *Segmentation of Noisy* Images. PhD thesis, Delft University of Technology, 1988.
7. Davi Geiger, Alok Gupta, Luiz A. Costa, and John Vlontzos. Dynamic programming for detecting, tracking and matching deformable contours. *IEEE Transactions on Pattern Analysis and Machine Intelligence,* 17(3):294–302, Mar 1995.
8. Dimitri P. Bertsekas. *Dynamic Programming.* Prentice-Hall, Inc., 1987.

Automatic Statistical Identification of Neuroanatomical Abnormalities between Different Populations

Alexandre Guimond[1], Svetlana Egorova[1], Ronald J. Killiany[2],
Marilyn S. Albert[3], and Charles R. G. Guttmann[1]

[1] Center for Neurological Imaging, Brigham and Women's Hospital, Harvard Medical School
{guimond,egorova,guttmann}@bwh.harvard.edu
[2] Department of Anatomy and Neurobiology, Boston University
rkilliany@cajal-1.bu.edu
[3] Departments of Phychiatry and Neurology, Massachusetts General Hospital, Harvard Medical School, albert@psych.mgh.harvard.edu

Abstract. We present a completely automatic method to identify abnormal anatomical configurations of the brain resulting from various pathologies. The statistical framework developed here is applied to identify regions that significant differ from normal anatomy in two groups of patients, namely subjects who subsequently converted to Alzheimer's Disease (AD) and subjects with mild AD. The regions identified are consistent with post-mortem pathological findings in AD.

1 Introduction

An important tool used to diagnose abnormal anatomical variations are medical atlases [1]. Traditional ones, such as by Talairach & Tournoux [2] or Schaltenbrand & Wahren [3], are presented in textbooks, but computerized atlases comprising information in a more practical and quantitative manner are becoming available [4–16]. They usually include information obtained from a set of subjects, as opposed to a single individual in most paper atlases, making them more representative of a population. For example, the Montreal Neurological Institute used 305 normal subjects to build an atlas comprising intensity variations after affine registration in the stereotaxic space defined by Talairach & Tournoux [8]. These methods also enable the calculation of normal shape variations [17–19].

Still, most of the clinical work regarding the identification of abnormal brain anatomy due to particular diseases involves manual intervention by skilled anatomists [20, 19]. The following work aims at developing a fully automated method that identifies regions in which the anatomy is significantly different between two given populations. We describe a statistical framework to perform such an analysis based on statistics obtained from displacement fields resulting from deformable registration. In the following section we describe the method developed to identify such regions. The groups of subjects used to test our procedure are then detailed, followed by results and a brief discussion.

2 Methodology

Affine registration based on the correlation ratio [21,22] is performed between the images from the groups under study and a reference image. Deformable registration based

T. Dohi and R. Kikinis (Eds.): MICCAI 2002, LNCS 2488, pp. 785–792, 2002.

on the demons' algorithm [23, 24], an intensity based registration method, is then performed to assess non-linear anatomical variations present between the reference image and each image of the two groups. The displacement fields resulting from the deformable registration are then used to assess significant anatomical differences between the groups of subjects. The statistical analysis performed to identify these differences follows.

Let $u_{ij}(x)$ be the three-dimensional displacement found by deformable registration at an anatomical location x in the reference scan to the corresponding anatomical location in image j of group i. Two important statistics that can be computed from these displacements are the groups' sample mean vector $\bar{u}_i(x)$ and covariance matrix $S_i(x)$,

$$\bar{u}_i(x) = \frac{1}{N_i} \sum_{j=1}^{N_i} u_{ij}(x), \tag{1}$$

$$S_i(x) = \frac{1}{N_i - 1} A_i, \tag{2}$$

where N_i is the number of subjects in group i, and A_i is the matrix of sums of squares and cross products of deviations about the mean for group i,

$$A_i = \sum_{j=1}^{N_i} [u_{ij}(x) - \bar{u}_i(x)] [u_{ij}(x) - \bar{u}_i(x)]'. \tag{3}$$

The following aims at identifying significant anatomical differences due to shape variations of the various structures composing the human brain. This will be done by assessing significant differences between the average displacements $\bar{u}_i(x)$ found for each group. Assuming that the displacements found for group i $(u_{i1}(x), \ldots, u_{iN_i}(x))$ are samples from a normal distribution $N(\mu_i, \Sigma_i)$, two common tests based on the T^2 statistic to assess whether the mean of one population a is equal to the mean of another population b are available. The use of one test or the other depends on the equality of the covariance matrices of each population.

In the case that both populations have the same covariance ($\Sigma_a = \Sigma_b$), it can be shown [25] that

$$\frac{N_a N_b (N_a + N_b - 4)}{3(N_a + N_b)(N_a + N_b - 2)} [\bar{u}_a(x) - \bar{u}_b(x)]' S^{-1} [\bar{u}_a(x) - \bar{u}_b(x)], \tag{4}$$

where

$$S = \frac{1}{N_a + N_b - 2} A, \tag{5}$$

$$A = A_a + A_b, \tag{6}$$

follows an F distribution with 3 and $N_a + N_b - 4$ degrees of freedom.

If both populations have different covariances ($\Sigma_a \neq \Sigma_b$), another test is used [25]. In this case, assuming without loss of generality that $N_a \leq N_b$,

$$\frac{N_a (N_a - 3)}{3(N_a - 1)} [\bar{u}_a(x) - \bar{u}_b(x)]' S^{-1} [\bar{u}_a(x) - \bar{u}_b(x)] \tag{7}$$

where

$$S = \frac{1}{N_a - 1} \sum_{j=1}^{N_a} [y_j(x) - \bar{y}(x)] [y_j(x) - \bar{y}(x)]', \tag{8}$$

$$y_j(x) = u_{aj}(x) - \sqrt{N_a/N_b} u_{bj}(x), \quad j = 1, \ldots, N_a, \tag{9}$$

$$\bar{y}(x) = \sum_{j=1}^{N_a} y_j(x), \tag{10}$$

follows an F distribution with 3 and $N_a - 3$ degrees of freedom.

When comparing displacement fields from populations that are afflicted by different diseases, assuming the equality of covariance matrices might not be the proper choice. To answer this question, we use another criterion designed to test the equality of different covariance matrices. By defining

$$\lambda = \left[\left(\frac{1}{k_a}\right)^{k_a} \left(\frac{1}{k_b}\right)^{k_b} \right]^{\frac{3}{2}n} \frac{|A_a|^{\frac{1}{2}n_a} |A_b|^{\frac{1}{2}n_b}}{|A|^{\frac{1}{2}n}}, \tag{11}$$

where $n_a = N_a - 1$, $n_b = N_b - 1$, $n = n_a + n_b$, $k_a = n_a/n$, and $k_b = n_b/n$, it can be shown [25] that the asymptotic expansion of the distribution of $-2\rho \log \lambda$ is

$$\Pr\{-2\rho \log \lambda \leq z\} = \Pr\{\chi_6^2 \leq z\} + \omega \left[\Pr\{\chi_{10}^2 \leq z\} - \Pr\{\chi_6^2 \leq z\} \right] + O\left(n^{-3}\right), \tag{12}$$

where

$$\rho = 1 - \frac{13}{12} \left(\frac{1}{n_a} + \frac{1}{n_b} - \frac{1}{n} \right), \tag{13}$$

$$\omega = \frac{5 \left(\frac{1}{n_a^2} + \frac{1}{n_b^2} - \frac{1}{n^2} \right) - 3(1-\rho)^2}{2\rho^2}. \tag{14}$$

Note that for a large n or for large values in A, the power calculations for the determinants of Eq. 11 will create overflows on most computers. To solve this problem, we identify the whitening transformation [26] for A and apply it to A, A_a, and A_b prior to calculating Eq. 11. Although this transformation changes the matrices, since the same linear transformation is applied to all of them, there is no effect on the result of the criterion of Eq. 11.

The whitening transformation for A is $\Phi \Lambda^{-1/2}$, where Φ is the matrix of eigenvectors of matrix A and Λ is the diagonal matrix consisting of its eigenvalues. This transformation makes A the identity matrix and the power calculations for the determinants of A_a and A_b fall within range on our computers[4]. Using this method, Eq. 11 becomes:

$$\lambda = \left[\left(\frac{1}{k_a}\right)^{k_a} \left(\frac{1}{k_b}\right)^{k_b} \right]^{\frac{3}{2}n} |\tilde{A}_a|^{\frac{1}{2}n_a} |\tilde{A}_b|^{\frac{1}{2}n_b}, \tag{15}$$

---

[4] Although this strategy was sufficient for our purposes, for very large n ($n \gg 200$) the same problem will occur and other strategies will have to be explored.

where

$$\tilde{A}_a = [\Phi\Lambda^{-1/2}]'A_a[\Phi\Lambda^{-1/2}], \tag{16}$$

$$\tilde{A}_b = [\Phi\Lambda^{-1/2}]'A_b[\Phi\Lambda^{-1/2}]. \tag{17}$$

Using Eq. 15, we can calculate p-value maps (or p-maps) that correspond to the probability that the covariance of the displacements from any two groups a and b are equal at a given anatomical position x in the reference scan. By setting the significance level at 0.95, and thus rejecting the null hypothesis that the covariances are equal for p-values smaller than 0.05, we can assess whether there is sufficient evidence from the displacements found at x for groups a and b to assume that the covariance of the displacements for both groups are different at that point.

If we accept the null hypothesis (the covariances from both groups are equal), Eq. 4 is used to test whether the mean displacement from both groups are equal. If the null hypothesis is rejected, Eq. 7 is used to perform the same test. In either case, we set the significance level at 0.95. This process is performed for each voxel x of the reference scan to identify anatomical position where there is significant evidence showing different average displacement between the two groups. In practical terms, this means that brain anatomy at position x for the two groups differs. If one of the groups is the normal group, these results show strong evidence that the identified regions correspond to pathological variations due to the disease affecting the other group.

3   Data

Detailed information regarding the subjects and data used in this study can be found in [20]. Briefly, the subjects in this study consisted of elderly individuals. All subjects were 65 or older, free of significant underlying medical, neurological, or psychiatric illness, and meet the Clinical Dementia Rating (CDR) [27] criteria described below. The CDR scale was designed to stage individuals according to their functional ability, from 0 representing normal function, to 5 representing the terminal phase of dementia.

A total of 74 subjects were used in this study. At the time of the MR acquisition, 37 of them were identified as normals (CDR=0), 20 as "questionable AD" (CDR=0.5) who converted to AD according to clinical research criteria for probable AD [28] after a 3 year follow-up, and 16 as "mild AD" according to the same criteria (CDR=1.0). These 3 groups will be referred to as normals, converters, and mild AD respectively in the following. Another elderly subject identified as normal (CDR=0) was also used and served as a reference image for the following work.

The MRI data used in this study consisted of three-dimensional T1-weighted gradient echo scans of the brain (TR = 35ms, TE = 5ms, FOV = 240cm^2, flip angle = 45°, slice thickness = 1.5mm, matrix size = 256 × 256). 124 coronal slices covering the entire brain were acquired for each subject. The resulting data volumes were composed of 256 × 256 × 124 voxels, each of size 0.9375 × 0.9375 × 1.5mm^3.

4   Results and Discussion

p-maps were generated as described in the previous section to identify anatomical locations where brain anatomy between two groups of subjects differed. In Fig. 1-a, we present regions identified as significantly different (p=0.05) between the normal and converter groups. Fig. 1-b, presents the result of the same test using the normal and mild AD groups. Of particular interest are the larger regions which lie in the inferior parietal lobule region (arrow in Fig. 1-a) and close to the hippocampal area (arrow in Fig. 1-b). These regions of the association and heteromodal cortex are known to be strongly affected by the characteristic plaques and tangles in AD [29]. Fig. 1-c shows a 3D rendering of pathological regions as identified by our method for the converter group. Note that most small regions lie inside the grey matter, in the posterior half of the brain, where grey matter atrophy has been reported for AD patients [29].

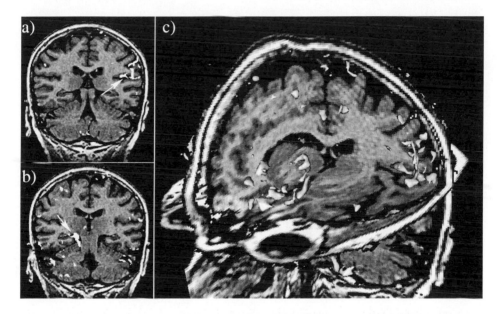

Fig. 1. Pathological regions as identified by our method between a) normal controls and patients who converted to AD 3 years after the MRI was performed, and b) normal controls and patients with mild AD. Also shown in c) is a 3D rendering of pathological regions (in red) as identified by comparing the normal and converter groups.

Although the statistical methods presented here to analyze displacements are independent of the registration method used, the confidence we have in the regions identified as pathological is based on the assumption that registration provided appropriate correspondence fields between the anatomical locations of the reference image and subjects under study. As mentioned previously, our deformable registration method is intensity-based, and as for most registration methods, one underlying assumption is the equivalence of brain topology between the images registered. As displayed in Fig. 2, this is not strictly the case when registering our reference image with AD patients. In this figure, we show corresponding coronal slices from the T1-weighted images of the reference subject (Fig. 2-a) and an AD patient (Fig. 2-b). These images have been processed to emphasize the contrast inside the white matter. As can be seen, the white matter of the reference subject is noisy, but represents a relatively uniform intensity region. In contrast, the white matter of the AD patient is much less uniform, with white matter signal abnormalities present at many locations (See arrows in Fig. 2-b). These abnormalities will tend to shrink to small regions during registration and the resulting displacement field will reflect this phenomenon. Hence, the statistics obtained from the displacement are encoding information regarding displacements that are due to brain shape differences, as well as white matter anomalies. Whether this is desired or not when building statistical brain models is probably disease and application dependant, and is currently under investigation in our group. A solution to solve a similar problem for multiple sclerosis patients is presented in [30].

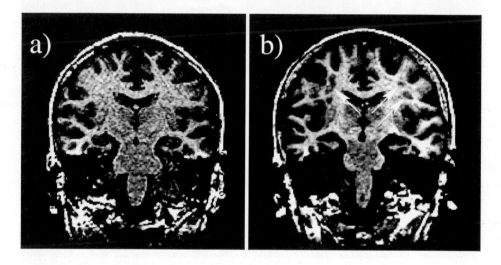

Fig. 2. T1-weighted MR images where contrast has been emphasized in the white matter: a) an elderly normal subject (the reference subject) and b) a patient with mild AD. Note the white matter signal abnormalities present in the patient (See arrows) but not in the reference subject.

Another aspect we are currently investigating is the incorporation of spatial information to compute the statistical maps produced with our method. The analysis presented here works on a voxel per voxel basis and does not take into account any information from neighboring voxels, but it is likely that information concerning abnormalities of neighboring voxels should be taken into account to calculate the p-value for a given anatomical position. To this end, we are currently investigating the incorporation of Markov Random Fields into our model in a way similar to that described in [31].

5   Conclusion

We have presented a statistical framework to analyze displacement fields obtained from deformable registration and identify anatomical regions that are significantly different between different populations. This technique was applied to identify such regions between normals controls and two groups of patients with memory impairments, namely subjects who subsequently converted to Alzheimer's Disease and subjects with a mild form of Alzheimer's Disease. Our method clearly identified brain regions known to be affected by this disease. It also singled-out small cortical regions mostly in the posterior part of the brain. Further analysis need to be performed to relate these last findings to clinical data.

Aside from validating and applying this technology to other diseases such as schizophrenia and multiple sclerosis, future work will focus on registration aspects to deal with white matter signal abnormalities present in MR scans obtained from diseased patients, and on the incorporation of spatial information into our statistical model.

References

1. Mazziotta, J.C., Toga, A.W., Evans, A., Fox, P., Lancaster, J.: A probabilistic atlas of the human brain: Theory and rationale for its development. Neuroimage **2** (1995) 89–101
2. Talairach, J., Tournoux, P.: Co-Planar Stereotaxic Atlas of the Human Brain. Thieme Medical Publishers, New York (1988)
3. Schaltenbrand, G., Wahren, W.: Atlas of Stereotaxy of the Human Brain. Georg Thieme Verlag, Stuttgart (1977)
4. Bajcsy, R., Kovačič, S.: Multiresolution elastic matching. Computer Vision, Graphics and Image Processing **46** (1989) 1–21
5. Greitz, T., Bohm, C., Holte, S., Eriksson, L.: A computerized brain atlas: Construction, anatomical content, and some applications. Journal of Computer Assisted Tomography **15** (1991) 26–38
6. Lemoine, D., Barillot, C., Gibaud, B., Pasqualini, E.: An anatomical-based 3D registration system of multimodality and atlas data in neurosurgery. Lecture Notes in Computer Science **511** (1991) 154–164
7. Höhne, K.H., Bomans, M., Riemer, M., Schubert, R., Tiede, U., Lierse, W.: A 3D anatomical atlas based on a volume model. IEEE Computer Graphics and Applications **12** (1992) 72–78
8. Evans, A.C., Kamber, M., Collins, D.L., Macdonald, D.: An MRI-based probabilistic atlas of neuroanatomy. In Shorvon, S., Fish, D., Andermann, F., Bydder, G.M., Stefan, H., eds.: Magnetic Resonance Scanning and Epilepsy. (1994) 263–274
9. Bookstein, F.L.: Landmarks, Edges, Morphometrics, and the Brain Atlas Problem. In: Functional Neuroimaging. Academic Press (1994)
10. Christensen, G., Miller, M.I., Vannier, M.W.: A 3D deformable magnetic resonance textbook based on elasticity. In: Spring Symposium: Applications of Computer Vision in Medical Image Processing, Stanford (CA), USA, American Association for Artificial Intelligence (1994)
11. Kikinis, R., Shenton, M.E., Iosifescu, D.V., McCarley, R.W., Saiviroonporn, P., Hokama, H.H., Robatino, A., Metcal, D., Wible, C.G., Portas, C.M., Donnino, R.M., Jolesz, F.A.: A digital brain atlas for surgical planning, model-driven segmentation, and teaching. IEEE Transactions on Visualization and Computer Graphics **2** (1996) 232–241

12. Le Briquer, L., Gee, J.C.: Design of a statistical model of brain shape. In Duncan, J.S., Gindi, G.R., eds.: Proceedings of the IPMI (IPMI'97), Vermont, USA, Springer-Verlag (1997)
13. Woods, R.P., Grafton, S.T., Watson, J.D.G., Sicotte, N.L., Mazziotta, J.C.: Automated image registration: Ii. intersubject validation of linear and nonlinear models. Journal of Computer Assisted Tomography **22** (1998) 153–165
14. Grenander, U., Miller, M.I.: Computational anatomy: An emerging discipline. Quarterly of Applied Mathematics **56** (1998) 617–694
15. Thompson, P.M., MacDonald, D., Mega, M.S., Holmes, C.J., Evans, A.C., Toga, A.W.: Detection and mapping of abnormal brain structure with a probabilistic atlas of cortical surfaces. Journal of Computer Assisted Tomography **21** (1998) 567–581
16. Subsol, G., Thirion, J.P., Ayache, N.: A scheme for automatically building three-dimensional morphometric anatomical atlases: Application to a skull atlas. Medical Image Analysis **2** (1998) 37–60
17. Guimond, A., Meunier, J., Thirion, J.P.: Average brain models: A convergence study. Computer Vision and Image Understanding **77** (1999) 192–210
18. Gee, J.C., Haynor, D.R., Briquer, L.L., Bajcsy, R.K.: Advances in elastic matching theory and its implementation. In Cinquin, P., Kikinis, R., Lavallee, S., eds.: Proceedings of CVRMed-MRCAS, Heidelberg, Springer-Verlag (1997)
19. Thompson, P.M., Toga, A.W.: Detection, visualization and animation of abnormal anatomic structure with a deformable probabilistic brain atlas based on random vector field transformations. Medical Image Analysis **1** (1997) 271–294
20. Killiany, R.J., Gomez-Isla, T., Moss, M., Kikinis, R., Sandor, T., Jolesz, F.A., Tanzi, R., Jones, K., Hyman, B.T., Albert, M.S.: Use of structural magnetic resonance imaging to predict who will get alzheimer's disease. Annals of Neurology **47** (2000) 430–439
21. Roche, A.: Recalage d'images médicales par inférence statistique. PhD thesis, Université de Nice Sophia-Antipolis (2001)
22. Roche, A., Malandain, G., Pennec, X., Ayache, N.: The correlation ratio as a new similarity measure for multimodal image registration. In Wells, W.M., Colchester, A., Delp, S., eds.: Proceedings of MICCAI. (1998) 1115–1124
23. Guimond, A., Roche, A., Ayache, N., Meunier, J.: Three-dimensional multimodal brain warping using the demons algorithm and adaptive intensity corrections. IEEE Transactions in Medical Imaging **20** (2001) 58–69
24. Thirion, J.P.: Image matching as a diffusion process: an analogy with Maxwell's demons. Medical Image Analysis **2** (1998) 243–260
25. Anderson, T.W.: An Introduction to Multivariate Statistical Analysis. Second edn. Probability and Mathematical Statistics. John Wiley & Sons (1984)
26. Fukunaga, K.: Introduction to Statistical Pattern Recognition. Second edn. Computer science and scientific computing. Academic Press (1990)
27. Hughes, C.P., Berg, L., Danziger, W.L., Coben, L., Martin, R.: A new clinical scale for the staging of dementia. British Journal of Psychiatry **140** (1982) 566–572
28. McKhann, G., Drachman, D., Folstein, M., Kaltzman, R., Price, D., Stadlan, E.: Clinical diagnosis of alzheimer's disease: Report of the nincds-adrda work group under the auspices of department of health and human services task force on alzheimer's disease. Neurology **39** (1984) 939–944
29. Kemper, T.L.: Neuroanatomical and Neuropathological Changes in Normal Aging and in Dementia. In: Clinical Neurology of Aging. Oxford University Press, New-York (1984) 9–52
30. Guimond, A., Wei, X., Guttmann, C.R.G.: Building a probabilistic anatomical brain atlas for multiple sclerosis. In: Proceedings of ISMRM. (2002) In Print.
31. Kapur, T.: Model based three dimensional Medical Imaging Segmentation. PhD thesis, Massachusetts Institute of Technology (1999)

Example-Based Assisting Approach for Pulmonary Nodule Classification in 3-D Thoracic CT Images

Yoshiki Kawata[1], Noboru Niki[1], Hironobu Ohmatsu[2], Noriyuki Moriyama[3]

[1] Dept. of Optical Science, Univ. of Tokushima, Tokushima, 770-8506, Japan
{kawata, niki}@opt.tokushima-u.ac.jp
[2] National Cancer Center East Hospital, Chiba, Japan
[3] National Cancer Center Hospital , Tokyo, Japan

Abstract. This paper describes an example-based assisting approach for classifying pulmonary nodules in 3-D thoracic CT images. In this approach the internal and surrounding structures of the nodule are characterized by the distribution pattern of CT density and 3-D curvature indexes. Each nodule is represented by means of a joint histogram using the distance value from the nodule center. When given an indeterminate nodule image, the images of lesions with known diagnoses (e.g. malignant vs. benign) are retrieved from a 3-D nodule image database. The malignant likelihood of the indeterminate case is estimated by the difference between the representation patterns of the indeterminate case and the retrieved lesions. In the present study, we adopt the Mahalanobis distance as the difference measure and then, explore the feasibility of the classification based on patterns of similar lesion images.

1 Introduction

The detection rate of small pulmonary nodules has recently increased due to the advances in imaging technology [1]. It is important to increase the positive predictive value (i.e. ratio of the number of lung cancers found to the total number of biopsies) without reducing the sensitivity of lung cancer detection. Computer-aided diagnosis (CAD) has the potential to increase the diagnostic accuracy by reducing the false-negative rate while increasing the positive predictive values of abnormalities in three-dimensional (3-D) thoracic images. The interpretation of the pulmonary nodule images often involves the matching features extracted from a database of the nodules with associated clinical information. When the matching procedure is performed well, the database can provide physicians with more information concerning the diagnosis and prognosis of the queried nodule. Moreover, the corresponding structures retrieved from the database may help to design the CAD scheme for the distinction between benign and malignant nodules.

In this paper, we formulate the nodule-classification problem as one of learning to recognize nodule patterns from examples. Each nodule pattern is represent by the extracted internal and surrounding features based on CT density and 3-D curvature indexes. We use a database of nodule images to search similar malignant and benign lesion patterns and construct a distribution-based local lesion model in a high-

T. Dohi and R. Kikinis (Eds.): MICCAI 2002, LNCS 2488, pp. 793–800, 2002.

dimensional image vector space of the nodule representation. We then estimate the likelihood of the malignancy by computing the difference between representation patterns of the indeterminate case and the retrieved lesions. We first describe the representation method used as a pre-process of the data and then give the definition of the similarity criteria. We are then showing results of similar nodule images and estimation the malignant likelihood.

2   Materials and Methods

2.1   3-D Nodule Data

The 3D chest image used in this paper was a stack of thin-section CT images obtained by the helical CT scanner (Toshiba TCT900S Superhelix and Xvigor). The thin-section CT images were measured under the following conditions; beam width: 2mm, table speed: 2mm/sec, tube voltage: 120kV, tube current : 250mA or 200mA. The range of pixel size in each square slice of 512 pixels was between 0.3x0.3 mm^2 and 0.4x0.4 mm^2, and the slice contains an extended region of the lung area. The 3D chest image was reconstructed from the thin-section CT images by a linear interpolation technique to make each voxel isotropic. The data set in this study included 263 3-D chest images from 263 patients provided by National Cancer Center Hospital East, Tochigi Cancer Center, and Kanagawa Cancer Center. Of the 263 cases, 194 contained malignant nodules, and 69 contained benign nodules.

2.2 Nodule Representation

We build a 3-D nodule image database from the data set. The database consists of two types elements, such as text-based elements and image-based elements. The text-based elements of the database are as follows, ID number, measurement conditions, sex, age, diagnosis result, nodule diameter and volume that compute from the segmented nodule image. The image-based elements are as follows, the 3-D ROI image with a nodule of interest, the segmented nodule image, the representation of local density pattern inside the nodule and nodule surroundings. Since the internal and surrounding structures of the nodule are important cues to distinct malignancy from benign cases, we concentrate on the feature representation inside the nodule and the nodule surroundings. As pre-processing of the 3-D nodule image database, we perform the following nodule segmentation, feature extraction, and representation procedures.

2.2.1 Segmentation of the nodule and its surroundings
The segmentation of the 3D pulmonary nodule image consists of three steps [2]; 1) extraction of lung area, 2) selection of the region of interest (ROI) including the nodule region, and 3) nodule segmentation based on a deformable surface approach.

The ROI including the nodule was selected interactively. A pulmonary nodule was segmented from the selected ROI image by the deformable surface approach. The nodule surrounding region was computed by the distance from the nodule surface. The distance was obtained by applying the Euclidean distance transformation approach proposed by Saito et al. [6] to the nodule surrounding region.

2.2.2 Feature extraction

Each voxel in the region of interest (ROI) including the pulmonary nodule is locally represented by CT density and curvature index. By assuming that each voxel in the ROI lies on the surface which has the normal corresponding to the 3-D gradient at the voxel, we computed directly the curvatures on each voxel from the first and the second derivatives of the gray level image of the ROI. At each voxel two principal curvatures and directions of principal curvatures are computed by using the approach proposed by Thirion [3]. As the curvature index at each voxel in the ROI image, we use the shape index that is computed from two principal curvatures [4],[5]. The continuous surface type is mapped on the interval [0, 1] of the shape index value.

To quantify the relationship between the nodule and its surrounding structure such as vessel and pleura, we focus on two indicators of malignancy, which are denoted as vascular convergence and pleural retraction. In the 3-D thoracic CT images, these findings are observed so that the vessel and pleura images are drawn in the nodule. We assumed that the shape of the vessel and the pleura images are similar to cylindrical or conic structures. Therefore, we measure an amount of the vascular convergence and pleural retraction by computing the absolute value of the inner product of the directions of cylindrical or conic structures and the normal directions of the nodule surface. For the representation of the directions, we compute two vector fields that consist of the directions of the maximum principal curvature and normal vector of the nodule surface. The vector field is denoted as the maximum principal curvature vector (MPV) field. The normal directions of the nodule surface at the vicinity of the nodule are estimated by a diffusion procedure proposed by Xu [7]. The approach is to keep the desirable property of the gradients near the nodule edges, but to expand the gradient away from the edges into homogeneous regions of the nodule surrounding using the computational diffusion process. The vector field obtained by the normal vector of the nodule surface is denoted as gradient vector (GV) field.

2.2.3 Joint-histogram based representation

In order to characterize the distribution pattern of the CT density and the shape index inside nodule, we compute two types of joint histogram using the distance value from the nodule center. Since the distance value depends on the nodule size, the first type is directly derived from the distance value and used to search similar lesions. Once obtained similar lesions, the variation of internal structure provides more important information to classify nodule patterns rather than the nodule size. Therefore, the second type is derived from the normalized distance value which ranges between zero and one value and used to evaluate the likelihood of the malignancy. To compute the distance value at each voxel, we apply the Euclidean distance transformation technique [6] to the segmented nodule image and obtain the maximum distance value

(D_M) inside the nodule. Since the distance value (v_d) at each voxel is the distance from the nodule surface, the maximum distance value seems to be assigned to the voxel at the nodule center area. To obtain the distance from the nodule center, we compute the value $(D_M - v_d)$ at each voxel inside the nodule. Let $I(\mathbf{x})$ and $D(\mathbf{x})$ be respectively the CT density value and the distance value at the voxel $\mathbf{x}$ in the nodule image. The first type of joint histogram of $I(\mathbf{x})$ and $D(\mathbf{x})$ is expressed as

$$H(d_1 = \frac{k_1}{B_1}, d_2 = \frac{k_2}{B_2}) = \frac{1}{N} \sum_{i=1}^{N} K_{k_1, k_2}(I(\mathbf{x}_i), D(\mathbf{x}_i)) \tag{1}$$

with

$$K_{k_1, k_2}(t_1, t_2) \begin{cases} 1 & \frac{k_1-1}{B_1} \leq t_1 < \frac{k_1}{B_1}, \frac{k_2-1}{B_2} \leq t_2 < \frac{k_2}{B_2} \\ 0 & otherwise \end{cases} \tag{2}$$

where B_1 and B_2 are the numbers of bins for the CT density value and the distance value, respectively, and N is the number of voxels inside the nodule. Statistically, the normalized joint histogram denotes the joint probability of the CT density value and the distance value. It measures how the CT density value distributes inside the nodule with respect to the distance from the nodule center. The similar equation for the first type of joint histogram of the shape index value and the distance value is obtained. In the preliminary study, the domain of CT density, distance value, and shape index values were specified to [-1000, 500] (HU), [0, 50] (voxels), [0, 1], respectively. The number of bins was set to 50 for each value. The second type of joint histograms is computed by substituting the normalized distance value by D_M for the distance value. For the second type of joint histogram, the number of bins was set to 20 for each value.

For the representation of the nodule surrounding region, we compute the absolute value (F) of the inner product between MPV and GV fields at each voxel in surrounding region of the nodule. Then, we represent the nodule surrounding by using the joint histogram of the distance value from the nodule surface and the absolute value of the inner product. To select the part of cylindrical or conic structures in the surrounding region, we specified two threshold values T_{SH}..for the shape index value (SH) and then obtained the region consisting of voxels which satisfied with a condition of $SH < T_{SH}$. The value of T_{SH} was set to 0.5. This process means that the surface types of cylindrical or conic structures are extracted by the shape index value. Two types of joint histogram are computed for the selected region in the similar equation of the computation the joint histogram of the CT density value and the distance value.

2.3 Similarity measure for retrieving lesions

It is a possible way to directly apply a similarity measure to the 3-D nodule image. However, this approach requires solving the registration between two images. In this study, we apply a simple similarity measure, which is the correlation coefficient (CC) to the nodule representation based on the joint histogram.

$$CC = \frac{\sum\limits_{n=1}^{B_1} \sum\limits_{m=1}^{B_2} (H_1(n,m) - \overline{H}_1)(H_2(n,m) - \overline{H}_2)}{\sqrt{\sum\limits_{n=1}^{B_1} \sum\limits_{m=1}^{B_2} (H_1(n,m) - \overline{H}_1)^2 \sum\limits_{n=1}^{B_1} \sum\limits_{m=1}^{B_2} (H_2(n,m) - \overline{H}_2)^2}} \tag{3}$$

where $\overline{H}_1$ and $\overline{H}_2$ are the mean value of the joint histograms, H_1 and H_2, respectively.

At the first glance of a given nodule image, it is thought of that the nodule size and nodule density are important indexes for the visual assessment. Then, the features with respect to the local intensity structure are examined in detail to search similar patterns. In this study, we generate the list of similar nodule image by the searching process based on the similarity. We apply the similarity measure to the joint histogram of the CT density value and the distance value and then sort the CC value from more to less of similar patterns.

2.4 Difference Measure for Classifying Nodule Patterns

We select respectively the M examples from each list of the malignant and benign similar pattern to construct local two malignant and benign clusters that are similar to the indeterminate case concerning the CT density distribution pattern and the nodule size. The second type of the joint-histogram is used to model the distributions of the retrieved malignant and benign examples. Each malignant and benign example is represented by two 20x20 pixel images of the joint histograms regarding the shape index and F values and treated as 800-dimensional feature vector space. The Mahalanobis distance is used as a distance measure between the indeterminate pattern and each local model. In this preliminary study, we classify the indeterminate case into the cluster with small Mahalanobis distance.

3 Experimental Results

We considered the benign and malignant nodules shown in Fig. 1 as indeterminate cases and applied our approach to these cases.

Fig. 2 presents the first joint histogram-based representations of the malignant and benign cases shown in Fig. 1. Compared malignant with benign cases, it is observed that there is a few difference pattern between the joint histogram based representations with respect to CT density and distance except for the different expansion along the distance axis. While, it can be observed that there are difference patterns of the joint histogram-based representations concerning the shape index and the F value. Compared the malignant case with the benign case, the benign case has extremely high frequency of the shape index value around zero. This means that peak surface type occupies the inner structure of the benign case. Owning to the component of vessels and speculations, it seems that malignant case has larger amount of the component radiating from the nodule than the benign case.

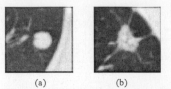

(a)   (b)

Fig. 1. ROI slice images including benign and malignant nodules. (a) Benign case. (b) Malignant case.

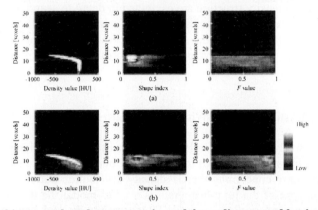

Fig. 2. Joint histogram-based representations of the malignant and benign cases shown in Fig. 1. (a) Benign case. (b) Malignant case. From left to right, representation with respect to the CT density value, shape index value, and *F* value, respectively.

Fig. 3 presents the searching similar images of the indeterminate cases shown in Fig.1 (a). This figure shows sorting results of similar images obtained from benign and malignant groups in our database. Fig. 4 presents the joint histogram-based representations of the most similar benign and malignant nodules to the indeterminate case. Compared these results with the representation result of the indeterminate case shown in Fig.2 (a), it can be observed that the indeterminate nodule pattern is similar to the benign one shown in Fig.4 (a). The Maharanobis distance of the indeterminate case was more close to the benign cluster. Fig. 5 presents the searching similar images of the indeterminate cases shown in Fig.1 (b). Fig. 6 presents the joint histogram-based representations of the most similar benign and malignant nodules to the indeterminate case. Compared these results with the representation result of the indeterminate case shown in Fig.2 (b), it can be observed that the indeterminate nodule pattern is similar to the malignant one shown in Fig.6 (b). The Maharanobis distance of the indeterminate case was more close to the malignant cluster.

4. Conclusion

We have presented an example-based assisting approach for classifying pulmonary nodules in 3-D thoracic CT images. The main idea is to formulate the nodule-classification problem as one of learning to recognize nodule patterns from examples.

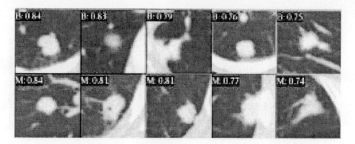

Fig. 3. Similar image of the case shown in Fig.1 (a). First row: similar image obtained from the benign group (B). Second row: similar images obtained from the malignant group (M). From left to right: sorting result from more to less similar pattern. The fraction number denotes the *CC* value in Eq. (3).

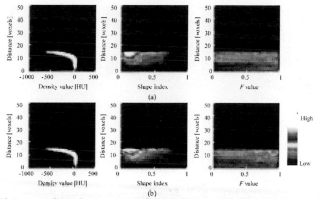

Fig. 4. Joint histogram-based representation of the most similar benign and malignant patterns of the case shown in Fig. 1(a). (a) Most similar benign pattern. (b) Most similar malignant pattern. From left to right, representation with respect to the CT density value, shape index value, and *F* value, respectively.

We have presented the application results of the searching similar images for an indeterminate nodule and then estimated the likelihood of the malignancy by computing the difference between representation patterns of the indeterminate case and the retrieved lesions. More research requires building a classifier between malignant and benign cases based on the similar patterns feature spaces. Still, we believe that the searching similar image approach would provide a better understanding for any given nodule in assisting physician's diagnostic decisions.

References

[1] M. Kaneko, K. Eguchi, H. Ohmatsu, R. Kakinuma, T. Naruke, K. Suemasu, N. Moriyama : Peripheral lung cancer: Screening and detection with low-dose spiral CT versus radiography. Radiology, vol.201 (1996) 798-802.

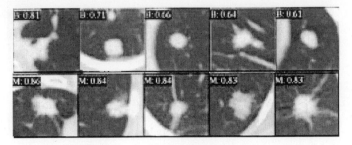

Fig. 5. Similar image of the case shown in Fig.1 (b). First row: similar image obtained from the benign group (B). Second row: similar images obtained from the malignant group (M). From left to right: sorting result from more to less similar pattern. The fraction number denotes the *CC* value in Eq. (3).

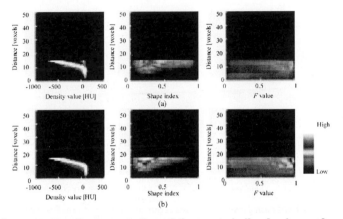

Fig. 6. Joint histogram-based representation of the most similar benign and malignant patterns of the case shown in Fig. 1(b). (a) Most similar benign pattern. (b) Most similar malignant pattern. From left to right, representation with respect to the CT density value, shape index value, and *F* value, respectively.

[2] Y. Kawata, N. Niki, H. Ohmatsu, R. Kakinuma, K. Eguchi, M. Kaneko, N. Moriyama : Quantitative surface characterization of pulmonary nodules based on thin-section CT images. IEEE Trans. Nuclear Science, vol. 45 (1998) 2132-2138.

[3] J.-P, Thirion and A. Gourdon : Computing the differential characteristics of isointensity surfaces. Computer Vision and Image Understanding, vol.61 (1995) 190-202.

[4] J. J. Koenderink and A. J. V. Doorn : Surface shape and curvature scales. Image and Vision Computing, vol.10 (1992) 557-565.

[5] Y. Kawata, N. Niki, H. Ohmatsu : Curvature based internal structure analysis of pulmonary nodules using thoracic 3-D CT images. IEICE Trans., vol.J-83-D-II (2000) 209-218.

[6] T. Saito and J. Toriwaki : Euclidean distance transformation for three-dimensional digital images. Trans. IEICE, vol.J76-D-II (1993) 445-453.

[7] C. Xu and J.L. Prince : Snake, shape, and gradient vector flow. IEEE Trans. Image Processing, vol. 7 (1998) 359-369.

Author Index

Lecture Notes in Computer Science

For information about Vols. 1–2404
please contact your bookseller or Springer-Verlag